Stilianos E. Kountakis · Joseph B. Jacobs · Jan Gosepath (Eds.)

Revision Sinus Surgery

Stilianos E. Kountakis · Joseph B. Jacobs
Jan Gosepath (Eds.)

Revision Sinus Surgery

With 274 Figures and 41 Tables

Springer

Stilianos E. Kountakis, MD, PhD
Department of Otolaryngology –
Head and Neck Surgery
Medical College of Georgia
1120 Fifteenth Street, Suite BP-4136
Augusta, GA 30912-4060
USA
Email: skountakis@mail.mcg.edu

Joseph B. Jacobs, MD
New York University Medical Center
Department of Otolaryngology
530 First Avenue, Suite 3C
New York, NY 10016-6402
USA
Email: joseph.jacobs@med.nyu.edu

Jan Gosepath, MD, PhD
Department of Otolaryngology –
Head and Neck Surgery
Dr. Horst Schmidt Kliniken
Ludwig-Erhard-Straße 100
65199 Wiesbaden
Germany
Email: jan.gosepath@hsk-wiesbaden.de

ISBN 978-3-662-51832-8 ISBN 978-3-540-78931-4 (eBook)

DOI 10.1007/978-3-540-78931-4

Softcover reprint of the hardcover 1st edition 2008

Cover design: Frido Steinen-Broo, eStudio Calamar, Spain
Production, reproduction and typesetting: le-tex publishing services oHG, Leipzig, Germany

Printed on acid-free paper

9 8 7 6 5 4 3 2 1

springer.com

Dedication

To the Memory of my mother, Eftihia Kountakis.
To my wife Eleni, our children and our new baby girl Alexandra Elena.
To my sister Maria Kountakis for her support during the difficult years.
To my Rhinology Fellows for a lifetime of learning.

Stilianos E. Kountakis, MD

To the Memory of my mother, Helen Jacobs.
To my wife Patti and my children Stacy and Allison.
To my sons-in-law Rich and Jeff.
To my granddaughter Ava.
To the department of Otolaryngology at New York University.

Joseph B. Jacobs, MD

To my wife Anja
To my academic teacher Professor Wolf J. Mann

Jan Gosepath, MD, PhD

Preface

The field of rhinology has rapidly advanced over the last two decades, enabling surgeons to utilize endoscopic techniques and instrumentation to perform the majority of operations within the paranasal sinuses. Despite significant progress with medical management and surgical instrumentation, however, many patients who suffer from chronic sinonasal disease develop recurrences of symptomatic disease requiring revision endoscopic sinus surgery.

Anatomic alteration due to prior sinus surgery, mucosal scarring and associated chronic mucosal inflammation all increase the complexity of such procedures. Therefore, even in the hands of experienced sinus surgeons, increased risk of negative outcomes exists. This project was undertaken to develop a concise reference that provides an exhaustive source of information relating to the complex pre- and post-operative management of the revision sinus surgery patient. *Revision Sinus Surgery* is the first textbook available dedicated to this topic.

International leading rhinologic experts were invited to author the book. Pertinent topics include specific surgical indications and techniques, pre- and post-operative medical management and recognition and treatment of surgical complications. Chapters are arranged with bulleted tips and pearls, as well as numerous illustrations to highlight the text. A DVD accompanies the book, containing videos that demonstrate actual procedures performed by the contributing authors. This book is a comprehensive volume that can be used as a complete reference source by all otolaryngologists.

Stilianos E. Kountakis, MD, PhD
Joseph B. Jacobs, MD
Jan Gosepath, MD

Contents

Contributors

Vijay K. Anand, MD
772 Park Ave
New York, NY 10021
USA
Email: vijayanandmd@aol.com

Pete S. Batra, MD
Section of Nasal and Sinus Disorders
Head and Neck Institute
Cleveland Clinic Foundation
9500 Euclid Ave, A71
Cleveland, OH 44195
USA
Email: batrap@ccf.org

Benjamin Bleier, MD
Department of Otorhinolaryngology
University of Pennsylvania
3400 Spruce Street
Philadelphia, PA 19104
USA
Email: benjamin.bleier@uphs.upenn.edu

Ulrike Bockmühl, MD, PhD
Department of Otorhinolaryngology – Head and Neck Surgery
University Hospital Gießen
Klinikstraße 29
35392 Gießen
Germany
Email: ulrike.bockmuehl@hno.med.uni-giessen.de

Seth M. Brown, MD, MBA
12 North Main St., Suite 30
West Hartford, CT 06107
USA
Email: sethmbrown@msn.com

Roy R. Casiano, MD
University of Miami
1475 NW 12th Ave
Suite 4025
Miami, FL 33136-1002
USA
Email: rcasiano@med.miami.edu

Yvonne Chan, MD, FRCSC
Georgia Nasal and Sinus Institute
4750 Waters Avenue
Suite 112
Savannah, GA 31404-6220
USA
Email: y.chan@utoronto.ca

Rakesh K. Chandra, MD
Northwestern Sinus and Allergy Center
Department of Otolaryngology – Head and Neck Surgery
Northwestern University
Feinberg School of Medicine
675 N. St. Clair St.-Galter 15-200
Chicago, IL 60611
USA
Email: rickchandra@hotmail.com

Dennis F. Chang, MD
Loma Linda University Sinus and Allergy Center
Department of Otolaryngology – Head and Neck Surgery
Loma Linda University Medical Center
11234 Anderson Street #2586A
Loma Linda, CA 92354
USA
Email: dfchang@llccp.net

Alexander G. Chiu, MD
Division of Rhinology
Department of Otorhinolaryngology
University of Pennsylvania
3400 Spruce Street
Philadelphia, PA 19104-4283
USA
Email: alexander.chiu@uphs.upenn.edu

Martin J. Citardi, MD
Department of Otorhinolaryngology – Head and Neck Surgery
University of Texas Medical School at Houston
6431 Fannin, MSB 5.202
Houston, TX 77030
USA
Email: martin.j.citardi@uth.tmc.edu

David B. Conley, MD
Department of Otolaryngology
Northwestern University
Feinberg School of Medicine
303 East Chicago Avenue
Chicago, IL 60611-3008
USA
Email: dbcentmd@northwestern.edu

Subinoy Das, MD
Department of Otolaryngology – Head and Neck Surgery
Medical College of Georgia
1120 Fifteenth Street, Suite BP-4136
Augusta, GA 30912-4060
USA
Email: sdas@mcg.edu

John M. DelGaudio, MD
Department of Otolaryngology
The Emory Clinic
1365 Clifton Road, NE
Atlanta, GA 30322
USA
Email: john.delgaudio@emoryhealthcare.org

Martin Desrosiers, MD, FRCSC
Montreal General Hospital, Room A2-141
1650 Cedar Avenue
H3G 1A4 Montreal, Quebec
Canada
Email: desrosiers_martin@hotmail.com

Wolfgang Draf, MD, Hon MD, PhD, FRCSC
INI International Neuroscience Institute
ENT Department
Rudolf-Pichlmayr-Straße 4
30625 Hannover
Germany
Email: wdraf@aol.com

Berrylin J. Ferguson, MD
Division of Sino-Nasal Disorders and Allergy
Department of Otolaryngology
University of Pittsburgh School of Medicine
Eye and Ear Institute
200 Lothrop Street, Suite 500
Pittsburgh, PA 15213-2546
USA
Email: fergusonbj@upmc.edu

Ramon E. Figueroa, MD
Department of Radiology
Medical College of Georgia
1120 Fifteenth Street, Suite BA-1414
Augusta, GA 30912
USA
Email: rfiguero@mcg.edu

João Flávio, MD
Hospital Prof. Edmundo Vasconcelos
Rua Borges Lagoa, 1450
Vila Clementino
CEP 04038-905, Sao Paulo
Brazil

Adam J. Folbe, MD
Department of Otolaryngology – Head and Neck Surgery
Wayne State University
4201 St. Antoine
5E UHC
Detroit, MI 48201
USA
Email: afolbe@med.wayne.edu

Wytske J. Fokkens, MD
Department of Otorhinolaryngology
Academic Medical Centre
University of Amsterdam
Postbus 22660
1100 DD Amsterdam
The Netherlands
Email: w.j.fokkens@amc.nl

Marvin P. Fried, MD
Albert Einstein College of Medicine
Department of Otolaryngology
3400 Bainbridge Avenue, 3rd Floor
Bronx, NY 10467
USA
Email: mfried@montefiore.org

Christos Georgalas, MD
Academic Medical Centre
University of Amsterdam
Postbus 22660
1100 DD Amsterdam
The Netherlands

Andrew N. Goldberg, MD, MSCE, FACS
University of California, San Francisco
Department of Otolaryngology – Head and Neck Surgery
San Francisco, CA 94143
USA
Email: agoldberg@ohns.ucsf.edu

Jan Gosepath, MD, PhD
Department of Otolaryngology – Head and Neck Surgery
Dr. Horst Schmidt Kliniken
Ludwig-Erhard-Straße 100
65199 Wiesbaden
Germany
Email: gosepath@hno.klinik.uni-mainz.de

Timothy Haegen, MD
Head and Neck Surgery
Naval Hospital Camp Pendleton
PSC 477 Box 555191
Camp Pendleton, CA 92055
USA
Email: timothy.haegen@med.navy.mil

Richard J. Harvey, MD
Medical University of South Carolina
Department of Otolaryngology
PO Box 250550
135 Rutledge Ave., Suite 1130
Charleston, SC 29425
USA
Email: richard@richardharvery.com.au

Peter H. Hwang, MD
Department of Otolaryngology
Stanford University
801 Welch Road
Stanford, CA 94304
USA
Email: phwang@ohns.stanford.edu

Joseph B. Jacobs, MD
New York University Medical Center
Department of Otolaryngology
530 First Avenue, Suite 3C
New York, NY 10016-6402
USA
Email: joseph.jacobs@med.nyu.edu

Larry Kalish, MBBS (Hons), MS, MMed (Clin Epi), FRACS
Department of Otorhinolaryngology
Concord Repatriation Hospital
Concord, Sydney
NSW Australia
Email: lhkalish@mac.com

Seth J. Kanowitz, MD
Ear, Nose, Throat – Head and Neck Surgery
Advanced Sinus and Nasal Surgery
95 Madison Avenue, Suite 105
Morristown, NJ 07960
USA
Email: sethkanowitzmd@gmail.com

David W. Kennedy, MD
Department of Otolaryngology
University of Pennsylvania
3400 Spruce Street
5th Floor – Ravdin Building
Philadelphia, PA 19104-4283
USA
Email: kennedyd@uphs.upenn.edu

Robert C. Kern, MD
Department of Otolaryngology
Northwestern University
Feinberg School of Medicine
303 East Chicago Avenue
Chicago, IL 60611-3008
USA
Email: rkern@nmff.org

Todd T. Kingdom, MD
Department of Otolaryngology
University of Colorado
AO-1, 12631E 17th Ave, B205
P.O. Box 6511
Aurora, CO 80045
USA
Email: todd.kingdom@uchsc.edu

Karen A. Kölln, MD
G0412 Neurosciences Hospital
101 Manning Drive
Chapel Hill, NC 27599-7070
USA
Email: kkolln@unch.unc.edu

Stilianos E. Kountakis, MD, PhD
Department of Otolaryngology – Head and Neck Surgery
Medical College of Georgia
1120 Fifteenth Street, Suite BP-4136
Augusta, GA 30912-4060
USA
Email: skountakis@mail.mcg.edu

Biana G. Lanson, MD
Department of Otolaryngology
New York University
462 First Avenue
NBV 5E5
New York, NY 10016
USA
Email: bgl201@med.nyu.edu

Richard A. Lebowitz, MD
Department of Otolaryngology
New York University Medical Center
530 First Avenue, Suite 3C
New York, NY 10016-6402
USA
Email: richard.lebowitz@nyumc.org

W. Derek Leight, MD
Department of Otolaryngology – Head and Neck Surgery
The University of North Carolina at Chapel Hill
G0412 Neurosciences Hospital, CB #7070
Chapel Hill, NC 27599
USA

Valerie J. Lund MS FRCS FRCSEd
Institute of Laryngology and Otology
University College London
Royal National Throat Nose and Ear Hospital
330 Grays Inn Road
London WC1X 8DA
United Kingdom
Email: v.lund@ucl.ac.uk

Elisa M. Lynskey, MD
Department of Otolaryngology
New York University
462 First Avenue, NBV 5E5
New York, NY 10016
USA
Email: elisa.lynskey@med.nyu.edu

Patricia A. Maeso, MD
Department of Otolaryngology – Head and Neck Surgery
Medical College of Georgia
1120 Fifteenth Street, Suite BP-4136
Augusta, GA 30912-4060
USA
Email: pmaeso@mcg.edu

Li-Xing Man, MD, MSc
Department of Otolaryngology
Unversity of Pittsburgh School of Medicine
Eye and Ear Institute
200 Lothrop Street, Suite 500
Pittsburgh, PA 15213-2546
USA
Email: manl@upmc.edu

William H. Moretz III, MD
Department of Otolaryngology – Head and Neck Surgery
Medical College of Georgia
1120 Fifteenth Street, Suite BP-4136
Augusta, GA 30912-4060
USA
Email: wmoretz@mcg.edu

Iman Naseri, MD
Department of Otolaryngology
The Emory Clinic
1365 Clifton Road, NE
Atlanta, GA 30322
USA

Metin Önerci, MD
Department of Otorhinolaryngology – Head and Neck Surgery
University of Hacettepe
06100 Sıhhıye, Ankara
Turkey
Email: metin@tr.net

Richard R. Orlandi, MD, FACS
Division of Otolaryngology – Head and Neck Surgery
University of Utah School of Medicine
50 North Medical Drive, 3C120
Salt Lake City, UT 84132
USA
Email: richard.orlandi@hsc.utah.edu

James N. Palmer, MD
Hospital University of Pennsylvania
3400 Spruce Street
5th floor, Ravdin Building
Philadelphia, PA 19104
USA
Email: james.palmer@uphs.upenn.edu

David M. Poetker, MD, MA
Department of Otolaryngology
and Communication Sciences
Medical College of Wisconsin
9200 W. Wisconsin Ave
Milwaukee, WI 53226
USA
Email: dpoetker@mcw.edu

Hassan H. Ramadan, MD
Department of Otolaryngology
West Virginia University
PO Box 9200
Morgantown, WV 26506-9200
USA
Email: hramadan@hsc.wvu.edu

Vijay R. Ramakrishnan, MD
Department of Otolaryngology
University of Colorado
AO-1, 12631E 17th Ave, B205
P.O. Box 6511
Aurora, CO 80045
USA

Joseph Raviv, MD
Department of Otolaryngology – Head and Neck Surgery
Northwestern University Feinberg School of Medicine
Evanston, IL
USA
Email: j-raviv@enh.org

Ryan M. Rehl, MD
Arizona Sinus Center
1515 North 9th Street, Suite B
Phoenix, AZ 85006
USA
Email: rrehl@arizonasinus.com

Scott M. Rickert, MD
Department of Otorhinolaryngology
Weill Cornell Medical College
1305 York Avenue, 5th Floor
New York, NY 10021
USA
Email: smr139@columbia.edu

Bas Rinia, MD
Department of Otorhinolaryngology
Academic Medical Centre
University of Amsterdam
Postbus 22660
1100 DD Amsterdam
The Netherlands

Frederick C. Roediger, MD
University of California, San Francisco
Department of Otolaryngology – Head and Neck Surgery
San Francisco, CA 94143
USA
Email: froediger@ohns.ucsf.edu

Raymond Sacks, MD, Bch FCS, ORL FRACS
Head of Department of Otorhinolaryngology
Concord Repatriation Hospital
Suite12, Level 1, The Madison
25–29 Hunter Street
Hornsby
NSW Australia 2075
Email: rsacks@commander360.com

Rodney J. Schlosser, MD
Department of Otolaryngology
Medical University of South Carolina
PO Box 250550
135 Rutledge Ave., Suite 1130
Charleston, SC 29425
USA
Email: schlossr@musc.edu

John Scianna, MD
Department of Otolaryngology
Loyola University
2160 South First Avenue
Maywood, IL 60153-3304
USA

Brent A. Senior, MD, FACS
Department of Otolaryngology – Head and Neck Surgery
The University of North Carolina at Chapel Hill
G0412 Neurosciences Hospital, CB #7070
Chapel Hill, NC 27599
USA
Email: brent_senior@med.unc.edu

Michael J. Sillers, MD, FACS
Alabama Nasal and Sinus Center
7191 Cahaba Valley Road
Birmingham, AL 35242
USA
Email: michaelsillers@charter.net

Timothy L. Smith, MD, MPH
Oregon Sinus Center
Department of Otolaryngology/Head and Neck Surgery
Oregon Health and Science University (OHSU)
3181 SW Sam Jackson Park Rd., PV-01
Portland, OR 97239
USA
Email: smithtim@ohsu.edu

Aldo C. Stamm, MD, PhD
Director of ENT Sao Paulo Center
Rua Alfonso Bras 525 - Cj 13
04511-010 Sao Paulo
Brazil
Email: cof@centrodeorl.com.br

James Stankiewicz, MD
Department of Otolaryngology
Loyola University
2160 South First Avenue
Maywood, IL 60153-3304
USA
Email: jstank@lumc.edu

Michael G. Stewart, MD, MPH
Department of Otorhinolaryngology
Weill Cornell Medical College
1305 York Avenue, 5th Floor
New York, NY 10021
USA
Email: mgs2002@med.cornell.edu

Abtin Tabaee, MD
10 Union Square East
Suite 4J
New York
USA
Email: atabaee@hotmail.com

Marc A. Tewfik, MD
Montreal General Hospital, Room A2-141
1650 Cedar Avenue
H3G 1A4 Montreal, Quebec
Canada
Email: marc.tewfik@mail.mcgill.ca

Winston C. Vaughan, MD
Stanford Sinus Center
Stanford University
R-135 Edwards Building
300 Pasteur Drive
Stanford, CA 94305
USA
Email: sinusmd@aol.com

Mark C. Weissler, MD, FACS
University of North Carolina
G0412 Neurosciences Hospital
CB 7070
Chapel Hill, NC 27599
USA
Email: mark_weissler@med.unc.edu

Sarah K. Wise, MD
Department of Otolaryngology
Medical University of South Carolina
PO Box 250550
135 Rutledge Ave., Suite 1130
Charleston, SC 29425
USA
Email: wisesa@musc.edu

Bradford A. Woodworth, MD
Division of Otolaryngology
Department of Surgery
University of Alabama – Birmingham
BDB 563, 1530 3rd Ave S
Birmingham, AL 35294
USA
Email: bwoodwo@hotmail.com

Chapter 1

Imaging Anatomy in Revision Sinus Surgery

1

Ramon E. Figueroa

Core Messages

- An intimate knowledge of sinus anatomy and a clear understanding of the baseline postsurgical anatomy are required for safe and effective revision sinus surgery.
- Appropriate utilization of computer-assisted surgical navigation with CT crossregistration improves safety margins on revision sinus surgery.
- Rhinologists should evaluate each side of the face as a completely independent anatomic, functional, and surgical entity.
- Familiarity with anatomic variants in the frontal recess is required for safe anterior skull base and frontal recess surgery.
- Persistent mucosal polypoid changes in a surgical site on follow-up postsurgical computed tomography, retained surgical surfaces (uncinate process, agger nasi, frontal bulla cells), or new bone formation are negative prognostic signs.

Contents

Introduction

The resulting imaging anatomy of the paranasal sinuses following initial functional endoscopic sinus surgery (FESS) must be thoroughly evaluated to establish the new postsurgical baseline of the sinonasal anatomy. These postsurgical changes may vary from subtle remodeling of anatomy to extensive resection with loss of sinus landmarks, frequently resulting in widely open sinus spaces into the nasal cavity. The great variability of the postsurgical changes is a reflection of the variety of accepted surgical techniques, the surgeon's perception of the specific problem prior to FESS, and the individualized surgical approach to the resolution of the identified problem. The detailed assessment of the postsurgical changes must emphasize which structures have been resected and which anatomy is still intact. In addition, it must identify the presence of any scar tissue formation, retraction of mucosal surfaces, and unresolved sinus drainage issues. In cases were revision surgery is needed to solve persistent sinus obstruction or postsurgical synechiae, a detailed presurgical mapping of the anatomy must be performed with emphasis on the identification of endoscopic landmarks related to the anatomic surgical targets, especially if the surgical target is close to the lamina papyracea, cribriform plate, or sphenoid sinus walls.

The recent introduction of multidetector helical scanning with its seamless high-resolution imaging databases and the wide availability of computer-assisted surgical navigation workstations allow today a real-time mapping of the progress through the surgical procedure, even in postsurgical fields devoid of residual endoscopic anatomic landmarks. The combination of improved imaging clarity from surgical navigation with computed tomography (CT) crossregistration and recent development of new powered instruments and modern endoscopic devices is effectively extending the surgical safety margin, allowing the rhinologist to solve more complex sinonasal and skull-base problems.

Caldwell-Luc and Nasoantral Windows

The Caldwell-Luc operation, named after the American physician George Caldwell and the French laryngologist Henry Luc, was first described in the late nineteenth century as a surgical decompressive technique to remove diseased mucosa from the maxillary sinus, be it infectious or tumor [1]. The procedure is performed via direct trocar puncture through the anterior maxilla above the second molar tooth, allowing for initial decompression of the maxillary disease, followed by the opening of a nasoantral window at the inferior meatus to connect the maxillary sinus lumen to the nasal cavity. This procedure is recognized on sinus CT by the associated focal defect of the anterior maxillary wall above the alveolar process and the opening within the inferior meatus into the lumen of the maxillary sinus (Fig. 1.1). This operation, which has been used widely over the last century, is being performed with less frequency today, having been replaced by the more physiologic endoscopic middle meatal antrostomy. Still, this surgery is considered safe and effective when removal of all of the diseased maxillary sinus mucosa is desired.

Imaging Anatomy in Post-FESS Ostiomeatal Complex

The postsurgical CT anatomy of the ostiomeatal complex will reflect the presurgical anatomic problems leading to surgery combined with the surgical management chosen by the surgeon to address the patient's clinical problem. An almost infinite variety of surgical changes result from the appropriately tailored surgical approach selected by experienced rhinologists, who must carefully individualize the extent of the procedure to the specific patient's problem (Fig. 1.2). These surgical changes, alone or in combinations, may include septoplasty, turbinate remodeling/resection, uncinectomy, middle meatal antrostomy, internal ethmoidectomy, sphenoidotomy, and/or frontal recess/frontal bulla cell/agger nasi decompression [2, 3].

- The first step in a comprehensive evaluation of a postsurgical nasal cavity is to determine which structures have been previously resected and which structures remain, thus establishing the new anatomic baseline of the nasal cavity.
- The second step in this evaluation is to determine the relationship between the postsurgical changes and the patient's current symptoms.
- The third and final step is to review the danger zones of the nasal cavity in the light of the distorted postsurgical anatomy prior to any revision surgery.

This relationship is inferred by the presence of acute sinus fluid levels, sinus opacity, or persistent sinus mucosal dis-

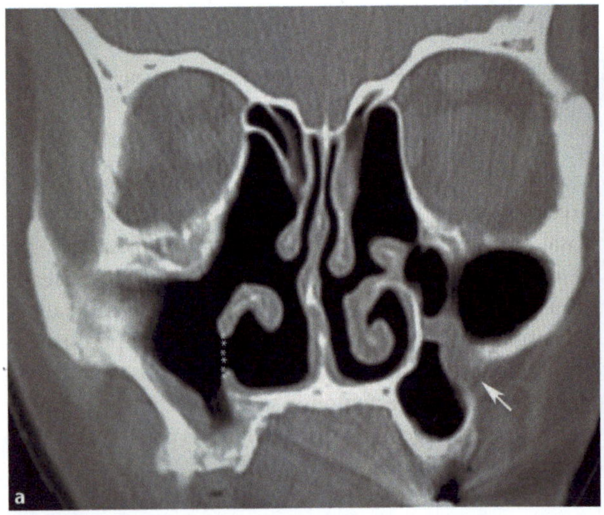

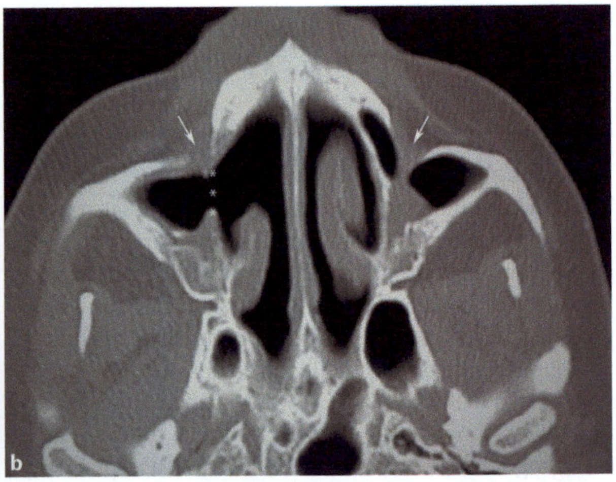

Fig. 1.1a,b Caldwell-Luc procedure. Coronal and axial computed tomography (CT) images at the level of the maxillary sinuses, showing bilateral anterior maxillary sinus-wall defects (*arrows* in **a** and **b**) as a result of Caldwell-Luc surgery, combined with inferior meatal nasoantral windows (*asterisks*). Notice also the right middle meatal antrostomy and right inferior turbinectomy

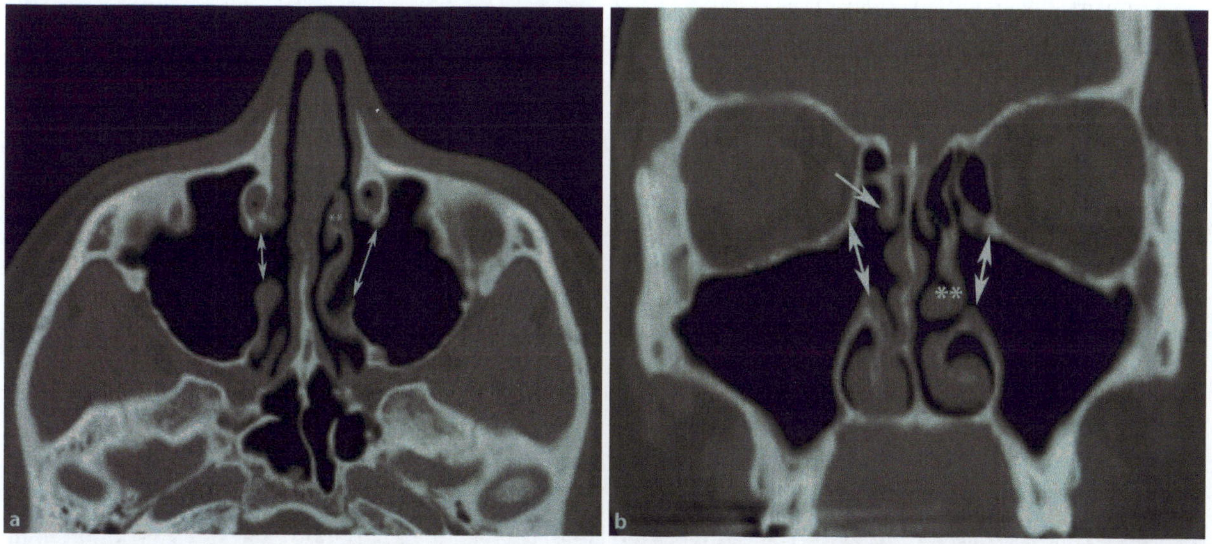

Fig. 1.2 **a** and **b** Middle meatal antrostomies. There are bilateral middle meatal antrostomies (*double-headed arrows*), with a right-sided middle turbinectomy (*arrow* in **b**). Notice the complete resection of the uncinate processes and the wide pattern of communication with the middle meatus. There is also a left paradoxical middle turbinate

ease. Soft-tissue density within the surgical ostia is an important postsurgical finding, suggesting the presence of scar tissue formation, polyps and/or hyperplasic mucosal changes, all of which are indistinct by CT findings.

Septoplasty

Septoplasty is a common adjunct finding in FESS due to the frequency of septal deviations producing asymmetric nasal cavity narrowing, occasionally to the point of laterally deflecting the middle and/or inferior turbinates. After septoplasty, the nasal septum will appear unusually vertical and straight, with a thin mucosa and no apparent nasal spurs. Postsurgical complications such as septal hematomas or septal ischemia may lead to triangular cartilage chondronecrosis, resulting in nasal septal perforations or saddle-nose deformity.

Turbinectomies

Partial resection of the inferior turbinate is seen frequently in patients with symptoms of chronic nasal congestion and polyposis, with the reduction of turbinate surface increasing meatal diameters, thus increasing the total air volume through the nose. Inferior turbinectomy is recognized on coronal CT as a foreshortened "stumped" inferior turbinate (Fig. 1.3).

Partial or subtotal resection of the middle turbine may be necessary whenever a concha bullosa or a lateralized middle turbinate is producing a mass effect toward the lateral nasal wall. Whenever truly indicated, middle turbinate surgical remodeling must be carefully performed to the minimal degree that solves the clinical problem, taking into consideration the fact that its mucosa is critical for olfactory function. Its basal lamella is one of the most important surgical landmarks for safe endonasal navigation, maintaining turbinate stability by function of its three-planar attachments (vertical attachment to the cribriform plate, coronal attachment to the lamina papyracea, and axial attachment to the medial maxillary sinus wall at the prechoanal level). The iatrogenic fracture of the middle turbinate vertical attachment is a dreaded complication, resulting in the risks of cerebrospinal fluid fistula at the cribriform plate, floppy middle turbinate behavior, and postsurgical lateralization and scaring. Thus, the resulting postsurgical appearance of the middle turbinate may vary from a barely perceptible thinning of its bulbous portion, to a small residual upper basal lamella stump in cases of subtotal resection.

- Lateralization of the middle turbinate is an important postsurgical finding, since it secondarily narrows the middle meatus, potentiates synechia formation, and predisposes to recurrent obstruction of the underlying drainage pathways by granulation tissue and scaring (Fig. 1.4).

successful. The previous endoscopic drainage procedure is extended by resecting the frontal sinus floor from the nasal septum to the lamina papyracea. The dissection also removes the anterior face of the frontal recess to enlarge the frontal sinus ostium to its maximum dimension. The Draf II procedure looks very similar to the Draf I procedure on coronal images, requiring the evaluation of sequential axial or sagittal images to allow the extensive removal of the anterior face of the frontal recess and the frontal sinus floor. Endoscopic frontal sinusotomy (Draf II) procedure can also be easily distinguished from the Draf III procedure (see below) by the lack of resection of the superior nasal septum and the entire frontal sinus floor.

Median Frontal Drainage (Modified Lothrop Procedure or Draf III)

The modified Lothrop procedure, or Draf III procedure, first described in the mid-1990s, is indicated for the most severe forms of chronic frontal sinusitis, where the only other choice is an osteoplastic flap with frontal sinus obliteration. This procedure involves the removal of the inferior portion of the interfrontal septum, the superior part of the nasal septum, and both frontal sinus floors. The lamina papyracea and posterior walls of each frontal sinus remain intact. This procedure results in a wide opening into both frontal sinuses (Fig. 1.8).

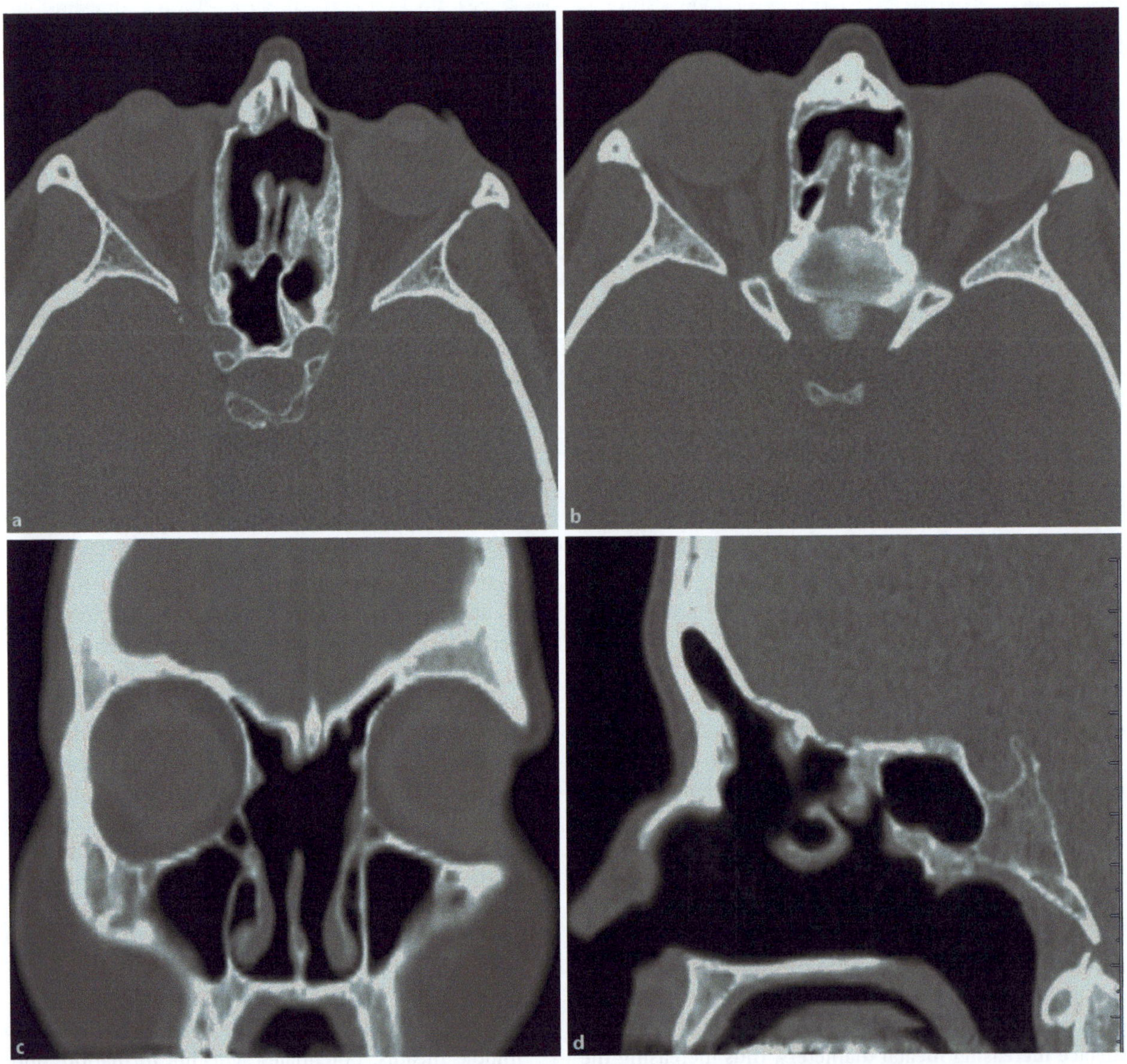

Fig. 1.8a–d Draf III (modified Lothrop) procedure. Axial (**a**,**b**) coronal (**c**), and sagittal CT images

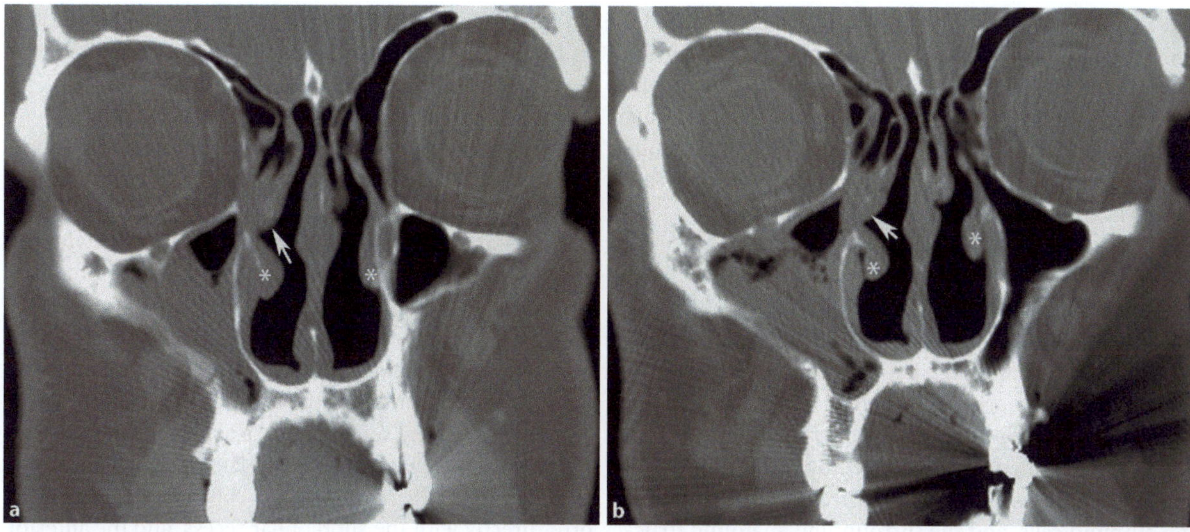

Fig. 1.4a,b Lateralized middle turbinate in a patient 4 months after FESS, with recurrent facial pain and fever. These sequential coronal images show lateralization of the right middle turbinate (*arrow*) obstructing the middle meatal antrostomy, already with active mucosal disease in the right maxillary sinus. Note also subtotal resection of both inferior turbinates (*asterisk*)

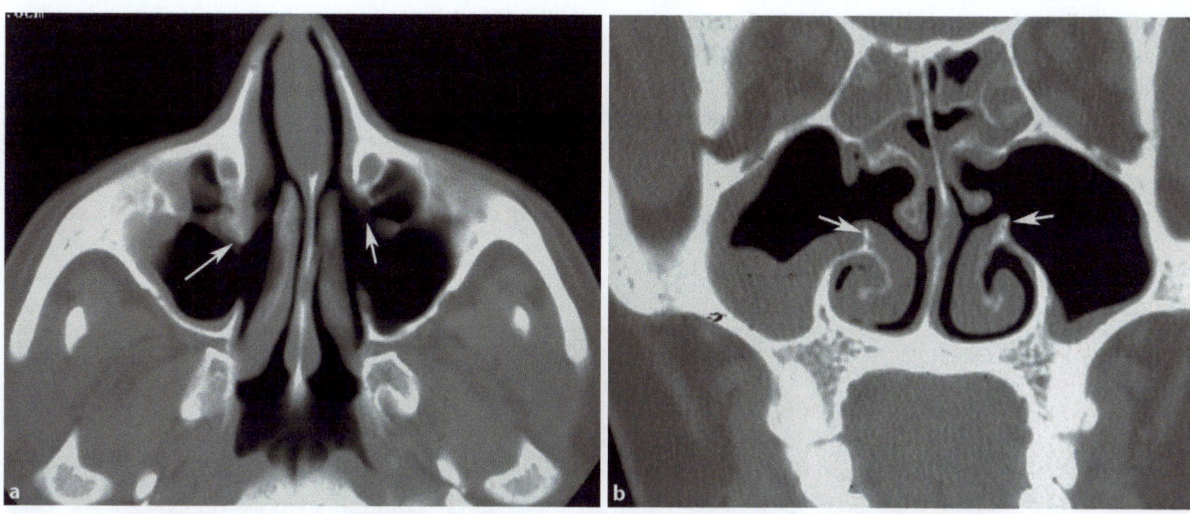

Fig. 1.5a,b Residual uncinate process. Axial (**a**) and coronal (**b**) CT images demonstrate persistent uncinate processes (*arrows*) bilaterally in spite of previous FESS. Note the persistent active mucosal thickening in both maxillary sinuses, which is worse on the right side

tium, which would result in a maxillary sinusotomy not bearing mucociliary clearance.

Internal Ethmoidectomy

The internal ethmoidectomy is an intranasal endoscopic procedure that is performed to manage mucosal disease within the anterior ethmoidal air cells. It requires the initial resection of the bulla ethmoidalis followed by resection of the ethmoidal cells, located anterior and inferior to the basal lamella of the middle turbinate. If a posterior ethmoidectomy is also needed, the basal lamella of the middle turbinate is then penetrated to decompress the posterior ethmoidal air cells. This approach is also extendable to the sphenoid sinus (transethmoidal sphenoidotomy). An internal ethmoidectomy appears by CT as a wide ethmoidal cavity that is devoid of septations

(Fig. 1.6). It is important that residual opaque ethmoidal air cells are identified, since they may be an indicator for recurrent sinus disease. The presence of mucosal polypoid changes and mucosal congestion within any residual ethmoidal cells is also a concern as they obscure the underlying anatomic landmarks that are necessary for safe surgery near the skull base.

Frontal Sinus Drainage Surgery

The frontal sinus drainage pathway is one of the most complex anatomic areas of the skull base. Its drainage pathways, the frontal sinus ostium and the frontal recess, are modified, shifted, and narrowed by the pneumatized agger nasi, anterior ethmoid cells, frontal cells, supraorbital ethmoid cells, and the surrounding anatomic structures (vertical insertion of the uncinate process and bulla lamella) [4]. The complexity of the frontal sinus variable drainage pathway starts at the frontal sinus ostium, which is oriented nearly perpendicular to the posterior sinus wall, indented anteriorly by the nasal beak. Its caliber is modified by the presence and size of pneumatized agger nasi and/or frontal cells. When markedly pneumatized, agger nasi cells can cause obstruction of the frontal sinus drainage pathway and thus have surgical implications. A second group of frontal recess cells, the frontal cells, are superior to the agger nasi cells. Bent and Kuhn described the frontal cells grouping them into four patterns [5]:

1. Type 1: a single cell above the agger nasi.
2. Type 2: a tier of two or more cells above the agger cell.
3. Type 3: a single cell extending from the agger cell into the frontal sinus.
4. Type 4: an isolated cell within the frontal sinus.

The frontal sinus ostium may also be narrowed by supraorbital ethmoid cells arising posterior to the frontal sinus and pneumatizing the orbital plate of the frontal bone. The frontal sinus ostium communicates directly with the frontal recess inferiorly, a narrow passageway bounded anteriorly by the agger nasi, laterally by the orbit, and medially by the middle turbinate. The posterior limit of the frontal recess varies depending upon the ethmoid bulla or bulla lamella, reaching to the skull base. When the bulla lamella reaches the skull base, it provides a posterior wall to the frontal recess. When the bulla lamella fails to reach the skull base, the frontal recess communicates posteriorly, directly with the suprabullar recess, and the anterior ethmoidal artery may become its only discrete posterior margin. The frontal recess opens inferiorly to either the ethmoid infundibulum or the middle meatus depending on the uncinate process configuration. When the anterior portion of the uncinate process attaches to the skull base, the frontal recess opens to the ethmoid infundibulum, and from there to the middle meatus via the hiatus semilunaris. When the uncinate process attaches to the lamina papyracea instead of the skull base, the frontal recess opens directly to the middle meatus [6].

- Each pneumatized sinus space grows independently, with its rate of growth, final volume, and configuration being determined by its ventilation, drainage, and the

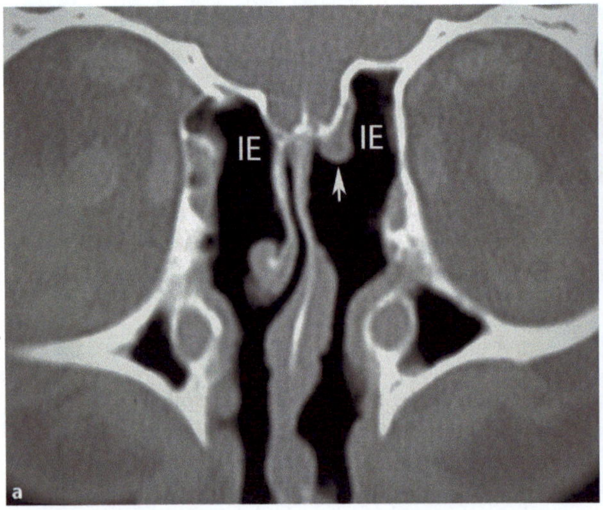

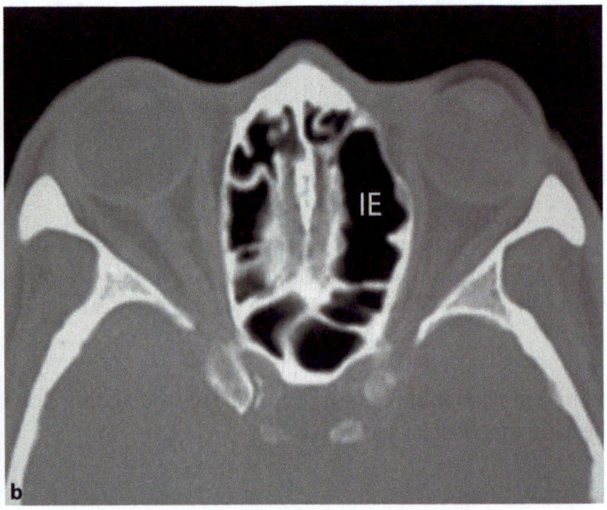

Fig. 1.6a,b Internal ethmoidectomy. **a** Coronal image showing bilateral internal ethmoidectomies (*IE*) and left middle turbinectomy (*arrow*). **b** Axial image at the level of the orbit shows the asymmetric lack of internal septations in the left ethmoid labyrinth internal ethmoidectomy

corresponding growth (or lack of it) of the competing surrounding sinuses and skull base.

This independent and competing nature of the structures surrounding the frontal recess adds an additional dimension of complexity to the frontal sinus drainage pathway. It is thus understandable why chronic frontal sinusitis secondary to impaired frontal recess drainage is so difficult to manage surgically, as reflected by the wide range of surgical procedures devised for frontal sinus decompression over the years. The spectrum of treatment options ranges from surgical ostiomeatal complex decompression combined with conservative long-term medical management, to endoscopic frontal recess exploration, the more recent endoscopic frontal sinus modified Lothrop procedure, external frontal sinusotomy, osteoplastic fat obliteration, or multiple variations of all of these [7].

Most endoscopic frontal sinus procedures are performed in patients who had previous ostiomeatal complex surgery in whom long-term conservative medical management failed. In these patients, it is not uncommon to find frontal recess scarring, osteoneogenesis, and incompletely resected anatomic variants, particularly incomplete removal of obstructing agger nasi cells and/or frontal cells leading to chronic frontal sinusitis (Fig. 1.7). Modern endoscopic surgical techniques and instruments, combined with image-guided three-dimensional navigation techniques have resulted in increased endoscopic management of most frontal sinus pathology. Endoscopic approaches tend to preserve the sinus mucosa, with less scar tissue than external approaches, resulting in less mucosal shrinkage and secondary obstruction. If the endoscopic approach fails to provide long-term drainage of the frontal sinus, then an external approach with obliteration of the frontal sinus still remains as a viable surgical alternative.

Endoscopic Frontal Recess Approach (Draf I Procedure)

Dr. Wolfgang Draf popularized a progressive three-stage endoscopic approach to the management of chronic frontal sinus drainage problems for patients in whom classic ostiomeatal endoscopic sinus surgery is unsuccessful [8]. The Draf type I procedure, or endoscopic frontal recess approach, is indicated when frontal sinus disease persists in spite of more conservative ostiomeatal and anterior ethmoid endoscopic approaches. The Draf I procedure involves complete removal of the anterior ethmoid cells and the uncinate process up to the frontal sinus ostium, including the removal of any frontal cells or other obstructing structures to assure the patency of the frontal sinus ostium.

Endoscopic Frontal Sinusotomy (Draf II Procedure)

The endoscopic frontal sinusotomy, or Draf II procedure, is performed in severe forms of chronic frontal sinusitis for which the endoscopic frontal recess approach was un-

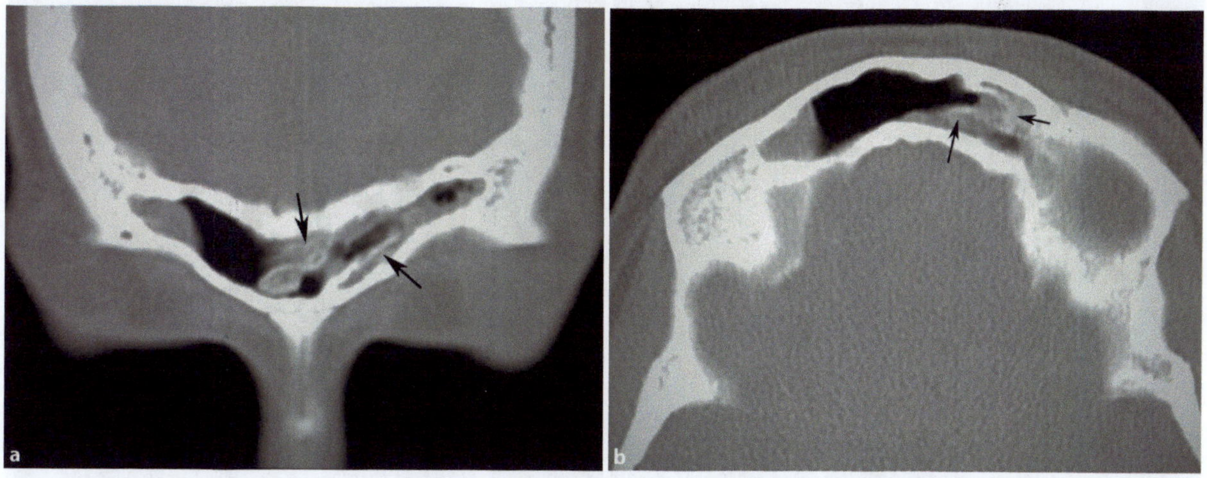

Fig. 1.7a,b Postinflammatory osteoneogenesis. Coronal (**a**) and axial (**b**) sinus CT sections at the level of the frontal sinuses show osteoneogenesis with persistent frontal sinus inflammatory mucosal engorgement (*black arrows*)

successful. The previous endoscopic drainage procedure is extended by resecting the frontal sinus floor from the nasal septum to the lamina papyracea. The dissection also removes the anterior face of the frontal recess to enlarge the frontal sinus ostium to its maximum dimension. The Draf II procedure looks very similar to the Draf I procedure on coronal images, requiring the evaluation of sequential axial or sagittal images to allow the extensive removal of the anterior face of the frontal recess and the frontal sinus floor. Endoscopic frontal sinusotomy (Draf II) procedure can also be easily distinguished from the Draf III procedure (see below) by the lack of resection of the superior nasal septum and the entire frontal sinus floor.

Median Frontal Drainage (Modified Lothrop Procedure or Draf III)

The modified Lothrop procedure, or Draf III procedure, first described in the mid-1990s, is indicated for the most severe forms of chronic frontal sinusitis, where the only other choice is an osteoplastic flap with frontal sinus obliteration. This procedure involves the removal of the inferior portion of the interfrontal septum, the superior part of the nasal septum, and both frontal sinus floors. The lamina papyracea and posterior walls of each frontal sinus remain intact. This procedure results in a wide opening into both frontal sinuses (Fig. 1.8).

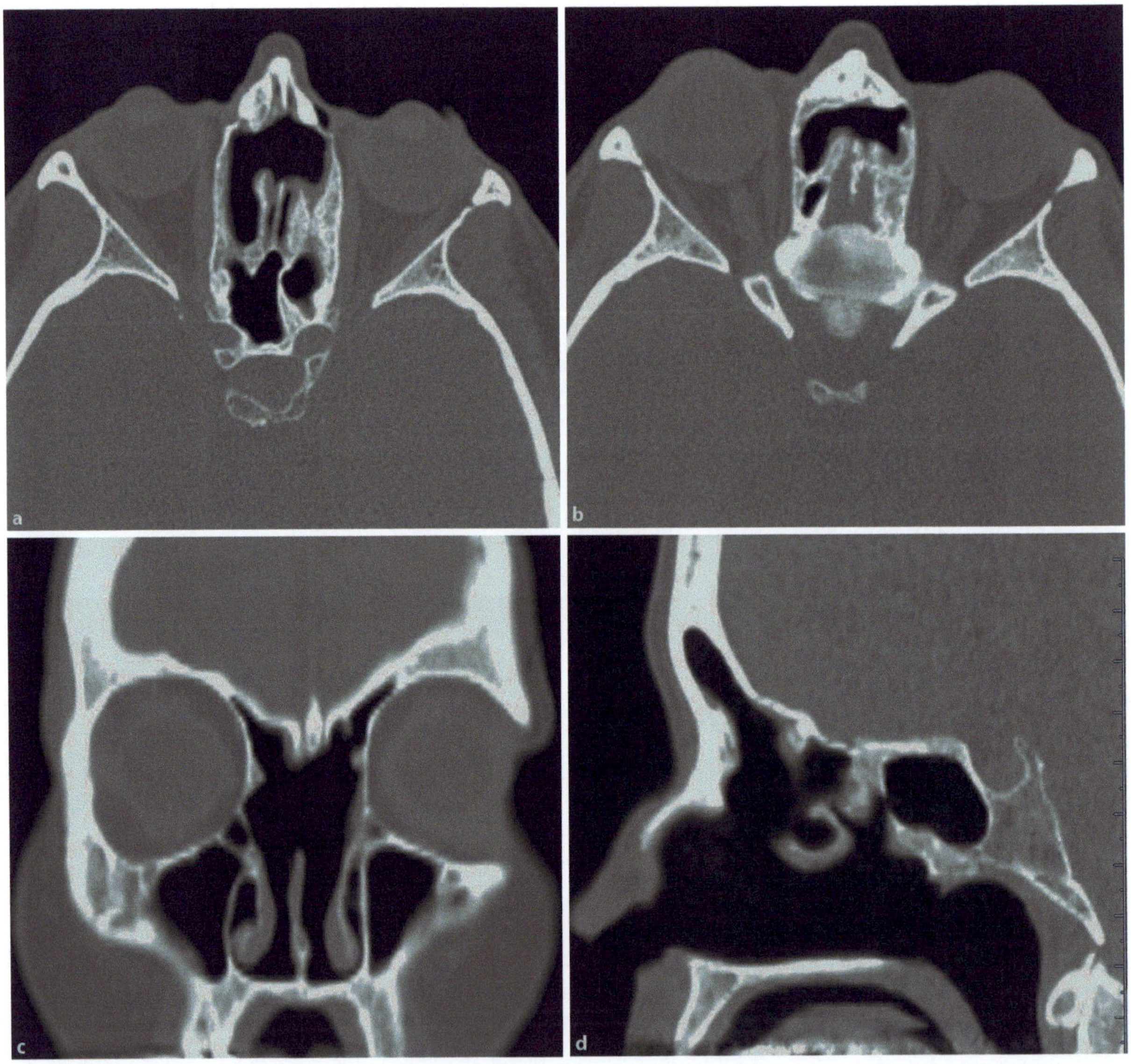

Fig. 1.8a–d Draf III (modified Lothrop) procedure. Axial (**a**,**b**) coronal (**c**), and sagittal CT images

- The surgical defect component in the superior nasal septum after a Draf III procedure should not be mistaken for an unintended postoperative septal perforation.

Frontal Sinus Trephination

The trephination procedure is a limited external approach for frontal sinus drainage. An incision is made above the brow and a hole is drilled through the anterior wall of the frontal sinus taking care to avoid the supratrochlear and supraorbital neurovascular bundles (see Chap. 33). The inferior wall of the frontal sinus is devoid of bone marrow, which may lessen the risk of developing osteomyelitis. Frontal sinus trephination is indicated in complicated acute frontal sinusitis to allow the release of pus and irrigation of the sinus to prevent impending intracranial complications. It can also be used in conjunction with endoscopic approaches to the frontal sinus in chronic frontal sinusitis or frontal sinus mucoceles, where the trephination helps to identify the frontal recess by passing a catheter down the frontal recess, also allowing it to be stented and to prevent its stenosis. This approach provides fast and easy access to the frontal sinus to place an irrigation drain in the sinus. Its main disadvantages are the risks of associated scarring, sinocutaneous fistula formation, and injury to the supraorbital nerve bundle and the trochlea, which can cause diplopia [9]. Image guidance is critical for accurate trephine placement in particularly small frontal sinuses or to gain access to isolated type 4 frontal sinus disease.

Osteoplastic Flap with Frontal Sinus Obliteration

- Long-term stability of the mucociliary clearance of the frontal sinus must be maintained for endoscopic surgery of the frontal sinus to be successful. If this is not achieved, an osteoplastic flap procedure with sinus obliteration may be the only remaining option.

The indications for this procedure include chronic frontal sinusitis in spite of prior endoscopic surgery, mucopyocele, frontal bone trauma with fractures involving the drainage pathways, and resection of frontal tumors near the frontal recess. The outline of the sinus can be determined by using a cut template made from a 6-foot (1.83 m) Caldwell x-ray, which approaches the exact size of the frontal sinus. Other methods include the use of a wire thorough an image-guidance-placed frontal sinus trephination to palpate the extent of the sinus. Beveled osteotomy cuts through the frontal bone prevent collapse of the anterior table into the sinus lumen upon postoperative closure. Frontal sinus obliteration requires all of the mucosa to be drill-removed and the frontal recess occluded. The sinus is then packed with fat, bone marrow, pericranial flaps, or synthetic materials, and then the bony flap is replaced.

The postoperative imaging appearance by CT and/or magnetic resonance imaging (MRI) is highly variable due to the spectrum of tissues used for sinus packing, with imaging behavior reflecting fat, chronic inflammatory changes, retained secretions, granulation tissue, and fibrosis. MRI may be of limited utility in distinguishing symptomatic patients with recurrent disease from asymptomatic patients with imaging findings related to scar tissue. Imaging is useful for the early detection of postoperative mucocele formation, which is recognized by its mass effect and signal behavior of inspissated secretions [10, 11].

Endoscopic Sphenoidotomy

The postsurgical appearance of the sphenoethmoidal recess following endoscopic sphenoidotomy varies depending upon whether the sphenoidotomy was transnasal, transethmoidal, or transseptal. Transnasal sphenoidotomy may be performed as a selective procedure, where the only subtle finding may be a selective expansion of the sphenoid sinus ostium in the sphenoethmoid recess. Transethmoidal sphenoidotomies, on the other hand, are performed in the realm of a complete functional endoscopic surgery, where middle meatal antrostomy changes, internal ethmoidectomy changes, and sphenoid sinus rostrum defects ipsilateral to the ethmoidectomy defects become parts of the imaging constellation (Fig. 1.9). Finally, transseptal sphenoidotomy changes are a combination of septal remodeling with occasional residual septal split appearance combined with a midline sphenoid rostrum defect and variable resection of the sphenoid intersinus septum. These changes are seen typically in the realm of more extensive sphenoid sinus explorations or surgical exposures for transsphenoidal pituitary surgery. The accurate imaging identification of the optic nerves, internal carotid arteries, maxillary division of the trigeminal nerve, and the vidian neurovascular package in reference to the pneumatized sphenoid sinus is even more important in postsurgical sphenoid re-exploration, since the usual anatomic and endoscopic sinus appearance may be significantly distorted by previous procedures, postsurgical scar and/or persistent inflammatory changes. Imaging guidance is thus critical for the safe and accurate depiction of all of neighboring structures of the sphenoid sinus.

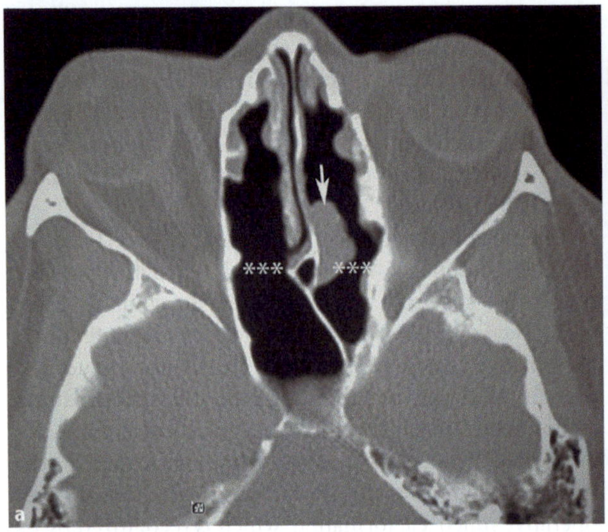

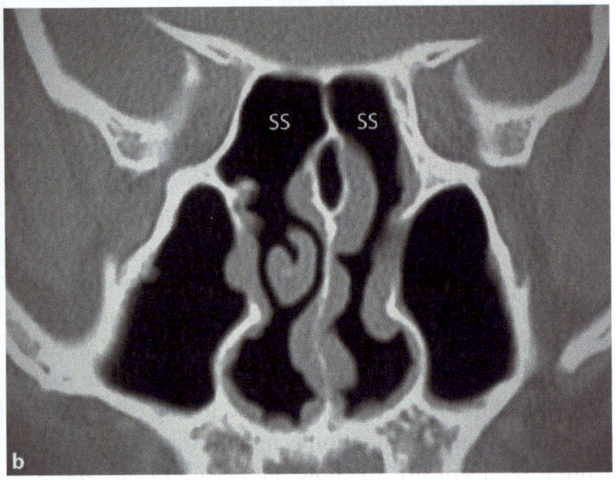

Fig. 1.9a,b Sphenoidotomy. **a** Axial CT showing bilateral internal ethmoidectomies and transethmoidal sphenoidotomies (*asterisks*). Note the persistent polypoid disease (*arrow*) in the left posterior ethmoid sinus. **b** Coronal CT at the level of the rostrum of the sphenoid showing open communication into the sphenoid sinus (*SS*), with no residual sphenoethmoid recess components. Note the absent left-middle and bilateral inferior turbinates from prior turbinectomies

Negative Prognostic Findings Post-FESS

There is a series of postsurgical imaging findings that imply a persistent underlying physiologic problem, with poor prognostic implications for recurrence of sinus disease. These CT findings may include a wide range of elements, such as incomplete resection of surgical structures (especially uncinate process, agger nasi, or frontal bulla cells), mucosal nodular changes at areas of prior surgical manipulation (mucosal stripping, granulation tissue, mucosal scarring, synechiae formation, polyposis), or postinflammatory increased bone formation (osteoneogenesis). All of these changes should be detectable in a good-quality postsurgical sinus CT, which should be performed ideally at least 8 weeks after the surgical trauma to allow for reversible inflammatory changes to resolve. These changes result in recurrent or persistent obstruction of the mucociliary drainage at the affected points, with increased potential for recurrent symptoms. Persistent nasal septal deviation leading to a narrowed nasal cavity and lateralization of the middle turbinate against the lateral nasal wall are two additional factors with poor prognostic implications for recurrent sinus disease. The relevance of these CT findings must be judged by the rhinologist based on the presence of mucosal congestion and/or fluid accumulation in the affected sinus space in combination with assessment of the patient's clinical behavior (persistent sinus pressure, pain and/or fever).

Conclusion

The postsurgical anatomy of the paranasal sinus drainage pathways and their surrounding structures must be evaluated in an integrated fashion, emphasizing the interrelationship between sinus anatomy and function. The presence of residual surgical structures, mucosal nodular changes at areas of prior surgical manipulation or postinflammatory new bone formation are poor prognostic factors for recurrent postsurgical sinus disease.

References

1. KE Matheny, JA Duncavage (2003) Contemporary indications for the Caldwell-Luc procedure. Curr Opin Otolaryngol Head Neck Surg 11:23–26
2. Stammberger HR, Kennedy DW, Bolger WE, et al. (1995) Paranasal sinuses: anatomic terminology and nomenclature. Ann Rhinol Otol Laryngol (Suppl) 167:7–16
3. Kayalioglu G, Oyar O, Govsa F (2000) Nasal cavity and paranasal sinus bony variations: a computed tomographic study. Rhinology 38:108–113
4. Daniels DL, Mafee MF, Smith MM, et al. (2003) The frontal sinus drainage pathway and related structures. AJNR Am J Neuroradiol 24:1618–1626
5. Bent JP, Cuilty-Siller C, Kuhn FH (1994) The frontal cell as a cause of frontal sinus obstruction. Am J Rhinol 8:185–191

6. Perez P, Sabate J, Carmona A, et al. (2000) Anatomical variations in the human paranasal sinus region studied by CT. J Anat 197:221–227
7. Benoit CM, Duncavage JA (2001) Combined external and endoscopic frontal sinusotomy with stent placement: a retrospective review; Laryngoscope 111:1246–1249
8. Draf W (1991) Endonasal micro-endoscopic frontal sinus surgery: the Fulda concept. Operative Tech Otolaryngol Head Neck Surg 4:234–240
9. Lewis D, Busaba N (2006) Surgical Management: Sinusitis; Taylor and Francis Group, Boca Raton, Florida, pp 257–264
10. Melhelm ER, Oliverio PJ, Benson ML, et al. (1996) Optimal CT evaluation for functional endoscopic sinus surgery. AJNR Am J Neuroradiol 17:181–188
11. Weber R, Draf W, Keerl R, et al. (2000) Osteoplastic frontal sinus surgery with fat obliteration: technique and long-term results using magnetic resonance imaging in 82 operations. Laryngoscope 110:1037–1044

Chapter 2

Indications for Revision Endoscopic Sinus Surgery

2

Marc A. Tewfik and Martin Desrosiers

Core Messages

- The goal of assessment of the patient with symptoms suggestive of persistent or recurrent sinus disease is to identify the presence of technical, mucosal, and systemic factors contributing to poor outcome by using appropriate investigations.
- The goal of surgery is to improve medical management by reducing disease load and improving access for continuing medical care for those with severe mucosal disease.
- Indications for revision endoscopic sinus surgery can be categorized as follows: (i) incomplete previous surgery, (ii) complications of previous surgery, (iii) recurrent or persistent sinus disease, and (iv) histological evidence of neoplasia. These criteria are not absolute and the decision to reoperate is most often based on clinician judgment and experience.
- The most common technical factors associated with failure of primary surgery are: (i) middle-meatal scarring and lateralization of the middle turbinate, and (ii) frontal sinus obstruction from retained agger nasi or anterior ethmoid cells. These common situations must be actively sought out with endoscopy and radiologic imaging.
- Given the multiple factors that contribute to the persistence of disease, combinations of both medical therapy and surgery may play a role in the continuum of management as the patient's disease condition evolves over time.
- The patient should be informed that further surgery may be necessary in the future.

Contents

Introduction

The management of chronic rhinosinusitis (CRS) can be quite challenging, even to the experienced rhinologist. This is particularly true for severe CRS that has not responded to an initial surgical attempt (refractory CRS). Revision surgery may have a role in the continuum of management of the patient's disease condition; however, the clinician should understand that different care may be required at different time points, depending on the underlying factors contributing to sinus disease.

The decision to reoperate on a patient with sinus disease is centered principally on the demonstration of a symptomatic obstruction to sinus drainage or the presence of significant disease load in the sinuses. This must be tempered by the clinician's judgment, experience, and comfort level. Given the nature of endoscopic sinus surgery (ESS) and the close proximity of numerous critical structures, special care must be taken to avoid serious intraoperative complications as a result of damage to adjacent structures [8,10,16]. Preoperative sinus imaging and a precise understanding of the patient's anatomy are thus of paramount importance.

Indications for revision sinus surgery can be grossly divided into four main categories:

1. Incomplete previous surgery.
2. Complications of previous surgery.
3. Recurrent or persistent sinus disease.
4. Histological evidence of neoplasia.

The first occurs when prior surgery has been incomplete. Such is the case when there is refractory CRS or recurrent acute sinusitis with persistence of ethmoid cells, or a deviated nasal septum not adequately repaired and causing obstruction to access or drainage. Incompletely resected cells can be identified by their typical appearance and position. Often, the agger nasi and anterior ethmoid cells have been left in place while surgery clears a straight-line back through the posterior ethmoids up to the skull base (Fig. 2.1). Unopened infraorbital ethmoid (Haller) cells can obstruct maxillary sinus outflow. The "missed ostium sequence," as described by Parsons et al. [13], occurs when there is incomplete removal of the most anterior portion of the uncinate process, thus obscuring the position of the natural maxillary sinus ostium. This prevents the middle meatal antrostomy from communicating with the natural ostium, resulting in a recirculation phenomenon. In this instance, mucociliary flow causes mucus to re-enter the sinus, causing a functional obstruction of the maxillary sinus and continued sinus disease.

Several series have looked at the causes of postsurgical persistent or recurrent disease, and provide information regarding the frequency of various anatomic findings. Chu et al. [7] evaluated 153 patients requiring revision ESS, and found that the most common surgical alteration associated with recurrent sinus disease was middle-meatal scarring and lateralization of the middle turbinate. This was usually the result of partial middle turbinectomy during the initial surgery.

Musy and Kountakis [11] reported that the most common postsurgical findings associated with primary surgery failure are:

1. Lateralization of the middle turbinate (78%).
2. Incomplete anterior ethmoidectomy (64%).
3. Scarred frontal recess (50%).
4. Retained agger nasi cell (49%).
5. Incomplete posterior ethmoidectomy (41%).
6. Retained uncinate process (37%).
7. Middle meatal antrostomy stenosis (39%).
8. Recurrent polyposis (37%).

Ramadan [14] reviewed 52 cases and found that the most common cause of failure was residual air cells and adhesions in the ethmoid area (31%), followed by maxillary sinus ostial stenosis (27%), frontal sinus ostial stenosis (25%), and a separate maxillary sinus ostium stenosis (15%). In their series of 67 patients requiring revision frontal sinus surgery, Chiu and Vaughn [6] identified residual agger nasi cell or ethmoid bulla remnants in 79.1% of cases, retained uncinate process in 38.8%, lateralized middle turbinate remnant in 35.8%, recurrent polyposis in 29.9%, unopened frontal recess cells in 11.9%, and neo-osteogenesis of the frontal recess in 4.5%. A maxim to guide the surgeon is that the patient can never truly be deemed a failure of therapy until all obstructions to drainage and ventilation (or irrigation) are corrected.

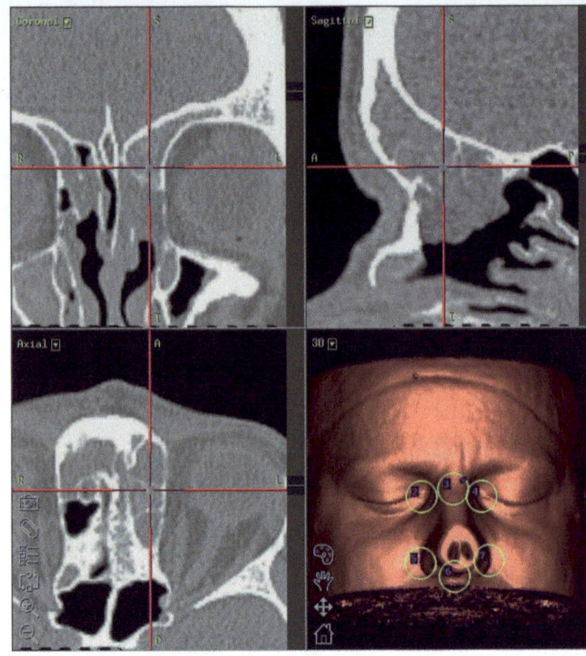

Fig. 2.1 Symptomatic frontal sinus obstruction. Screen shot from a computer-assisted navigation system demonstrating frontal sinus obstruction in three planes on computed tomography (CT). Persistent agger nasi cells and anterior ethmoid cells responsible for obstruction are best identified on a sagittal view (*top right*)

Indications for Surgery

Incomplete Previous Surgery

1. Persistence of symptoms and signs of CRS with or without nasal polyposis or recurrent acute sinusitis with persistent ethmoid cells on computed tomography (CT).
2. Deviated nasal septum not adequately repaired at primary surgery and causing obstruction.

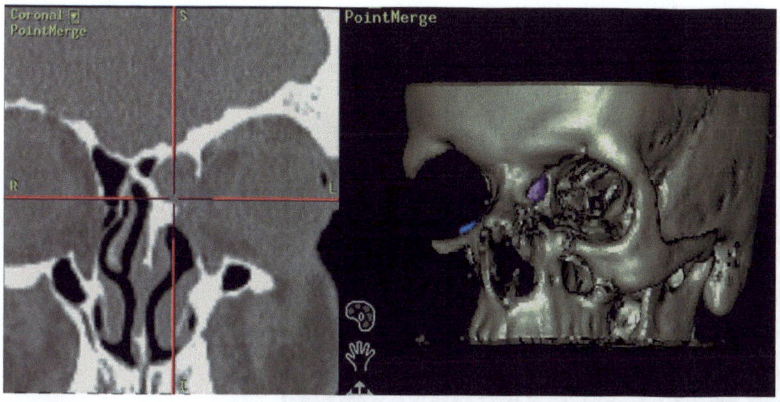

Fig. 2.2 Mucocele. Left frontal sinus mucocele presenting as a painless left exophthalmos. Note the circular, sphere-like form typical of mucoceles. A three-dimensional, computer-generated illustration of the lesion is also shown (*right*)

3. Persistent maxillary sinus disease in the setting of a retained uncinate process.

Complications of Previous Surgery

Complications of prior ESS constitute the second major group of indications for surgical revision. These include:

1. Suspected mucocele formation.
2. Suspected cerebrospinal fluid (CSF) leak for which conservative management was unsuccessful.
3. Synechiae causing obstruction of the nasal passage or sinus outflow tract.

Due to its narrow anatomic outflow pathway, the frontal sinus is particularly susceptible to this group of complications, and thus is often the target of revision sinus surgery. A mucocele can be suspected on CT when there is smooth, round enlargement of a completely opacified sinus cell with associated bony remodeling and thinning (Fig. 2.2). It is useful to follow a graded approach to the frontal sinus; a discussion of frontal sinus techniques is presented later on.

The surgeon should always be alert to the risk of pre-existing CSF leaks, which may have gone unnoticed during previous surgery. A significant proportion of CSF leaks are iatrogenic in origin. They occur most commonly in the areas of the olfactory fossa and fovea ethmoidalis (Fig. 2.3). The skull-base bone in these areas can be extremely thin, and may be penetrated by direct instrumentation or cauterization for control of bleeding [15]. In some cases, bony remodeling expose the once-protected vital structures to trauma during surgery.

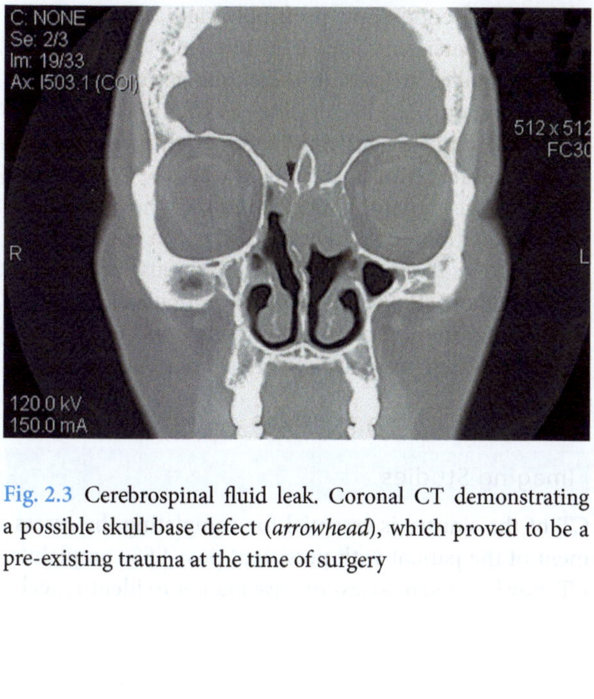

Fig. 2.3 Cerebrospinal fluid leak. Coronal CT demonstrating a possible skull-base defect (*arrowhead*), which proved to be a pre-existing trauma at the time of surgery

Recurrent or Persistent Sinus Disease

Recalcitrant inflammatory sinus disease is the third category of indications for revision ESS. This includes:

1. Recurrent acute sinusitis.
2. CRS with or without nasal polyps.
3. Allergic fungal rhinosinusitis (Fig. 2.4).

Another indication included in this category is in the management of patients with nasal polyposis who have an intolerance or contraindication to oral corticosteroids. It remains, as a whole, a poorly understood group of diseases. Considerable research efforts are currently focused on improving the management of these difficult patients. Although discussions of these entities and of medical management are presented in depth in later chapters, a guiding principal is that an adequate trial of maximal medical therapy must be attempted preoperatively and documented in the chart.

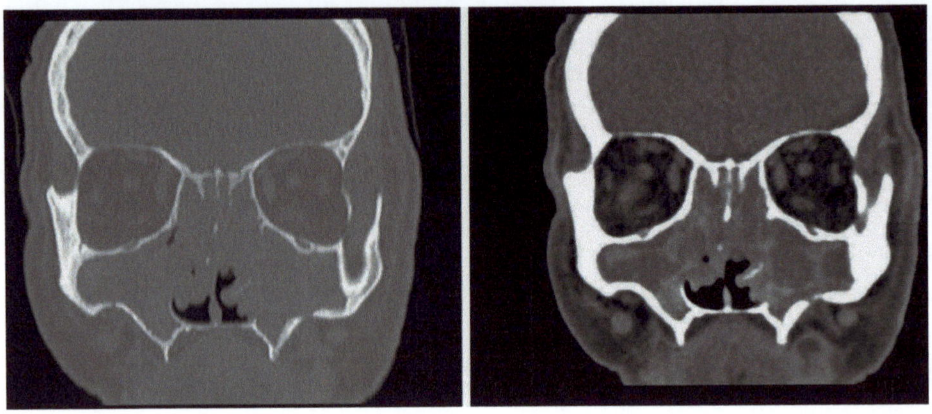

Fig. 2.4 Allergic fungal rhinosinusitis. Involvement of all of the sinus cavities is shown on CT in the bone window (*left*); examination in the soft-tissue window (*right*) shows evidence of allergic fungal sinusitis/eosinophilic mucinous rhinosinusitis in all sinuses

Histological Evidence of Neoplasia

1. Unexpected diagnosis of neoplasia on pathological analysis with subtotal resection.
2. Localized severe disease suspicious for neoplasia, such as inverted papilloma.

Once diagnosed, these patients are reoperated for complete removal of the tumor. These most commonly consist of inverted papillomas [12,17,18]; however, they may be any of a variety of benign or malignant nasal or paranasal sinus tumors [2].

Preoperative Workup

Assessment of the Patient with Post-ESS Symptoms

The clinician should attempt to elicit the patient's symptoms and classify them according to their severity. The goal of the medical workup is to identify the mucosal, systemic, and environmental factors responsible for poor outcome. A history of underlying immune deficiency, connective tissue disorder, malignancies, or genetic disorder such as cystic fibrosis or primary ciliary dyskinesia should be sought. A complete immune workup, and possibly a vaccine response, should be ordered to rule out immune deficiency if it is suspected. Blood work is also helpful to rule out other systemic disorders such as Wegener's granulomatosis and sarcoidosis. Defects in functional immune response not evident in static testing have been identified in certain patients who have refractory CRS. In the absence of a response to all other therapies, a 6-month trial of intravenous immunoglobulin may be warranted [5]. This option should be discussed with the patient before administration.

It is important to consider the potential contribution of allergy to symptoms or disease, as a significantly higher percentage of these patients will have allergies as compared to the general population. A total serum IgE level, as well as a hemogram with differential cell count to detect serum eosinophilia, may be useful to further characterize patients. Allergy testing and management should be included in their care to minimize the contribution of allergy to the disorder. Allergen reduction or avoidance, medications, and possibly immunotherapy may play a role in management.

Cigarette smoking has been associated with statistically worse outcomes after ESS based on disease-specific quality-of-life measures [4].

Sinonasal endoscopy, preferably rigid, is essential in evaluating persistent disease. It may help identify structural anomalies, masses, or secretions not seen on anterior rhinoscopy. The bacteriology of CRS may vary in an individual patient over time. Obtaining endoscopically guided cultures from the middle meatus or the sphenoethmoid recess (not the nasal cavity) will help in the selection of antibiotic therapy, particularly in cases that are unresponsive to empiric therapy. Care must be taken to avoid contact with the nasal wall or vestibule to minimize contamination, and to sample directly within purulent secretions when present, rather than adjacent areas.

Imaging Studies

CT of the sinuses is essential for completing the assessment of the patient with persistent post-ESS complaints. CT may be used to assess disease load or to identify technical factors that may not be revealed on endoscopy, such as residual ethmoid cells, obstructions to sinus drainage, or mucocele formation. Disease load can be determined by identifying the number of sinuses involved with disease and the extent of their involvement (mucosal thickening vs. opacification). The Lund-MacKay staging system is an effective method of standardizing reporting of radiologic severity of disease [3,9]. Care must be exercised in the face of exuberant local disease out of proportion to the rest of the sinus cavities to ensure against a missed diagnosis of neoplasm such as inverted papilloma.

When frontal sinus involvement is suspected, helical CT with three-dimensional reconstruction is needed for analysis of the anatomy of the frontal recess. Frontal sinus opacification is often noted on CT. However, this radiologic finding also needs to be assessed in terms of clinical context by assessing the patient's symptoms. For example, it is not unusual in extensive sinonasal polyposis for patients to demonstrate a significant amount of frontal sinus involvement. Thus, in patients with nasal polyposis, frontal sinus opacification in the absence of frontal symptoms or bony remodeling is not in and of itself an indication for revision.

The Role of Image-Guided Surgery

When ordering imaging studies, consideration should be given to the possibility of image-guided surgery as part of the initial evaluation of the potential surgical patient. The rationale for this is that normal anatomy is invariably altered in previously operated patients, and the usual anatomic landmarks – including the middle turbinate, uncinate process, and basal lamella – may have been removed. Formal indications for computer-aided surgery endorsed by the American Academy of Otolaryngology – Head and Neck Surgery are [1]:

1. Revision sinus surgery.
2. Distorted sinus anatomy of development, postoperative, or traumatic origin.
3. Extensive sinonasal polyposis.
4. Pathology involving the frontal, posterior ethmoid, and sphenoid sinuses.
5. Disease abutting the skull base, orbit, optic nerve, or carotid artery.
6. CSF rhinorrhea or conditions where there is a skull-base defect.
7. Benign and malignant sinonasal neoplasms.

Other Causes

In patients with post-ESS symptoms where no origin for their symptoms can be identified, other causes of sinonasal symptoms should be considered. In the case of facial pain: neuralgia, migraine equivalent (midfacial headache), or dental problems may be responsible. The axial CT should be used to carefully assess the possibility of a small periapical dental abscess producing pain. In individuals with a history of migraine or multiple surgeries, a trial of amitriptyline may be warranted.

Surgery

The role of revision surgery is principally to improve medical management, and surgery should be planned and executed to optimize this. This is achieved by either reducing disease load, by removing recurrent nasal polyps or hypertrophic sinonasal mucosa (Fig. 2.5), or improving access for continuing medical care in the form of topical solutions. Wide antrostomies are created for problem sinuses in order to provide better access for irrigating solutions. Continued postoperative medical therapy is essential and can be considered an integral part of surgical care.

Tips and Pearls

1. Ensure an adequate trial of maximal medical therapy before planning surgery.
2. Surgery is indicated only after failure of appropriate medical management.
3. Be wary of pain as a sole presenting symptom in the absence of other physical findings.
4. Know when and how to use navigation.
5. Know your limitations as a surgeon – be realistic.

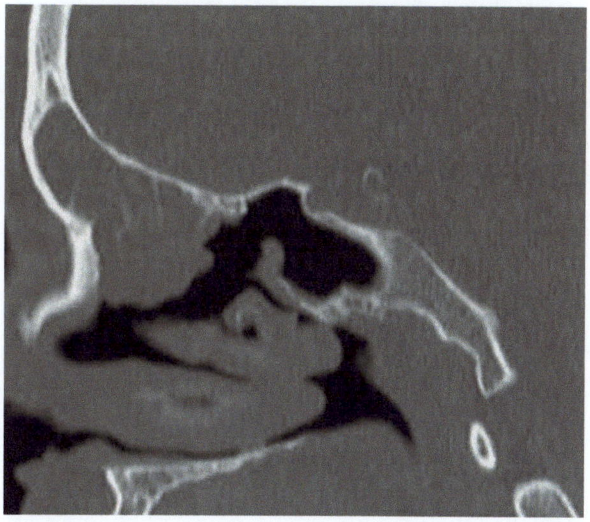

Fig. 2.5 Recurrence of sinonasal polyposis. Sagittal CT showing extensive soft-tissue changes and polypoid disease in the region of the frontal recess. Note is made of the persistence of the anterior ethmoid cells, which indicates that previous surgery has not addressed these areas

2

References

1. AAO-HNS Policy on Intra-Operative Use of Computer-Aided Surgery (2005) American Academy of Otolaryngology-Head Neck Surgery. http://www.entlink.net/practice/rules/image-guiding.cfm
2. Batra PS, Citardi MJ (2006) Endoscopic management of sinonasal malignancy. Otolaryngol Clin North Am 39:519–637, x–xi
3. Bhattacharyya N (1999) Computed tomographic staging and the fate of the dependent sinuses in revision endoscopic sinus surgery. Arch Otolaryngol Head Neck Surg 125:994–999
4. Briggs RD, Wright ST, Cordes S, et al. (2004) Smoking in chronic rhinosinusitis: a predictor of poor long-term outcome after endoscopic sinus surgery. Laryngoscope 114:126–128
5. Chee L, Graham SM, Carothers DG, et al. (2001) Immune dysfunction in refractory sinusitis in a tertiary care setting. Laryngoscope 111:233–235
6. Chiu AG, Vaughan WC (2004) Revision endoscopic frontal sinus surgery with surgical navigation. Otolaryngol Head Neck Surg 130:312–318
7. Chu CT, Lebowitz RA, Jacobs JB (1997) An analysis of sites of disease in revision endoscopic sinus surgery. Am J Rhinol 11:287–291
8. Dessi P, Castro F, Triglia JM, et al. (1994) Major complications of sinus surgery: a review of 1192 procedures. J Laryngol Otol 108:212–215
9. Kountakis SE, Bradley DT (2003) Effect of asthma on sinus computed tomography grade and symptom scores in patients undergoing revision functional endoscopic sinus surgery. Am J Rhinol 17:215–219
10. Maniglia AJ (1991) Fatal and other major complications of endoscopic sinus surgery. Laryngoscope 101:349–354
11. Musy PY, Kountakis SE (2004) Anatomic findings in patients undergoing revision endoscopic sinus surgery. Am J Otolaryngol 25:418–422
12. Oikawa K, Furuta Y, Itoh T, et al. (2007) Clinical and pathological analysis of recurrent inverted papilloma. Ann Otol Rhinol Laryngol 116:297–303
13. Parsons DS, Stivers FE, Talbot AR (1996) The missed ostium sequence and the surgical approach to revision functional endoscopic sinus surgery. Otolaryngol Clin North Am 29:169–183
14. Ramadan HH (1999) Surgical causes of failure in endoscopic sinus surgery. Laryngoscope 109:27–29
15. Schlosser RJ, Bolger WE (2004) Nasal cerebrospinal fluid leaks: critical review and surgical considerations. Laryngoscope 114:255–265
16. Stankiewicz JA (1989) Complications of endoscopic sinus surgery. Otolaryngol Clin North Am 22:749–758
17. Wormald PJ, Ooi E, van Hasselt CA, et al. (2003) Endoscopic removal of sinonasal inverted papilloma including endoscopic medial maxillectomy. Laryngoscope 113:867–873
18. Zhang G, Rodriguez X, Hussain A, et al. (2007) Outcomes of the extended endoscopic approach for management of inverted papilloma. J Otolaryngol 36:83–87

Chapter 3

Predictors of Failure of Primary Surgery

3

Iman Naseri and John M. DelGaudio

Core Messages

- Surgical success should be defined as significant symptom improvement or resolution, in addition to improvement of mucosal inflammation and sinus obstruction.
- Identification and maximal medical management of coexisting disease factors must be considered prior to ensuing surgical treatment to improve the results of endoscopic sinus surgery.
- Smoking has been found to increase the likelihood of a poor surgical outcome, and reflux disease is more common in surgically refractory patients with chronic rhinosinusitis.
- Significant nasal polyposis and advanced Lund-MacKay scores increase the chance of long-term failure of primary surgery.

Contents

Introduction

Endoscopic sinus surgery (ESS) is the preferred treatment for patients with chronic rhinosinusitis (CRS) that has failed to respond to maximal medical treatment. ESS has been found to be effective in up to 90% of patients, with long-term symptomatic improvement in up to 98% of patients [7, 16, 17, 24, 37, 39].

Multiple factors are implicated in the increased the risk for failure of primary ESS. These include [6, 7, 16, 39]:

1. Allergies.
2. Tobacco use.
3. Gastroesophageal reflux (GER) disease.
4. Previous open sinus procedures.
5. Severe mucosal disease.
6. Stage of sinus disease.
7. Inadequate postoperative care.
8. Scarring and synechiae.
9. Inadequate surgery.

The overall success rate of primary endoscopic sinus surgery ranges from 80 to 97% based on several criteria used to measure success [4, 9, 12, 13, 16, 24, 28, 36, 37, 43, 44]. It was shown that the extent of the disease measured preoperatively by computed tomography (CT) may dictate the surgical outcome [16]. CT scans and endoscopic examinations are used as outcome measurements in conjunction with subjective symptom evaluations. Among the staging systems that utilize CT scans, the Lund-MacKay staging system has been recommended by the Task Force on rhinosinusitis of the American Academy of Otolaryngology – Head and Neck Surgery [27, 45]. Two tests have been used most in clinical practice for symptom evaluation, the sinonasal outcome test (SNOT-20) and the symptom score instrument [26, 35].

Prior to discussing the factors that predispose to increased risk of failure of ESS we need to define what would be considered a failure.

- If the goal of sinus surgery is to improve or resolve sinonasal symptoms, sinus obstruction, and mucosal inflammation, then failure to accomplish these goals should be considered a failure.

By using this definition of failure, we can divide the predictors of failure into several categories, including patient selection factors, comorbidities, disease factors, and anatomic and surgical factors.

Patient Selection Factors

A successful surgical procedure begins with appropriate indications. ESS is indicated for CRS refractory to maximal medical therapy, mucoceles, extrasinus extension of CRS, and tumors.

- Sinus surgery may not be effective in resolving symptoms of postnasal drip (PND) or headache, even if the surgical procedure is technically perfect and the sinonasal mucosa is healthy in the postoperative period.

Also, the extent of surgery performed should be dictated by the degree of sinus disease observed on a preoperative CT scan. Failure to address involved sinuses at the primary procedure is likely to result in failure.

PND is a common symptom that can be found in patients with a myriad of sinonasal diseases. In patients with PND as the primary symptom, especially when there is minimal sinus disease on CT scan, the surgeon should be careful to treat other conditions that may be more likely to cause the PND prior to recommending surgery. Wise and DelGaudio found that in patients with and without CRS, those with a complaint of PND were significantly more likely to have pathologic reflux at the level of the nasopharynx and the hypopharynx [47]. Appropriate medical treatment of reflux should be performed prior to attributing this symptom to CRS, especially in the absence of purulent nasopharyngeal drainage.

- Sinus surgery may not be effective as a treatment for headache in the absence of sinus CT findings that correlate with the location of the headache

Multiple studies have found that over 90% of patients with a diagnosis of sinus headache and a normal CT scan of the sinuses meet the International Headache Society criteria for migraine headache [38]. DelGaudio has found that approximately 90% of patients presenting with a diagnosis of sinus headache and a normal or minimally diseased CT scan of the sinuses have reduction or resolution of their headaches with treatment with triptans (personal communication). Patients with sinus disease on CT scan and headache should be counseled that the sinus surgery may not resolve their headaches, especially if the headache location does not correlate to the area of sinus involvement.

Comorbidities

Reflux disease has been implicated to be associated with CRS, and has specifically been shown to be associated with a worse prognosis for ESS. Chambers et al. retrospectively reviewed 182 patients who had undergone ESS to determine the prognostic factors for poor outcome [7]. They found that a history of GER was the only historical factor that was a predictor of poor symptom outcome after ESS. DelGaudio showed that patients with persistent symptoms of CRS and sinonasal inflammation after ESS have significantly greater degrees of reflux at all levels of the aerodigestive tract, especially the nasopharynx, when compared to controls.

- This study is the first to demonstrate that direct nasopharyngeal reflux of gastric acid is found in adults with surgically refractory CRS at a significantly higher frequency than in control patients

The likely mechanism of effect on the nasal mucosa is mucosal edema and impaired mucociliary clearance. As acid travels up the digestive tract it reaches areas with less ability to protect against the acid and digestive enzymes present in the refluxate. It is likely that the nasopharyngeal and nasal mucosa have a lower threshold for injury from gastric contents. These results support the possibility that even more minor pH drops can cause harmful effects in the upper aerodigestive tract as a result of acid or pepsin exposure [11].

The role of reflux in CRS is especially evident in the pediatric population [34]. Treatment of GER in these patients leads to improvement of their sinus disease. Studies have also shown that medically refractory chronic sinusitis patients have improvement after treatment for GER [1]. Similarly, a significant reduction in the need for sinus surgery was also seen in such patients who underwent treatment for their reflux. Thus, one must recognize that reflux may play a role in worsening of symptoms of sinus disease, and the sinus surgeon should be wary of advocating surgery without proper diagnosis and treatment for this condition.

The deleterious effects of tobacco smoke on the aerodigestive tract are well documented. Despite the strong associations, there is a lack of controlled trials demonstrating the deleterious effects of tobacco smoke on sinonasal structures. Cigarette smoking has been shown to impede mucociliary transport and increase nasal resistance [3]. Although not a contraindication for ESS, patients who continue to smoke postoperatively are at a higher risk for complications and a worse outcome [6, 39]. This is most likely due to chronic mucosal irritation from the smoke, resulting in mucosal edema, poor mucosal healing, and increased postoperative scarring and synechiae formation. Little is known about the impact of smoking cessation and the reversal of these effects. Patients should be counseled on the effects of tobacco use on the success of ESS [8].

Many systemic diseases can affect the health of the sinonasal mucosa and negatively impact the results of ESS. Diseases such as sarcoidosis and Wegener's granulomatosis affect the respiratory tract and cause nasal mucosal inflammation, crusting, and dryness, which have a significant negative impact on healing after surgery. These patients have extensive edema and crusting postoperatively that frequently results in scarring and synechiae formation. ESS should only be performed in these patients if absolutely necessary, and only after maximal medical therapy has failed and the underlying systemic inflammatory condition has been controlled as much as possible.

Disease Factors

The most important factors that determine whether a patient is likely to have a poorer long-term outcome from ESS are related to the underling sinonasal disease factors. Like other chronic conditions, the worse the disease at the time of surgery, the greater the likelihood of persistence or recurrence. Factors that have been shown to predict failure of primary ESS include nasal polyps, ciliary dysmotility, advanced Lund-MacKay score, hyperostosis of the sinonasal bones, and asthma.

Nasal polyps, regardless of their underlying etiology, represent an advanced stage of mucosal inflammation. In addition to causing sinonasal obstruction, the polypoid mucosa inhibits normal mucociliary clearance [46]. Since the treatment of inflammation is predominantly a medical endeavor, it is not surprising that patients with polyps have a lower long-term success rate with ESS when compared to CRS patients without polyps.

- Sinus surgery in patients with polyps is directed at reducing the obstructive symptoms and reducing the inflammatory load so that medical therapy has a greater likelihood of controlling the underlying disease

There is an established relationship between nasal polyposis and the need for revision ESS [15, 20, 23]. There is also a higher rate of revision surgery in the polyp versus CRS patients [10]. Liu et al. demonstrated that sinus surgery in patients with bilateral maxillary rhinosinusitis from polyps has a 20.5% success rate [25]. Overall, patients with nasal polyposis typically have worse postoperative outcomes both objectively and subjectively when compared to CRS alone. Higher preoperative Lund-MacKay scores seen in the presence of nasal polyposis may be attributed to the bulk and mass effect of the polyps on imaging. Subjectively, patients with polyps have higher SNOT-20 scores than those with CRS. Deal et al. postulate that higher degrees of nasal obstruction in addition to the sequelae from decreased mucociliary transport may explain such observations [10].

As expected, patients with nasal polyposis have worse postoperative endoscopic findings and symptom scores than their CRS counterparts. Even at 1 year postoperatively, they have been found to have more severe disease, as evidenced by CT and endoscopy [45]. When bilateral nasal polyposis exists along with allergies, various immune interactions exist to cause a significant increase in their recurrence rates after surgery [40–42]. Thus, it is important to identify such patients and maximize their treatment for allergies.

- Asthma has been indicated for causing a significant increase in the need for revision surgery, and some would argue that it is the most important prognostic indicator for surgical failure [20, 22].

The frequency increases to 36–96% in aspirin-sensitive patients with asthma [2, 21]. Various reports have quoted the rate of nasal polyposis in asthmatics to be as high as 41% [22, 30]. Lawson et al. demonstrated a 50% success rate with asthmatics undergoing primary surgery, compared to 88% success among nonasthmatics [22]. Batra et al. demonstrated that improved postoperative sinonasal symptoms correlate directly with Lund-MacKay scores. In addition, aspirin-sensitive patients had higher Lund-MacKay scores pre- and postoperatively when compared with their aspirin-tolerant counterparts [2].

In patients with advanced disease, chronic use of systemic steroids has been associated with the need for revision ESS. These patients are likely to have hyper-reactive airway disease and must be properly identified because they are more likely to fail primary surgery and will require longer follow-up [31]. Strict control of asthma is strongly encouraged in the perioperative management of such patient groups.

- The correlation between asthma and CRS/nasal polyps most likely reflects the effect of an inflammatory process on the entire respiratory tract (the unified airway concept).

Recurrence rates are also higher in patients recognized to have Samter's triad (asthma, nasal polyps, and sensitivity to aspirin). Endoscopic sinus surgery for such patients has indicated a reduction of both upper- and lower-airway symptoms. This has been demonstrated by lower Lund-MacKay scores and improved pulmonary function tests [2]. Although not adopted as a standard regimen, the use of leukotriene inhibitors may have a role in the treatment of nasal polyposis, especially in the presence of Samter's triad.

3

Chronic rhinosinusitis is very common among patients with cystic fibrosis (CF). This population suffers from one of the highest rates of refractory CRS [32]. Because of the presence of ciliary dysmotility, these patients are at constant risk for life-threatening pulmonary infections. The deficiency of the CF transmembrane regulator protein causes chloride channel dysfunction at the epithelial cells of the upper respiratory tract. The resultant increase of sodium chloride in these cells leads to dehydration of the extracellular fluids and accumulation of thickened secretions in the sinonasal cavities [48]. Up to 50% of pediatric CF patients have nasal polyposis, and this patient population typically requires multiple surgeries throughout life. These patients should be treated aggressively both medically and surgically as they present a significant challenge because of the significant effect that the sinus disease has on pulmonary function. Nonetheless, all patients with CF require careful follow-up and frequent endoscopic examinations.

Sarcoidosis is a systemic disease that may cause inflammatory rhinosinusitis refractory to the traditional treatments. In a study from the Mayo clinic involving 2319 patients with sarcoidosis, 9% had head and neck manifestations, and 1% had sinonasal involvement [29]. The clinical signs may mimic chronic rhinitis or CRS with extensive crusting. These patients should be treated with high suspicion for the diagnosis of sinonasal sarcoidosis [5]. Definitive diagnosis should be made by endoscopy-guided biopsy of suspicious lesions to rule out chronic noncaseating granulomas. Extensive crusting and edema in the postoperative period can lead to synechiae and obstruction.

Osteitis has been shown to be present in the sinus bone of CRS specimens [14, 18, 33]. Kim et al. evaluated the effect of osteitis on surgical outcome in patients undergoing ESS for CRS. They found that the success rate of ESS for patients with preoperative CT scan evidence of osteitis was 51.9%, compared to a success rate of 75.9% in patients without CT evidence of osteitis [19]. The reason for this is unknown and requires further study. Longer treatment with antibiotics or anti-inflammatory agents may be necessary in the perioperative period in this group of patients.

Conclusion

Primary ESS has a very high rate of success, especially if the surgery is performed meticulously and for the appropriate indications. Predictors of failure include inappropriate patient selection, failure to medically address comorbidities, advanced sinonasal disease severity, and anatomic factors. Careful attention to each of these factors preoperatively may help to reduce failures.

References

1. Barbero GJ (1996) Gastroesophageal reflux and upper airway disease. Otolaryngol Clin North Am 29:27–38
2. Batra PS, Kern RC, Tripathi A, Conley DB, Ditto AM, et al. (2003) Outcome analysis of endoscopic sinus surgery in patients with nasal polyps and asthma. Laryngoscope 113:1703–1706
3. Benninger MS (1999) The impact of cigarette smoking and environmental tobacco smoke on nasal and sinus disease: a review of the literature. Am J Rhinol 13:435–438
4. Biedlingmaier JF (1993) Endoscopic sinus surgery with middle turbinate resection: results and complications. Ear Nose Throat J 72:351–355
5. Braun JJ, Gentine A, Pauli G (2004) Sinonasal sarcoidosis: review and report of fifteen cases. Laryngoscope 114:1960–1963
6. Briggs RD, Wright ST, Cordes S, Calhoun KH (2004) Smoking in chronic rhinosinusitis: a predictor of poor long-term outcome after endoscopic sinus surgery. Laryngoscope 114:126–128
7. Chambers DW, Davis WE, Cook PR, Nishioka GJ, Rudman DT (1997) Long-term outcome analysis of functional endoscopic sinus surgery: correlation of symptoms with endoscopic examination findings and potential prognostic variables. Laryngoscope 107:504–510
8. Das S, Becker AM, Perakis H, Prosser JD, Kountakis SE (2007) The effects of smoking on short-term quality of life outcomes in sinus surgery. Laryngoscope (in press)
9. Davis WE, Templer JW, LaMear WR (1991) Patency rate of endoscopic middle meatus antrostomy. Laryngoscope 101:416–420
10. Deal RT, Kountakis SE (2004) Significance of nasal polyps in chronic rhinosinusitis: symptoms and surgical outcomes. Laryngoscope 114:1932–1935
11. DelGaudio JM (2005) Direct nasopharyngeal reflux of gastric acid is a contributing factor in refractory chronic rhinosinusitis. Laryngoscope 115:946–957
12. Hoffman SR, Dersarkissian RM, Buck SH, Stinziano GD, Buck GM (1989) Sinus disease and surgical treatment: a results oriented quality assurance study. Otolaryngol Head Neck Surg 100:573–577
13. Hoffman SR, Mahoney MC, Chmiel JF, Stinziano GD, Hoffman KN (1993) Symptom relief after endoscopic sinus surgery: an outcomes-based study. Ear Nose Throat J 72:413–414
14. Jang YJ, Koo TW, Chung SY, Park SG (2002) Bone involvement in chronic rhinosinusitis assessed by 99mTc-MDP bone SPECT. Clin Otolaryngol Allied Sci 27:156–161
15. Jiang RS, Hsu CY (2002) Revision functional endoscopic sinus surgery. Ann Otol Rhinol Laryngol 111:155–159
16. Kennedy DW (1992) Prognostic factors, outcomes and staging in ethmoid sinus surgery. Laryngoscope 102:1–18

17. Kennedy DW, Wright ED, Goldberg AN (2000) Objective and subjective outcomes in surgery for chronic sinusitis. Laryngoscope 110:29–31
18. Khalid AN, Hunt J, Perloff JR, Kennedy DW (2002) The role of bone in chronic rhinosinusitis. Laryngoscope 112:1951–1957
19. Kim HY, Dhong HJ, Lee HJ, Chung YJ, Yim YJ, et al. (2006) Hyperostosis may affect prognosis after primary endoscopic sinus surgery for chronic rhinosinusitis. Otolaryngol Head Neck Surg 135:94–99
20. King JM, Caldarelli DD, Pigato JB (1994) A review of revision functional endoscopic sinus surgery. Laryngoscope 104:404–408
21. Larsen K (1996) The clinical relationship of nasal polyps to asthma. Allergy Asthma Proc 17:243–249
22. Lawson W (1991) The intranasal ethmoidectomy: an experience with 1,077 procedures. Laryngoscope 101:367–371
23. Lazar RH, Younis RT, Long TE, Gross CW (1992) Revision functional endonasal sinus surgery. Ear Nose Throat J 71:131–133
24. Levine HL (1990) Functional endoscopic sinus surgery: evaluation, surgery, and follow-up of 250 patients. Laryngoscope 100:79–84
25. Liu CM, Yeh TH, Hsu MM (1994) Clinical evaluation of maxillary diffuse polypoid sinusitis after functional endoscopic sinus surgery. Am J Rhinol 8:7–11
26. Lund VJ, Holmstrom M, Scadding GK (1991) Functional endoscopic sinus surgery in the management of chronic rhinosinusitis. An objective assessment. J Laryngol Otol 105:832–835
27. Lund VJ, Kennedy DW (1997) Staging for rhinosinusitis. Otolaryngol Head Neck Surg 117:S35–50
28. Matthews BL, Smith LE, Jones R, Miller C, Brookschmidt JK (1991) Endoscopic sinus surgery: outcome in 155 cases. Otolaryngol Head Neck Surg 104:244–246
29. McCaffrey TV, McDonald TJ (1983) Sarcoidosis of the nose and paranasal sinuses. Laryngoscope 93:1281–1284
30. McFadden EA, Woodson BT, Fink JN, Toohill RJ (1997) Surgical treatment of aspirin triad sinusitis. Am J Rhinol 11:263–270
31. Moses RL, Cornetta A, Atkins JP Jr, Roth M, Rosen MR, et al. (1998) Revision endoscopic sinus surgery: the Thomas Jefferson University experience. Ear Nose Throat J 77:190–195
32. Moss RB, King VV (1995) Management of sinusitis in cystic fibrosis by endoscopic surgery and serial antimicrobial lavage. Reduction in recurrence requiring surgery. Arch Otolaryngol Head Neck Surg 121:566–572
33. Perloff JR, Gannon FH, Bolger WE, Montone KT, Orlandi R, et al. (2000) Bone involvement in sinusitis: an apparent pathway for the spread of disease. Laryngoscope 110:2095–2099
34. Phipps CD, Wood WE, Gibson WS, Cochran WJ (2000) Gastroesophageal reflux contributing to chronic sinus disease in children: a prospective analysis. Arch Otolaryngol Head Neck Surg 126:831–836
35. Piccirillo JF, Merritt MG Jr, Richards ML (2002) Psychometric and clinimetric validity of the 20-Item Sino-Nasal Outcome Test (SNOT-20). Otolaryngol Head Neck Surg 126:41–47
36. Schaefer SD, Manning S, Close LG (1989) Endoscopic paranasal sinus surgery: indications and considerations. Laryngoscope 99:1–5
37. Schaitkin B, May M, Shapiro A, Fucci M, Mester SJ (1993) Endoscopic sinus surgery: 4-year follow-up on the first 100 patients. Laryngoscope 103:1117–1120
38. Schreiber CP, Hutchinson S, Webster CJ, Ames M, Richardson MS, et al. (2004) Prevalence of migraine in patients with a history of self-reported or physician-diagnosed "sinus" headache. Arch Intern Med 164:1769–1772
39. Senior BA, Kennedy DW, Tanabodee J, Kroger H, Hassab M, et al. (1998) Long-term results of functional endoscopic sinus surgery. Laryngoscope 108:151–157
40. Settipane GA (1996) Epidemiology of nasal polyps. Allergy Asthma Proc 17:231–236
41. Settipane GA (1996) Nasal polyps and immunoglobulin E (IgE). Allergy Asthma Proc 17:269–273
42. Settipane GA, Klein DE, Settipane RJ (1991) Nasal polyps. State of the art. Rhinol Suppl 11:33–36
43. Smith LF, Brindley PC (1993) Indications, evaluation, complications, and results of functional endoscopic sinus surgery in 200 patients. Otolaryngol Head Neck Surg 108:688–696
44. Stammberger H (1986) Endoscopic endonasal surgery – concepts in treatment of recurring rhinosinusitis. Part II. Surgical technique. Otolaryngol Head Neck Surg 94:147–156
45. Toros SZ, Bolukbasi S, Naiboglu B, Er B, Akkaynak C, at al. (2007) Comparative outcomes of endoscopic sinus surgery in patients with chronic sinusitis and nasal polyps. Eur Arch Otorhinolaryngol 264:1003–1008
46. Waguespack R (1995) Mucociliary clearance patterns following endoscopic sinus surgery. Laryngoscope 105:1–40
47. Wise SK, Wise JC, DelGaudio JM (2006) Association of nasopharyngeal and laryngopharyngeal reflux with postnasal drip symptomatology in patients with and without rhinosinusitis. Am J Rhinol 20:283–289
48. Yung MW, Gould J, Upton GJ (2002) Nasal polyposis in children with cystic fibrosis: a long-term follow-up study. Ann Otol Rhinol Laryngol 111:1081–1086

Chapter 4

Pathophysiology of Inflammation in the Surgically Failed Sinus Cavity

4

Wytske J. Fokkens, Bas Rinia and Christos Georgalas

Core Messages

- Chronic rhinosinusitis with or without polyps is an inflammatory disease. Treatment should always consist of a sandwich of optimal medical treatment, if necessary followed by surgery and than always followed by a (sometimes extensive) period of medical treatment.
- Both extrinsic and intrinsic patient factors may be associated with an unfavourable outcome after endoscopic sinus surgery.
- A careful assessment of these factors may serve as a helpful prognostic indicator of the outcome of endoscopic sinus surgery.
- Optimising the management of underlying systemic disease is vital in order to achieve a satisfactory outcome, especially in revision surgery.

Contents

Introduction

Chronic rhinosinusitis (CRS) with or without polyps is an inflammatory disease of the nose and the paranasal sinuses characterised by symptoms of nasal blockage/obstruction/congestion, nasal discharge (anterior/posterior nasal drip), facial pain/pressure, and deterioration or loss of the sense of smell [1]. Treatment should always consist of a sandwich of optimal medical treatment, if necessary followed by surgery and then always followed by a (sometimes extensive) period of medical treatment.

The primary goal of medical treatment is the reduction or resolution of the underlying inflammation. The primary goal of surgical treatment is to remove irreversibly diseased mucosa, to aerate the sinuses and to render them more accessible to medical treatment. Although most ear-nose-and-throat surgeons currently use sandwich therapy, approximately 10% of patients respond poorly to sinus surgery with concomitant medical therapy and eventually undergo a secondary surgical procedure [2]. In this chapter we will assess the role of inflammation in patients who fail sinus surgery, including the role of intrinsic patient factors and external factors that adversely influence surgical outcome.

4

Intrinsic factors

CRS most likely consists of different phenotypes. The different phenotypes of CRS are often lumped together as a single disease entity, because at this moment it seems impossible to clearly differentiate between them [1]. CRS with nasal polyps (NP) is one of the subgroups that has the most distinctive characteristics; some studies have attempted to use inflammatory markers in order to differentiate CRS with NP from the other subgroups [3–5]. Although some of these studies point to more pronounced eosinophilia and interleukin-5 expression in patients with NPs than in patients with CRS, these studies also suggest the existence of a continuum in which differences might be evident towards the ends of the spectrum, but no clear cut-off point exists between patients with NP and other forms of CRS. In this chapter we will refer to CRS as a single entity except when clear differences between different phenotypes are described in the literature.

There are several intrinsic factors that can give rise to, or affect the clinical course of CRS. They need to be recognised and considered because they can adversely influence sinus surgery outcome. Some of these factors may also require specific therapeutic interventions, in addition to sinus surgery.

Allergy and Atopy

- Although there is still no clear evidence of a causal link between allergy and CRS, the chances of symptomatic improvement after endoscopic sinus surgery (ESS) are optimised if the underlying allergy is addressed.

It is tempting to speculate that allergic inflammation in the nose predisposes the atopic individual to the development of CRS. Both conditions share the same trend of increasing prevalence [6] and frequently coexist in the same individual. It has been postulated that swelling of the nasal mucosa in allergic rhinitis at the site of the sinus ostia may compromise ventilation and even obstruct them completely, leading to mucus retention and infection. Furthermore, there is a growing consensus that the mucosa of the nasal airway is in a continuum with the paranasal sinuses, as reflected by the use of the term "rhinosinusitis" rather than "sinusitis".

However, critical analysis of the papers citing atopy as a risk factor for chronic rhinosinusitis reveals that whilst there appears to be a higher prevalence of allergy in patients presenting with symptoms consistent with sinusitis than would be expected in the general population, this may be the result of selection bias, as the doctors involved often had an interest in allergy [7, 8]. Among CRS patients undergoing sinus surgery, the prevalence of sensitisation ranges from 30 to 62% [9–11], of which the majority (60%) are sensitive to multiple allergens [11]. Just like in asthma, there are some indications that in patients with more severe forms of CRS, allergy is less important [11]. Notwithstanding the lack of hard epidemiologic evidence of a clear causal relationship between allergy and CRS, it is obvious that failure to address allergy as a contributing factor to CRS diminishes the chances of success of surgical intervention [12]. Half of the patients who have had sinus surgery before, believed that the surgery alone was not sufficient to completely resolve the recurrent episodes of infection [12]. However, the rate of revision surgery was not significantly different between atopic and non-atopic patients [9].

Asthma

Asthma is frequently associated with CRS and NP. In patients with concomitant asthma, a trend to suffer from more severe forms of sinus disease is observed [13]. In addition, CRS is self-reported in a very high percentage (70%) of patients suffering from asthma [14]. Asthmatic patients with concomitant CRS had more asthma exacerbations, worse asthma scores, worse cough and worse sleep quality than those without CRS.

At the cellular level the difference between asthmatic and non-asthmatic patients suffering from CRS/NP becomes evident: Patients with NP who have concomitant asthma tend to have a more prominent eosinophilic infiltration . This suggests a more aggressive inflammatory response, especially in the subgroup with aspirin-intolerant asthma [15–22].

These data clearly support a strong link between the lower and the upper airways. Medical and/or surgical treatment of the upper airways of asthmatics with CRS/NP, positively influences the course of bronchial asthma. Several studies report asthma symptom improvement, less asthma attacks, less steroid use (topical and systemic) and improvement in peak expiratory flow after surgery and medical treatment of the upper airways [23–25]. There is no clear evidence that CRS/NP patients with asthma benefit less from sinus surgery than patients without asthma [13, 26, 27]. Nevertheless, post-operative endoscopic findings were worse in patients with concomitant asthma [28–30], and patients with asthma did require significantly more revision sinus procedures overall [31].

Acetylsalicylic Acid intolerance

- Patients with asthma and acetylsalicylic acid (ASA) intolerance tend to have worse outcomes following functional ESS (FESS) and require revision surgery more often.

Already in 1922, Widal described a triad of symptoms, which later came to be known as the Samter's triad: intolerance to ASA compounds (e.g. aspirin), bronchial asthma and (often severe) CRS with NP. The mechanism of the hypersensitivity reaction to aspirin is not immunological, but may be related to the inhibition of cyclo-oxygenase (COX-1 and COX-2), an enzyme responsible for prostaglandin synthesis, by aspirin.

Symptoms of this ASA triad usually commence around the 20th year of life. Initially, patients present with nasal blocking, rhinorrhea and hyposmia followed in a couple of years by the formation of NPs and (often steroid dependent) asthma. Ingestion of aspirin (or another non-steroidal anti-inflammatory drug, NSAID) results in an exacerbation of rhinitis and asthma, but independent of the exposure to NSAIDs, the disease will continue lifelong. Patients suffering from CRS and/or NP with ASA intolerance tend to suffer from more extensive sinus disease. They benefit from sinus surgery, but to a lesser extent than patients without ASA intolerance [32]. However, they are more prone to disease recurrence and more frequently have to undergo revision surgery than ASA-tolerant CRS/NP patients [32–34].

"Osteitis" – the Role of Bone

Areas of increased bone density and irregular bony thickening are frequently seen on CT in areas of chronic inflammation in patients with CRS and may be a marker of the underlying chronic inflammatory process [35–37]. Although to date bacterial organisms have not been identified in the bone of either humans or animal models of CRS, it has been suggested that this irregular bony thickening is a sign of bony involvement, which might in turn maintain mucosal inflammation [35–37].

Cystic Fibrosis and Primary Ciliary Dyskinesia

Both cystic fibrosis (CF) and primary ciliary dyskinesia (PCD) manifest, among other things, with recurrent upper and lower respiratory tract infections. Patients with CF almost without exception suffer from CRS, and develop NP in approximately 50% of cases. CRS is also almost always present in patients with PCD, but the prevalence of NP in this group of patients is only about 5%. Both CF and PCD are autosomal recessive genetic diseases and should be considered in children with CRS with or without NP.

When suspected, CF can be diagnosed by means of a sweat test or DNA analysis. Ciliary activity in PCD can be investigated in a mucosa biopsy from the upper or lower airways, if necessary after culturing. A nasal brush is also a possibility as a way of collecting nasal epithelial cells.

Long-term antibiotics and local/systemic steroids are the cornerstones of treatment. Multiple surgical procedures are often needed in order to achieve symptomatic relief of the upper, as well as the lower, airways. Since mucociliary clearance is compromised in both diseases, simple FESS is often not sufficient. In addition to nasal lavages, radical sinus surgery is often unavoidable [38, 39]. Perioperative morbidity is assumed to be higher in CF patients, due to underlying medical issues, such as acquired coagulopathies and advanced pulmonary disease.

Immune Disorders

Several acquired and non-acquired immunodeficiencies can cause CRS (with or without NP). They may gravely affect the patient's clinical course and influence the responsiveness of CRS to standard medical and surgical treatment. They should always be considered in cases of recalcitrant sinus disease.

- In cases of recalcitrant disease that is resistant to both medical and surgical treatment, the patient must be assessed for the presence of underlying congenital immunodeficiencies. However, with the exception of humoral deficiency, which may necessitate treatment with intravenous immunoglobulin, the significance of subtle immunodeficiencies is uncertain.

Non-acquired Immunodeficiency Disorders

A high percentage of patients with severe CRS, refractory to medical treatment, seem to suffer from impaired T-cell function, impaired granulocyte function [40], some form of immunoglobulin deficiency and common variable immunodeficiency [41–43]. The prognostic value of these findings, nevertheless, is limited [44–46].

Non-acquired immunodeficiencies may affect humoral, cellular and frequently both immune response pathways. These patients are at an increased risk of developing CRS [47–49]. Some examples include common variable immunodeficiency, ataxia telangiectasia and X-linked agammaglobulinaemia. Currently, there is not enough data to evaluate the role of sinus surgery in this group of patients. In patients with an identified humoral deficiency, there may be a role for concomitant intravenous immunoglobulin therapy [50].

Specific Mucosal Diseases

A few systemic inflammatory conditions are associated with CRS. Three of the most frequently encountered include Wegener's granulomatosis (WG), sarcoidosis and

Churg-Straus syndrome. These can cause severe nasal and paranasal sinus complaints and need to be recognised, because they need specific therapeutic interventions.

Wegener's Granulomatosis

- The role of surgery in active WG is essentially limited to providing a sample of diseased mucosa for histological diagnosis.

WG is a multisystem disease with a complex genetic background, characterised by vasculitis with multi-organ involvement. The most common features include granulomatous inflammation of the upper and lower respiratory tracts and glomerulonephritis. It usually presents at age 30–50 years, and affects males approximately 1.5 times more often than females. In up to 95% of the patients, the head and neck region is the first to be affected [51].

Nasal involvement becomes evident mostly as persistent purulent rhinorrhoea and sinusitis, sometimes with ulcerating lesions of the nasal and sinus mucosa. Findings on nasal examination may range from a purulent infection with no obvious mucosal abnormalities to (destructive/necrotising) granulomatous lesions of the septal and lateral nasal wall mucosa (Fig. 4.1). Destruction of the septum may result in the characteristic saddle-nose deformity (Fig. 4.2).

A positive (c)anti-neutrophil cytoplasmic antibody test and a raised erythrocyte sedimentation rate together with a characteristic clinical picture are highly suggestive of WG. However, the diagnosis is confirmed with histology and, if the nose is affected, a biopsy sample should be taken from the affected mucosa while the patient is not using corticosteroids. There is no point in taking a biopsy sample from macroscopically healthy mucosa.

Untreated WG is usually fatal. Patients should be jointly managed with a clinical immunologist. In gener-

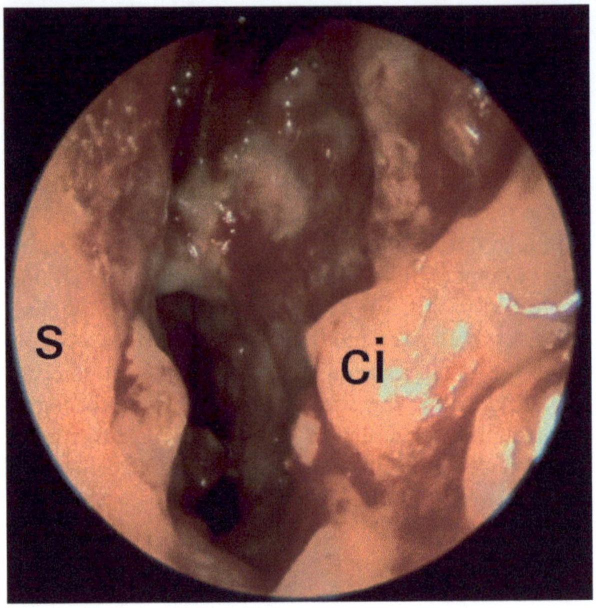

Fig. 4.1 Patients with nasal granulomatosis. This figure shows destructive/necrotising granulomatous inflammation of the septal and lateral nasal wall mucosa. *ci* Concha inferior, *S* septum

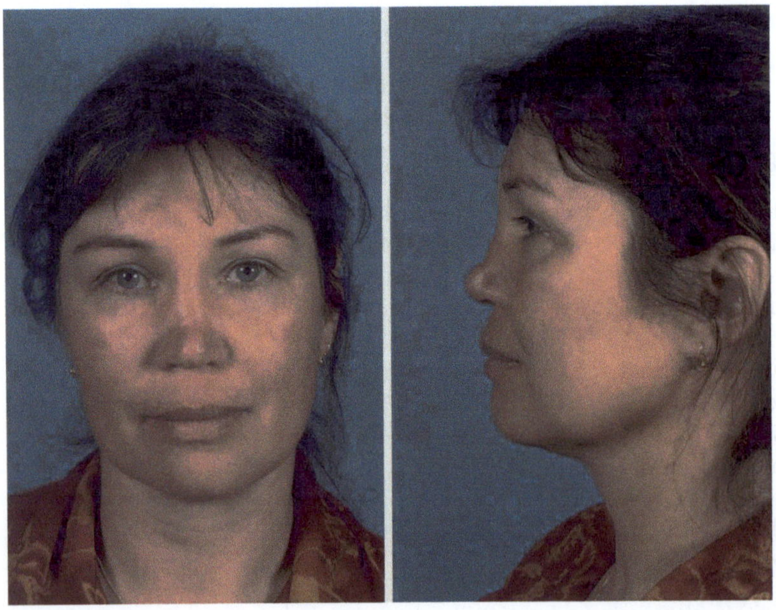

Fig. 4.2 Patient with nasal deformity due to destruction of the septum

alised disease, the induction treatment is systemic and consists of cytostatics (e.g. cyclophosphamide) combined with steroids [51, 52] After achieving remission, maintenance therapy usually consists of azathioprine (an immunosuppressant) 2 mg/kg daily. When WG is localised only to the nose, the treatment can consist of cotrimoxazol 960 mg daily and topical steroid drops or steroid ointment applied to the nasal mucosa with a cotton bud. The outcome of FESS in these cases is frequently disappointing and therefore surgery should be avoided. Reconstruction of the saddle deformity should only be considered if the disease is in complete remission. Even then, nasal surgery could induce disease recurrence [51].

Sarcoidosis

Sarcoidosis is a chronic noncaseating granulomatous disease of unknown aetiology, principally affecting the (lower) respiratory tract. The overall incidence is approximately 6–10 per 100,000 [53]. Sinonasal involvement is rare, with reported incidences of 0.7–6% in the literature [54].

Most frequent complaints suggestive of nasal involvement are reduced airflow, rhinorrhoea, anosmia and crusting. Findings on examination of the nose may range from mild mucosal changes such as turbinate hypertrophy and a strawberry-like appearance of the nasal mucosa, to severe crusting, septal perforation and even a saddle-nose deformity (Fig. 4.3) [54].

A diagnosis of sarcoidosis is made on the basis of clinical findings, a plain chest X-ray (showing bilateral hilar lymphadenopathy), raised angiotensin-converting enzyme titre in serum and a biopsy of the affected mucosa.

Sarcoidosis patients with sinonasal involvement tend to have lower remission rates and to require more often long-term systemic treatment [54]. Treatment of the nose with local steroids is often not effective, and systemic treatment, in the form of oral steroids, immunosuppressants such as methotrexate (a folic acid antagonist) or azathioprine is necessary. Surgery for sinonasal sarcoidosis is controversial; although it may alleviate symptoms on the short-term, surgery alone does not eradicate the disease or prevent recurrence [55].

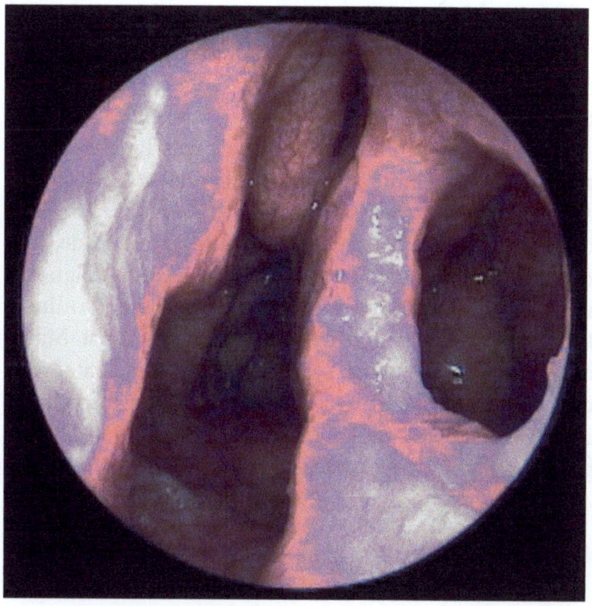

Fig. 4.3 Patient with nasal septal perforation

Churg-Strauss Syndrome

- In sarcoidosis, as in Churg-Strauss syndrome, the role of surgery is controversial: It may occasionally be used concurrently with steroids and immunosuppressants; however, its effects seem to be limited to short-term symptomatic improvement.

Churg-Strauss syndrome (CSS) is a rare necrotising granulomatous vasculitis of unknown aetiology. It affects small- to medium-sized blood vessels. The most frequently involved organs are the nose, paranasal sinuses, lungs and peripheral nervous system. Many other organs can also be involved, such as the heart, kidneys, skin and gastrointestinal tract. The American College of Rheumatology established six criteria for the diagnosis of CSS:

1. A history of asthma.
2. Eosinophilia > 10%.
3. Mononeuropathy or polyneuropathy.
4. Non-fixed pulmonary infiltrates.
5. Paranasal sinus abnormalities.
6. Biopsy showing extravascular eosinophils.

The diagnosis of CSS is made when four or more of these criteria are present.

Clinically, the disease process can be divided into three phases: The prodromal phase, consisting of asthma possibly associated with allergic rhinitis and often complicated by sinonasal polyposis and recurrent rhinosinusitis. The second phase is characterised by peripheral blood eosinophilia and/or eosinophilic tissue infiltrates (i.e. eosinophilic pneumonia or gastroenteritis). The third phase is dominated by manifestations resulting from systemic vasculitis (i.e. polyneuropathy).

Nasal involvement is seen in approximately 69–75% of patients [56, 57]. Presenting nasal symptoms are those related to allergic rhinitis, rhinosinusitis, NP and crusting lesions throughout the nose.

The diagnosis can be confirmed by laboratory testing (leukocytosis with more than 10% eosinophils) and tissue biopsy sampling (necrotising vasculitis, extravascular necrotising granulomas and tissue eosinophilia).

Since the first phase of the disease is barely distinguishable from common chronic (allergic) rhinosinusitis and polyposis, patients frequently undergo FESS. This does not negatively influence the disease outcome, but revision surgery is usually needed. Once the diagnosis is made, treatment options should again be determined in close consultation with a clinical immunologist. Many of these patients require systemic steroids and in severe cases, azathioprine or cyclophosphamide for a long period of time. Some patients might benefit from immunoglobulin or interferon-α treatment [58, 59].

External Factors

Microbiology

Bacteria and Biofilms

- The recent focus on *Staphylococcus aureus* enterotoxins (SAEs) and biofilms as central factors in the pathophysiology of CRS may serve as a helpful paradigm in explaining some cases of medical and surgical failure. Novel forms of treatment that would potentially target them are required.

The role of bacteria in chronic sinus disease is far from clear. Bhattacharyya [60] showed that aerobic as well as anaerobic species could be cultured from both diseased and non-diseased sinuses. Polymicrobial colonisation is often found. The most frequently cultured "pathogens" in CRS appear to be coagulase-negative *Staphylococcus* species (24–80%), *S. aureus* (9–33%), *Streptococcus pneumoniae* (0–7%) and anaerobes (0–8%) [61]. *Pseudomonas aeruginosa* is also cultured in some cases [62–64]. Bacteriology in patients with CRS/NP who have been medically and surgically treated does not seem to differ much from that in untreated patients.

Gram-positive *S. aureus* bacteria have the innate capability of releasing classical and egc-locus-derived enterotoxins, which show superantigen activity and effectively modify the functions of T and B cells, eosinophils and other inflammatory and structural cells. The stimulation may lead to a type 2 T-helper (TH)-cell-polarised eosinophilic inflammation as well as a multiclonal immunoglobulin E (IgE) production, exacerbating airway disease in the upper and lower respiratory tracts. Recently, *S. aureus* has been demonstrated to reside intra-epithelially and potentially to release superantigens into the tissue from within the epithelial cells. An immune defect, either in the innate or adaptive immunity, might be responsible for this phenomenon. Follicle-like structures and lymphocyte accumulations, specifically binding enterotoxins, can be found within the mucosal tissue. Interestingly, IgE antibodies to enterotoxins can be found in the majority of ASA-sensitive patients, including those with NP as well as severe asthma. However, therapeutic approaches are so far limited and empirical, and inadequate in dealing with this currently underestimated clinical challenge. In conclusion, these data suggest that SAEs are at least modifiers of disease in CRS with NP [65, 66].

Another interesting finding in CRS is the formation of bacterial biofilms [67, 68]. A biofilm is defined as an organised community of bacteria, adherent to a surface and contained in an extracellular polymeric substance produced by the bacteria themselves (containing polysaccharides, nucleic acids and proteins) [69]. Because of the protective function of this matrix and their low metabolism, bacteria in biofilms are less susceptible to both innate and adaptive host defence mechanisms, as well as to antibiotics. Biofilms allow bacteria to remain attached to the mucosa for months to years, with intermittent acute exacerbations. CRS possesses the hallmarks of a biofilm-mediated disease since it is a chronic disease that is characterised by acute exacerbations. The involved micro-organisms are often difficult to culture and define and are resistant to eradication, even with directed antibiotics. Bendouah et al. evaluated semi-quantitatively the bacterial ability to form biofilms in patients who had undergone an FESS procedure for CRS [70]. They conclude that there is a correlation between in vitro biofilm-producing capacity by both *S. aureus* and *P. aeruginosa* and unfavourable evolution after FESS, as determined by symptom scores and endoscopic signs. This suggests a possible role for biofilm production in chronic recalcitrant sinus disease. However, the relative importance of these biofilms, as well as possible therapeutic strategies against biofilms, requires further investigation.

Prophylactic antibacterial treatment should not differ much between primary and revision sinus surgery. In case of severe disease and/or many recurrences, perioperative treatment specifically targeted against cultured pathogens is suggested. Together with topical and/or systemic anti-inflammatory treatment, this maximises the chances of healing of the affected mucosa.

Fungus

- There is controversy regarding the role of fungi in the pathogenesis of common forms of CRS and evidence that treatment with topical antifungals is not effective.

There is increasing interest in the concept that the most common forms of sinus disease may be caused by the inflammation stimulated by airborne fungal antigens. In 1999 it was proposed that most patients with CRS exhibit eosinophilic infiltration and the presence of fungi by histology or culture [71]. This assertion was based on finding a positive fungal culture by using a new culture technique in 202 of 210 (96%) patients with CRS who were evaluated prospectively in a cohort study. Using this new culture technique, the same percentage of positive fungi cultures was found in normal controls [72].

Some authors suggest that non-IgE-mediated mechanisms underlying the response to fungal spores might be responsible for the eosinophilic inflammation seen in some individuals [73]. Shin et al. found that patients with CRS had an exaggerated humoral and TH1 and TH2 cellular response to common airborne fungi, particularly *Alternaria*. No increase in type I sensitivity was found in patients as compared with controls [74].

The fungal hypothesis, based of the premise of an altered local immune (non-allergic) response to fungal presence in nasal/sinus secretions resulting in the generation of chronic eosinophilic rhinosinusitis and NP [71], has led to the concept of treating CRS with and without NP with a topical antimycotic. The use of topical or systemic antifungal agents, however, has not consistently been shown to help patients with CRS [75, 76].

Environmental Factors

Cigarette smoking was shown to be associated with a higher prevalence of rhinosinusitis in Canada [77], whereas this observation was not confirmed in a nationwide survey in Korea [78]. Other lifestyle-related factors are undoubtedly involved in the chronic inflammatory processes of rhinosinusitis. For instance, low income was associated with a higher prevalence of CRS [77]. Despite in vitro data demonstrating the toxicity of pollutants on respiratory epithelium, there is no convincing evidence of a causal link between pollutants and toxins, such as ozone, and CRS.

Acquired Immunodeficiency Disorders

- Patients with acquired immunodeficiency (patients with AIDS and bone marrow transplant recipients) tend to present with CRS associated with atypical pathogens. Targeted antibiotics against the causative pathogens is the mainstay of treatment, with surgery preserved only with those patients who fail medical management. However, in those patients who present with invasive fungal disease, early and aggressive surgical and medical treatment is mandatory.

Human Immunodeficiency Virus

The most common causes of acquired immunodeficiencies in patients suffering from CRS are human immunodeficiency virus (HIV) infection and bone marrow transplantation (BMT).

Patients with HIV have a higher risk of developing CRS, especially at CD4 counts below 50 cells/mm^3, with reported prevalence ranging from 10 to 70% [79–81]. Many pathogens can be identified in the sinuses of HIV-positive patients with CRS. Most frequently these are *Staphylococcus* (coagulase negative), *P. aeruginosa*, *Streptococcus* and *Aspergillus fumigates* [81]. Clearly, first-line treatment of CRS in HIV-positive patients should be directed against the identified organism. If this targeted medical treatment fails, FESS has been reported to be beneficial in retrospective studies [79, 82].

Bone Marrow Transplantation

BMT is also a frequent cause of acquired immune deficiency. Allogeneic BMT in particular is notorious for being associated with impairment of cellular as well as humoral immunity, due to the necessity of intensive immunosuppression. Approximately 40–50% of allogeneic BMT recipients develop CRS [79, 83]. The sinus microbiology of patients with CRS after BMT reveals predominantly Gram-negative bacteria (56.7%; including *P. aeruginosa* and *Searratia marescens*), followed by Gram-positive bacteria (26.7%) and various fungi (16.6%) [84]. Again, treatment should be directed primarily against the causative pathogens. This suggests that a culture swab from the middle meatus, or a biopsy sample if necessary, should be performed in all BMT patients suffering from sinus disease. Limited surgical approaches with intensive post-operative care seems appropriate in a selected group of BMT patients with CRS who are refractory to medical treatment [85]. Nevertheless, there is insufficient data to allow us to adequately assess the role of FESS in BMT patients suffering from CRS.

Both HIV and BMT patients are at risk of developing invasive fungal rhinossinusitis, a condition that carries a high mortality rate. If this condition is detected early, combined surgical and antifungal treatment may be beneficial [86, 87].

4

Helicobacter pylori and Laryngopharyngeal Reflux

Helicobacter pylori DNA has been detected in between 11% [88] and 33% [89] of sinus samples from patients with CRS, but not from controls. Although this suggest a link, no causal relationship has been established.

Immunopathophysiology

- A better understanding of the pathophysiology of mucosal inflammation in patients with CRS, including the role of matrix metalloproteinase (MMP)-9 in healing may help us in the future in selecting patients who are more likely to benefit from surgery.

So far, there are only a few reports concerning underlying immunologic processes and their relation with disease intensity and sinus surgery outcome.

Both CRS and NP are characterised by abundant mucosal infiltration by inflammatory cells. In CRS these are predominantly neutrophils and eosinophils. NP is typified by a uniquely eosinophilic inflammation. In both CRS and NP the eosinophilic influx is higher in asthmatic patients when compared with non-asthmatic patients [15–18, 21]. This difference in eosinophilic influx is even more marked in ASA-intolerant patients [19, 20, 22, 90]. Eosinophilia seems to be correlated with disease severity [91] and prognosis [92]. This correlation between the extent of eosinophilia and disease severity is also seen in the lower airways of patients with asthma. Patients with a higher degree of eosinophilia have significantly more severe symptoms and residual airway obstruction after bronchodilatory therapy [93–95].

These differences also become apparent at an immunoglobulin level. IgE levels are significantly higher in CRS patients with and without NP compared to controls [96, 97]. In CRS, the pre-operative total IgE level seems to correlate with the extent of disease as assessed on pre-operative CT scans of the paranasal sinuses [98]. In NP, local production of IgE is a characteristic feature, with a more then ten-fold increase of IgE-producing plasma cells in patients with NP versus controls. Analysis of specific IgE revealed a multiclonal IgE response in NP tissue and IgE antibodies to SAEs in about 30–50% of the patients. In NP patients with concomitant asthma or ASA intolerance this is even higher: 60–80% [99]. Patients with high IgE levels also have significantly more extensive eosinophilic inflammation [15].

MMP-9 is an endopeptidase that degrades gelatin types 1 and 4, and collagen types 4 and 5. By actively degrading those extracellular matrix components it may be involved in tissue-remodelling processes in chronic sinus disease [100]. In CRS and NP, MMP-9 is significantly higher compared to healthy controls. Also, the pre-operative level of MMP-9 is related to the healing process after surgery, with patients with lower MMP-9 levels demonstrating better mucosa healing. This holds true for MMP-9 concentration in nasal lavages [101], as well as MMP-9 expression in the extracellular matrix [100]. After sinus surgery, the level of MMP-9 rises. Again, the lowest increases are seen in patients with better healing mucosa. MMP-9 might be a potential factor to predict and monitor mucosal healing quality after sinus surgery. Inflammatory cells represent the major source of increased MMP-9 expression, which is linked to poor healing quality.

Conclusion

It appears that the "inflammatory state" of the paranasal sinus mucosa is negatively correlated with the outcome after sinus surgery. More extensive inflammation, which is seen for example in (ASA-intolerant) asthmatic patients, significantly reduces the healing quality of the mucosa. In order to reduce the need for revision sinus surgery to a minimum, it is thus crucial to simultaneously reduce tissue inflammation at the time of FESS. This can be achieved by topical steroid treatment, nasal lavages and if necessary, systemic steroids, combined with systemic antibiotics.

References

1. Fokkens W, Lund V, Mullol J; European Position Paper on Rhinosinusitis and Nasal Polyps Group (2007) European position paper on rhinosinusitis and nasal polyps 2007. Rhinol Suppl. (20):1–136
2. Bhattacharyya N (2004) Clinical outcomes after revision endoscopic sinus surgery. Arch Otolaryngol Head Neck Surg 130:975–978
3. Bachert C, Van Cauwenberge PB (1997) Inflammatory mechanisms in chronic sinusitis. Acta Otorhinolaryngol Belg 51:209–217
4. Hamilos DL, Leung DY, Wood R, Bean DK, Song YL, Schotman E, et al. (1996) Eosinophil infiltration in non-allergic chronic hyperplastic sinusitis with nasal polyposis (CHS/NP) is associated with endothelial VCAM-1 upregulation and expression of TNF-alpha. Am J Respir Cell Mol Biol 15:443–450
5. Berger G, Kattan A, Bernheim J, Ophir D (2002) Polypoid mucosa with eosinophilia and glandular hyperplasia in chronic sinusitis: a histopathological and immunohistochemical study. Laryngoscope 112:738–745

6. Jones NS, Carney AS, Davis A (1998) The prevalence of allergic rhinosinusitis: a review. J Laryngol Otol 112:1019–1030
7. Slavin RG (1988) Sinusitis in adults and its relation to allergic rhinitis, asthma, and nasal polyps. J Allergy Clin Immunol 82:950–956
8. Rachelefsky GS, Goldberg M, Katz RM, Boris G, Gyepes MT, Shapiro MJ, et al. (1978) Sinus disease in children with respiratory allergy. J Allergy Clin Immunol 61:310–314
9. Robinson S, Douglas R, Wormald PJ (2006) The relationship between atopy and chronic rhinosinusitis. Am J Rhinol 20:625–628
10. Gutman M, Torres A, Keen KJ, Houser SM (2004) Prevalence of allergy in patients with chronic rhinosinusitis. Otolaryngol Head Neck Surg 130:545–552
11. Emanuel IA, Shah SB (2000) Chronic rhinosinusitis: allergy and sinus computed tomography relationships. Otolaryngol Head Neck Surg 123:687–691
12. Lane AP, Pine HS, Pillsbury HC 3rd (2001) Allergy testing and immunotherapy in an academic otolaryngology practice: a 20-year review. Otolaryngol Head Neck Surg 124:9–15
13. Kennedy DW (1992) Prognostic factors, outcomes and staging in ethmoid sinus surgery. Laryngoscope 102:1–18
14. Dixon AE, Kaminsky DA, Holbrook JT, Wise RA, Shade DM, Irvin CG (2006) Allergic rhinitis and sinusitis in asthma: differential effects on symptoms and pulmonary function. Chest 130:429–435
15. Bachert C, Gevaert P, Holtappels G, Johansson SG, van CP (2001) Total and specific IgE in nasal polyps is related to local eosinophilic inflammation. J Allergy Clin Immunol 107:607–614
16. Bateman ND, Shahi A, Feeley KM, Woolford TJ (2005) Activated eosinophils in nasal polyps: a comparison of asthmatic and non-asthmatic patients. Clin Otolaryngol 30:221–225
17. Dhong HJ, Kim HY, Cho DY (2005) Histopathologic characteristics of chronic sinusitis with bronchial asthma. Acta Otolaryngol 125:169–176
18. Haruna S, Nakanishi M, Otori N, Moriyama H (2004) Histopathological features of nasal polyps with asthma association: an immunohistochemical study. Am J Rhinol 18:165–172
19. Jankowski R, Bouchoua F, Coffinet L, Vignaud JM (2002) Clinical factors influencing the eosinophil infiltration of nasal polyps. Rhinology 40:173–178
20. Kowalski ML, Lewandowska-Polak A, Wozniak J, Ptasinska A, Jankowski A, Wagrowska-Danilewicz M, et al. (2005) Association of stem cell factor expression in nasal polyp epithelial cells with aspirin sensitivity and asthma. Allergy 60:631–637
21. Ragab A, Clement P, Vincken W (2006) Correlation between the cytology of the nasal middle meatus and BAL in chronic rhinosinusitis. Rhinology 43:11–17
22. Olze H, Forster U, Zuberbier T, Morawietz L, Luger EO (2006) Eosinophilic nasal polyps are a rich source of eotaxin, eotaxin-2 and eotaxin-3. Rhinology 44:145–150
23. Senior BA, Kennedy DW (1996) Management of sinusitis in the asthmatic patient. Ann Allergy Asthma Immunol 77:6–15
24. Dunlop G, Scadding GK, Lund VJ (1999) The effect of endoscopic sinus surgery on asthma: management of patients with chronic rhinosinusitis, nasal polyposis, and asthma. Am J Rhinol 13:261–265
25. Ikeda K, Tanno N, Tamura G, Suzuki H, Oshima T, Shimomura A, et al. (1999) Endoscopic sinus surgery improves pulmonary function in patients with asthma associated with chronic sinusitis. Ann Otol Rhinol Laryngol 108:355–359
26. Chambers DW, Davis WE, Cook PR, Nishioka GJ, Rudman DT (1997) Long-term outcome analysis of functional endoscopic sinus surgery: correlation of symptoms with endoscopic examination findings and potential prognostic variables. Laryngoscope 107:504–510
27. Wang PC, Chu CC, Liang SC, Tai CJ (2002) Outcome predictors for endoscopic sinus surgery. Otolaryngol Head Neck Surg 126:154–159
28. Kim HY, Dhong HJ, Chung SK, Chung YJ, Kim MG (2006) Clinical characteristics of chronic rhinosinusitis with asthma. Auris Nasus Larynx 33:403–408
29. Marks SC, Shamsa F (1997) Evaluation of prognostic factors in endoscopic sinus surgery. Am J Rhinol 11:187–191
30. Smith TL, Mendolia-Loffredo S, Loehrl TA, Sparapani R, Laud PW, Nattinger AB (2005) Predictive factors and outcomes in endoscopic sinus surgery for chronic rhinosinusitis. Laryngoscope 115:2199–2205
31. Seybt MW, McMains KC, Kountakis SE (2007) The prevalence and effect of asthma on adults with chronic rhinosinusitis. Ear Nose Throat J 86:409–411
32. McFadden EA, Woodson BT, Fink JN, Toohill RJ (1997) Surgical treatment of aspirin triad sinusitis. Am J Rhinol 11:263–270
33. Amar YG, Frenkiel S, Sobol SE (2000) Outcome analysis of endoscopic sinus surgery for chronic sinusitis in patients having Samter's triad. J Otolaryngol 29:7–12
34. Smith TL, Batra PS, Seiden AM, Hannley M (2005) Evidence supporting endoscopic sinus surgery in the management of adult chronic rhinosinusitis: a systematic review. Am J Rhinol 19:537–543
35. Cho SH, Min HJ, Han HX, Paik SS, Kim KR (2006) CT analysis and histopathology of bone remodeling in patients with chronic rhinosinusitis. Otolaryngol Head Neck Surg 135:404–408
36. Lee JT, Kennedy DW, Palmer JN, Feldman M, Chiu AG (2006) The incidence of concurrent osteitis in patients with chronic rhinosinusitis: a clinicopathological study. Am J Rhinol 20:278–282

4

37. Kennedy DW, Senior BA, Gannon FH, Montone KT, Hwang P, Lanza DC (1998) Histology and histomorphometry of ethmoid bone in chronic rhinosinusitis. Laryngoscope 108:502–507
38. Videler WJ, van Drunen CM, van der Meulen FW, Fokkens WJ (2007) Radical surgery: effect on quality of life and pain in chronic rhinosinusitis. Otolaryngol Head Neck Surg 136:261–267
39. Videler WJ, Wreesmann VB, van der Meulen FW, Knegt PP, Fokkens WJ (2006) Repetitive endoscopic sinus surgery failure: a role for radical surgery? Otolaryngol Head Neck Surg 134:586–591
40. Kalkman PM, Fokkens WJ, de Wit HJ, van de Merwe JP, Hooijkaas H, van Haarst JM, et al. (2002) A hampered chemoattractant-induced cytoskeletal rearrangement in granulocytes of patients with unexplained severe chronic and relapsing infections of the upper and lower airways. In vitro restoration by G-CSF exposure. Clin Exp Immunol 127:115–122
41. Chee L, Graham SM, Carothers DG, Ballas ZK (2001) Immune dysfunction in refractory sinusitis in a tertiary care setting. Laryngoscope 111:233–235
42. Scadding GK, Lund VJ, Darby YC, Navas-Romero J, Seymour N, Turner MW (1994) IgG subclass levels in chronic rhinosinusitis. Rhinology 32:15–19
43. Sethi DS, Winkelstein JA, Lederman H, Loury MC (1995) Immunologic defects in patients with chronic recurrent sinusitis: diagnosis and management. Otolaryngol Head Neck Surg 112:242–247
44. Buckley RH (2002) Immunoglobulin G subclass deficiency: fact or fancy? Curr Allergy Asthma Rep 2:356–360
45. Maguire GA, Kumararatne DS, Joyce HJ (2002) Are there any clinical indications for measuring IgG subclasses? Ann Clin Biochem 39:374–377
46. Seppanen M, Suvilehto J, Lokki ML, Notkola IL, Jarvinen A, Jarva H, et al. (2006) Immunoglobulins and complement factor C4 in adult rhinosinusitis. Clin Exp Immunol 145:219–227
47. Buehring I, Friedrich B, Schaaf J, Schmidt H, Ahrens P, Zielen S (1997) Chronic sinusitis refractory to standard management in patients with humoral immunodeficiencies. Clin Exp Immunol 109:468–472
48. Cunningham-Rundles C, Bodian C (1999) Common variable immunodeficiency: clinical and immunological features of 248 patients. Clin Immunol 92:34–48
49. Rose MA, Schubert R, Schmitt-Grohe S, Reichenbach J, Zielen S (2006) Immunoglobulins and inflammatory cytokines in nasal secretions in humoral immunodeficiencies. Laryngoscope 116:239–244
50. Lusk RP, Polmar SH, Muntz HR (1991) Endoscopic ethmoidectomy and maxillary antrostomy in immunodeficient patients. Arch Otolaryngol Head Neck Surg 117:60–63
51. Gottschlich S, Ambrosch P, Kramkowski D, Laudien M, Buchelt T, Gross WL, et al. (2006) Head and neck manifestations of Wegener's granulomatosis. Rhinology 44:227–233
52. Hellmich B, Lamprecht P, Gross WL (2006) Advances in the therapy of Wegener's granulomatosis. Curr Opin Rheumatol 18:25–32
53. Braun JJ, Gentine A, Pauli G (2004) Sinonasal sarcoidosis: review and report of fifteen cases. Laryngoscope 114:1960–1963
54. Aubart FC, Ouayoun M, Brauner M, Attali P, Kambouchner M, Valeyre D, et al. (2006) Sinonasal involvement in sarcoidosis: a case-control study of 20 patients. Medicine (Baltimore) 85:365–371
55. Marks SC, Goodman RS (1998) Surgical management of nasal and sinus sarcoidosis. Otolaryngol Head Neck Surg 118:856–858
56. Bacciu A, Bacciu S, Mercante G, Ingegnoli F, Grasselli C, Vaglio A, et al. (2006) Ear, nose and throat manifestations of Churg-Strauss syndrome. Acta Otolaryngol 126:503–509
57. Olsen KD, Neel HB, III, Deremee RA, Weiland LH (1980) Nasal manifestations of allergic granulomatosis and angiitis (Churg-Strauss syndrome). Otolaryngol Head Neck Surg 88:85–89
58. Danieli MG, Cappelli M, Malcangi G, Logullo F, Salvi A, Danieli G (2004) Long term effectiveness of intravenous immunoglobulin in Churg-Strauss syndrome. Ann Rheum Dis 63:1649–1654
59. Hellmich B, Gross WL (2004) Recent progress in the pharmacotherapy of Churg-Strauss syndrome. Expert Opin Pharmacother 5:25–35
60. Bhattacharyya N (2005) Bacterial infection in chronic rhinosinusitis: a controlled paired analysis. Am J Rhinol 19:544–548
61. Araujo E, Palombini BC, Cantarelli V, Pereira A, Mariante Al (2003) Microbiology of middle meatus in chronic rhinosinusitis. Am J Rhinol 17:9–15
62. Kingdom TT, Swain RE Jr (2004) The microbiology and antimicrobial resistance patterns in chronic rhinosinusitis. Am J Otolaryngol 25:323–328
63. Nadel DM, Lanza DC, Kennedy DW (1998) Endoscopically guided cultures in chronic sinusitis. Am J Rhinol 12:233–241
64. Yildirim A, Oh C, Erdem H, Kunt T (2004) Bacteriology in patients with chronic sinusitis who have been medically and surgically treated. Ear Nose Throat J 83:836–838
65. Bachert C, Gevaert P, van Cauwenberge P (2002) *Staphylococcus aureus* enterotoxins: a key in airway disease? Allergy 57:480–487
66. Zhang N, Gevaert P, van Zele T, Perez-Novo C, Patou J, Holtappels G, et al. (2005) An update on the impact of *Staphylococcus aureus* enterotoxins in chronic sinusitis with nasal polyposis. Rhinology 43:162–168
67. Cryer J, Schipor I, Perloff JR, Palmer JN (2004) Evidence of bacterial biofilms in human chronic sinusitis. ORL J Otorhinolaryngol Relat Spec 66:155–158
68. Sanclement JA, Webster P, Thomas J, Ramadan HH (2005) Bacterial biofilms in surgical specimens of patients with chronic rhinosinusitis. Laryngoscope 115:578–582

69. Harvey RJ, Lund VJ (2007) Biofilms and chronic rhinosinusitis: systematic review of evidence, current concepts and directions for research. Rhinology 45:3–13
70. Bendouah Z, Barbeau J, Hamad WA, Desrosiers M (2006). Biofilm formation by *Staphylococcus aureus* and *Pseudomonas aeruginosa* is associated with an unfavorable evolution after surgery for chronic sinusitis and nasal polyposis. Otolaryngol Head Neck Surg 134:991–996
71. Ponikau JU, Sherris DA, Kern EB, Homburger HA, Frigas E, Gaffey TA, et al. (1999) The diagnosis and incidence of allergic fungal sinusitis. Mayo Clin Proc 74:877–884
72. Braun H, Stammberger H, Buzina W, Freudenschuss K, Lackner A, Beham A (2003) Incidence and detection of fungi and eosinophilic granulocytes in chronic rhinosinusitis. German. Laryngorhinootologie 82:330–340
73. Sasama J, Sherris DA, Shin SH, Kephart GM, Kern EB, Ponikau JU (2005) New paradigm for the roles of fungi and eosinophils in chronic rhinosinusitis. Curr Opin Otolaryngol Head Neck Surg 13:2–8
74. Shin SH, Ponikau JU, Sherris DA, Congdon D, Frigas E, Homburger HA, et al. (2004) Chronic rhinosinusitis: an enhanced immune response to ubiquitous airborne fungi. J Allergy Clin Immunol 114:1369–1375
75. Weschta M, Rimek D, Formanek M, Polzehl D, Podbielski A, Riechelmann H (2004) Topical antifungal treatment of chronic rhinosinusitis with nasal polyps: a randomized, double-blind clinical trial. J Allergy Clin Immunol 113:1122–1128
76. Ebbens FA, Scadding GK, Badia L, Hellings PW, Jorissen M, Mullol J, et al. (2006) Amphotericin B nasal lavages: not a solution for patients with chronic rhinosinusitis. J Allergy Clin Immunol 118:1149–1156
77. Chen Y, Dales R, Lin M (2003) The epidemiology of chronic rhinosinusitis in Canadians. Laryngoscope 113:1199–1205
78. Min YG, Jung HW, Kim HS, Park SK, Yoo KY (1996) Prevalence and risk factors of chronic sinusitis in Korea: results of a nationwide survey. Eur Arch Otorhinolaryngol 253:435–439
79. Murphy C, Davidson TM, Jellison W, Austin S, Mathews WC, Ellison DW, et al. (2000) Sinonasal disease and olfactory impairment in HIV disease: endoscopic sinus surgery and outcome measures. Laryngoscope 110:1707–1710
80. Porter JP, Patel AA, Dewey CM, Stewart MG (1999) Prevalence of sinonasal symptoms in patients with HIV infection. Am J Rhinol 13:203–208
81. Tami TA (1995) The management of sinusitis in patients infected with the human immunodeficiency virus (HIV). Ear Nose Throat J 74:360–363
82. Sabini P, Josephson GD, Reisacher WR, Pincus R (1998) The role of endoscopic sinus surgery in patients with acquired immune deficiency syndrome. Am J Otolaryngol 19:351–356
83. Savage DG, Taylor P, Blackwell J, Chen F, Szydlo RM, Rule SA, et al. (1997) Paranasal sinusitis following allogeneic bone marrow transplant. Bone Marrow Transplant 19:55–59
84. Imamura R, Voegels R, Sperandio F, Sennes LU, Silva R, Butugan O, et al. (1999) Microbiology of sinusitis in patients undergoing bone marrow transplantation. Otolaryngol Head Neck Surg 120:279–282
85. Sterman BM (1999) Sinus surgery in bone marrow transplantation patients. Am J Rhinol 13:315–317
86. Anselmo-Lima WT, Lopes RP, Valera FC, Demarco RC (2004) Invasive fungal rhinosinusitis in immunocompromised patients. Rhinology 42:141–144
87. Hunt SM, Miyamoto RC, Cornelius RS, Tami TA (2000) Invasive fungal sinusitis in the acquired immunodeficiency syndrome. Otolaryngol Clin North Am 33:335–347
88. Morinaka S, Ichimiya M, Nakamura H (2003) Detection of *Helicobacter pylori* in nasal and maxillary sinus specimens from patients with chronic sinusitis. Laryngoscope 113:1557–1563
89. Ozdek A, Cirak MY, Samim E, Bayiz U, Safak MA, Turet S (2003) A possible role of Helicobacter pylori in chronic rhinosinusitis: a preliminary report. Laryngoscope 113:679–682
90. Kowalski ML, Grzegorczyk J, Pawliczak R, Kornatowski T, Wagrowska-Danilewicz M, Danilewicz M (2002) Decreased apoptosis and distinct profile of infiltrating cells in the nasal polyps of patients with aspirin hypersensitivity. Allergy 57:493–500
91. Szucs E, Ravandi S, Goossens A, Beel M, Clement PA (2002) Eosinophilia in the ethmoid mucosa and its relationship to the severity of inflammation in chronic rhinosinusitis. Am J Rhinol 16:131–134
92. Zadeh MH, Banthia V, Anand VK, Huang C (2002) Significance of eosinophilia in chronic rhinosinusitis. Am J Rhinol 16:313–317
93. Bumbacea D, Campbell D, Nguyen L, Carr D, Barnes PJ, Robinson D, et al. (2004) Parameters associated with persistent airflow obstruction in chronic severe asthma. Eur Respir J 24:122–128
94. Miranda C, Busacker A, Balzar S, Trudeau J, Wenzel SE (2004) Distinguishing severe asthma phenotypes: role of age at onset and eosinophilic inflammation. J Allergy Clin Immunol 113:101–108
95. Pumputiene I, Emuzyte R, Dubakiene R, Firantiene R, Tamosiunas V (2006) T cell and eosinophil activation in mild and moderate atopic and nonatopic children's asthma in remission. Allergy 61:43–48
96. Carney AS, Tan LW, Adams D, Varelias A, Ooi EH, Wormald PJ (2006) Th2 immunological inflammation in allergic fungal sinusitis, nonallergic eosinophilic fungal sinusitis, and chronic rhinosinusitis. Am J Rhinol 20:145–149
97. Donovan R, Johansson SG, Bennich H, Soothill JF (1970) Immunoglobulins in nasal polyp fluid. Int Arch Allergy Appl Immunol 37:154–166

98. Lal D, Baroody FM, Weitzel EK, deTineo M, Naclerio RM (2006) Total IgE levels do not change 1 year after endoscopic sinus surgery in patients with chronic rhinosinusitis. Int Arch Allergy Immunol 139:146–148
99. Van ZT, Gevaert P, Watelet JB, Claeys G, Holtappels G, Claeys C, et al. (2004) *Staphylococcus aureus* colonization and IgE antibody formation to enterotoxins is increased in nasal polyposis. J Allergy Clin Immunol 114:981–983
100. Watelet JB, Demetter P, Claeys C, van CP, Cuvelier C, Bachert C (2005) Neutrophil-derived metalloproteinase-9 predicts healing quality after sinus surgery. Laryngoscope 115:56–61
101. Watelet JB, Claeys C, van CP, Bachert C (2004) Predictive and monitoring value of matrix metalloproteinase-9 for healing quality after sinus surgery. Wound Repair Regen 12:412–418

Chapter 5

Medical Management after Primary Surgery Failure and Preoperative Medical Management

5

Jan Gosepath

Core Messages

- Despite growing evidence of common pathways in underlying immunologic deficiencies or sensitizations, medical therapy has still to address a spectrum of potentially causative etiologic factors of chronic rhinosinusitis (CRS).
- A complete etiological workup is the key to defining an individualized medical treatment protocol suitable to prevent or reduce the risk of repeated recurrence after primary surgery failure.
- In postoperative medical management, effective topical treatment should be combined with well-tolerated, long-term systemic therapy as the causative mechanisms in CRS always represent a systemic disease.
- Disturbances of the arachidonic acid pathway and consecutive pathologic leukotriene release have been identified as a common pathway and frequent driving force behind mucosal inflammatory disease of the upper as well as the lower airway, especially, but not only, in patients with aspirin intolerance.
- Aspirin desensitization can be performed successfully and, using a novel low-dose protocol, can be applied as a life-long treatment. As this is effective at the enzyme level of the arachidonic acid pathway, it is more causative and, based on clinical trials, more effective than leukotriene antagonists.

Contents

Introduction

A difficult challenge in treating chronic rhinosinusitis (CRS) is to offer patients with recurrent disease after previous surgical treatment a therapeutic concept that addresses individually relevant etiological factors, but is based on well-standardized criteria and validated pathways of medical therapy. So far, regardless of the surgical technique applied, a fair amount of patients, especially those with polypoid changes, will at some point in time present with recurrent disease.

Until today, we have not succeeded in elaborating a universal causative medical treatment for recurrent – especially polypous – CRS that would reverse the disease process and make a surgical revision obsolete. The goal therefore is to evaluate the individual constellation of pathophysiological aspects of a patient. An emerging development with increasing relevance for the future is the application of in vitro assays validated to individually test patients for the relevance of single etiologic factors. This will help to better target medical treatment both pre- and postoperatively in an effort to reduce the risk of yet another recurrence after the necessary surgical revision.

Etiological Evaluation and Preoperative Medical Treatment

Exploration of patients suffering from CRS is complex. It is crucial to evaluate the relevance of several possible etiological factors and pinpoint those that play a role in the individual pathogenetic development. A complete workup should include taking the following aspects into consideration:

1. Inhalant allergies.
2. Ciliary dysfunction.
3. Aspirin intolerance (AI).
4. Immunodeficiency.
5. An immunologic reaction to fungi.
6. Presence of bacteria that are resistant to the applied antibiotic treatment.

Testing for inhalant allergies includes prick, intracutaneous, and running anaerobic sprint testing followed by nasal provocation testing, if clinically indicated [11]. The relevant sensitization-specific immunotherapy or the increasingly accepted sublingual immunotherapy should be performed for 3 years continuously. Although this is not a causative treatment option for CRS, it may reduce one relevant concomitant inflammatory stimulus rendering the mucosa prone to recurrent disease, and in some patients may help to prevent the development of allergic bronchial asthma.

Dysfunction of mucociliary clearance can be detected using the clinical test for saccharin transit time (STT), where a piece of saccharin is placed on the head of the inferior turbinate and the time taken until a sweet sensation is clearly felt in the pharynx is measured. Physiologically, a sweet sensation will be noticed after between 8 and 20 min. The functional integrity of the ciliary cells as motor units can be further evaluated with the help of video-interference contrast microscopy. In the case of a prolonged STT, this is a very valuable method to rule out syndromes of primary ciliary dyskinesia.

- Any impairment of mucociliary transport can be clinically relevant, as persistent stasis of the mucus blanket will trigger recurrent rhinosinusitis.

In a study published in 1997 we showed that patients suffering from recurrent CRS often do have a prolonged STT, but rarely a significant decrease in ciliary activity [14]. These observations could be explained either by poor coordination of ciliary activity in these patients and/or alterations of the nasal mucus in terms of viscosity and its content of enzymes, inflammatory mediators, and toxic proteins released from eosinophilic granulocytes. However, this study was able to show that endonasal sinus surgery may improve mucociliary transport time, as measured by STT, in patients with severe CRS.

One critical group in the range of patients suffering from CRS, and especially in the subgroup with nasal polyposis, are individuals with AI. It was understood early on that this particular entity is associated with a very high risk of recurrence of sinonasal polyposis independent of the number and kind of previous surgical interventions [7]. The diagnosis of AI is not always associated with the full clinical picture of the aspirin triad, which consists of: (1) nasal polyposis, (2) intrinsic bronchial asthma, and (3) aspirin-induced worsening of asthmatic symptoms,

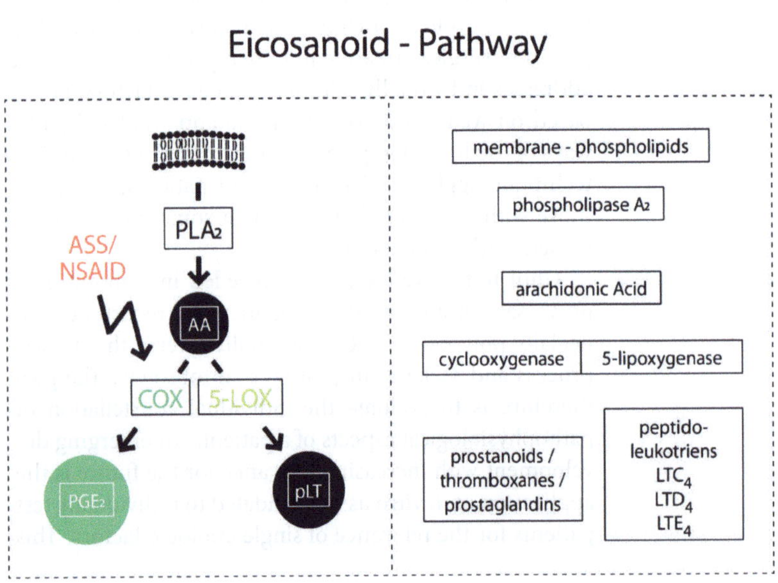

Fig. 5.1 Interaction between nonsteroidal anti-inflammatory drugs (*NSAIDs*) and the arachidonic acid pathway. *AA* Arachidonic acid, *ASS* acetylsalicylic acid, *COX* cyclooxygenase, *5-LOX* 5-lipoxygenase, *LTC_4* leukotriene C_4, *LTD_4* leukotriene D_4, LTE_4 leukotriene E_4, *PLA_2* phospholipase A_2, *pLT* peptidoleukotriene

often along with naso-ocular symptoms [23]. However, in sensitive individuals even very small single doses of aspirin may cause rhinorrhea, bronchiolar constriction, and pseudoanaphylactic shock symptoms related to a non-IgE-mediated pharmacological hypersensitivity reaction [24]. Not only aspirin, but most other nonsteroidal anti-inflammatory drugs interact with the eicosanoid pathway (Fig. 5.1). All patients diagnosed with AI have a considerable chance of clinical improvement or decreased risk of recurrence if adaptive desensitization therapy is performed.

- A low-dose, low-risk, aspirin-desensitizing protocol using a maintenance dose of only 100 mg of oral aspirin per day is effective in the management of patients with Samter's (aspirin) triad [8].

This low dosage, along with its minimal risk of adverse side effects, offers the option of a long-term and, if possible, life-long treatment, which is ultimately mandatory as a lasting effect of the desensitization.

In 143 patients characterized in a retrospective investigation we diagnosed AI in 55 (38.5%) [15]. Patients diagnosed with AI revealed to be the subgroup with (1) the highest rate of revision surgeries performed over time and (2) the shortest interval between the respective operations. According to the definition of AI it is obvious, that the subgroup of CRS patients with nasal polyps is likely to have the highest incidence of AI.

In vitro analysis of eicosanoid release from mixed leukocyte cultures using a functional enzyme immunoassay offers a new tool not only to help establish the diagnosis of AI, but also to individually monitor the effect and verify the success of a desensitization therapy over time. Long-term follow up over at least 3 years in a group of

Table 5.1 Clinical parameters after a 2-year course of low-dose aspirin desensitization with a daily maintenance dose of 100 mg ($n = 18$ patients). *FEV1* forced expiratory volume in 1s

Free of recurrent nasal polyps	15/18
Improved FEV1	7/12
Improved sense of smell (sniffin' sticks)	11/18
Revision due to recurrent polyps	1/18

patients undergoing desensitization using a daily maintenance dose of as little as 100 mg of aspirin revealed the treatment to be effective both clinically as well as in vitro (Table 5.1, Fig. 5.2) [10]. Eicosanoid levels shifted back to a normal release pattern during therapy, with an increase of prostaglandin in relation to leukotriene release. This underlines a prominent role of cyclo-oxygenase (COX)-dependant mediators, which is in keeping with findings in recurrent nasal polyposis of aspirin-tolerant patients. Immunohistochemical staining of polypoid tissue revealed a downregulation of COX-2 in these tissues as compared to normal nasal mucosa [13]. This unveils a possible mechanism of increased proinflammatory leukotriene release in nasal polyps, since COX-mediated prostaglandin E_2 (PGE_2) release inhibits leukotriene release in the nasal mucosa of normal controls.

The exact etiologic mechanisms underlying the formation of nasal polyps remain obscure. However, this entity of chronic inflammatory disease of the nasal respiratory mucosa is associated with remarkable edema. Vascular permeability/vascular endothelial growth factor (VPF/VEGF) plays an important role in inducing angiogenesis

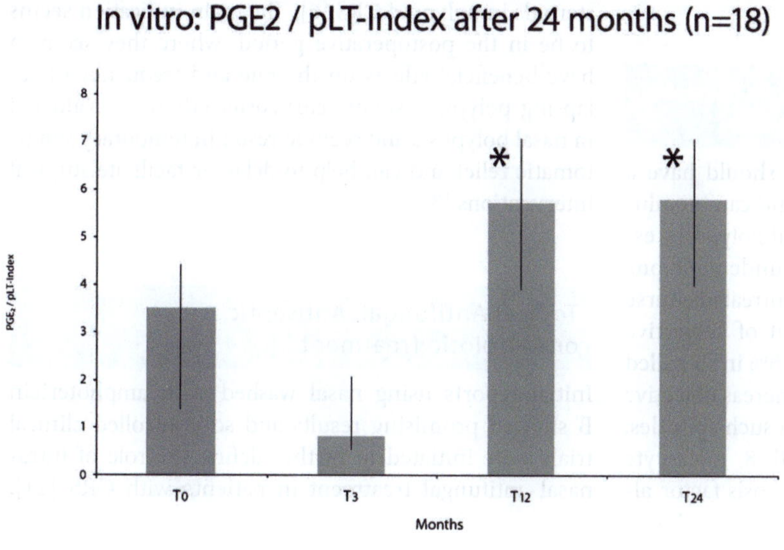

Fig. 5.2 The corresponding in vitro parameters of the same group of patients ($n = 18$) shown in Table 5.1 after 2 years of low-dose aspirin desensitization with a daily maintenance dose of 100 mg. *PGE₂* Prostaglandin E_2

and/or modulating capillary permeability. We investigated the expression and localization of VPF/VEGF in nasal polyps as compared to healthy controls in order to evaluate its significance in the pathophysiology of nasal polyps. The expression of VPF/VEGF in specimens of nasal polyps was markedly stronger than in specimens of healthy nasal mucosa of controls [12]. VPF/VEGF labeling in polypous tissue was located in vascular endothelial cells as well as in basilar membranes and epithelial cells. The observed expression pattern in nasal polyps as opposed to controls of healthy nasal mucosa suggests that VPF/VEGF might play a significant role in the etiology of nasal polyposis. These findings need to be discussed with respect to the differential expression of COX isoenzymes -1 and -2 (COX-1 and COX-2, respectively) in nasal polyps, where COX-1 is upregulated and COX-2 is downregulated, following immunohistochemical analysis. Studies involving intestinal hyperplastic polyps suggest that COX-1 in particular can upregulate VPF/VEGF [25]. This mechanism might play a key role in polyp growth and edema formation in nasal polyposis.

Preoperative Medical Treatment

When patients present with moderate symptoms and limited mucosal changes after primary surgery, a combination of nasal irrigations, culture-guided antibiotics if purulent secretions, as well as topical and/or short-term oral steroids can reduce or even resolve symptoms and endoscopic findings. There is evidence that in some patients a long-term course of low-dose macrolides can help to reduce the presence of biofilm and inflammatory mediators [27]. In the majority of patients with recurrent nasal polyps, however, medical preoperative treatment can only serve to control the inflammatory reaction as much as possible and to optimize conditions until the necessary surgical revision is performed.

Postoperative Care and Long-Term Medical Management to Prevent Recurrence

Certain applications of medical therapy should have a prominent role in the treatment of CRS and can be valuable in reducing the risk of recurrent nasal polyposis, especially in patients who have previously undergone one or multiple surgical interventions. In an untreated course of CRS, patients may show improvement of subjective symptoms to an extent of approximately 25% in so-called "stable episodes" over a 4-week period, whereas objective clinical parameters vary insignificantly. In such episodes, mRNA of interleukin (IL)-1beta, IL-6, IL-8, monocyte chemoattractant protein-1 and tumor necrosis factor-alpha as well as peptidoleukotriene (pLT) and PGE_2 levels are still detectable and appear to play a role in the persistence of inflammation in CRS [16].

- Initial postoperative medical management should focus on the support of immediate wound healing and the prevention of scarring, synechiae formation, and wound infections.

The preferred protocol to achieve these goals varies to a certain extent between surgeons and is mostly based on topical applications of irrigations and solutions including creams, decongestants, and steroids. Patients are usually seen in the office at weekly intervals for endoscopic follow up and crust removal from the surgical cavity, as necessary.

The goal of long-term medical treatment in the postoperative phase is to achieve a steady decrease of relevant inflammatory mediators and thus to prevent the formation of recurrent disease. Common regimens to accomplish this include:

1. Topical and systemic steroids.
2. Topical antifungal, antiseptic, or antibiotic treatment.
3. Systemic antibiotics and antihistamines.
4. Aspirin desensitization.

Topical and Systemic Steroids

Steroids, used topically or systemically or both generally have a strong anti-inflammatory effect and can reduce eosinophilia as they directly interact with several chemokines and cytokines involved in the inflammatory process. In particular, the suppressive effect on the T-cell production of IL-5 is an important aspect in this regard [1]. A large number of symptomatic clinical reports as well as prospective studies involving objective measurement of nasal function have established the role of topical steroids in polypoid CRS [6]. The main indication seems to be in the postoperative period, where they seem to have beneficial effects on the rate and frequency of relapsing polyps. Systemic corticosteroids were evaluated in nasal polyposis and seem to result in temporary symptomatic relief and can help to delay or facilitate surgical interventions [3].

Topical Antifungal, Antiseptic, or Antibiotic Treatment

Initial reports using nasal washed with amphotericin B showed promising results and so controlled clinical trials were initiated to further define the role of intranasal antifungal treatment in patients with CRS [21].

Heterogeneous experiences on the effectiveness of this treatment option have been published [5, 27]. Practical clinical experience suggests that the individual response to antifungal agents appears to be unpredictable, but the chance of a positive effect on the course of CRS seems to increase with the duration of treatment. Some of the existing studies reporting ineffectiveness were unblinded after only short-term applications of 8–12 weeks and suffered from a preselection of patients with massive polyposis. The latter certainly should be a criterion to take caution with any topical intranasal treatment as solutions and/or nebulized substances will not even penetrate into the paranasal cavities. However, further evaluation of this treatment modality in prospective, placebo-controlled trials will help to shed more light on its place in our armamentarium and on patient selection criteria.

- Whenever applying topical solutions intranasally, potential side effects on mucociliary clearance should not be overlooked.

In an in vitro study on primary human nasal respiratory cell cultures we evaluated the effects of different concentrations of several topical solutions on mucociliary clearance, as measured by ciliary beat frequency (CBF) over time [9]. In controls, perfused with cell culture medium (RPMI) only, CBF was measured at an average of 9.5±1.7 Hz, which remained constant over more than 12 h. Perfusion with a 5% solution of ofloxacin as an antibiotic solution led to an average CBF of 8 Hz, but ciliary activity ceased after 7 h. With a 50% ofloxacin solution, the average CBF was only 7.5 Hz and stopped after 6 h 30 min. Using antiseptic solutions, perfusion with 5% of Betadine revealed an average CBF of 7 Hz, which was kept up for 1 h 30 min; however, with 10% it was down to 4.5 Hz and lasted for only 30 min. Hydrogen peroxide was used in a 1% and in a 3% solution and seemed less ciliotoxic than Betadine, as 1% led to an average CBF of 7 Hz, which was kept up for over 8 h, and 3% to 6 Hz for 5 h 30 min. Using antifungal solutions, amphotericin B revealed only little ciliotoxicity in low concentrations, as CBF was measured at 9 Hz for 8 h at a concentration of 2.5% and at 8 Hz for 7 h at 5%. After increasing the concentration to a 10% solution, CBF dropped to 3.5 Hz and lasted only 2 h. Interestingly, no dose-dependent effect was observed after perfusion with clotrimazole at all three chosen concentrations of 10%, 20%, and 50%. CBF remained at a constant average frequency of 9 Hz, but stopped after no more than 30 min in all experiments. The strongest dose dependence was seen for itraconazole: at a concentration of 0.25%, a CBF of 6 Hz lasted for 7 h 45 min; at 0.5%, ciliary activity lasted only 1 h 15 min at 6 Hz and at 1% it was only 3 Hz for 30 min.

Systemic Antibiotics and Antihistamines

Antibiotic treatment has not been established as an effective treatment in patients with CRS. A prominent pathogenic role of bacteria seems to be limited to acute forms of rhinosinusitis and is doubtful in CRS [18, 19]. Thus antibiotic treatment has mostly been proven effective in acute sinusitis [4]. There are only limited data from controlled studies on antibiotic treatment in CRS, and in most of these, a long-term effect on the course of CRS could not be shown [17]. Long-term applications of macrolides for at least 3 months may, however, have beneficial effects on clinical and in vitro parameters of CRS [26]. In addition to the antimicrobial mode of action, these drugs are known to have direct anti-inflammatory effects and may improve the viscoelasticity of the mucous blanket [20]. An inhibitory effect on biofilm production of *Pseudomonas aeruginosa* has also been described [2].

Antihistamines are known to play a role in the adjuvant treatment of sinusitis, but no efficacy has been established for antihistamines in CRS without allergic rhinitis being present as an underlying condition [22].

Aspirin Desensitization

The best timing to initiate a scheduled aspirin desensitization after sinus surgery is following the initial wound healing, at around the 3rd or 4th, but no later than the 6th postoperative week, before edematous or polypoid changes recur. To start desensitization therapy, patients need to be hospitalized for 2 days for close monitoring for potential pseudoanaphylactic reactions. Oral aspirin is given in increasing dosages over these 2 days (day 1: increase up to 100 mg, day 2: increase up to 500 mg). Doses are slowly increased only after a repeated check of airway resistance and forced expiratory volume in 1 s (FEV1), excluding a decrease in FEV1 of 25% or greater after the respective preceding dose. Should that occur, the previous dose is repeated without further increase at the time of the next application until lung function has recovered. On the 3rd day aspirin is reduced to 100 mg/day for long-term maintenance. In prospective trials, clinical reassessments as well as the functional in vitro assay were repeated at each follow-up visit of every patient, in an attempt to identify changes in the release of eicosanoids over time and to correlate these with the clinical course [10]. Since there is a relative overproduction of pLT in aspirin-sensitive individuals, it is desirable to achieve an increase in the "PGE_2/pLT index" over time. We observed a significant improvement of in vitro findings, which was positively correlated to the individual clinical course and the recurrence rate of nasal polyps observed in this group of patients [8].

The data underline the role of the in vitro assay and indicate the effectiveness of a desensitization protocol that can be maintained as a long-term treatment without adverse side effects. The excellent compliance and low rate of adverse effects associated with a dose of 100 mg of aspirin per day was sufficiently validated in large cohorts of cardiovascular and neurological patients, using equivalent dosages for prevention protocols. Results suggest that the recurrence rate of nasal polyps after surgical therapy can be reduced; however, only long-term treatment can secure a beneficial outcome over time.

Future Directions

As our understanding of pathophysiological mechanisms evolve, we will be able to develop more sophisticated and more effective medical treatment modalities for inflammatory diseases such as CRS. It will be crucial to define antigens and endogenous causative factors triggering the underlying immune response, especially at a genetic level. A therapeutic concept of the future will individually tailor a therapeutic strategy to a respective risk profile of a patient. Research will be dominated by identifying missing links between in vitro and in vivo parameters and between chronic inflammation of the upper and lower airway as their systemic parameters are most likely identical to a large extent. A next step, which will be of utmost relevance for any healthcare system confronted with disorders as prevalent as CRS, will be screening strategies characterizing patient profiles, ultimately leading to individualized prevention protocols.

Tips and Pearls

1. An individual workup including all relevant etiological factors is mandatory to tailor a medical management protocol to the needs of a patient suffering from recurrent CRS after previous surgery.
2. Analysis of mucociliary transport by the STT, and if abnormal, measurement of the CBF, assesses a crucial functional parameter in a time- and cost-efficient manner, and should be performed routinely.
3. Although inhalant allergies have no causative role in CRS, they represent a relevant stimulus for eosinophilic mucosal inflammation and should be addressed appropriately.
4. The use of topical and/or systemic steroids, as well as the use of antibiotics or antifungal medications, should be tailored to the individual pathology.
5. Adaptive desensitization therapy can be performed successfully in patients with AI; however, only long-term treatment can secure a beneficial outcome over time. Using a novel low-dose aspirin-desensitizing protocol, this treatment can be maintained long term without adverse side effects.
6. Pathologic eicosanoid release patterns similar to those of patients suffering from AI have been demonstrated in patients with recurrent nasal polyposis and are currently being evaluated as therapeutic targets in these patients.

References

1. Bachert C, Geveart P (1999) Effect of intranasal corticosteroids on release of cytokines and inflammatory mediators. Allergy 54:116–123
2. Baumann U, King M, App EM, Tai S, Konig A, Fischer JJ, Zimmermann T, Sextro W, von der Hardt H (2004) Long term azithromycin therapy in cystic fibrosis patients: a study on drug levels and sputum properties. Can Respir J 11:151–155
3. Bonfils P (1998) Medical treatment of paranasal sinus polyposis: a prospective study in 181 patients. Ann Otolaryngol Chir Cervicofac 115:202–214
4. Buchem FL van, Knottnerus JA, Schrijnemaekers VJ, Peeters MF (1997) Primary-care-based randomised placebo-controlled trial of antibiotic treatment in acute maxillary sinusitis. Lancet 349:683–687
5. Ebbens FA, Scadding GK, Badia L, Hellings PW, Jorissen M, Mullol J, Cardesin A, Bachert C, van Zele TP, Dijkgraaf MG, Lund V, Fokkens WJ (2006) Amphotericin B nasal lavages: not a solution for patients with chronic rhinosinusitis. J Allergy Clin Immunol 118:1149–1156
6. Filiaci F, Passali D, Puxeddu R, Schrewelius C (2000) A randomized controlled trial showing efficacy of once daily intranasal budesonide in nasal polyposis. Rhinology 38:185–190
7. Gosepath J, Hoffmann F, Schafer D, Amedee RG, Mann WJ (1999) Aspirin intolerance in patients with chronic sinusitis. ORL J Otorhinolaryngol Relat Spec 61:146–150
8. Gosepath J, Schaefer D, Amedee RG, Mann WJ (2001) Individual monitoring of aspirin desensitization. Arch Otolaryngol Head Neck Surg 127:316–321
9. Gosepath J, Grebneva N, Mossikhin S, Mann WJ (2002) Topical antibiotic, antifungal, and antiseptic solutions decrease ciliary activity in nasal respiratory cells. Am J Rhinol 16:25–31
10. Gosepath J, Schaefer D, Mann WJ (2002) Aspirin sensitivity: long term follow up after up to 3 years of adaptive desensitization using a maintenance dose of 100 mg of aspirin a day. Laryngorhinootologie 81:732–738
11. Gosepath J, Amedee RG, Mann WJ (2005) Nasal provocation testing as an international standard for evaluation of allergic and non-allergic rhinitis. Laryngoscope 115:512–516

12. Gosepath J, Brieger J, Lehr HA, Mann WJ (2005) Expression, localization and significance of vascular permeability/vascular endothelial growth factor (VPF/VEGF) in nasal polyps. Am J Rhinol 19:7–13
13. Gosepath J, Brieger J, Mann WJ (2005) New immunohistologic findings on the differential role of cyclooxygenase-1 (Cox-1) and Cox-2 in nasal polyps. Am J Rhinol 19:111–116
14. Hafner B, Davris S, Riechelmann H, Mann WJ, Amedee RG (1997) Endonasal sinus surgery improves mucociliary transport in severe chronic sinusitis. Am J Rhinol 11:271–274
15. Kaldenbach T, Schafer D, Gosepath J, Bittinger F, Klimek L, Mann WJ (1999) Significance of eosinophilic granulocytes in relation to allergy and aspirin intolerance in patients with sinusitis polyposa Laryngorhinootologie 78:429–434
16. Kühnemund M, Ismail C, Brieger J, Schaefer D, Mann WJ (2004) Untreated chronic sinusitis, a comparison of symptoms and mediator profiles. Laryngoscope 114:561–565
17. Legent F, Bordure P, Beauvillain C, Berche P (1994) A double-blind comparison of ciprofloxacin and amoxycillin/clavulanic acid in the treatment of chronic sinusitis. Chemotherapy 40:8–15
18. Nadel DM, Lanza DC, Kennedy DW (1998) Endoscopically guided cultures in chronic sinusitis. Am J Rhinol 12:233–241
19. Nadel DM, Lanza DC, Kennedy DW (1999) Endoscopically guided sinus cultures in normal subjects. Am J Rhinol 13:87–90
20. Nagata T, Mukae H, Kadota J, Hayashi T, Fujii T, Kuroki M, Shirai R, Yanagihara K, Tomono K, Koji T, Kohno S (2004) Effect of erythromycin on chronic respiratory infection caused by *Pseudomonas aeruginosa* with biofilm formation in an experimental murine model. Antimicrob Agents Chemother 48:2251–2259
21. Ponikau JU, Sherris DA, Kita H, Kern EB (2002) Intranasal antifungal treatment in 51 patients with chronic rhinosinusitis. J Allergy Clin Immunol 110:862–866
22. Renvall U, Lindquist N (1974) A double blind clinical study with Monydrin tablet in patients with non allergic chronic rhinitis. J Int Med Res 7:235–292
23. Samter M, Zeitz HJ (1978) The aspirin triad and the prostaglandins. In: Samter M (ed) Immunological Diseases, 3rd edn. Little and Brown, Boston, pp 900–927
24. Schäfer D, Schmid M, Göde UC, Baenkler HW (1999) Dynamics of eicosanoids in peripheral blood cells during bronchial provocation in aspirin intolerant asthmatics. Eur Respir J 13:638–646
25. Tsujii M, Kawano S, Tsuji S, Sawaoka H, Hori M, DuBois RN (1996) Cyclooxygenase regulates angiogenesis induced by colon cancer cells. Cell 87:803–809
26. Wallwork B, Coman W, MacKay-Sim A, Greiff L, Cervin A (2006) A double-blind, randomized, placebo-controlled trial of macrolide in the treatment of chronic rhinosinusitis. Laryngoscope 116:189–193
27. Weschta M, Rimek D, Formanek M, Polzehl D, Podbielski A, Riechelmann H (2004) Topical antifungal treatment of chronic rhinosinusitis with nasal polyps: a randomized, double-blind clinical trial. J Allergy Clin Immunol 113:1122–1128

Chapter 6

New Technologies for Revision Sinus Surgery

6

Elisa M. Lynskey, Richard A. Lebowitz,
Joseph B. Jacobs, and Marvin P. Fried

Core Messages

- Technological advances continue to enhance endoscopic sinus surgical procedures. The development and utility of these techniques and devices continues to evolve and at this time the final chapter cannot yet be written. New technologies should enhance preoperative, intraoperative, and postoperative surgical treatment and care. Our ability to treat inflammatory as well as neoplastic disease will benefit from the availability of such devices.
- Intraoperative computed tomography as well as magnetic resonance imaging are presently available. There are several devices that have the capability of demonstrating surgical anatomic change, and such data can be transferred to update image guidance. This exciting development should enhance surgical procedures for both inflammatory and neoplastic disease.
- Endoscopic sinus surgery simulation facilitates educational opportunities for resident training and education as well as increasing skill set development for practitioners. These computerized systems provide a novel interactive scenario during which a specific surgical procedure can be programmed for simulation prior to a definitive procedure.
- The development of balloon sinus ostial dilation provides an alternative method for the treatment of localized anatomic and mucosal obstruction of sinus outflow tracts. Initial experience confirms the feasibility and safety of the technique, and early results suggest improved sinus function.

Contents

Introduction

The advent of endoscopic sinus surgery has revolutionized the surgical management of sinus disease. This minimally invasive approach was initially based on the development of illuminated endoscopes and video systems, which occurred simultaneously with enhancements in computed tomography (CT) scanning techniques. Refinement in surgical equipment, such as powered shavers and cutting instrumentation, permitted careful and meticulous removal of diseased mucosa and anatomic structures with minimal surgical trauma. The advent of image guidance enabled rhinologic surgeons to accurately localize surgical instruments while performing paranasal sinus and skull-base surgery for chronic inflammatory processes as well as neoplastic disease. Further development of these image-guidance systems and the related instrumentation has extended the indications for endoscopic procedures involving the base of skull. However, despite the accuracy of current image-guided systems, they are limited by the utilization of preoperative scan data, which do not reflect the surgical changes that occur as bone and soft tissue are removed. Several exciting and revolutionary intraoperative imaging systems have been developed that can provide intraoperative images, which can be used to update the image-guided system.

Surgical simulation training is currently being used in several surgical specialties.

- The endoscopic sinus surgery simulator (ES3) is an interactive computer-based platform, adapted from military flight simulation, which provides a virtual surgery experience for surgical education.

Several different modes, reflecting various skill sets and levels of difficulty, are available for training purposes. The ES3 has been validated by a multi-institutional study, and with the increasing focus on outcomes and assessment tools, may become an integral part of resident training and physician credentialing.

Balloon sinus catheterization has been introduced for the treatment of frontal, sphenoid, and maxillary sinus outflow obstruction. Initial published results are promising in the setting of mucosal and anatomic obstruction. Additional studies including long-term outcome results are needed to define the role of this technology in the treatment of rhinosinusitis.

Intraoperative Imaging

Intraoperative imaging may prove to be one of the most important advances in image-guided revision endoscopic sinus surgery, particularly in the setting of neoplastic disease, and surgery at the skull base.

- Intraoperative imaging allows the surgeon to identify the limits of the skull base and orbit with greater accuracy, and to determine the extent of surgical resection and its potential effect on the anatomic relationship between the surrounding vital structures.

Stereotactic image-guided surgery was first introduced in conjunction with neurosurgical procedures to guide ablation of discrete areas; these initial cases were calibrated using plain films, anatomic landmarks, and anatomic atlases [2]. From that point, a series of framed stereotactic systems was developed. In 1986, Roberts and associates published reports of a frameless navigation system that utilized radiopaque glass beads as fiducial markers [11]. Since then, computer-aided surgery has undergone dramatic advances and become increasingly more available and user-friendly.

- Stereotactic image-guidance systems are still limited by their reliance on images obtained preoperatively. As surgery progresses and anatomy is altered, the images remain static and do not reflect the surgical changes.

Recent innovations have allowed for intraoperative updating of the images used in stereotactic surgery. Fluoroscopy has been used extensively in the operating room for neurosurgical, orthopedic, and vascular procedures. More recently, the C-arm has been used to create reconstructed images for three-dimensional navigation by neurosurgeons and orthopedists [7, 10]; recently, Brown and colleagues investigated utilizing this technology during endoscopic sinus surgery [4]. In their initial experience with 14 patients, image quality was poor, but adjustments were made and for the final 6 patients they were able to produce images that allowed for evaluation of disease and anatomical structures with navigation accuracy similar to that found with CT images (within 2 mm). Limitations included image distortion and artifact caused by nasal packing and blood in the sinuses, as well as reduced image quality in patients with extensive nasal polyposis (Figs. 6.1 and 6.2).

One concern about intraoperative imaging is that of radiation exposure for the patient, the physician, and the operating room personnel. Traditional stereotactic surgical techniques utilize the preoperative CT scan data and therefore do not require intraoperative imaging with the associated radiation exposure. Manarey's group investigated the amount of radiation exposure during FluoroCAT fluoroscopy to reconstruct triplanar images for stereotactic surgery [9]. Cumulative radiation exposures were measured for two separate scans in all three modes. The maximum surface and central radiation exposure (range 1.89–10.7 mG, depending on fluoroscopic mode) was significantly less than that of a sinus CT with image-guidance protocol (85.4 mG).

Current technology also allows for intraoperative magnetic resonance imaging (MRI). This modality provides superior soft-tissue imaging without radiation exposure. The soft-tissue detail is particularly beneficial in cases of endoscopic resection of tumors of the anterior skull base. Disadvantages of MRI include expense, longer scanning time, and the necessity of specialized, nonfer-

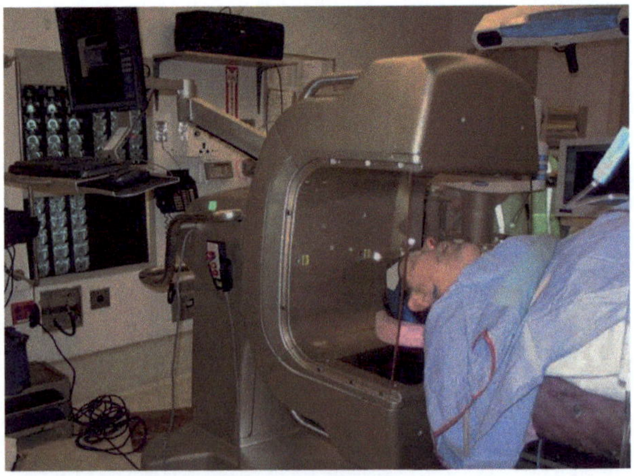

Fig. 6.1 Xoran X-cat intraoperative computed tomography (CT) scanner in use

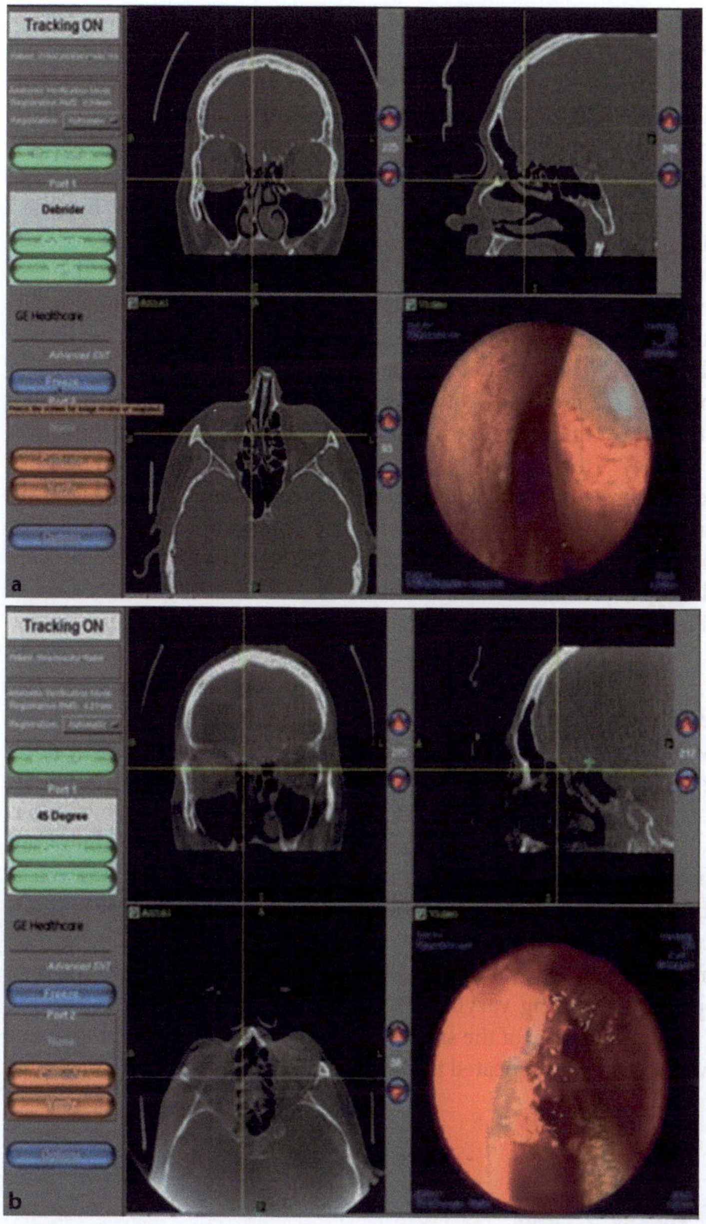

Fig. 6.2 Preoperative CT images (**a**) and intraoperative updated images (**b**) showing a mucocele before and after drainage, respectively

romagnetic operating room equipment and instruments. Early experience utilizing intraoperative MRI was been reported, and demonstrated the feasibility and accuracy of this modality [8]. More recently, Anand et al. published their experience with intraoperative MRI during endoscopic transsphenoidal resections of pituitary tumors. Residual tumor was identified in three out of ten patients using intraoperative MRI. Additional endoscopic resection was performed and there were no intraoperative complications [1].

Ultimately, the utility of intraoperative imaging will be judged based on its benefits, technical difficulties and limitations, and potential risks.

Endoscopic Sinus Surgery Simulator

Endoscopic sinus surgery requires the ability to work with both hands in a small space around delicate structures. Varied anatomy and the close proximity of vital structures such as the orbit and skull base contribute to the difficulty in gaining proficiency in these procedures. Residents typically acquire these skills through a process that begins with observation and progresses to operative experience under the supervision of attending surgeons. Practice on cadaver models is available, but is limited by the cost and availability of cadaveric specimens. In response to the need for repeated practice to develop these skills, the idea of a surgical simulator was explored. The field of aviation has used simulators for years to train and improve the skills of both commercial and military pilots. As a Department of Defense contractor, Lockheed Martin has been responsible for the development and implementation of many of these flight simulators and assembled a team to engineer a surgical training device.

The result of these efforts is the endoscopic sinus surgery simulator (ES3), which utilizes both visual and haptic (force) feedback in a virtual reality environment. There are four principle components of this system: (1) a Silicon Graphics Inc. Octane workstation, which serves as the simulation host platform, (2) a personal computer (PC)-based haptic controller, which provides control and coordination between an instrument handle and a set of virtual surgical instruments, (3) a PC-based voice recognition-enabled instructor, which operates the simulator based on spoken commands, and (4) an electromechanical platform, which includes a replica of an endoscope, a surgical tool handle, and a mannequin head (Figs. 6.3 and 6.4).

- The endoscopic sinus surgery simulator collects and analyzes performance data in real time to provide immediate feedback to the participant regarding performance errors.

The system also archives data for end-results analysis. It provides an opportunity for residents to practice maneuvers repeatedly to gain proficiency without the risk of patient harm. It also allows for residents to repeat a specific scenario as needed, and since the perioperative aspects of patient care have been eliminated, the simulator allows for more procedures to be completed within a set period of time. All of these factors will help to accelerate the learning curve for students and residents, while enhancing patient safety. The simulator also provides an objective assessment of surgical skill and would help to standardize residency training programs with regard to endoscopic sinus procedures.

In a prospective, multi-institutional study by Fried and associates, 10 expert otolaryngologists, 14 residents, and 10 medical students were evaluated using the ES3 [6]. They each performed 23 trials with the simulator, beginning at novice mode and ending at advanced mode. Their findings show that in the novice mode, there is a significant difference in the starting point between all three groups, but as the number of repetitions increases, the scores improve and the gap between attending physicians, residents and medical students closes, with all three groups achieving the same endpoint after ten repetitions. After completing the novice trials, exercises performed in the intermediate and advanced modes did not show any statistically significant differences between the three groups' total scores. The results in the novice mode clearly demonstrate three different skill levels at the beginning, with all three levels ultimately ending at a level of high performance. Moreover, the variations seen at the outset in all three groups were significantly narrowed, indicating that the performance was comparable between the members of each group. Thus, simulator training can bring individuals to a higher level of proficiency as well as decrease the variability within each group. These findings support prior data published by Weghorst and her group, which validates the ability of the simulator to distinguish among varying levels of initial expertise, as well as the ability of the simulator to increase the level of proficiency with repeated trials [12].

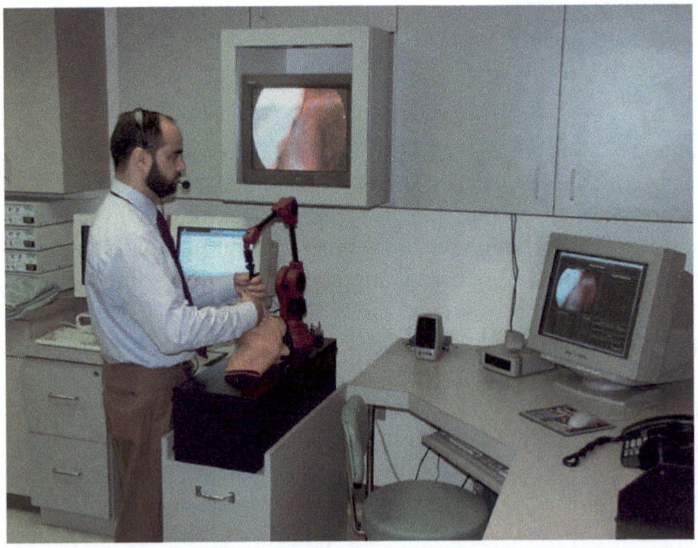

Fig. 6.3 The endoscopic sinus surgery simulator in use

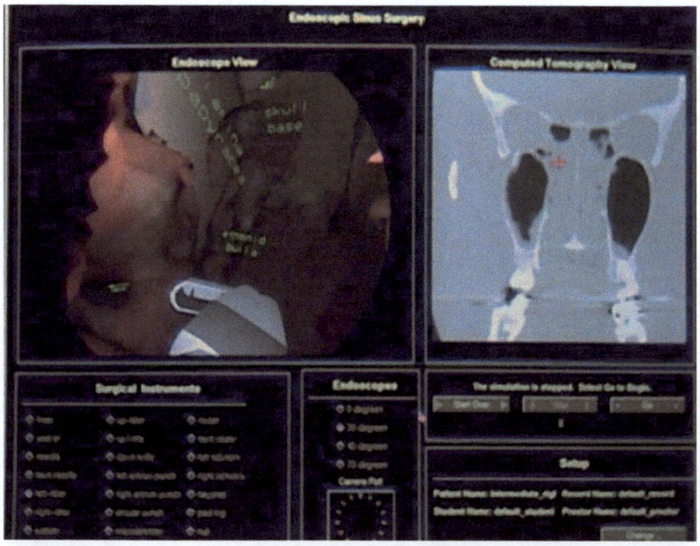

Fig. 6.4 The video monitor of the endoscopic sinus surgery simulator

A study by Edmond takes the assessment of surgical skills one step further by addressing the impact of the surgical simulator on operating room performance [5]. In this setting, some of the junior residents were trained using the surgical simulator and others were not. Surgical performance in the operating room was then rated by senior surgeons watching videotapes. The two residents who were trained with the simulator were consistently rated better across all measures than the two residents who weren't. Although this study size was small, it was the first to look at how endoscopic sinus simulation experience would translate to surgical skill. It shows that the simulator appears to have a positive impact on residents' operative skill. A controlled multi-institutional study involving larger groups of trainees is currently underway to confirm the ability of the ES3 to enable skills that can be transferred from the simulation laboratory to the operating room.

Balloon Sinus Ostial Dilatation

A recent introduction to endoscopic sinus surgery is the use of balloon catheters for dilation of sinus ostia. This approach was introduced based on the concept of catheter dilation used in other disciplines such as cardiology and urology. It is hypothesized that this procedure will reduce mucosal trauma as compared to typical endoscopic surgery techniques, thus reducing the formation of scar tissue and restenosis at sinus ostia.

Balloon sinus ostial dilation involves the cannulation of the maxillary ostia, sphenoid ostia, or frontal sinus outflow tract by a balloon catheter. A hollow cannula is placed near the sinus ostia under endoscopic visualization. Under fluoroscopic guidance, a sinus guide wire is fed through the cannula into the sinus and the balloon catheter is then advanced over the guide wire. The proximal and distal portions of the balloon are radiopaque to allow for visualization and correct placement within the ostia; the distal mark should be visualized within the sinus and the proximal mark should be external to the sinus. The balloon is then inflated with a radiopaque fluid to apply 6–10 atm (608–1013 kPa) of pressure. The balloon should remain inflated for a few seconds and may then be deflated, repositioned, and reinflated if necessary. After dilation, the guide wire may also be used to position a sinus lavage catheter. Upon completion of the procedure, endoscopic visualization of the sinus ostia should confirm its patency (Fig. 6.5).

This procedure has its limitations, however, and cannot be used in patients with sinonasal polyposis or extensive sinonasal osteoneogenesis. Extensive scar tissue from prior surgical procedures may also limit the ability to dilate the sinus drainage pathways. Due to the nature of this procedure and the anatomy of the ethmoid sinuses, traditional endoscopic surgery techniques are necessary to facilitate drainage of this area. Because of these limitations, the patient and surgeon must always be prepared to proceed with debridement using traditional techniques. The balloon catheter technique also requires fluoroscopic guidance, which exposes both the patient and operating room staff to radiation. Bolger et al. found that the average amount of radiation exposure during surgery was approximately 730 mrem (16 μC/kg), comparable to the amount of radiation exposure during a chest CT scan (800 mrem, or 17 μC/kg) [3]. Although precautions such as radiological shields should be worn, the cumulative dose to the surgeon and operative staff is a concern and

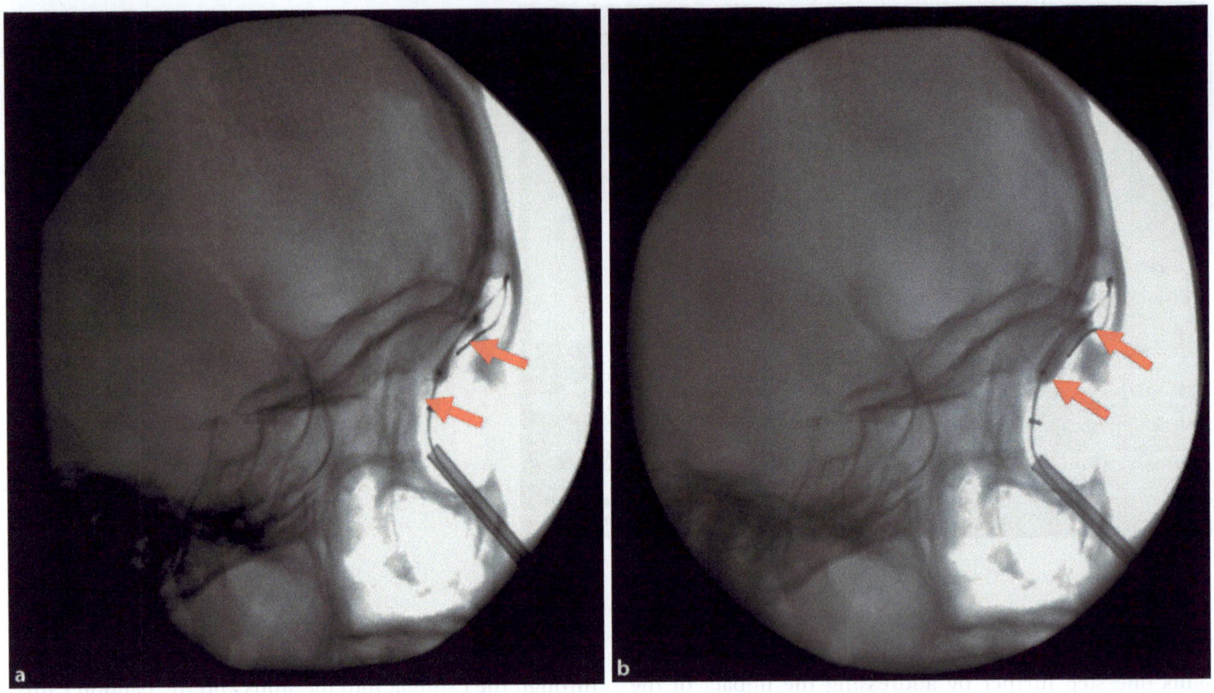

Fig. 6.5 Fluoroscopic views of balloon catheter dilation of the frontal sinus outflow tract. The proximal and distal radiopaque markers of the balloon can be visualized (*arrows*)

the benefit of the procedure must outweigh the risk and additional cost involved.

A prospective, multicenter study conducted by Bolger and colleagues followed 109 patients for 6 months after endoscopic balloon catheter sinusotomy [3]. They were able to successfully cannulate and dilate 96.9% of sinus ostia and there were no serious adverse postoperative sequelae (cerebrospinal fluid rhinorrhea, orbital injury, or epistaxis requiring packing). At the end of the 6-month follow-up period, endoscopy revealed that 80.5% of the dilated sinus ostia remained patent, 1.6% were nonpatent, and 17.9% could not be adequately visualized. A quality-of-life questionnaire also revealed statistically significant improvement in patient symptoms after balloon dilation. Revision surgery was required in three patients (2.75%); appropriate patient selection criteria appear to be essential to successful outcomes with balloon sinuplasty.

- Balloon catheter dilation appears to be a promising new tool in the quest for minimally invasive interventions.

Based on current reports, balloon catheter dilation could potentially provide durable results and improvement. It remains to be seen, however, whether or not these dilated ostia will remain patent over longer periods of time. This technique may be particularly advantageous in the dilation of frontal sinus outflow tracts, where minimal mucosal trauma is highly desirable to prevent scar tissue and stenosis.

References

1. Anand VK, Schwartz TH, Hiltzik DH (2006) Endoscopic transphenoidal pituitary surgery with real-time intraoperative magnetic resonance imaging. Am J Rhinol 20:401–405
2. Anon JB (1998) Computer-aided endoscopic sinus surgery. Laryngoscope 108:949–961
3. Bolger WE, Brown CL, Church CA, et al. (2007) Safety and outcomes of balloon catheter sinusotomy: a multicenter 24-week analysis in 115 patients. Otolaryngol Head Neck 137:10–20
4. Brown SM, Sadoughi B, Cuellar H, et al. (2007) Feasibility of near real-time image-guided sinus surgery using intraoperative fluoroscopic computed axial tomography. Otolaryngol Head Neck 136:268–273
5. Edmond CV Jr (2002) Impact of the endoscopic sinus surgical simulator on operating room performance. Laryngoscope 112:1148–1158

6. Fried MP, Sadoughi B, Weghorst SJ, et al. (2007) Construct validity of the endoscopic sinus surgery simulator: II. Assessment of discriminant validity and expert benchmarking. Arch Otolaryngol 133:350–357
7. Holly LT, Foley KT (2003) Three-dimensional fluoroscopy-guided percutaneous thoracolumbar pedicle screw placement. Technical note. J Neurosurg 99:324–329
8. Hsu L, Fried MP, Jolesz FA (1998) MR-guided endoscopic sinus surgery. Am J Neuroradiol 19:1235–1240
9. Manarey CR, Anand VK (2006) Radiation dosimetry of the FluoroCAT scan for real-time endoscopic sinus surgery. Otolaryngol Head Neck 135:409–412
10. Richter M, Geerling J, Zech S, et al. (2005) Intraoperative three-dimensional imaging with a motorized mobile c-arm (SIREMOBIL ISO-C-3D) in foot and ankle trauma care: a preliminary report. J Orthop Trauma 19:259–266
11. Roberts DW, Strohbehn JW, Hatch JF, et al. (1986) A frameless stereotaxic integration of computerized tomographic imaging and the operating microscope. J Neurosurg 65: 545–549
12. Weghorst S, Airola C, Oppenheimer P (1998) Validation of the Madigan ESS simulator. Stud Health Technol Inform 50:399–405

Chapter 7

Surgical Anatomy in Revision Sinus Surgery

7

Adam J. Folbe and Roy R. Casiano

Core Messages

- Revision sinus surgery depends on knowing constant bony anatomical landmarks that are unaltered by prior surgery or advanced pathology.
- A wide maxillary antrostomy exposes the posterior lamellae and the medial orbital floor (MOF).
- The superior margin of the maxillary sinusotomy (junction of the inferior aspect of the lamina papyracea and MOF) forms a "bony ridge," which delineates the anterior ethmoid cells (medially) from the orbital floor (laterally).
- The posterior margin of the maxillary sinusotomy (posterior fontanelle remnant), delineates the middle turbinate/sphenopalatine foramen (medially) from the posterior wall of the maxillary sinus (laterally).
- The relationship between the MOF and adjacent structures can help guide the surgeon.
- The posterior ethmoid cells lie superior to the posterior orbital floor adjacent and medial to the ridge of the antrostomy.
- The sphenoid sinus lies inferior to the MOF, adjacent to the nasal septum, approximately 7 cm from the columella.
- The nasolacrimal duct runs anterior, but parallel to the direction of the frontal recess and infundibulum.

Contents

Introduction

The understanding of anatomy is crucial during any operation. Once the anatomy has been understood, the surgeon can proceed using designated landmarks to direct the surgery. However, during sinus surgery, because much of the paranasal sinus contents are thin bone structures with overlying soft tissue, some landmarks (i.e., the uncinate, ethmoid bullae, the basal or ground lamellae, middle turbinate) may be removed or scarred in different locations, making revision surgery more difficult.

Correlating computed tomography (CT) scan anatomy with endoscopic anatomy is very important. As discussed in other chapters, the use of navigational systems during surgery can aid the surgeon during revision sinus surgery. However, there is a margin of error with the systems and they require precise calibration. The surgeon should not substitute good fundamental knowledge of the anatomy with a navigational system. Because the paranasal sinuses are in such close proximity to the orbit and brain, the changes in anatomy surrounding them can result in dreaded complications. For example, by not properly identifying the medial orbital wall, inadvertent penetration through the periorbita can result in an orbital hematoma or blindness. In another example, if the surgeon encounters the posterior ethmoids and thinks it is the sphenoid sinus, they may inadvertently penetrate the skull base causing a cerebrospinal fluid leak or brain injury.

This chapter will focus on bony landmarks, knowledge of measurements from the columella, and relationships with adjacent sinus structures. With the understanding of these items, the "difficult" anatomy of revision sinus surgery will become more easily understandable. Throughout the chapter, it will become apparent that the orbital floor along with adjacent structures, are key landmarks for understanding sinus anatomy.

Nasal Cavity

Structures visualized in the nonoperated nasal cavity include the inferior turbinate, uncinate, middle turbinate, ethmoid bullae, and the septum. These are valuable landmarks for primary sinus surgery. However, these structures are often modified or removed during surgery. Fortunately, some structures in the nasal cavity are fairly constant (Fig. 7.1). The bulge or convexity on the anterior lateral nasal wall created by the nasolacrimal duct is a constant landmark pre- or postoperatively. As will be mentioned later, this is a valuable landmark by which to locate the maxillary sinus ostium as well as the frontal sinus recess. Often, the anterior/superior attachments of the uncinate and middle turbinate are left intact, and provide additional landmarks for the frontal recess. More posteriorly, the nasopharynx and its surrounding structures can be visualized. The choanal arch and the relationship between the posterior nasal septum, eustachian tube, tail of the inferior turbinate, posterior extent of middle turbinate at the basal lamellae, and nasal floor can be appreciated. Even in revision surgery, the tail of the inferior turbinate and the tail and horizontal attachment of the middle turbinate, are commonly left untouched.

- The posterior fontanelle is located superior to the lateral attachment of the posterior one-third of the inferior turbinate.
- The sphenopalatine foramen is located at the coronal plane and slightly superior to the tail of the middle turbinate.
- Both can be used as landmarks to identify the level of the middle meatus [3, 7, 10].

Maxillary Sinus

The maxillary sinus is the first sinus to develop in the infant. It is shaped like a pyramid, with the base being the posterior wall; the peak is associated with the facial surface of the maxilla. The posterior wall of the maxillary sinus consists of thin bone that separates the pterygomaxillary fossa medially and the infratemporal fossa laterally. The floor is the alveolar process of the maxilla and the hard palate. The roof of the maxillary sinus corresponds to the floor of the orbit. Along the roof, the maxillary division of the trigeminal nerve (V2) can often be seen running in anterolateral direction toward the infraorbital

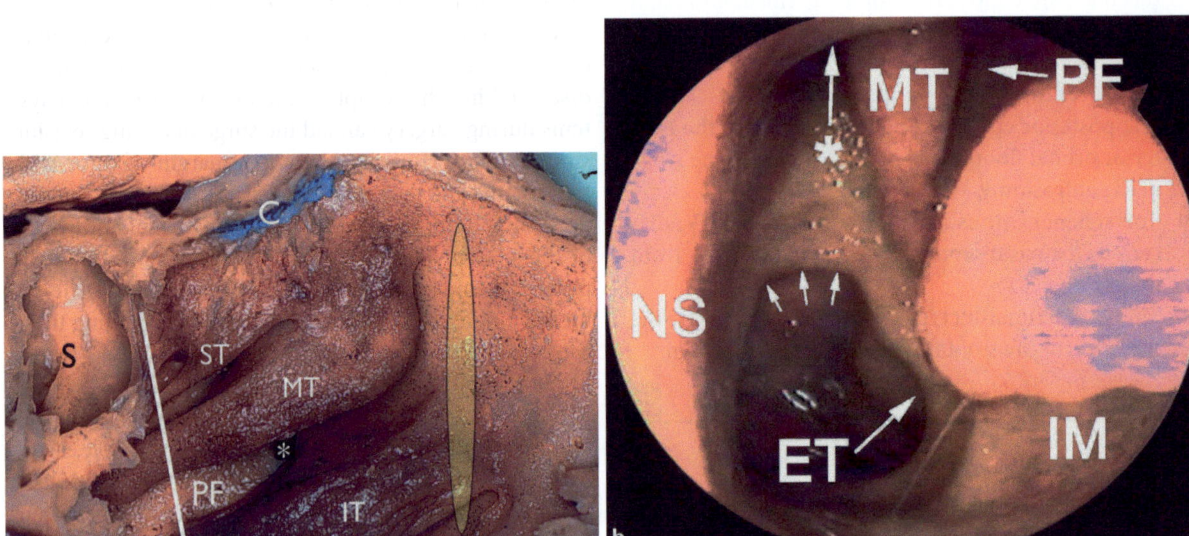

Fig. 7.1 **a** Sagittal view of lateral nasal wall starting anteriorly, the approximate location of the nasolacrimal duct is highlighted in *yellow*. The *white line* along the anterior face of sphenoid sinus lies 7 cm from the columella. It also demarcates the posterior wall of the maxillary sinus and the coronal plane just anterior to the level of the sphenopalatine foramen and anterior wall of sphenoid sinus. A secondary ostium is denoted by the *white asterisk*. *C* Cribriform, *S* sphenoid sinus, *PF* posterior fontanelle, *ST* superior turbinate, *MT* middle turbinate, *IT* inferior turbinate. **b** The structures around the posterior nasopharynx remain fairly constant in revision sinus surgery. The choanal arch is denoted by the *small white arrows*. The sphenoethmoidal recess can be seen behind a septal spur (*white asterisk*). *ET* Eustachian tube, *IT* tail of the inferior turbinate, *MT* tail of the middle turbinate, *NS* posterior nasal septum

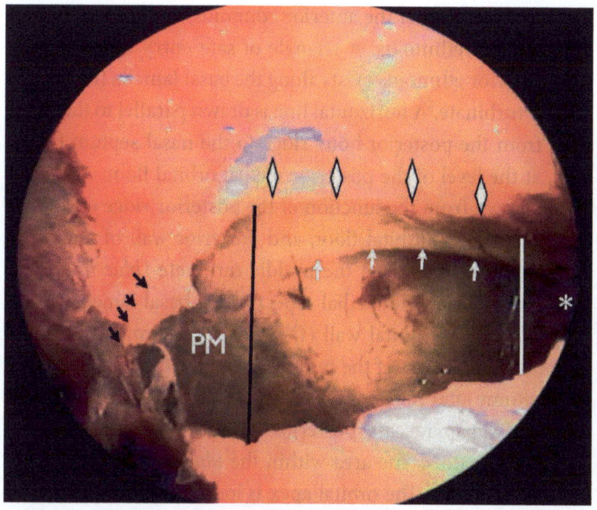

Fig. 7.2 Endoscopic view of large maxillary antrostomy viewed with a 30° telescope: the distance between the orbital floor and the lateral attachment of the inferior turbinate is greater over the posterior one-third of the inferior turbinate (*black line*) than over the anterior one-third of the inferior turbinate (*white line*). The maxillary division of the trigeminal nerve (V2) runs along the roof of the maxillary sinus (*white arrows*). The horizontal bony ridge of the antrostomy (*white diamonds*) lies medially, and the medial orbital floor and medial orbital wall lie laterally. The *asterisk* indicates the location of the natural ostium. The posterior maxillary wall (*PM*) lies in the coronal plane with the face of the sphenoid sinus and sphenopalatine artery, which lie medial to the vertical ridge of the antrostomy (*black arrows*)

foramen (Fig. 7.2). The medial maxillary wall makes up the lateral walls of the middle and inferior meati. The posterior fontanelle is located between the posterior one-third of the middle and inferior turbinate. Often, a secondary maxillary ostium may be observed in this area (Fig. 7.1a). The distance between the orbital floor, which inclines anteroinferiorly, as one proceeds anterior along the middle meatus, and lateral attachment of the inferior turbinate, is much greater here. This anatomical relationship can be utilized to enter the maxillary sinus when the natural ostium is obscured by disease, scarring, or previous surgery. The surgeon merely finds the posterior fontanelle area above the posterior one-third of the inferior turbinate and enters blindly into the maxillary sinus with minimal chance of inadvertent orbital penetration. The natural ostium of the maxillary sinus may be found posterolateral to the uncinate process, and inferolateral to the ethmoid bulla.

- The superior margin of the maxillary ostium is also the junction of the medial orbital floor and the inferomedial orbital wall (infundibulum).
- Therefore, anteroposterior resection of the uncinate with a sickle knife or microdebrider may inadvertently enter above the level of the natural ostium and result in orbital penetration.

Also, in revision surgery, these structures are usually absent or scarred. As mentioned previously, the use of the posterior fontanelle and the bony nasolacrimal duct can help outline the maxillary sinus sinusotomy, while ensuring incorporation of the natural ostium within the surgical sinusotomy. During surgery, the margin of the orbital floor is followed anteriorly until the surgical antrostomy is connected with the area of the natural ostium, just posterior to the nasal lacrimal duct, and inferior to the level of the orbital floor. Care should be taken not to dissect too far inferiorly, in order to avoid transecting the lateral attachment of the inferior turbinate and inadvertent entry into the inferior meatus (Fig. 7.3). With a wide antrostomy, a bony "ridge," as described by May et al. in 1994, is formed [9]. This ridge demarcates the remnant of the posterior fontanelle, and is a critical landmark in determining the approximate location of the anterior and posterior ethmoid sinuses. The ethmoid sinuses are located medial to this ridge, whereas the maxillary sinus and medial orbital floor (MOF) are located lateral to the ridge. The MOF is a key landmark that will help guide the surgeon through the rest of the anatomy.

- The posterior wall of the maxillary sinus demarcates the approximate level of the anterior sphenoid sinus wall in the coronal plane, as one proceeds posteriorly through the ethmoid labyrinth.

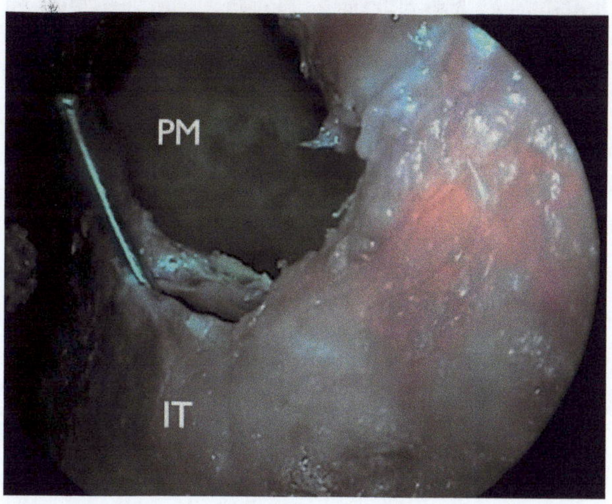

Fig. 7.3 Endoscopic view of maxillary sinus antrostomy. If dissection is carried to far inferiorly, the superior aspect of the inferior turbinate (*IT*) may be cut, and the inferior meatus may be inadvertently entered. The ostium seeker is directed through the defect in the superior aspect of the inferior turbinate

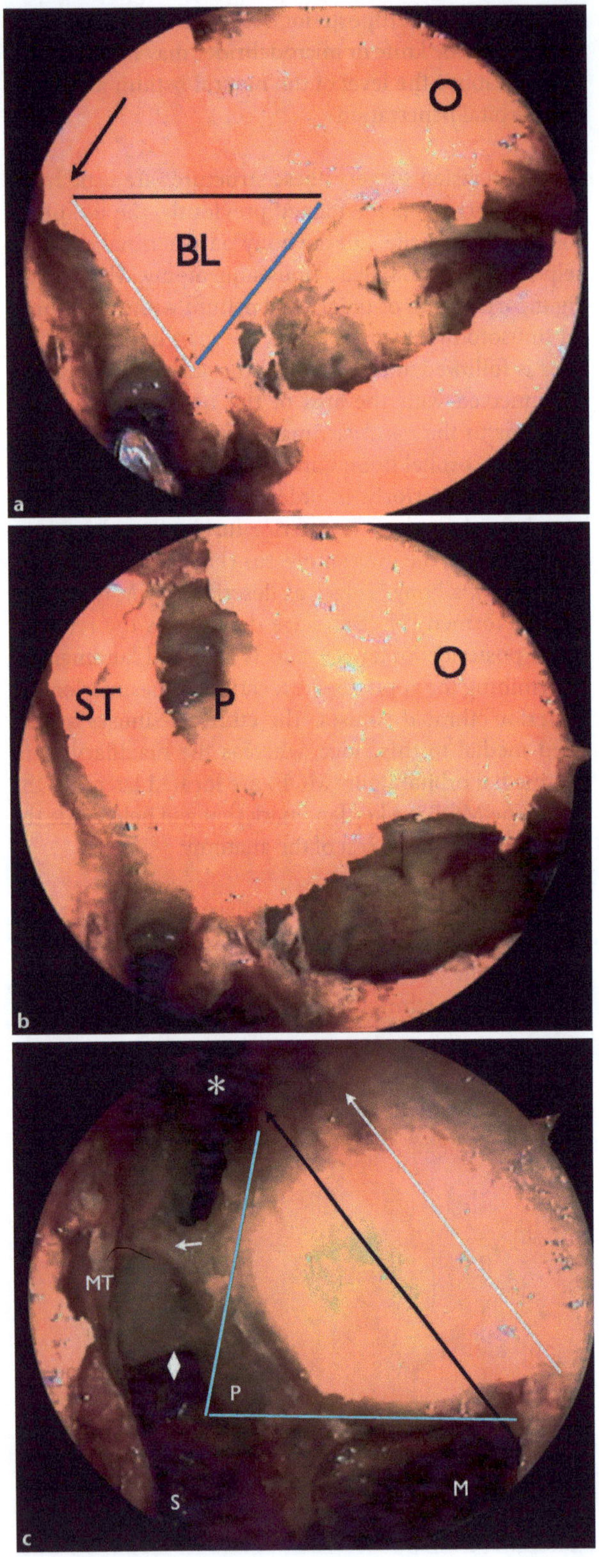

Fig. 7.4 **a** Borders of the anterior ethmoids, and safe entry into the posterior ethmoids. A triangle of safe entry into the inferior posterior ethmoids exists along the basal lamella (*BL*) of the middle turbinate. A horizontal line is drawn parallel to the nasal floor from the posterior bony ridge to the nasal septum (*black line*), at the level of the posterior medial orbital floor. A second line is drawn from the junction of the posterior ridge of the antrostomy, medial orbital floor, and posterior wall of maxillary antrostomy to the tail of the middle turbinate (*blue line*). The third line is along the medial aspect of the basal lamella (*white line*) and medial orbital wall (*O*). The *black arrow* demarcates the posterior lamella of the middle turbinate. **b** Completed ethmoidectomy after removal of the "safe triangle." *O* Medial orbital wall/lamina papyracea, *P* posterior ethmoids, *ST* remnant of superior turbinate. **c** The area within the *blue triangle* represents the orbital "cone." The orbital apex is located at the apex of the cone, at the coronal plane of the posterior wall of maxillary sinus and approximately 7–8 cm from the columella. The anterior ethmoid artery is denoted by the *white arrow*; the posterior ethmoid artery is denoted by the *white diamond*; the frontal sinus is denoted by the *asterisk*. The vertical lamellae of the middle turbinate (*MT*) at its attachment to the skull base is lateral to the olfactory cleft. The *black line* (base of orbital cone triangle) reflects the trajectory into the frontal infundibulum from the most anterior point of the maxillary antrostomy/natural ostium to a point a few millimeters behind the anterior attachment of middle turbinate, and parallel to the convexity of the nasolacrimal duct (*white line*). *M* Maxillary sinus, *P* posterior ethmoids, *S* sphenoid sinus

Ethmoid Labyrinth

The anterior ethmoids are comprised of multiple cells of variable dimensions and thin bone. Because of the variable and complex relationships of these cells within the ethmoid bullae, the anterior ethmoid sinuses are also called the ethmoid labyrinth [2]. The most anterior cells are called the agger nasi cells. These will be discussed further in the frontal sinus section, because they lie along the anterior border of the frontal recess. The anterior ethmoid cavity is bordered medially by the vertical lamellae of middle turbinate inserting into the skull base and lateral cribriform plate, laterally by the lamina papyracea or medial orbital wall, and posteriorly by the horizontal attachment of the middle turbinate to the lateral nasal wall and orbit. The latter structure is also referred to as the basal or ground lamellae of the middle turbinate (Fig. 7.4). The basal lamella divides the anterior and posterior ethmoid cells. Superiorly, the ethmoids are bound by the fovea ethmoidalis or roof of the ethmoid sinus. The anterior and posterior ethmoid arteries run from a lateral-to-medial direction along the ethmoid roof. The ethmoid roof is bony and runs in an inferomedial direction towards the cribriform plate. In 1965, Keros described three classifications for the depth of the cribriform in relation to the roof of the ethmoids. As can be seen, the bone is typically thicker on the lateral side, adjacent to the orbital wall.

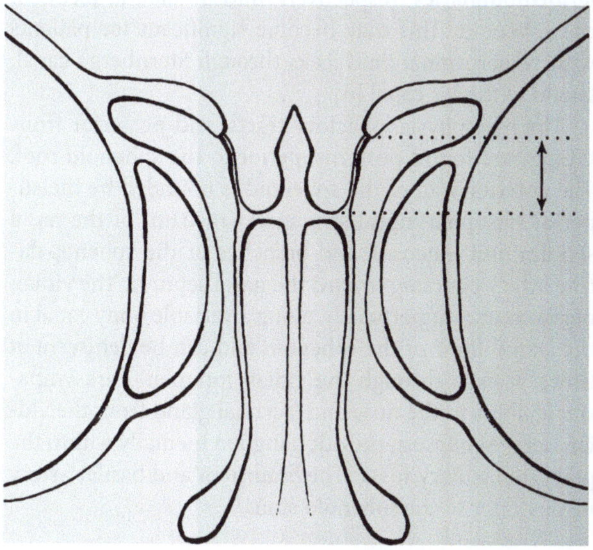

Fig. 7.5 Coronal view of the olfactory clefts and fossae. The *double-headed arrow* indicates the length of the lateral lamella of the cribriform plate, defining the type of olfactory fossa according to Keros. Type 1 corresponds to an olfactory fossa 1–3 mm deep in relation to the roof of the ethmoids. Type 2 is 4–7 mm deep. Type 3 is a depth of 8 mm and above

- Surgeons should exercise extreme care when dissecting or probing medially along the ethmoid roof, in order to minimize the risk of inadvertent intracranial penetration (Fig. 7.5).

As mentioned earlier, the three important lamellae when discussing surgery and ethmoid anatomy are the uncinate process, ethmoid bulla, and basal or ground lamellae. These are valuable landmarks in sinus surgery. However, these landmarks are commonly removed or altered during primary sinus surgery. As a result, they are not necessarily dependable for revision sinus surgery anatomy.

Dependable anatomical structures in the ethmoid region during revision sinus surgery are:
1. MOF.
2. Bony ridge of the maxillary antrostomy.
3. Superior attachment of the middle turbinate.

The MOF helps demarcate several important regions [5]. First, it helps identify the lateral extent of the surgeon's dissection. Second, it exposes the level of the skull base at the posterior ethmoids, which should lie superior to the MOF, as described previously in Figs. 7.4 and 7.6. Finally, it provides a level for safe entry into the sphenoid sinus or posterior ethmoid sinuses, giving the surgeon greater space to navigate posteriorly into the nose and paranasal sinuses, and define the superior and lateral limits of

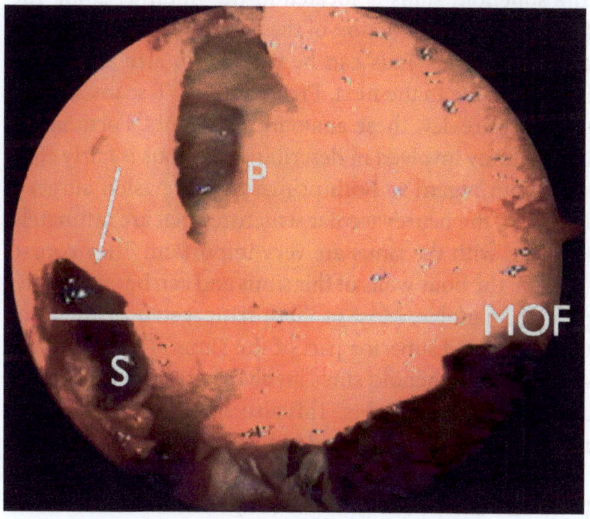

Fig. 7.6 Locations of sphenoid sinus (*S*) and posterior ethmoids (*P*) in relation to the medial orbital floor (*MOF*). Most of the posterior ethmoid air cells are located superior to the MOF while most of the sphenoid sinus is mostly inferior to it (*white line*) and adjacent to the nasal septum. This line also transects the approximate level of natural ostium of the sphenoid sinus superomedial to the tail of the superior turbinate (*white arrow*)

dissection. The bony ridge of the maxillary antrostomy, along with the MOF, gives the surgeon the proper trajectory when working in an anterior-to-posterior direction while dissecting the ethmoid cavity. Finally, the vertical attachment of the middle turbinate to the skull base is a good landmark to demarcate the medial aspect of the dissection of the superior ethmoid cells. The olfactory cleft will be found medial to this attachment.

Two special ethmoid cells deserve mention because they can distort the anatomy and confuse an unsuspecting surgeon. First, the Onodi cells (sphenoethmoid cells) are sphenoethmoid recess cells, and can vary in their pneumatization. These cells can extend superior and lateral to the sphenoid sinus. As a result, they can expose the optic nerve, which can run through the cell. If not identified on preoperative CT scans, an optic nerve injury may result with dissection in this area. Second, the supraorbital ethmoid cells are superior ethmoid cells that can arise posterior to the frontal recess and extend over the orbit (supraorbital extension). They can interfere with frontal sinus drainage posteriorly in a similar way that the agger nasi cells can act anteriorly. Often, these cells are confused with the frontal sinus [11]. Transillumination of these cells typically causes illumination of the medial canthal area, and not the frontal bone.

Sphenoid Sinus

The sphenoid sinus is located in the midline, along the skull base, at the junction of the anterior and middle cranial fossae. The sinus can be variable in size and shape from one side to the next. Preoperative CT scans are important to review these anatomical variants. Fortunately, the anatomy involved in describing the sinus is fairly constant with regard to both primary and revision surgery. However, the neurovascular structures that are intimately involved with the sinus are very important. They course through the bony walls of this sinus and can be fairly complex and variable. Most of these critical structures are in the lateral and superior part of the sinus. Therefore, safe access to the sphenoid sinus involves entry into this cavity as far medial as possible. This also assures that the sphenoid ostium is incorporated in the surgical sinusotomy.

There are several landmarks that can be used to identify a safe entry point into the sinus. The anterior wall of the sphenoid is approximately 7 cm from the columella at a 30° angle from the nasal floor (Fig. 7.7). As described extensively in the literature, the natural ostium lies superior and medial to the tail of the superior turbinate [4]. If the tail of the superior turbinate has been removed or distorted from prior surgery, the combination of using the MOF and the septum can be used to identify the location of the sphenoid ostium (Fig. 7.6). When viewed through a 0° or 30° telescope, the natural ostium of the sphenoid, and therefore safest area to enter, is always at the level the posterior MOF, adjacent to the nasal septum. The posterior wall of the sphenoid sinus is the skull base and usually measures approximately 9 cm from the columella. The intersinus septum can be variable in position. Often, the septum curves laterally and attaches at the face of the bone covering the carotid artery. Care should be taken not to inadvertently avulse this bony insertion onto the anteromedial face of the carotid artery, with resultant life-threatening hemorrhage.

- By opening the sphenoid and identifying the level of the skull base and lateral wall, at this level, the surgeon can confidently continue their dissection in an anterior direction to open up the superior and lateral aspects of the posterior and anterior ethmoid sinuses.

The lateral wall of the sphenoid sinus has several critical structures that should be recognized. Based on the degree of pneumatization, some structures may be more pronounced than others (Fig. 7.8). Four prominences along the wall that should be identified from superior to inferior are the optic nerve, internal carotid artery, second branch of the trigeminal nerve as it travels toward the foramen rotundum, and the vidian nerve [8]. In sinuses with a significant degree of lateral pneumatization, V2 and the vidian nerve can mark the superior and inferior boundaries, respectively, into the lateral recess of the sphenoid. This may become significant for patients with cerebrospinal fluid leaks through Sternberg's canal, lateral to the V2 canal [6].

The hypophysis, olfactory tracts, and posterior frontal gyri are found posterosuperior to the sphenoid roof. The anterior wall of the sphenoid is bounded by the superior nasopharyngeal structures (rostrum of the nasal septum and mucosa), and branches of the sphenopalatine artery coursing toward the nasal septum. The vidian nerve courses superficially, along a variable bony canal in the lateral floor of the sphenoid and can be dehiscent at times. It exits through the vidian foramen. Parasympathetic fibers to the nose and lacrimal gland from the vidian nerve synapse at the otic ganglion medially within the pterygomaxillary fossa. The brainstem and basilar artery lie posterior to the sphenoid sinus

Frontal Sinus

Similar to the sphenoid sinus, the frontal sinus can be variable in its degree of development. The frontal sinus drains via the frontal recess, which is very narrow and hourglass shaped. In primary surgery, useful landmarks to find the frontal sinus recess include the anterior eth-

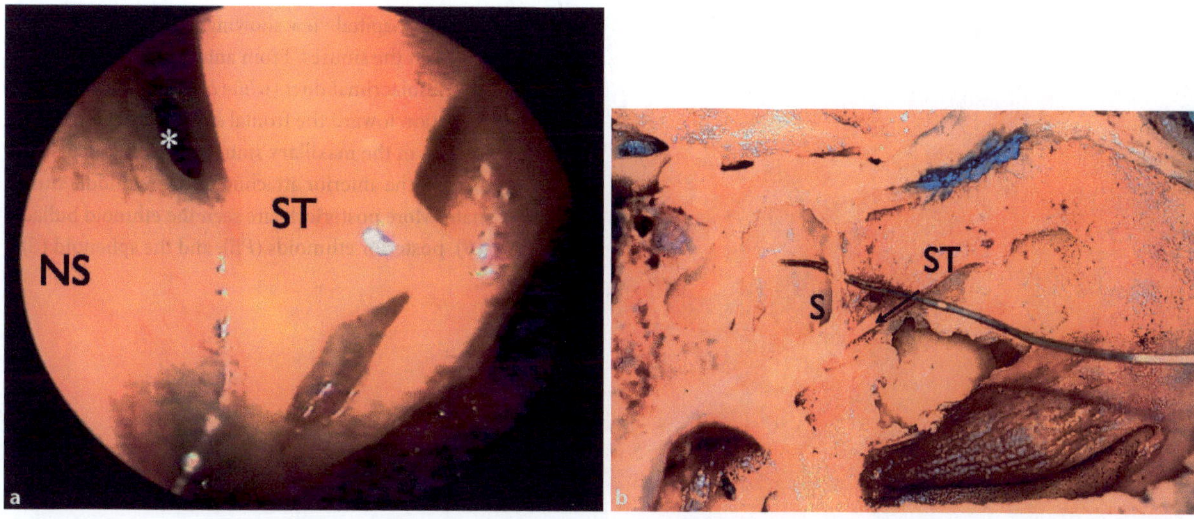

Fig. 7.7 **a** The location of the natural ostium of the sphenoid (*asterisk*) is located between the nasal septum (*NS*) and the tail of the superior turbinate (*ST*). **b** Sagittal view with the middle turbinate removed, showing the location of the sphenoid ostium. Wire is placed in the ostium. The superior turbinate (*ST*) and tail (*arrow*) show the relationship between the ostium and the ST

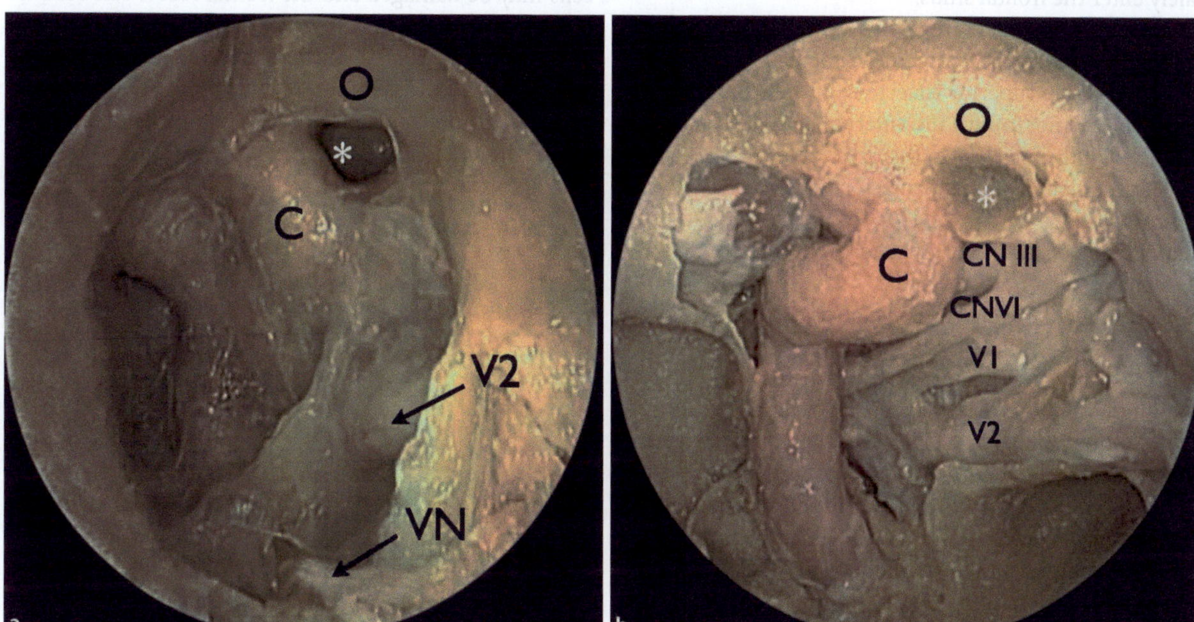

Fig. 7.8 **a** Endoscopic view from a cadaveric dissection showing the detailed anatomy of the lateral wall of the sphenoid sinus. Three convexities make up the lateral wall of the sphenoid sinus. The optic carotid recess is denoted by the *white asterisk*. *C* Cavernous portion of the carotid artery, *O* optic nerve, *VN* vidian nerve, *V2* maxillary division of the trigeminal nerve. Photographs courtesy of Islam Herzallah, MD. **b** Lateral wall of the sphenoid after removal of the bony wall and medial dural sheath of the cavernous sinus. *C* Carotid artery, *CN III* cranial nerve III, *CN VI* cranial nerve 6, *O* optic nerve, *VI* ophthalmic division of trigeminal nerve, *V2* maxillary division of trigeminal nerve. Photos courtesy of Islam Herzallah, MD [8]

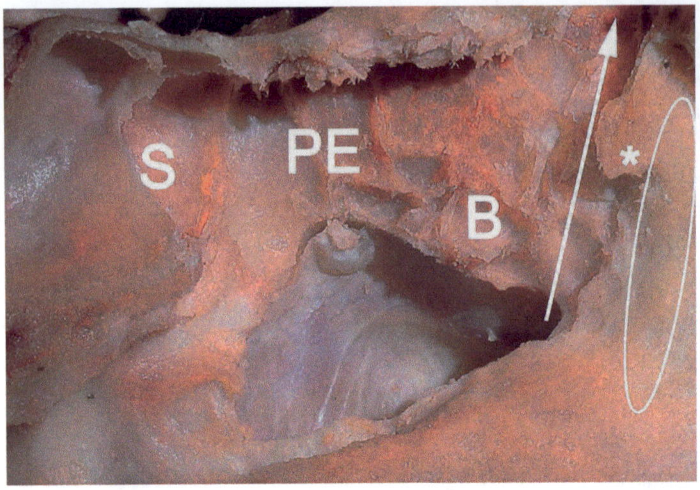

Fig. 7.9 Sagittal view showing the relationship between the sinuses. From anterior to posterior, the nasolacrimal duct (*white oval*) is parallel to the direction toward the frontal sinus from the natural ostium of the maxillary sinus (*white arrow*), just behind the anterior attachment of the middle turbinate. More posteriorly are seen the ethmoid bullae (*B*), posterior ethmoids (*PE*), and the sphenoid (*S*)

moid cells, anterior superior attachments of the middle turbinate, and the uncinate process. However, in revision surgery, these structures are usually altered or removed. As a result, other landmarks have been sought after to safely enter the frontal sinus.

The key to revision frontal surgery is to have some landmark directing the surgeon in the general direction and appropriate superior trajectory of the frontal infundibulum, and not toward the anterior skull base, which is located slightly posterior to this area. These are:

1. Natural ostium or most anterior portion of maxillary antrostomy.
2. Remnant of the anterior attachment and vertical lamella of the middle turbinate.
3. Convexity of the nasolacrimal duct [5].

Starting at the anterior maxillary antrostomy (or preferably the natural ostium of the maxillary sinus), and following a line parallel to the nasolacrimal duct, the frontal recess can be confidently accessed using a small probe, a few millimeters behind the anterior attachment of the middle turbinate (Figs. 7.4c and 7.9). In well-pneumatized frontal sinuses, a supraturbinal (laterally) or transeptal (medial) penetration, anterior to the coronal plane of the frontal infundibulum and anterior attachment of the middle turbinate, may be possible. Posterior landmarks also exist. By following the roof of the ethmoids anteriorly, the surgeon can identify the anterior ethmoid artery as it runs along the posterior aspect of the frontal recess and infundibulum. Once the anterior ethmoid artery is seen, the surgeon identifies the area of the frontal infundibulum by also following the medial orbital wall superiorly, as it defines the lateral extent of this opening into the frontal sinus. Medially, the border of the frontal infundibulum is the vertical lamella of the middle turbinate. Anteriorly lie the agger nasi cell and variable frontal sinus cells, as described later. As mentioned earlier, the amount of pneumatization of the agger nasi can affect the outflow of the frontal sinus [12]. Posteriorly, supraorbital cells can obscure the recess. In previous surgery, the suprabullar cells may be damaged and the frontal recess can become scarred with bone and debris. The recognition and removal of these cells is critical for confident entry into the frontal sinus and resolution of the patient's symptoms.

In the frontal sinus itself, there can be variable structures. The intersinus septum can be midline or laterally

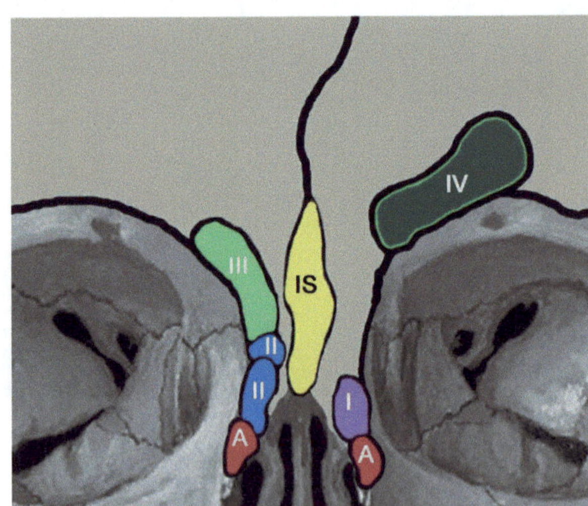

Fig. 7.10 Type I is a single air cell above the agger nasi. Type II is a group of small air cells above the agger nasi, but below the orbital roof. Type III is a single air cell extending from the agger nasi into the frontal sinus. Finally, type IV is an isolated air cell within the frontal sinus not contiguous with the agger nasi. *A* Agger nasi cell, *IS* inner sinus septum

displaced in either direction. It can also be pneumatized and become an isolated air cell. Bent and Kuhn classified frontal cells into four types [1]. During revision surgery, some or all of these intersinus cells can be present. Type I is a single air cell above the agger nasi. Type II is a group of small air cells above the agger nasi, but below the orbital roof. Type III is a single air cell extending from the agger nasi into the frontal sinus. Finally, type IV is an isolated air cell within the frontal sinus not contiguous with the agger nasi (Fig. 7.10).

Conclusion

With a sound understanding of the intricate sinus anatomy, a surgeon can confidently perform revision sinus surgery. The navigational systems are not a substitute for anatomical knowledge. They can provide a false sense of security and may lead the surgery beyond the limits at which the surgeon feels comfortable. However, the landmarks discussed in this chapter are reliable, and recognizable by any surgeon, and should supersede any navigational system.

References

1. Bent J, Kuhn FA, Cuilty C (1994) The frontal cell in frontal recess obstruction. Am J Rhinol 8:185–191
2. Bodino C, Jankowski R, Gringnon B, et al. (2004) Surgical anatomy of the turbinal wall of the ethmoidal labyrinth. Rhinology 42:73–80
3. Bolger WE (2001) Anatomy of the paranasal sinuses. In: Kennedy DW, Bolger WE, Zinreich J (eds) Diseases of the Sinuses, Diagnosis and Management. Decker, Hamilton, Ontario, pp 1–12
4. Bolger WE, Keyes A (2001) Use of superior meatus/turbinate in the endoscopic approach to the sphenoid sinus. Otolaryngol Head Neck Surg 120:308–313
5. Casiano RR (2001) A stepwise surgical technique using the medial orbital floor as the key landmark in performing endoscopic sinus surgery. Laryngoscope 111: 964–974
6. Castelnuovo P, Dallan I, Pistochini A, et al. (2007) Endonasal endoscopic repair of Sternberg's canal cerebrospinal fluid leaks. Laryngoscope 117:345–349
7. Graney DO, Rice DH (1998) Paranasal sinus anatomy. In: Cummings CW, Fredrickson JM, Harker LA, et al. (eds) Otolaryngology – Head and Neck Surgery, 3rd edn. Mosby, St. Louis, pp 1059–1064
8. Herzallah IR, Casiano RR (2007) Endoscopic endonasal study of the internal carotid artery course and variations. Am J Rhinol 21:262–270
9. May M, Schaitkin B, Kay SL(1994) Revision endoscopic sinus surgery: six friendly surgical landmarks. Laryngoscope 104:766–767
10. Polavaram R, Devaiah AK, Sakai O, et al. (2004) Anatomic variants and pearls – functional endoscopic sinus surgery. Otolaryngol Clin North Am 37: 221–242
11. Stammberger HR, Kennedy DW (1995) Paranasal sinuses: anatomic terminology and nomenclature. The Anatomic Terminology Group. Ann Otol Rhinol Laryngol Suppl 167:7–16
12. Wormald PJ (2003) The agger nasi cell: the key to understanding the anatomy of the frontal recess. Otolaryngol Head Neck Surg 129:497–507

Chapter 8

Surgical Instruments in Revision Endoscopic Sinus Surgery

8

Vijay R. Ramakrishnan and Todd T. Kingdom

Core Messages

- Continued development and refinement of available surgical instrumentation for endoscopic sinus surgery (ESS) remains important.
- The patient undergoing revision ESS may present a unique set of anatomic and surgical challenges requiring unique instrument solutions.
- New developments and refinements have improved visualization (videoscopic equipment), our ability to precisely handle soft tissue (microdebriders, through-cutting instruments), our ability to remove bone efficiently (high-speed burs), and our access (angled and malleable instrumentation) during ESS.
- The revision ESS surgeon must be experienced with these current and evolving instruments in order to optimize outcome and safety.

Contents

Introduction and Background

On a basic level, surgical instrumentation and surgical concepts are similar for both primary endoscopic sinus surgery (ESS) and revision ESS. However, unique situations and challenges will present during revision ESS, requiring the surgeon to be familiar with a wide range of surgical techniques and instrumentation. The surgeon must be knowledgeable, comfortable, and facile with the available surgical equipment options. The goal of this chapter is to review current surgical instruments of value for use in revision ESS.

Historically, surgical concepts behind the management of sinus disease have centered around "radical" therapy for "irreversible" mucosal disease. Messerklinger's work, which began in the 1950s, introduced new concepts of reversible mucosal disease, mucosal sparing approaches, and the development of functional surgical techniques. The stated goals of the Messerklinger technique were to remove the obstructing anatomic variations causing disease and to resect only the most severely diseased mucosa in key locations [7]. To achieve these goals, the surgeon must be able to accurately visualize and diagnose endonasal disease, limit the scope of dissection as indicated, and precisely manipulate variable anatomy. This required a basic change in instrument design concepts that have only recently been widely available. Refinements in the videoscopic chain have enhanced visualization of the surgical field, the development of fine through-cutting instruments has provided the opportunity for mucosal sparing procedures, and the introduction of powered instrumentation has expanded the rhinologist's armamentarium greatly. These developments have been critical to the evolution of both primary and revision ESS.

Mucosal preservation has been emphasized as an important objective for both successful primary and revision sinus surgery. Much of the technology presented in this chapter focuses on this important concept – precision dissection and mucosal preservation. Clinical experience suggests that surgical efficiency, mucosal recovery, and patient outcomes are improved with mucosal preservation. Meticulous removal of soft tissue and attempted mucosal preservation ought to be goals of the sinus surgeon in both primary and revision cases.

- Mucosal preservation is an important objective for both primary and revision ESS.
- New instrument design focuses on the surgeon's need for precision in a variety of clinical situations.
- The operating surgeon must be aware of increasing distortion and disorientation and decreasing illumination with increasing telescopic angle of the endoscope.

Videoscopy and Visualization

With the use of assorted endoscopes, the surgeon is capable of direct visualization of most sites within the surgical field. The zero-degree endoscope is preferred because of its optimal lighting and minimal optical distortion and disorientation; however, it may be inadequate in meeting the needs of many revision procedures. Angled endoscopes, including 30, 45, and 70°, have been designed to facilitate visualization around "corners" and to extend the surgeon's "reach" (Fig. 8.1). Current technology has improved the width of view and degree of illumination for angled telescopes, but the operating surgeon must still consider the increasing distortion and disorientation associated with increasing telescopic angle [3]. Revision ESS often requires extended visualization and access, thus surgeon comfort with angled endoscopes is essential. Several attempts at creation of a three-dimensional endoscope have provided a superior stationary image, but can be disorienting when rotated laterally, and have not been widely utilized [4].

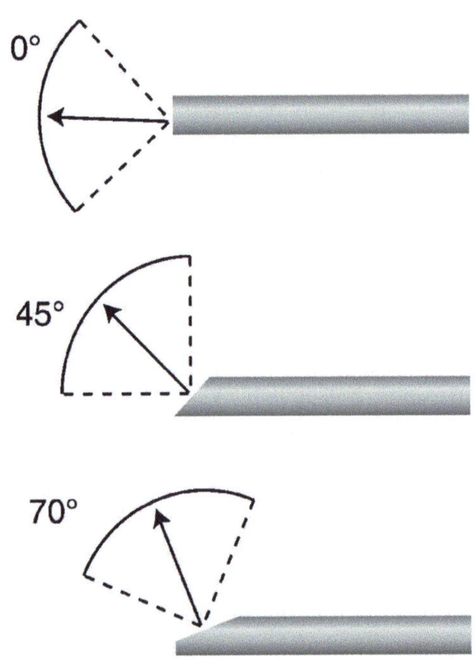

Fig. 8.1 Rigid nasal endoscopes with angles ranging from 0 to 70° (drawing by Scott Baird, adapted from Karl Storz Endoscopy America, Culver City, California)

Improvements in camera technology have addressed concerns of illumination, color rendition, and weight. Color rendition and depth perception on the videoscopic projection are less accurate than that of the direct endoscopic view, yet current technology has mitigated these concerns. In addition, operating from the projection screen facilitates the four-handed technique, which may be of benefit in difficult revision cases and endoscopic skull-base procedures [4]. High-definition (HD) video technology is the latest evolution in endoscopic visualization. HD-compatible video camera systems provide 1920 × 1080 pixels of resolution in a native 16:9 aspect ratio. Potential advantages include higher input resolution delivering more detail and depth of focus, larger viewing format with the 16:9 aspect ratio supported by widescreen monitors, and enhanced color brilliance. Though in its infancy, HD videoscopic technology should prove valuable in the differentiation between soft-tissue types and further augment extended rhinologic surgical approaches.

Mucosal-Sparing Instrumentation

Although mucosal preservation has been a tenet of primary and revision ESS since Messerklinger's early work, appropriate instrumentation had not been widely available for many years. Until recently, ESS surgical instruments were too large and promoted more of a "rip and tear" technique when removing mucosal disease. Mucosal loss and bone exposure has been associated with increased scarring and mucosal sequestration, decreased ciliary function, chronic inflammation, neo-osteogenesis, and a propensity toward persistent pain [5,8]. Although intuitive, the true value of mucosal sparing techniques has not been objectively established. A prospective, randomized, controlled study in 24 patients with chronic rhinosinusitis comparing the use of microdebriders to conventional instrumentation found no statistical difference in symptoms, saccharin transport times, or endoscopic findings of synechiae and ostial reocclusion at 3-, 6-, and 13-month follow up [9]. Vauterin et al. performed a prospective, randomized, double-blinded experiment comparing the use of through-cutting forceps to noncutting forceps. At 3-week and 12-month follow up, there was no statistical difference in patient symptoms or endoscopic findings of parameters including adhesions, polyps, edema, crusting, and secretions [11]. Certainly, further studies are needed to define the effects of mucosal preservation on microscopic and clinical outcome. As of today, however, mucosal preservation and meticulous soft-tissue removal ought to be fundamental goals of the sinus surgeon. Consequently, instrument design and technique development focuses on the concept of mucosal preservation and minimally-invasive surgical principles.

A wide array of instruments for ESS is now available from several manufacturers. Fine, through-cutting instruments with straight and up-biting jaws have been designed for both mucosal dissection and removal of thin bone. The cutting width of these tools ranges from submillimeter to 4 mm in size. These instruments also come in a variety of angles, with the operating portion angled up, down, or curved to the side (Fig. 8.2). The design of the cutting end of these instruments can include a microscissor blade and linear or circular cutting punches (Fig. 8.3). In addition, there are differences in the strength of these cutting instruments.

- Instrument shaft and handle lengths vary depending on the intended objective: 13–15 cm for standard ESS, extending to 18 cm for endoscopic skull-base approaches.

The current selection of mucosal sparing instrumentation allows the surgeon to match the instrument to the tissue type to be removed and the access needed to accomplish the task. Quite literally, there are numerous instruments to choose from to fit the surgeon's goals and objectives. Several chapters within this textbook will be devoted to revision maxillary, ethmoid, sphenoid, and frontal sinus surgery. To avoid redundancy only brief comments on frontal sinus instrumentation will be included in this section. The evolution of mucosal sparing frontal sinus instruments represents one of the most significant advances in revision ESS. The frontal sinus surgeon can now select from a variety of fine, angled instruments to manipulate the frontal recess and to access the frontal sinus. Circular punches and through-cutting forceps

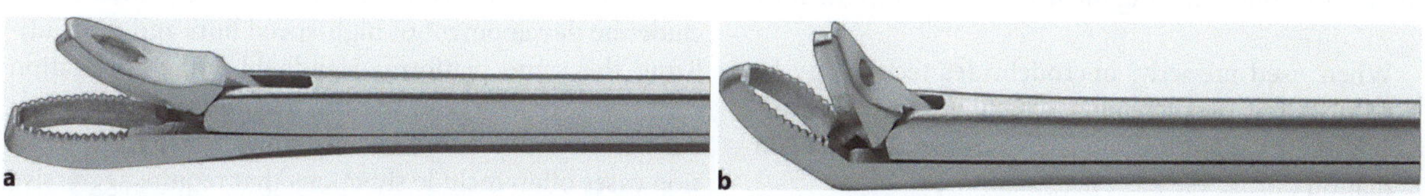

Fig. 8.2 Through-cutting, mucosal sparing forceps: **a** straight, **b** upturned 45° (Karl Storz Endoscopy America, Culver City, California, USA)

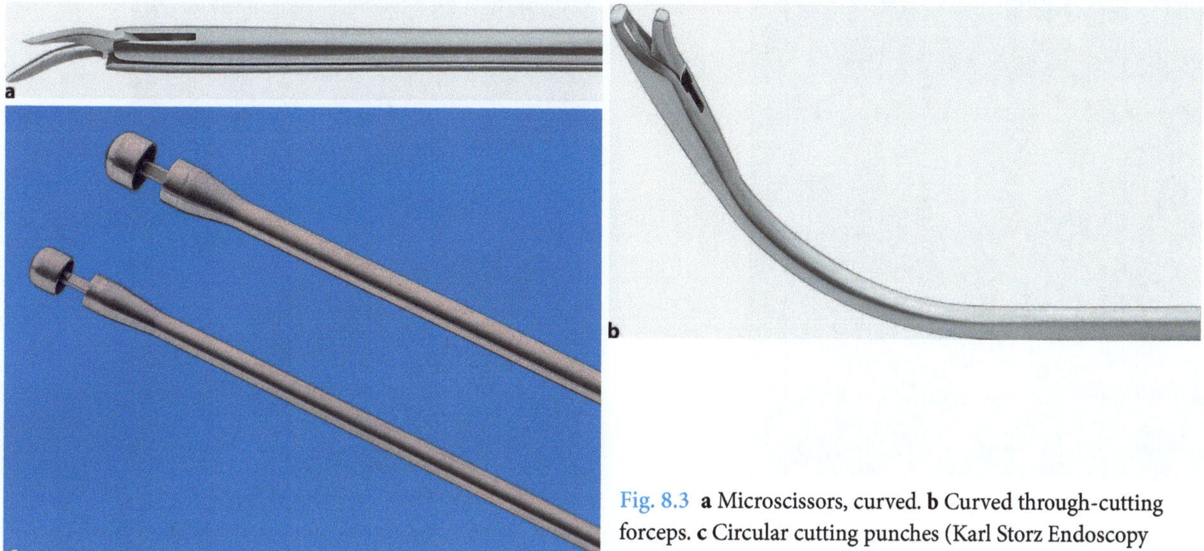

Fig. 8.3 **a** Microscissors, curved. **b** Curved through-cutting forceps. **c** Circular cutting punches (Karl Storz Endoscopy America)

with shaft angles ranging from 45 to 110° facilitate precise mucosa-sparing dissection (Fig. 8.4). More robust punches with 70 and 90° angled shafts are available for precise yet aggressive bone removal in the frontal recess region (Fig. 8.5). In addition, a variety of angled curettes, picks, and probes are available to augment this type of dissection.

- Wide selections of mucosal sparing ESS instruments are available to the surgeon, including options in shaft length, angle, size, and cutting action.

Powered Instrumentation

8

Powered instrumentation has aided tremendously in the challenges of revision sinus surgery, especially in the treatment of recurrent polyposis, synechiae, and osteitic bone. Microdebriders have been used intranasally for over 10 years [10]. Their use allows for rapid sharp dissection, reduced bleeding, constant suction and irrigation, and immediate tissue removal from the field. This provides excellent continuous visualization, allowing the surgeon to operate without removing the instrument from the nose.

- When used properly, microdebrider technology has reduced mucosal stripping, which has been shown to accelerate wound healing and decrease synechiae formation.

In a retrospective, nonblinded analysis, Krouse reported more rapid mucosal healing, with reduction in crusting, synechiae formation, and ostial occlusion, in patients who underwent ESS with a microdebrider when compared to standard techniques [6]. Bernstein's findings echoed these conclusions in a retrospective, uncontrolled analysis with a mean follow-up of 16 months [1].

The basic components of a microdebrider system are the power source, irrigation system, suction source, handpiece, and interchangeable disposable blades. The irrigation flow rate is adjustable to suit the surgeon's preference, and the linear suction path has been tailored to reduce the amount of clogging. Blade speed may be adjusted to maximize tissue cutting without system plugging. Microdebrider blades contain a fenestrated, blunt outer sheath to minimize tissue trauma, and a mobile inner blade with the cutting surface. This design eliminates avulsion of adjacent tissue to be preserved, which may occur with traditional instrumentation. Angled microdebrider blades up to 120 ° are now available and have facilitated surgery in areas of difficult access, such as the far reaches of the frontal and maxillary sinuses (Fig. 8.6). In addition, short-radius curved blades and rotating blade heads have made surgery in these areas easier. Video 8.1 demonstrates the use of the microdebrider for the removal of nasal polyps.

Microdebrider technology has been extended to include the development of high-speed burs and drills utilizing the same platform. Handheld suction-irrigation drills allow the surgeon to drill, irrigate, and utilize suction while under direct visualization of the target. Revision cases often include situations that require aggressive removal of osteitic bone or removal of bone for extended access. Angled burs allow for access to the frontal sinus with focused removal of bone from the frontal process

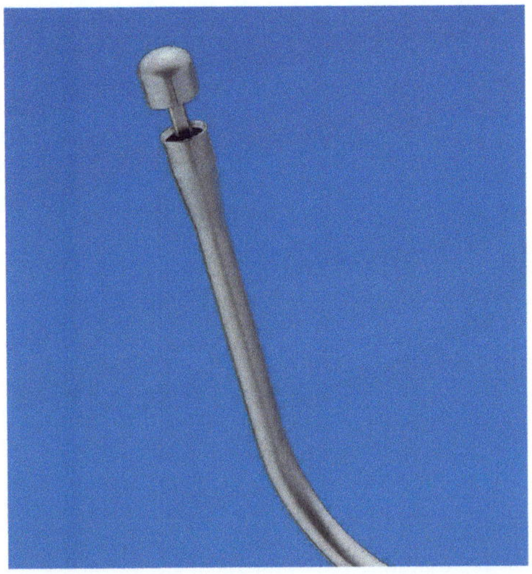

Fig. 8.4 Mucosal sparing and cutting frontal sinus instruments 65° circular cutting punch (Karl Storz Endoscopy America)

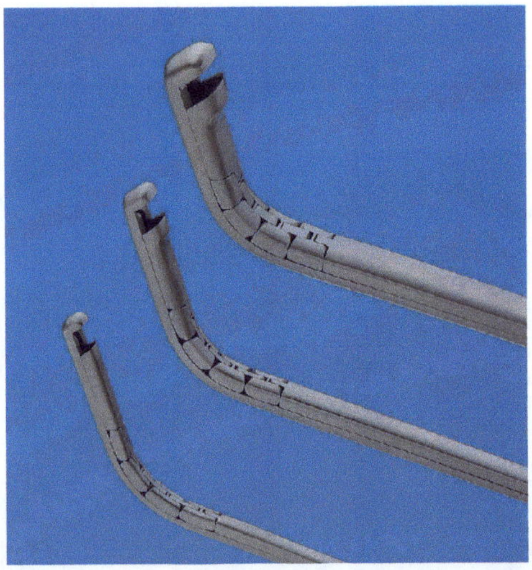

Fig. 8.5 70° cutting frontal sinus punches (Karl Storz Endoscopy America)

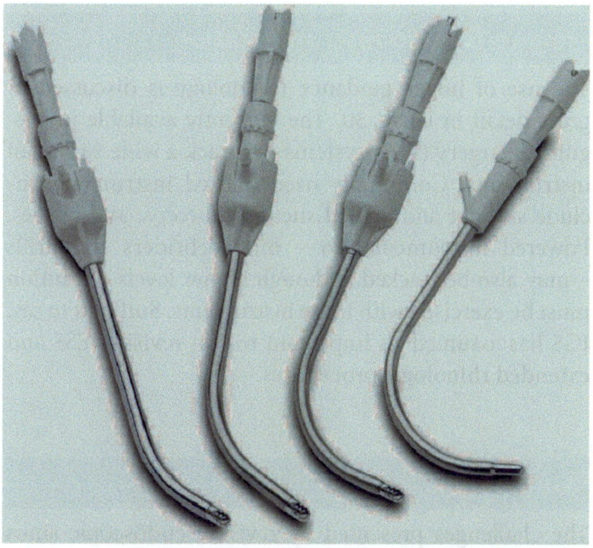

Fig. 8.6 Microdebrider blades with rotating cutting openings and shaft angles of 40, 60, 90, and 120° (Medtronic, Jacksonville, Florida, USA)

of the maxilla while keeping the amount of postoperative bone exposure to a minimum (Fig. 8.7). Chandra et al. reported on their experience using a 70° diamond bur for Draf IIb and Draf III procedures [2]. They emphasized the precise and efficient bone removal afforded with this device. The continuous irrigation helps to maintain bone viability by minimizing thermal damage, while the drill design resists skipping in such a tight area. Recent developments have focused on the design of high-speed burs for extended skull-base approaches in the region of the sella, sphenoid sinus, and clivus. Devices with a variety of shaft lengths and angles, and bur sizes and types are currently under development (Fig. 8.8).

The application of powered instrumentation for soft-tissue and bone removal in revision ESS has proven to be an invaluable advancement. However, one must remember that extensive removal of mucosa, skull-base penetration, and orbital injury are possible and potentially disastrous with the use of powered instrumentation. Video 8.2 demonstrates the use of a high-speed diamond bur for bone removal during an optic nerve decompression.

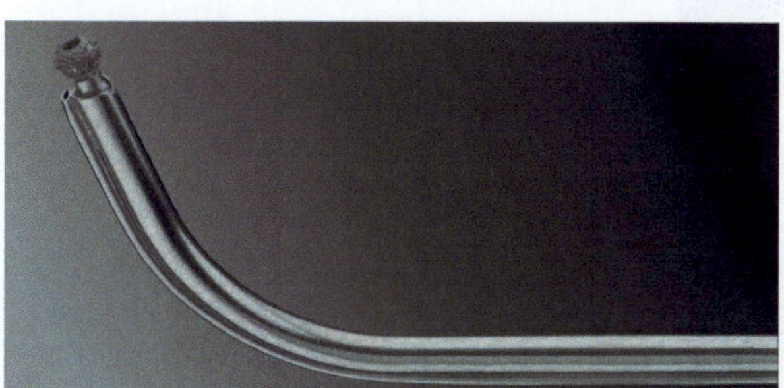

Fig. 8.7 70° degree high-speed diamond bur (Medtronic)

- A variety of blades for soft-tissue removal and burs for bone removal are available based on the same power platform.
- The surgeon must be aware of the potential hazards associated with the use of powered instrumentation in sinus surgery.

Modifications of Traditional Instruments

Traditional instruments have also been modified to increase their utility and efficacy. Visualization is fundamental to all intranasal procedures, and thus it seems intuitive to modify traditional instruments with the addition of suction.

- Suction instrumentation facilitates surgical precision and efficiency.

Suction elevators are particularly useful for endoscopically limited or revision septoplasty. A selection of suction curettes, elevators, punches, probes, hooks, and picks exist, and are extremely useful for difficult frontal

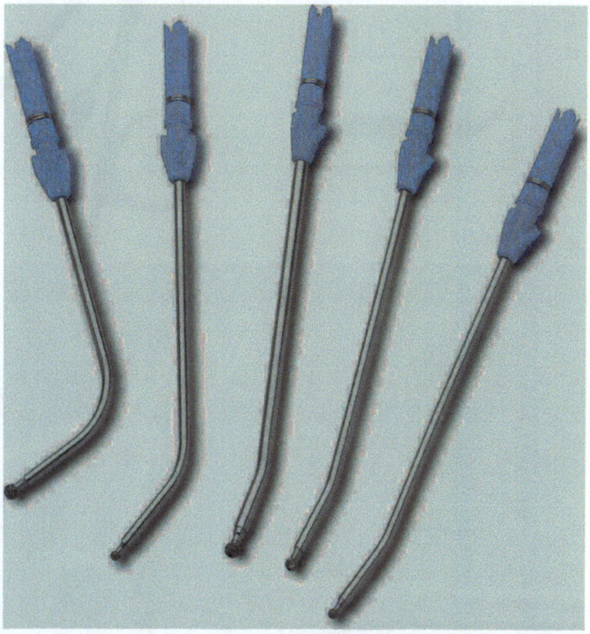

Fig. 8.8 High-speed skull-base burs with shaft angles ranging from 15 to 90° degrees. Diamond and cutting burs are available with fluted or round designs (Medtronic)

recess dissections, tumor removal, and extended revision procedures. Malleable suction probes, elevators, and curettes have been created to aid surgical access; these instruments have a working length of 11 cm, with the last 4 cm being of a malleable nature. Malleable instruments each have a predetermined strength appropriate for their individual uses, but have a finite lifespan due to intrinsic metallic properties.

The ability to control hemorrhage becomes more relevant in revision ESS cases and extended rhinologic procedures. Endoscopic cautery devices have been developed to assist with this challenge. Bipolar cautery, combined with small size, suction, and angled tips are ideal design goals. Several options are available that satisfy many of these objectives and have proven useful during endoscopic procedures (Fig. 8.9). In addition, endoscopic vascular clip appliers have been developed by several manufacturers to aid in the control of intranasal hemorrhage (Fig. 8.10). Although still of limited value due to design limitations, these instruments can be quite useful in select situations. Video 8.3 demonstrates the use of bipolar cautery, the vascular clip applier, and microscissors during endoscopic tumor removal.

Image-Guided Instrumentation

The use of image guidance technology is discussed in great detail in Chap. 30. The currently available image-guided surgery (IGS) systems can track a wide variety of instruments. Commonly used tracked instruments include straight and angled suctions, forceps, and probes. Powered instrumentation – microdebriders and drills – may also be tracked, although higher levels of caution must be exercised with these instruments. Suffice it to say, IGS has assumed an important role in revision ESS and extended rhinologic procedures.

Summary

The challenges presented by revision endoscopic sinus surgery – difficult anatomy, synechiae formation, bone removal, and precision soft-tissue removal – may be assuaged by the use of refined instrumentation. Mucosal preservation is stressed, and is also enhanced with the surgeon's knowledge of currently available technology and instrumentation. Visualization may be improved

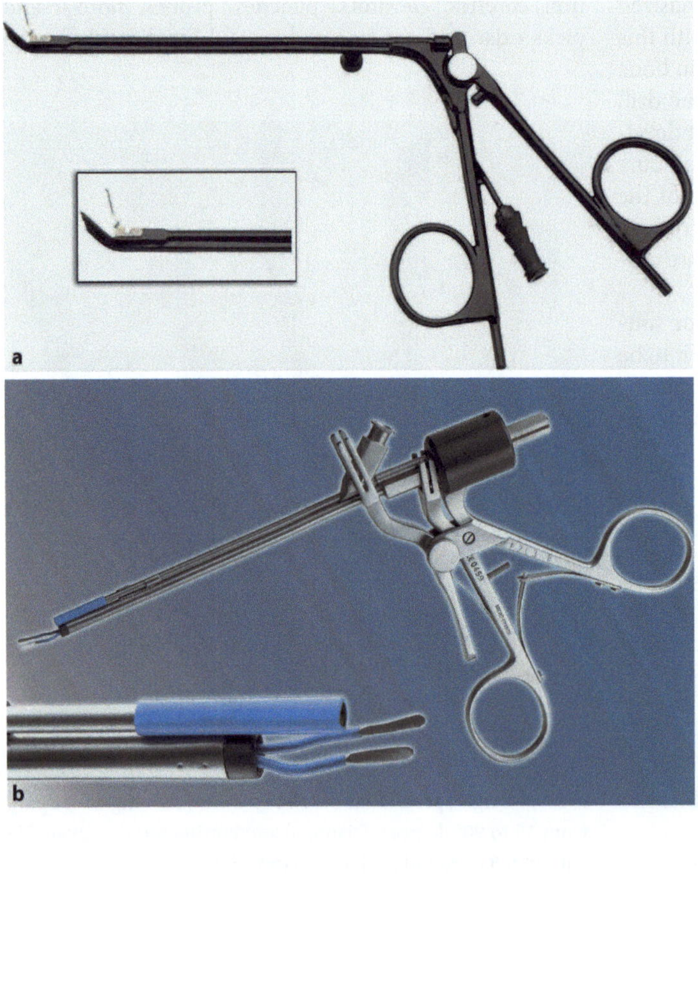

Fig. 8.9 **a** Stammberger endoscopic bipolar device (Karl Storz Endoscopy America). **b** Wormald endoscopic bipolar device (Medtronic)

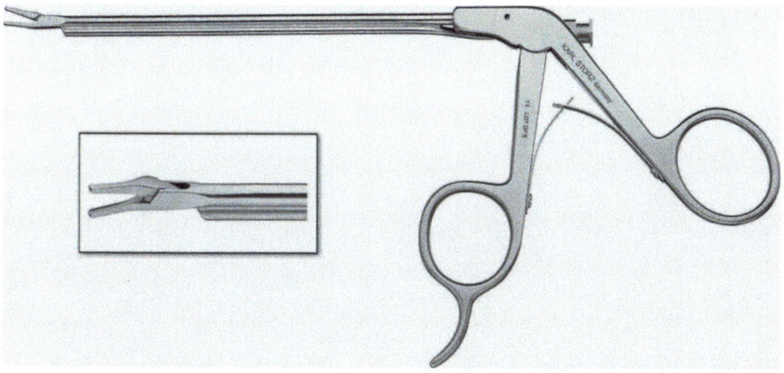

Fig. 8.10 Endoscopic clip applier (Karl Storz Endoscopy America; recommended clips: ligating clip cartridge, medium titanium clips. Ligaclip Extra by Ethicon, Cincinnati, OH, USA)

with use of angled telescopes, improved cameras and monitors, and the introduction of HD technology. Speed, hemostasis, and precision are hallmarks of powered instrumentation. Through-cutting instruments and refinements of existing instruments also help to address the unique challenges presented in difficult revision cases. The sinus surgeon who embarks upon complicated revision cases must have a complete knowledge of the available instruments, and feel comfortable with their use in the appropriate circumstance.

References

1. Bernstein JM, Lebowitz RA, Jacobs JB (1998) Initial report on postoperative healing after endoscopic sinus surgery with the microdebrider. Otolaryngol Head Neck Surg. 118:800–803
2. Chandra RK, Schlosser R, Kennedy DW (2004) Use of the 70-degree diamond burr in the management of complicated frontal sinus disease. Laryngoscope 114:188–192
3. Kang SK, White PS, Lee MS, et al. (2002) A randomized control trial of surgical task performance in frontal recess surgery: zero degree versus angled telescopes. Am J Rhinol 16:33–36
4. Kennedy DW (2007) Technical innovations and the evolution of endoscopic sinus surgery. Ann Otol Rhinol Laryngol Suppl 196:3–12
5. Kennedy DW (2000) Functional endoscopic sinus surgery: concepts, surgical indications, and instrumentation. In: Kennedy DW, Zinreich SJ, Bolger W (eds) Diseases of the Sinuses: Diagnosis and Endoscopic Management. Decker, Hamilton, Canada, pp 197–210
6. Krouse JH, Christmas DA Jr (1996) Powered instrumentation in functional endoscopic sinus surgery. II: A comparative study. Ear Nose Throat J 75:42–44
7. Messerklinger W (1978) Endoscopy of the Nose. Baltimore: Urban Schwarzenberg
8. Moriyama H, Yanagi K, Ohtori N, et al. (1996) Healing process of sinus mucosa after endoscopic sinus surgery. Am J Rhinol 10:61–66
9. Selivanova O, Kuehnemund M, Mann WJ, et al. (2003) Comparison of conventional instruments and mechanical debriders for surgery of patients with chronic rhinosinusitis. Am J Rhinol 17:197–202
10. Setliff RC III, Parsons DS (1994) The "hummer": new instrumentation for functional endoscopic sinus surgery. Am J Rhinol 8:275–278
11. Vauterin T, Vander Poorten V, Jorissen M (2006) Long term effects of cutting forceps in endoscopic sinus surgery. Rhinology 44:123–127

Chapter 9

Anesthetic Choices, Techniques, and Injections

9

W. Derek Leight and Brent Senior

Core Messages

- General anesthesia using total intravenous anesthesia (TIVA) with propofol and remifentanyl may improve endoscopic vision in the surgical field.
- TIVA may provide patients with a better postoperative recovery period due to the antiemetic effects of propofol and the decreased hangover effect due to the fast metabolism of these two drugs.
- If TIVA is unavailable, the use of inhaled anesthetics should be minimized to avoid vasodilation with reflex tachycardia, which may worsen the surgical field.
- Perioperative beta-blockers may also be useful in improving the quality of vision in the surgical field. The use of these drugs should be discussed preoperatively with an anesthesiologist.
- Both inhaled anesthetics and propofol infusions degrade platelet function, which may contribute to an overall worsening of the quality of vision in the surgical field over time.
- Local injections are safe and reliable methods to enhance visualization in the surgical field.

Contents

Introduction

Since its inception in the 1980s, functional endoscopic sinus surgery (FESS) has become an important tool in the treatment of sinonasal disease. Technological advances have improved surgical techniques, which in turn have led to a widening of the scope of surgically treatable diseases. In comparison to traditional otolaryngologic surgery, methods of anesthetic administration for FESS are more influential in determining the quality of the surgical field.

Anesthetic Choices

Local anesthesia with sedation has been a widely employed method for endoscopic sinus surgery. Several authors have reported this as the anesthetic method of choice, reporting fewer side effects, shorter operative times, and less perioperative bleeding.[5, 8] In addition, it is thought of as being theoretically safer, due to the fact that dissection in high-risk areas such as the anterior and posterior ethmoid bundles and lamina papyracea is more likely to induce pain and therefore allow the patient to alert the surgeon before an injury occurs [13]. Local anesthesia with sedation is more technically challenging for the anesthesiologist, as a balance must be achieved between patient comfort, respiratory drive, airway protection, surgical access, and positioning [13]. It is also dependent upon the patient's level of cooperation, which may tend to decrease over time. FESS under local anesthesia can produce patient anxiety, particularly during cases with heavy mucosal bleeding. Rising patient anxiety also tends to impact the surgeon and potentially the quality of the operation. Some groups use local anesthesia on a regular basis for straightforward cases; however, these are carefully selected beforehand [4]. In addition, the routine use of image-guidance systems makes the local anesthetic technique less feasible due to positioning factors and the necessity of patient immobility. The author's group believes that these limitations outweigh the theoretical anatomic advantage of local anesthesia.

General anesthesia consists of the following three phases: induction, maintenance, and emergence. The goal of general anesthesia is to safely produce, while maintaining physiologic stability:

9

1. Hypnosis.
2. Analgesia.
3. Amnesia.
4. Anesthesia.
5. Areflexia.
6. Anxiolysis.

General anesthesia for FESS is usually either a variant of balanced anesthesia, using a combination of sedative/hypnotics, inhaled anesthesia, opioids, and neuromuscular blocking agents, or total intravenous anesthesia (TIVA), using a combination of propofol and synthetic opioids.

Pharmacology of General Anesthesia

Volatile Anesthetics

Inhaled or volatile anesthetics are an important part of balanced anesthesia. They have been in use since the mid-nineteenth century and represent one of the most important advances in the history of medicine. Although their mechanism of action remains unclear, they are known to produce profound central nervous system depression resulting in unconsciousness and amnesia. They are also known to produce respiratory depression, myocardial depression, dose-dependent decreases in mean arterial blood pressure (MAP), and reflex tachycardia [12].

- Volatile anesthetics are traditionally used in the maintenance phase of general anesthesia and to improve the surgical field by producing "controlled hypotension."
- They produce dose-dependent hypotension with reflex tachycardia and profound vasodilation, which may worsen the surgical field when used alone.

Intravenous Anesthesia

Intravenous (IV) anesthesia using sedative/hypnotics such as barbiturates and benzodiazepines are important in the induction phase of general anesthesia. These drugs produce rapid-onset hypnosis and sedation. Since the introduction of propofol in the late 1980s, IV anesthetics have also become popular in the maintenance phase of anesthesia.

Propofol

Propofol, whose chemical name is isopropylphenol, represents a new class of IV anesthetics, the akylphenols. It is the most widely used IV induction agent in anesthetic practice. It is lipophilic, and almost completely insoluble in aqueous solution. It is therefore produced in a milky emulsion with lecithin, glycerol, and soybean oil. This formulation is a potential medium for bacterial growth, and must therefore be used with meticulous sterile technique and should be used within 6 h of opening the vial. Because lecithin comes from egg yolk, patients with egg allergies may be susceptible to allergic reactions. Because of its high lipophilic nature, propofol is rapidly partitioned across the blood-brain barrier upon injection. This accounts for the quick onset of its sedative and hypnotic effects. Plasma clearance and redistribution into skeletal muscle and fat is faster than its hepatic metabolism. The high plasma clearance rate combined with its action as an antiemetic is thought to contribute to its low "hangover effect," which makes it useful for outpatient surgery.

- Propofol:

1. Acts through potentiation of GABA receptors in the central nervous system.
2. Produces profound respiratory depression.
3. Produces systemic vasodilation at the level of arteries and veins.
4. Reduces cardiac preload and afterload.
5. Causes systemic hypotension with little or no reflex tachycardia due to inhibition of the baroreceptor reflex and therefore does not increase cardiac output.
6. Produces little or no analgesia [12].
7. Produces a small "hangover effect," which make it useful for outpatient surgery.

Opioid Agonists

Opioid agonists such as fentanyl produce analgesia without loss of touch, proprioception, or consciousness. Fentanyl, sufentanil, alfentanil, and remifentanyl are synthetic opioids that are derivatives of morphine. Fentanyl is approximately 100 times more potent than morphine. It has a more rapid onset and shorter duration of action. It is more lipid soluble than morphine, which determines its potency and onset. It is quickly redistributed into fat and skeletal muscle, with these sites becoming easily saturated. Therefore, during a continuous infusion the plasma clearance decreases significantly, causing a precipitous drop in clearance rates. This can lead to prolonged ventilatory depression and analgesia in cases of infusions longer than 2 h. Remifentanyl is a μ-selective opioid receptor agonist with an analgesic potency similar to that of fentanyl. It is more rapid acting than fentanyl, yet it is susceptible to hydrolysis by plasma and tissue esterases, which gives it a very quick offset. Its clearance is independent of liver and kidney function. The metabolites are inactive, and therefore produce noncumulative effects. In addition, remifentanyl is known to produce hypotension, whereas fentanyl does not [12, 15].

Balanced Anesthesia Versus TIVA

There is controversy regarding the method of choice for anesthetic delivery during FESS. The importance of obtaining the optimal surgical field in FESS has prompted several studies on the topic. In 1993, Blackwell et al. retrospectively showed a decrease in blood loss in patients undergoing ESS using propofol anesthesia compared to those using isoflurane [2]. Eberhart et al. showed an improvement in a visual analog scale assessment of the surgical field in patients treated with propofol and remifentanyl versus those treated with isoflurane and alfentanyl. There was no significant difference between groups in terms of MAP or estimated blood loss. Heart rate was significantly lower in the TIVA group [7]. Wormald et al. showed in a prospective randomized trial that TIVA using propofol and remifentanyl produced superior surgical fields when compared to traditional balanced anesthesia. This study found a positive correlation between surgical grade and MAP for both conditions, as well as an overall positive correlation with heart rate. When compared at specific MAPs, the TIVA group produced superior surgical grades. This suggests that TIVA produces a surgical field that is more sensitive to MAP than balanced anesthesia [15]. A recent study by Beule et al. compared anesthesia using propofol and fentanyl versus sevoflurane and fentanyl. This study found no significant difference in the amount of blood loss or quality of the surgical field as assessed by a visual analog scale. Several features of this study are potentially confounding, including the use of fentanyl instead of remifentanyl, and the overall high volumes of blood loss with large standard deviations reported in each group, which might have potentially confounded any statistical difference. Interestingly, they provide evidence of increased platelet dysfunction after 45 min in both groups, with the propofol group being significantly worse than the sevoflurane group [1].

With balanced anesthesia, the anesthesiologist attempts to improve the surgical field by increasing the concentration of inhaled anesthetic, which causes peripheral vasodilation, thereby lowering systemic vascular resistance and decreasing MAP. Inhaled anesthetics, however, do not decrease cardiac output, and in fact, increasing concentrations of common inhaled anesthetics result in a direct increase in heart rate. It has been postulated that lowering the blood pressure in this manner may actually worsen the surgical field [3, 15]. While propofol administration results in a drop in blood pressure through vasodilation, the venodilator effect produces a decrease in cardiac output by decreasing cardiac preload [9]. In addition, the baroreceptor reflex is blunted and there is no resultant increase in heart rate. Interestingly, these studies point to the potential importance of remifentanyl in improving the surgical field during TIVA. It is known that propofol combined with remifentanyl synergistically produces hypotension and bradycardia [14]. Using modern anesthesia techniques such as target-controlled infusion, TIVA with propofol and remifentanyl most likely produces a superior surgical field for FESS, with the added benefit of superior control of hypotension and heart rate due to the short-acting nature of these drugs. This produces a theoretical safety advantage as controlled hypotension may precipitate ischemic organ failure in rare instances [11].

Anesthesia for Sinus Surgery

Propofol and remifentanil used in combination produce significant hypotension and better blunting of hemodynamic responses to endotracheal intubation than any other combination of sedative/hypnotic and opioid [14].

Propofol and remifentanyl may produce a synergistic drop in MAP and heart rate, thereby significantly lowering cardiac output, which may be responsible for the improved surgical field with TIVA.

Pharmacology of Local Anesthetics

Key points:

1. Amino esters are more likely to produce allergic reactions.
2. Amino esters are metabolized by plasma cholinesterases and so are less likely to produce sustained plasma concentrations.

3. Amino amides are metabolized by the liver. Patients with liver disease or with decreased hepatic flow, such as in congestive heart failure, may experience increased plasma levels of anesthetics.
4. Administration of local vasoconstrictors such as epinephrine potentiate the duration of the effect while decreasing the systemic absorption.

The most commonly used local anesthetics are tertiary amines composed of a lipid-soluble benzene ring connected to an amine group by an alkyl group containing either an amide or ester linkage. This linkage divides the tertiary amines into two major groups: amino amides and amino esters. Tertiary amines are weak bases. They can exist in solution in two forms: an unprotonated, neutral (lipid soluble) form or a protonated, charged (water soluble) form. The main mechanism of action of tertiary amine local anesthetics is postulated to occur on the interior of the axon, by reversibly inhibiting voltage-gated sodium channels on the inner surface of the membrane. The lipid-soluble form is able to traverse the cell membrane easily, while the water-soluble form is responsible for binding to the sodium channel and blocking action-potential propagation. The specific properties of tertiary amines create important clinical differences in efficacy and potency. First, the dissociation constant is a measure of how likely the amine group is to be protonated (hydrophilic) or neutral (lipophilic) at a particular pH, which determines how quickly an anesthetic can traverse a membrane to exert an effect. Second, lipid solubility determines the likelihood of the anesthetic moving through myelin or other supporting cells. Consequently, anesthetics with higher lipid solubility tend to have increased time to onset and offset of effect due to increased sequestration in myelin. Increasing lipid solubility also tends to increase potency. For FESS, lidocaine is the most widely used local anesthetic. Discovered in 1948, it was the first amino amide local anesthetic. Its amide bond makes it more stable and less likely to cause allergic reactions than amino esters. Cocaine is a naturally occurring amino ester that has excellent anesthetic properties as well as vasoconstrictive properties, which make it ideal for FESS. It is the only tertiary amine that acts as a vasoconstrictor; all others are vasodilators. However, the euphoria and highly addictive nature of cocaine have made it one of the most widely abused recreational drugs. Therefore, it is now illegal in most countries and more difficult to use for legitimate medical purposes. Cocaine is also known to cause cardiac arrhythmias and many have recommended its abandonment for the use of safer mixtures [10].

Epinephrine, a human adrenergic catecholamine, is commonly added to local anesthetics at a variety of concentrations. Epinephrine induces peripheral vascular resistance via alpha-receptor-stimulated vasoconstriction. The authors commonly use 1% lidocaine with 1:100,000 epinephrine for injections.

9

Injections

Key points:
1. The greater palatine foramen injection is an effective method for controlling bleeding and providing anesthesia during endoscopic sinus surgery.
2. A combination of the sphenopalatine block with the greater palatine block leads to profound vasoconstriction in the posterior portion of the nasal cavity and significantly reduces bleeding.

The greater palatine foramen is located posteromedially to the third maxillary molar and anteromedially to the maxillary tuberosity and pterygoid hamulus (Fig. 9.1). The foramen opens into the greater palatine canal, which courses superiorly into the pterygopalatine fossa. Here, the third portion of the internal maxillary artery and its multiple branches supply the nose, paranasal sinuses, pharynx, orbit, palate, teeth, and facial skin. The closed space and bony walls of the pterygopalatine fossa make it ideal for local anesthesia. The optimal injection is delivered at the opening of the greater palatine canal, medial to the sphenopalatine foramen, where the terminal portion of the internal maxillary artery lies. Superiorly,

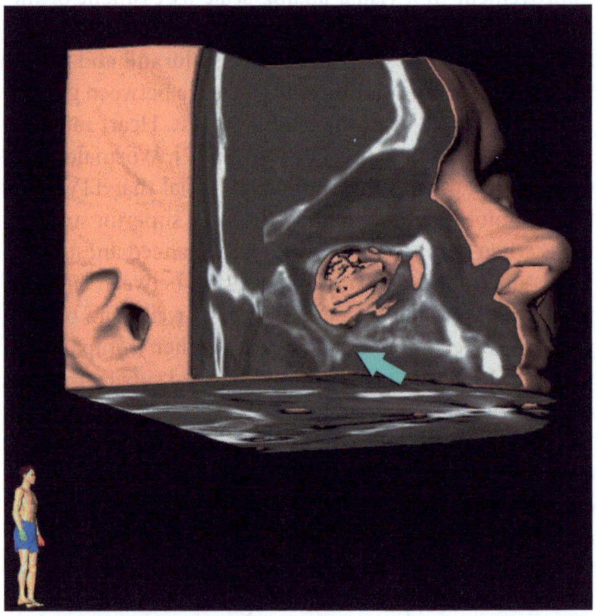

Fig. 9.1 The location and orientation of the greater palatine foramen and canal is clearly seen on this computed tomography scan (*arrows*)

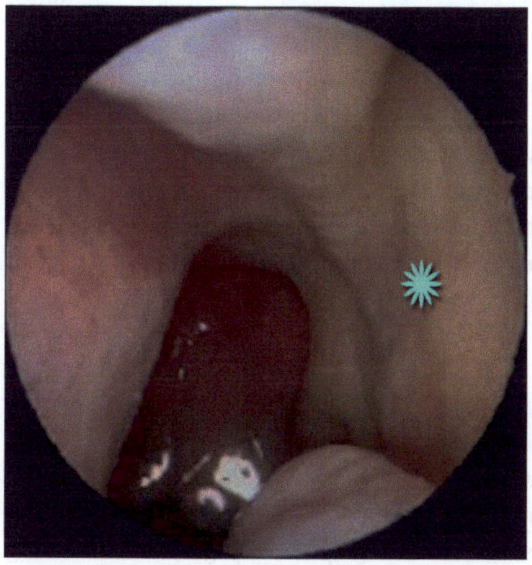

Fig. 9.2 The location of the sphenopalatine foramen at the posterior aspect of the middle turbinate is indicated by the *asterisk*

the pterygopalatine fossa is limited by the anterior basal portion of the greater wing of the sphenoid bone. The inferior orbital fissure is located anterosuperiorly in the pterygopalatine fossa and the superior orbital fissure and optic foramen lie just above it. The foramen rotundum is located posteriorly, superiorly, and laterally to the sphenopalatine foramen. The mean distance of the greater palatine foramen to the sphenopalatine foramen is 28 mm in men and 27 mm in women. The mean distance of the greater palatine foramen to the inferior orbital fissure is 40 mm in men and 37 mm in women [6]. The sphenopalatine foramen can also be injected transnasally. Here, the sphenopalatine artery and several branches of the maxillary nerve and pterygopalatine ganglion enter the nose just posterior to the posterior attachment of the middle turbinate (Fig. 9.2).

A combination of the sphenopalatine block with the greater palatine block leads to profound vasoconstriction in the posterior portion of the nasal cavity and significantly reduces bleeding.

Techniques

General Anesthesia

Prior to the start of each day, the overall anesthetic plans are reviewed with the anesthesiologist. The authors' preference is TIVA with propofol and remifentanyl when possible. The adjunctive use of beta blockade is discussed, but left up to the discretion of the anesthesiologist. In the preoperative suite, the patient is given oxymetazoline sprays in each nostril 2 h prior to surgery. After general endotracheal anesthesia is induced in the operating room, the patient is turned 90 degrees counterclockwise to facilitate the use of stereotactic computed tomography guidance. The patient is then placed in the beach chair position, which elevates the head approximately 10–20 degrees, as the reverse Trendelenburg position has been shown to reduce intracranial MAP without reducing cerebral perfusion pressure [14]. The CT guidance system is then registered and its accuracy confirmed.

Local Anesthesia

- The authors utilize bilateral greater palatine blocks in nearly all cases.

Three milliliters of 1% lidocaine with 1:100,000 of epinephrine are drawn into a Luerlock syringe. Before use, the expiration date and concentration of the lidocaine and epinephrine on the stock container are confirmed by the surgeon. A 25-gauge needle is measured with a ruler and bent to an angle of 60 degrees at a length of 25 mm for all adults (Fig. 9.3).

- The greater palatine foramen is usually located anterior to the junction of the hard and soft palate just medial to the second maxillary molar.

It can often be palpated, or seen as a subtle depression in the hard palate mucosa. The needle is placed into the greater palatine foramen and advanced to the bend of the needle. The needle is then aspirated for blood to prevent an intravascular injection. Then, 1.5 ml of anesthetic is injected. If the needle is properly placed, there is moderate resistance to the injection. If there is minimal resistance, it is likely that the needle is in the nasopharynx, and is

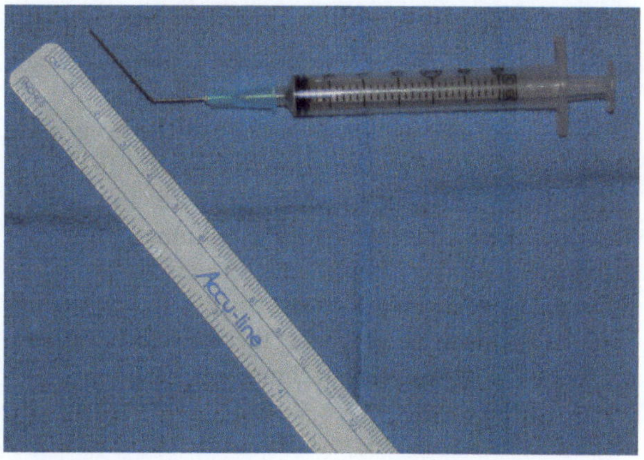

Fig. 9.3 A 25-gauge needle with a 60 angle at length 25 mm from the tip of the needle

not correctly placed in the canal. The same procedure is repeated for the contralateral canal (Video 9.1).

After the patient has been prepped and draped, a 0 degrees Hopkins rod is used to place oxymetazoline-soaked cotton pledgets in the nasal cavities. This is performed endoscopically to prevent the trauma to the septal mucosa or middle turbinate that can occur with blind placement and to prevent nuisance bleeding that could degrade the surgical field. Next, the remainder of the instrumentation is set up, including the image-guidance system, camera, monitors, DVD recording system, and microdebrider. The authors routinely use an endoscope irrigation system to wash away minor bleeding at the scope tip and always sit during the operation with an armrest for the left arm to help stabilize the scope.

9

- The sphenopalatine foramen is then injected under endoscopic guidance posterior and superior to the horizontal portion of the basal lamella at the posterior aspect of the middle turbinate (Video 9.2).

A solution of 1% lidocaine with 1:100,000 epinephrine is used. This is a technically difficult injection that is performed by placing a 30 bend in the first centimeter of a spinal needle or by using an angled tonsil needle. The tip of the needle is used to palpate the foramen. The needle is placed in an upward and lateral direction and used to inject the mucosa adjacent to the sphenopalatine foramen. Typically, blanching of the epithelium is already seen after a proper greater palatine block, and the sphenopalatine injection augments this blanching. If the foramen is unable to be reached, then a well-placed injection near the foramen will diffuse to the foramen and cause vasospasm of the sphenopalatine branches. Alternatively, the injection can be placed medially at the rostrum of the septum between the middle turbinate and the inferior turbinate to minimize bleeding from the posterior nasal artery.

- The lateral nasal wall is injected with 1% lidocaine with 1:100,000 of epinephrine.

A 25-gauge needle with a slight bend at the tip is used. The optimal injection is superior and anterior to the anterior attachment of the middle turbinate. The inferior border of the middle turbinate, the septum, the superior turbinate, and other supplemental injections can all be utilized depending on the disease process and type of operation. The uncinate process is then injected in several spots close to its superior attachment.

Conclusions

A thorough knowledge and understanding of the different options available for anesthesia and local anesthetic injections is critical to consistent operative success in endoscopic sinus surgery. A close, open working relationship with the anesthesia team is a key to safe, effective, and efficient delivery of anesthetic and better surgical outcomes.

References

1. Beule AG, Wilhelmi F, Kuhnel TS, Hansen E, Lackner KJ, Hosemann W (2007) Propofol versus sevoflurane: bleeding in endoscopic sinus surgery. Otolaryngol Head Neck Surg 136:45–50
2. Blackwell KE, Ross DA, Kapur P, Calcaterra TC (1993) Propofol for maintenance of general anesthesia: a technique to limit blood loss during endoscopic sinus surgery. Am J Otolaryngol 14:262–266
3. Boezaart AP, van der Merwe J, Coetzee A (1995) Comparison of sodium nitroprusside- and esmolol-induced controlled hypotension for functional endoscopic sinus surgery. Can J Anaesth 42:373–376
4. Danielsen A, Gravningsbraten R, Olofsson J (2003) Anaesthesia in endoscopic sinus surgery. Eur Arch Otorhinolaryngol 260:481–486
5. Danielsen A, Olofsson J (1996) Endoscopic endonasal sinus surgery. A long-term follow-up study. Acta Otolaryngol 116:611–619
6. Das S, Kim D, Cannon TY, Ebert CS Jr, Senior BA (2006) High-resolution computed tomography analysis of the greater palatine canal. Am J Rhinol 20:603–608
7. Eberhart LH, Folz BJ, Wulf H, Geldner G (2003) Intravenous anesthesia provides optimal surgical conditions during microscopic and endoscopic sinus surgery. Laryngoscope 113:1369–1373
8. Fedok FG, Ferraro RE, Kingsley CP, Fornadley JA (2000) Operative times, postanesthesia recovery times, and complications during sinonasal surgery using general anesthesia and local anesthesia with sedation. Otolaryngol Head Neck Surg 122:560–566
9. Goodchild CS, Serrao JM (1989) Cardiovascular effects of propofol in the anaesthetized dog. Br J Anaesth 63:87–92
10. Latorre F, Klimek L (1999) Does cocaine still have a role in nasal surgery? Drug Saf 20:9–13
11. Leigh JM (1975) The history of controlled hypotension. Br J Anaesth 47:745–749
12. Miller RD, Stoelting RK (2007) Basics of Anesthesia. 5th edn. Churchill Livingstone, Philadelphia

13. Thaler ER, Gottschalk A, Samaranayake R, Lanza DC, Kennedy DW (1997) Anesthesia in endoscopic sinus surgery. Am J Rhinol 11:409–413
14. Wilhelm W, Biedler A, Huppert A, et al. (2002) Comparison of the effects of remifentanil or fentanyl on anaesthetic induction characteristics of propofol, thiopental or etomidate. Eur J Anaesthesiol 19:350–356
15. Wormald PJ, van Renen G, Perks J, Jones JA, Langton-Hewer CD (2005) The effect of the total intravenous anesthesia compared with inhalational anesthesia on the surgical field during endoscopic sinus surgery. Am J Rhinol 19:514–520

Chapter 10

Tips and Pearls in Revision Sinus Surgery

10

Alexander G. Chiu and David W. Kennedy

Core Messages

- Successful revision endoscopic sinus surgery starts with proper patient selection and medical management of comorbidities and environmental influences.
- Preoperative planning in at least two and preferably three computed tomography planes is needed in order to plan the surgical approach and identify problem areas.
- A complete sphenoethmoidectomy is the best procedure for long-term success.
- A surgical approach is most safely done when identifying the medial orbital wall, roof of the maxillary sinus, and skull base posteriorly within the sphenoid sinus.
- All bony fragments should be removed from their attachment along the medial orbital wall, skull base, and frontal recess.
- As with primary surgery, the mucoperiosteum should be preserved.
- Nearly as important as a good technical surgery is meticulous long-term postoperative debridements and surveillance to ensure patency and mucosal health.

Contents

Introduction

Short- and long-term outcome studies have shown functional endoscopic sinus surgery (FESS) to be successful in over 90% of cases [3, 5]. Those patients who remain symptomatic following surgery often fall into three general categories:

1. Symptomatic due to persistent mucosal inflammation and purulence despite adequate technical surgery.
2. Symptomatic from isolated pathology within a selected sinus (i.e., the frontal sinus) that is secondary to scarring or closure of the individual natural ostium.
3. Symptomatic from persistent mucosal inflammation and purulence due to inadequate clearance of ethmoid cells and/or mucosal stripping from previous surgery.

The keys to success in performing a revision FESS are to correctly identify those patients in the latter two categories and address their revision procedure by managing their comorbidities perioperatively, thoroughly examining their preoperative radiography, and utilizing a meticulous mucosa-sparing technique in performing a complete sphenoethmoidectomy.

Patient Selection

When evaluating a patient for a revision FESS, it is important to review the patient's symptoms, associated comorbidities, and radiographic studies. Quality of life questionnaires, such as the Rhinosinusitis Outcome Measure and Sino-Nasal Outcome Test, are helpful in eliciting patient symptoms and importance to their overall quality of life.

Tips and Pearls

1. Managing the expectations of the patient is a critical part in the revision surgery process.
2. A patient who complains of clear, postnasal drainage with a significant history of allergic rhinitis and minimal mucosal disease on computed tomography (CT) scan is not likely to find relief in that symptom from a second surgery.
3. On the other hand, a patient with a chief complaint of thickened, purulent postnasal drainage and evidence of mucus recirculation on CT scan is likely to benefit from a revision surgery.

Before deciding on the necessity for any type of revision surgery, it is advisable to review the original CT scan before any surgery is performed. This helps the surgeon to evaluate the indications for the original surgery and is particularly important for the frontal sinus, where the primary surgical indication may be headache. In general, the symptom of headache correlates poorly with chronic rhinosinusitis and it is important to establish the presence or absence of disease in the frontal sinus prior to the first operation. If this remains the primary symptom, a revision surgery on asymptomatic iatrogenic mucosal change may be avoided.

As with the original CT scan, evaluating prior medical therapy, postoperative care, and medical compliance is important in selecting patients who will benefit from a revision surgery. Maximal medical therapy of a prolonged course of systemic oral steroids and culture-directed antibiotics should be performed prior to any surgical procedure. In many cases, a patient may remain symptomatic from an original surgery not for technical reasons, but for antibiotic-resistant bacteria commonly found in postsurgical patients, such as *Staphylococcus aureus* or *Pseudomonas aeruginosa*. Endoscopic-directed cultures can guide antimicrobial therapy and often resolve these infections without any additional surgery. Careful consideration should also be given to the environmental and general host factors that predispose to recurrent disease. Underlying factors such as allergic rhinitis, granulomatous disorders, and underlying immune deficiencies should be investigated, and where possible, managed before any revision surgery is undertaken. In general, elective revision sinus surgery should not be performed in patients who have not yet stopped smoking. Smoking postoperatively tends to cause significant scarring, has a major impact on outcomes, and is a major factor in surgical failure.

In order to evaluate whether the initial surgery(s) was technically inadequate, the initial preoperative report should be reviewed along with an examination of the pre- and post-surgical CT scans. An initial operative report that does not mention the dissection of superior ethmoid cells, agger nasi cells, and/or frontal recess cells may mean that a proper frontal recess dissection was never performed. Other details to look for include the description of the dissection of the skull base and sphenoid sinus. Reviewing postoperative CT scans is an appropriate next step, and is an objective aid in determining a cause for persistent disease. By understanding patient symptoms and expectations and correlating those with areas on nasal endoscopy and CT scan that may explain their symptoms, a calculated decision can be made on whether or not a patient will benefit from revision surgery.

Important Points to Consider when Deciding to Operate

1. Review indications for initial surgery.
2. Have a complete understanding of the patient's expectations.
3. Review the initial operative report.
4. Make sure maximal medical therapy has been performed.
5. Review initial and postoperative CT scans.

Nasal Endoscopy

Rigid or flexible nasal endoscopy is the most important part of the physical exam for a sinus surgeon. Using angled endoscopes during the initial patient evaluation will allow inspection of the maxillary sinus and natural ostium. Mucus recirculation in the maxillary sinus is one of the most common causes for revision surgery [4]. This is often secondary to a synechia that has developed between the natural ostium and antrostomy, or to a residual uncinate process. Both of these are difficult to ascertain from a straight-on examination using a 0° endoscope or sometimes even with a 30° telescope. A 45° or 70° endoscope is needed to completely eliminate this subtle finding (Fig. 10.1).

Endoscopy of the anterior nasal cavity will determine whether or not there are significant synechiae between the middle turbinate and medial orbital wall. Synechiae between the nasal septum and inferior turbinate can be a significant cause for nasal obstruction. Synechiae between the middle turbinate and lateral nasal wall can prevent examination of the ethmoid cavity and spheno-

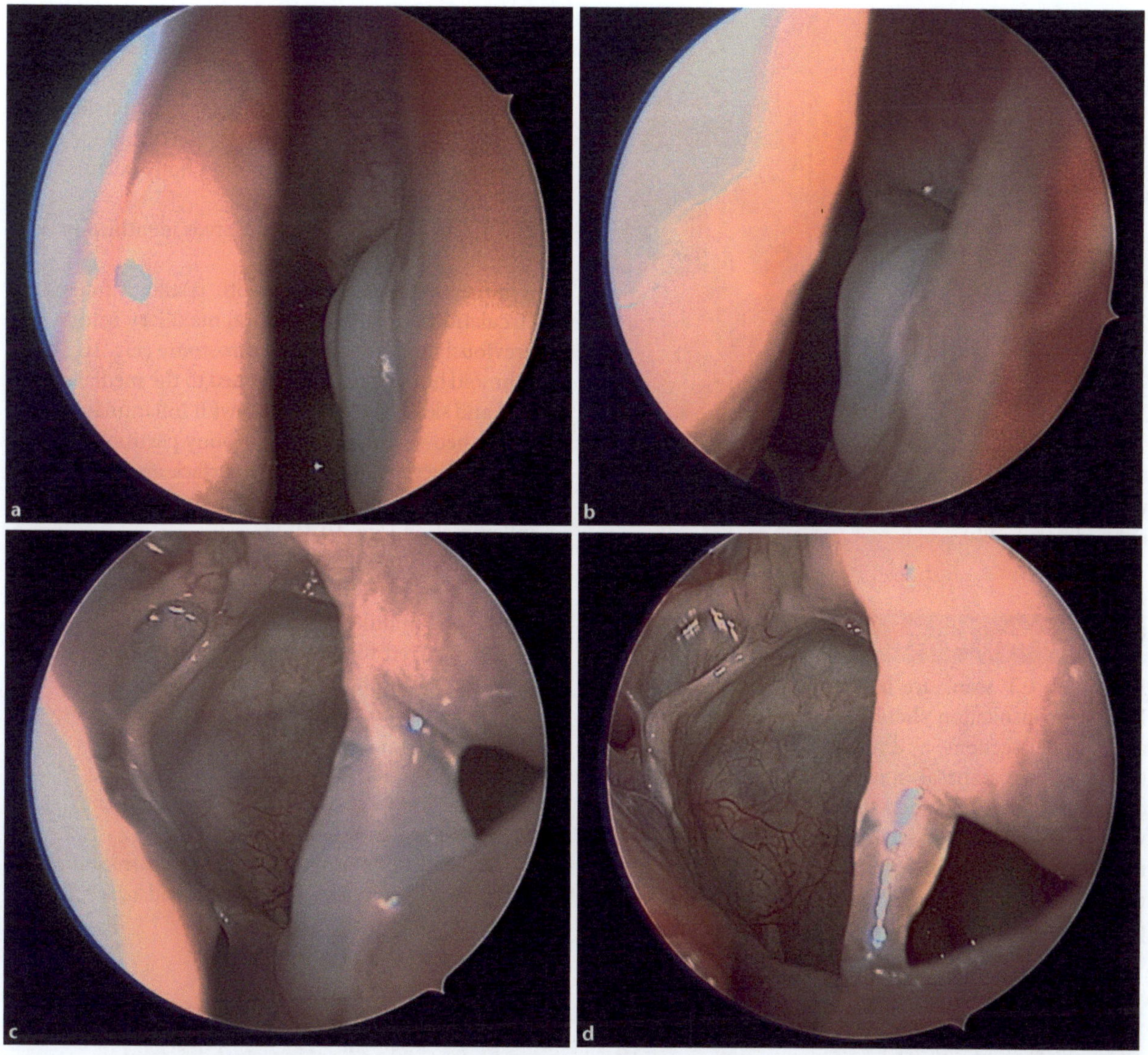

Fig. 10.1 Endoscopic view of a patient with mucus re-circulation following a functional endoscopic sinus surgery (FESS) procedure. A 0° endoscope shows thickened mucus at the antrostomy (**a**). Closer inspection with a 30° scope (**b**) and 70° scope (**c**) shows the scar band between the natural ostium and antrostomy that is creating the recirculation. Once the mucus is cleared, the scar band is clearly visualized (**d**)

ethmoid recess. These can often be lysed in clinic after topical analgesia, and a temporary spacer can be placed lateral to the middle turbinate to prevent the formation of additional synechiae.

The degree of mucosal edema and presence of mucopurulence should be determined in the endoscopic examination of the ethmoid cavity. Cultures should be taken of any purulence and examined for the presence of pathogenic aerobic, anaerobic, and fungal organisms. The sphenoid ostium should then be visualized and, if possible, examination of the sinus itself should be performed to determine the presence of mucus within the sinus. Allergic mucin or retained fungal elements in the inferior portion of the sphenoid sinus, as well as within the maxillary sinus, are a common source for persistent purulent rhinorrhea. Thick allergic mucus should also be submitted for pathology for examination with fungal stains and for the presence of Charcot-Leyden crystals.

Finally, the frontal recess should be examined with an angled endoscope. Signs to look for include the presence of polypoid edema, mucopurulence, and residual cells or bony partitions that may obstruct the frontal recess. Endoscopic findings should then be correlated with their radiographic appearance.

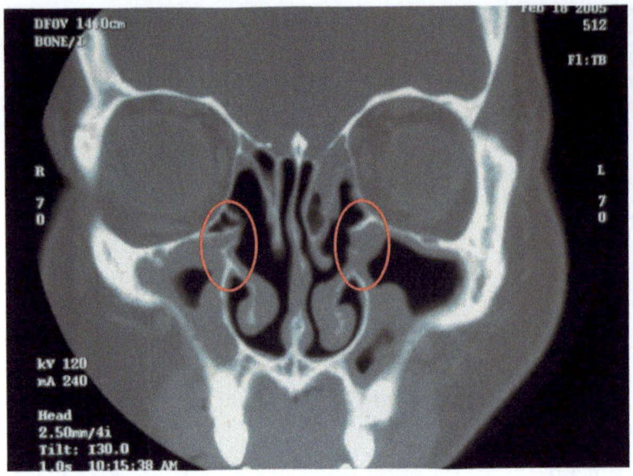

Fig. 10.2 Coronal computed tomography (CT) scan of a patient with a previous FESS who has a retained uncinate on the left and right sides (*red circle*)

CT Scan Review

Reviewing CT scans are best done in multiple planes. In-office consultation should result in a review of axial and coronal sections, at a maximum of 3-mm sections, through the paranasal sinuses. Many image-guidance companies now offer work-stations that allow for the review of CT scans in the sagittal plane, as well as the coronal and axial views. The coronal view is excellent in determining the presence of a remaining agger nasi, uncinate process, frontal recess, and/or supraorbital ethmoid cells. Sagittal and axial views are important in determining the anterior-to-posterior dimension of the frontal recess, and the identification of a supraorbital ethmoid, frontal recess, and/or interseptal frontal sinus air cell. Sagittal views are also instructive in demonstrating the vertical slope of the skull base and the degree of ethmoid bony partitions attached to the skull base.

The most common anatomical areas identified in revision surgery are the following:

1. Remnant uncinate process with resultant mucus recirculation between the natural maxillary ostium and previously made maxillary antrostomy (Fig. 10.2).
2. Ethmoid bony partitions attached to the medial orbital wall and skull base. In patients with inflammatory polyps or neo-osteogenesis, these bony partitions may be osteitic, serve to increase the surface area where polyps can grow, and as a nidus for persistent mucosal inflammation (Fig. 10.3).
3. Remnant infraorbital ethmoid cells that are obstructing the natural maxillary ostium.
4. Lateralized middle turbinate against the medial orbital wall or scarred to an agger nasi cell and/or ethmoid bulla remnant (Fig. 10.4).
5. Residual sphenoethmoidal (Onodi) cell or posterior ethmoid cell.
6. Remnant supraorbital or frontal recess cells.
7. Synechiae between the middle turbinate and lateral nasal wall and/or medical orbital wall.
8. Neo-osteogenesis of the skull base and frontal recess from previous mucosal stripping and/or prolonged mucosal inflammation

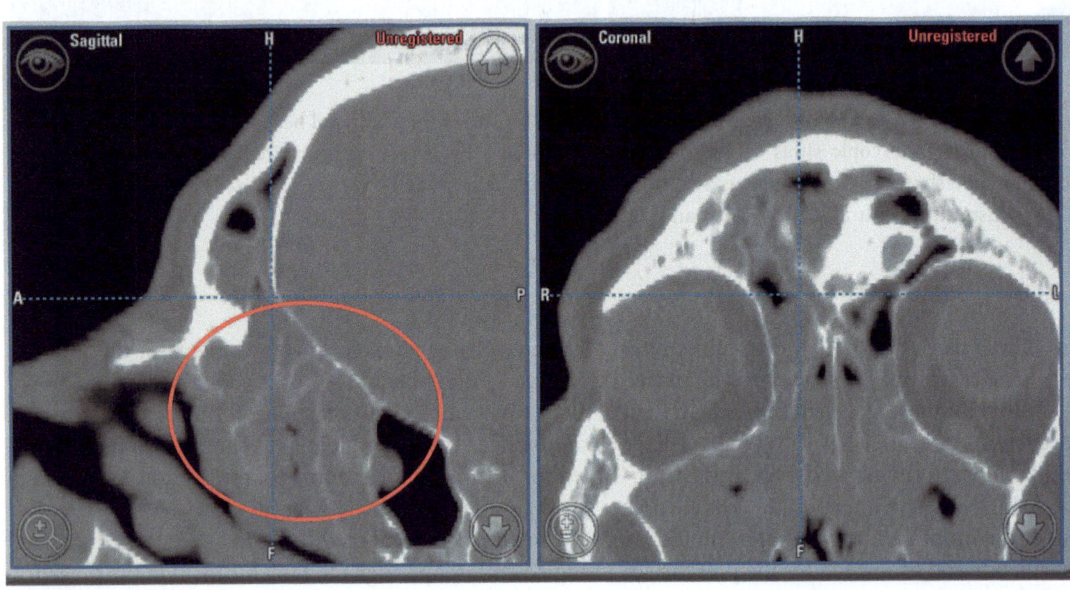

Fig. 10.3 Coronal and sagittal views of patient with nasal polyposis who had undergone a previous FESS. Note the multiple bony ethmoid partitions off the skull base on the sagittal view (*red circle*). Revision surgery will be aimed at removing these osteitic bony partitions

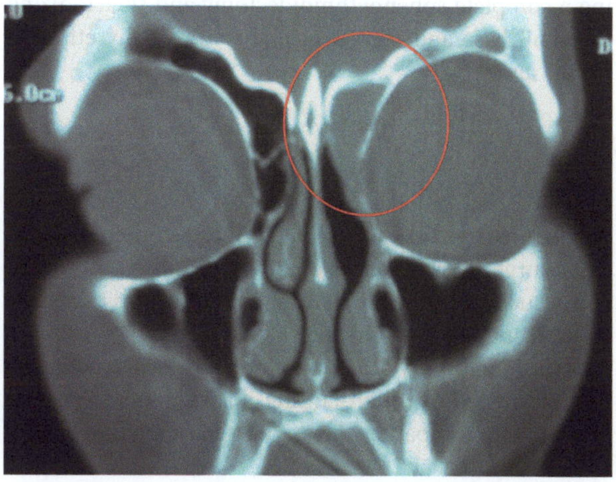

Fig. 10.4 Coronal CT scan of a patient with isolated left frontal recess disease. The left middle turbinate has lateralized against the medial orbital wall, resulting in the obstruction (*red circle*)

Preoperative Workup

Once the decision is made to perform a revision endoscopic procedure, it is imperative in the preoperative period to review each patient's anatomy, the amount of disease, and underlying comorbidities. CT scan and nasal endoscopy are the best modalities to use to assess the remnant bony partitions and areas of scarring that are obstructing the natural ostium of each sinus. Revision FESS is most often performed for recurrent nasal polyposis, persistent mucosal inflammation, mucoceles, or iatrogenic sinus disease. In each of these cases, mucosal inflammation should be kept at a minimum prior to the case in order to decrease surgical bleeding and improve endoscopic visualization.

Systemic steroids and oral antibiotics are helpful in stabilizing mucosal inflammation prior to surgery. Oral prednisone is started 1 week prior to surgery and continued for at least 2 weeks after surgery or until mucosal inflammation has resolved, as assessed by endoscopic examination. A prednisone dose of 0.6 mg/kg/day for 3 days followed by 0.4 mg/kg for 3 days is given starting 1 week prior to surgery. Along with this, culture-directed antibiotics are started 1 week prior to surgery. If no purulence is present, an empiric antibiotic such as a fluoroquinolone or combination of clindamycin and bactrim can be used to help stabilize the mucosa.

Patients are also instructed to stop aspirin or nonsteroidal anti-inflammatory drug use 1 week prior to surgery. Other agents that can potentially increase surgical bleeding, such as vitamin E and the herbal supplements ginger, gingko, and ginseng, are encouraged to be discontinued at least 3 weeks prior to surgery. In addition, active cigarette smoking should be stopped at least 3 weeks prior to surgery as well as in the 6 weeks following surgery to limit its deleterious effects on the nasal mucosa.

Patient comorbidities should also be optimized prior to surgery. In the case of FESS, asthma is the most common comorbidity and should be well controlled prior to surgery with inhalers and/or systemic steroids. Systemic hypertension should also be under good control, as poorly controlled intraoperative blood pressures can certainly worsen mucosal bleeding and complicate endoscopic visualization.

Prior to surgery, the informed consent process should also be carefully addressed. Compared to primary FESS, revision FESS often carries a greater risk for cerebrospinal fluid leaks, orbital injury, and postoperative drug-resistant infections. Major as well as minor complications should be discussed with the patients and it is prudent to have an FESS-specific consent form signed and witnessed prior to surgery [1].

Tips and Pearls

1. Preoperative oral steroids and antibiotics can often decrease mucosal edema and intraoperative bleeding.
2. The patient should refrain from cigarette smoking at least 3 weeks prior to surgery.
3. Obtain FESS-specific informed consent.

Surgical Equipment

Once the decision is made to perform a revision procedure, specialized instruments should be used to achieve a sound surgical technique of sparing mucosa while performing a complete sphenoethmoidectomy that removes osteitic ethmoid bony partitions.

Surgical Navigation Systems

With the advent of surgical navigation in the late 1980s, endoscopic surgeons have been increasingly utilizing this technology for intraoperative localization and preoperative planning. Fine-cut axial CT scans, often 1 mm in section, are reformatted into coronal and sagittal views and allow for a greater understanding of the anatomy, which has been distorted by previous surgery, polypoid mucosa, and/or anatomical variants. Preoperatively, image-guidance workstations can be used to plan out the dissection and identify areas that need to be addressed. Specifically, the frontal recess and the cells obstructing the frontal recess are best visualized utilizing the three views made available by the workstations, providing the surgeon with the ability to truly conceptualize the three-dimensional surgical anatomy prior to the procedure. In addition, osteitic bony partitions along the skull base and medial orbital wall are best seen using multiple views.

Intraoperatively, image guidance is useful in dissecting out remnant bony partitions while identifying the skull base and medial orbital wall. In many cases, previously operated and diseased ethmoid bone becomes osteitic and hardened, thus taking away the tactile difference between the skull base and ethmoid bone that is often appreciated and relied upon in primary surgery.

Some image-guidance systems also offer a virtual image update. Using computer software packages, a surgeon can trace their dissection and "virtually" eliminate the bony partitions and mucosal disease seen in the preoperative images (Fig. 10.5). This device can aid in performing a complete sphenoethmoidectomy and skeletonizing the skull base and medial orbital wall of bony ethmoid partitions.

Angled Endoscopes and Instruments

Angled instruments are essential in revision endoscopic sinus surgery. Endoscopes of 30°, 45°, and 70° allow direct visualization of the natural ostium of the maxillary sinus, frontal recess, and anterior skull base.

Revision surgery along the skull base necessitates the use of angled through-cutting instruments. Powered instrument companies have devised angled debrider

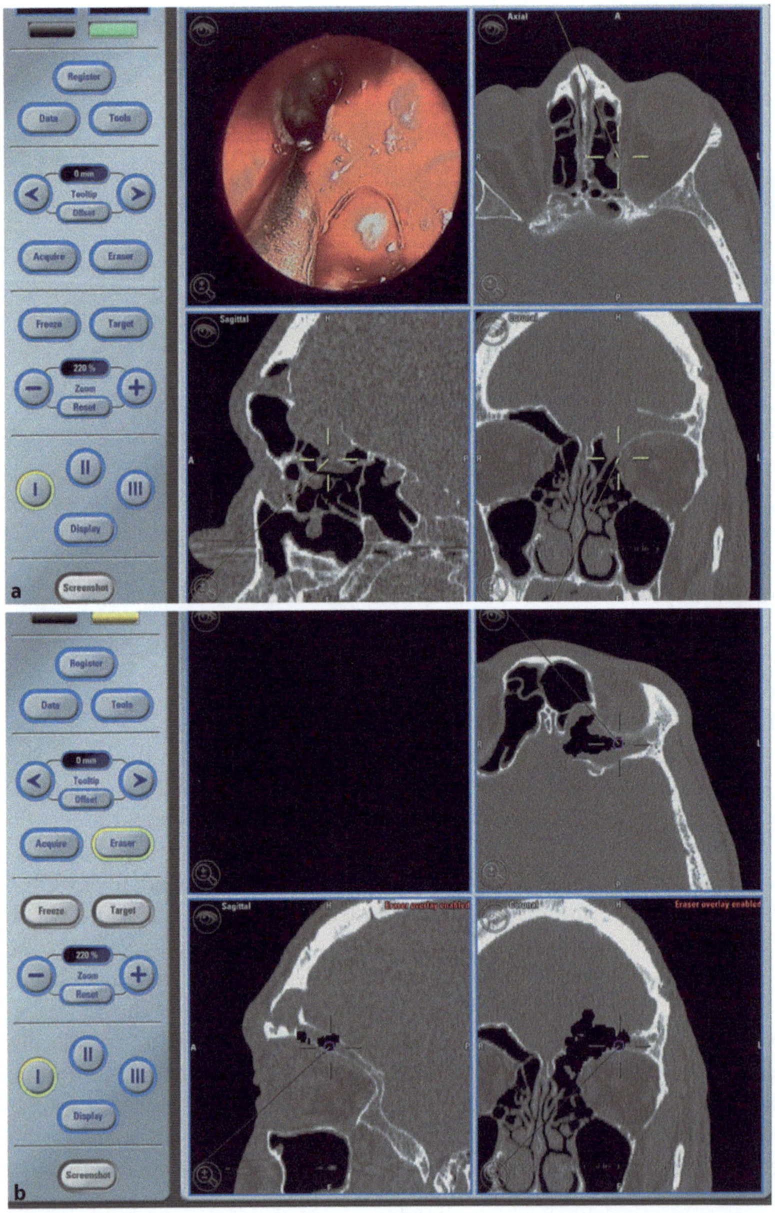

Fig. 10.5 An intraoperative endoscopic view with triplanar CT imaging of a patient with a left supraorbital ethmoid mucocele and corresponding skull base erosion (**a**). Upon entering the mucocele, the Eraser software program begins to digitally "erase" the mucocele based on the path of the instrument (**b**)

blades, as well as drills, diamond and cutting, that may be attached to hand-held microdebriders. The 70 diamond suction irrigation drill has, in particular, made a dramatic difference for revision frontal sinus surgery. In particular, the drill reduces the amount of trauma and exposed bone during an extended frontal recess approach [2]. There is a variety of 90° instruments designed to reach around the nasofrontal beak and into the frontal recess. These instruments, specifically designed for the frontal recess, are also useful in accessing pathology within the floor and anterior portion of the maxillary sinus. Fungal debris or mucus retention cysts along the floor of the sinus can be irrigated and instrumented out by using angled giraffe forceps and curettes. Revision procedures often become a methodic process of cut, remove, suction, and reexamine. These specialized instruments allow for the preservation of mucosa and removal of fine bony fragments, which if left behind, can serve as a nidus for scarring and infection along the maxillary sinus and anterior skull base.

Intraoperative CT Scans

A more recent development that is currently limited in accessibility but may become more prevalent in the future is the use of an intraoperative CT scanner to assess the thoroughness of revision surgery. Xoran Technologies (Ann Arbor, MI, USA) has developed a mobile intraoperative CT scanner that is able to perform 0.4-mm slice thickness scans of the paranasal sinuses while the patient is on the operating room table (Fig. 10.6). This allows the opportunity to assess the extent and thoroughness of the

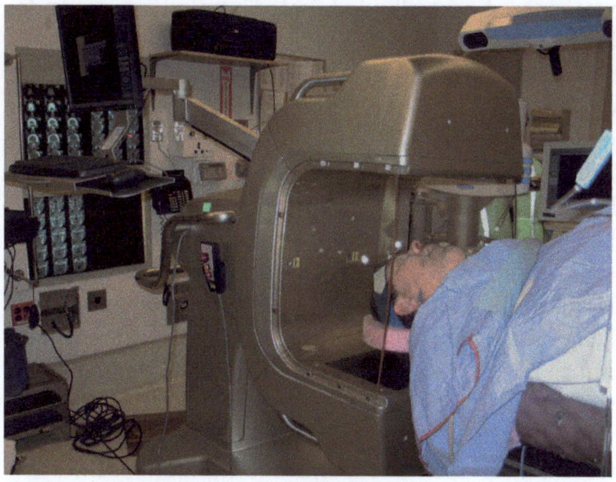

Fig. 10.6 Intraoperative CT with the xCAT™ – a mobile cone-beam scanner. A special head rest allows rotation of the gantry for image acquisition. CT scans are then transferred into the surgical navigation system of preference for a real-time update of the images

revision procedure, and these real-time pictures can be used to update image-guidance systems if additional surgery is needed.

Surgical Technique

General Principles

In revision surgical procedures the anatomy can be significantly distorted and landmarks such as the middle turbinate may be partially resected, making them unreliable for anatomic localization. Image guidance is a helpful tool, but should not be trusted blindly. Accurate identification of static anatomical landmarks that cannot be altered from previous surgery can help guide the revision procedure and minimize the risk of complications.

Tips and Pearls – I

1. Landmarks to be used include the roof of the maxillary sinus, the medial orbital wall, and the skull base.
2. The skull base is usually most easily identified in the posterior ethmoid or sphenoid sinuses, where it is more horizontal and the cells are larger.
3. The roof of the maxillary sinus is closely related to the approximate height of the sphenoid sinus. Staying at this vertical level of the maxillary sinus roof during dissection posteriorly keeps the surgeon from venturing into the anterior skull base.
4. Be careful where the skull base slopes down medially toward the attachment of the middle turbinate in the region of the anterior ethmoid artery. The ethmoid roof is at its thinnest in this area, and may even be membranous in part, making it particularly vulnerable to injury. As this area is approached, it is important to stay close and parallel to the medial orbital wall while remembering that the opening of the frontal sinus is most frequently medial, close to the attachment of the middle turbinate to the skull base.

Since revision FESS is most often performed for persistent mucosal edema and mucoceles, it is recommended that the procedure should be a complete sphenoethmoidectomy. For isolated mucus recirculation of the maxillary sinus or frontal sinus mucoceles, the procedure can be tailored to the specific sinus. But for the most part, a complete and thorough dissection removing remnant ethmoid bony partitions and skeletonizing the medial orbital wall and anterior skull base gives the patient their best opportunity for a lasting surgical procedure. Removing remnant osteitic bony partitions requires the use of through-cutting instruments. Additional mucosal stripping in a revision procedure can result in even more neo-osteogenesis, which can be particularly crippling in the sphenoid and frontal sinus. The steps to performing a revision FESS are identical to those of a primary FESS. The maxillary sinus is first identified, and the medial orbital wall is skeletonized free of ethmoid bony partitions. Dissection is then carried low and posterior through the inferior ethmoids and basal lamellae into the posterior ethmoids. The superior turbinate is then identified along with the natural os of the sphenoid sinus. Once the sphenoidotomy is enlarged, the skull base is identified and dissection is carried posterior to anterior along the skull base with angled endoscopes and instrumentation. Ethmoid bony partitions along the skull base are removed. The anterior ethmoid artery is identified and preserved and the frontal recess is dissected out.

Tips and Pearls – II

1. Be methodical in revision surgery. Remove all ethmoid bony partitions along the skull base and medial orbital wall.
2. Spare the mucosa and use through-cutting instruments.
3. Identify the skull base within the sphenoid sinus or posterior ethmoids.
4. Make a large antrostomy within the maxillary, sphenoid, and frontal sinus in patients with polypoid disease.

Maxillary Sinus

- Identifying a remnant uncinate process is the most critical step in revising a maxillary antrostomy.

Mucus recirculation is a common cause of recurrent symptoms following FESS and is due to a mucosal or bony partition between the natural ostium and the surgical antrostomy. Scarring can be a cause, as well as a remnant uncinate process. A back biter or angled ball-tip probe is a useful instrument to reach posterior to the uncinate process and resect anteriorly to its attachment along the lacrimal bone. Once the hard bone of the lacrimal is palpated, no further resection is performed to prevent a nasolacrimal duct injury. The superior attachment of the uncinate should also be removed. This attachment is often fused to the anterior face of the agger nasi cell, and can be a source for frontal recess obstruction following initial sinus surgery.

- Infraorbital ethmoid or Haller cells can also be a source of persistent obstruction of the maxillary sinus.

These cells are easily missed because they are often more anterior than expected. Using an angled endoscope, the bony walls of the infraorbital ethmoid cell can be visualized and removed using the combination of a ball tip probe, 90° forceps, and back-biter. Keep in mind its relation to the inferior orbital wall and infraorbital nerve as it courses along the roof of the maxillary sinus.

The floor of the maxillary sinus should be addressed in any revision procedure. Remnant fungal debris or mucus retention cysts should be identified and removed. Angled endoscopes such as the 45° or 70° are often needed to visualize these areas. Instruments normally used for the frontal recess, such as a 90° curette or giraffe forceps, are helpful in reaching down to the floor and removing debris. Irrigation with normal saline is also useful in removing thick allergic mucin or fungal debris from the sinus.

Inferior Ethmoid Sinus

Once the maxillary sinus antrostomy is revised, remnant ethmoid bony partitions off the medial orbital wall should be removed flush to the bone. The roof of the maxillary sinus can serve as a guide to the height of dissection through the ethmoid cavity as the surgeon moves posteriorly through the basal lamellae and into the posterior ethmoid cells. The basal lamella has an inferior, horizontal segment and a superior, vertical segment.

- Care should be taken to preserve the horizontal segment of the basal lamella to prevent postoperative lateralization of the middle turbinate.

Another specific area to address is the medial border of the ethmoid bulla. Often, this bony segment can be left untouched from a previous surgery in which the bulla was entered centrally and "cored" out with a microdebrider. The medial border can become osteitic, serve as a platform for polyp formation, and is best removed with a J-curette placed medial and posterior to the bony segment.

Once the dissection is carried through the basal lamellae and into the posterior ethmoid air cells, care should be taken to identify and remove any remaining ethmoid cells behind the maxillary sinus and against the posterior medial orbital wall or orbital apex. Often these retro maxillary cells can be left behind from a previous surgery and can again serve as a nidus for inflammation and polyposis.

The superior turbinate is then addressed. The superior turbinate serves as an anatomical landmark for the natural sphenoid os. Resecting the lower half of the superior turbinate allows visualization of the os while preserving olfactory function found in the superior portion of the superior turbinate. The basal lamellae of the superior turbinate as it attaches to the medial orbital wall can also be removed and debrided of inflammation and polyps.

Sphenoid Sinus

- The sphenoid sinus can be safely entered through the natural os of the sinus.

The os is located medially and inferior and can be entered with a straight J-curette. The thin bone of the anterior face of the sphenoid sinus often turns into hardened, osteitic bone in revision surgery. In addition, dissection in this area can be highly vascular and bleeding can easily obscure the visual field. Sphenopalatine artery injections of lidocaine with epinephrine can aid in decreasing mucosal bleeding and improving endoscopic visualization. This may be performed prior to dissection through a transpalatal injection through the greater palatine foramen, or transnasally by injecting in a region near the lateral insertion of the middle turbinate. In either case, sphenopalatine injections can greatly aid in performing a sphenoidotomy.

With bleeding under control, the anterior face of the sphenoid should be removed superiorly to the skull base and inferiorly to the level of the septal branch of the sphenopalatine artery.

- It is advantageous to create a large sphenoidotomy especially in a highly inflamed field, since the small surface area of the sphenoid makes it more likely to stenose in the postoperative period.

Heavy through-cutting hand instruments, such as the straight mushroom punch and Kerrison forceps, are often needed to cut through the thick bone of the sphenoid. The anterior face of the sphenoid should then be removed laterally to the orbital apex and medial orbital wall. An angled endoscope can then be used to view the floor of the sphenoid. Any remaining fungal debris or mucin should then be removed or irrigated from the sinus.

Sphenoethmoidal (Onodi) cells are ethmoid cells that lie superior and lateral to the sphenoid sinus. There is a typically an oblique bony partition that separates the cell from the sphenoid sinus. In maximally enlarging the sphenoid, this horizontal bony partition should be removed with a through-cutting forceps, while bearing in mind that it may be attached posteriorly to either the optic or carotid canal.

Superior Ethmoid Sinus

- The skull base can be safely identified along the roof of the sphenoid sinus. Once identified, dissection is carried from a posterior to anterior direction along the skull base to remove the superior ethmoid bony remnants attached to the skull base.

Again, the use of angled endoscopes and through-cutting forceps is recommended to improve visualization and remove ethmoid bony fragments while preserving the skull-base mucosa.

As the dissection along the skull base is carried forward, the anterior ethmoid artery typically lies in a superior extension of the anterior wall of the bulla ethmoidalis at, or somewhat below, the skull base, and courses anteriorly as it travels medially (Fig. 10.7). The openings of one, or more frequently two, supraorbital ethmoid cells often lie anterior to the vessel and extend laterally and superiorly.

Frontal Sinus

The opening to the frontal sinus is frequently not immediately evident, so it is important that the surgeon has conceptualized the location of the drainage pathway prior to the surgical procedure. Very fine malleable probes have been developed that can be utilized to gently probe the openings and help determine which of these ostia truly passes superiorly into the frontal sinus. Once the opening has been clearly identified, adjacent bony partitions may be fractured with specialized frontal sinus instruments to open the frontal sinus. Bony fragments are then teased out and redundant mucosa is trimmed with through-cutting instruments. Common areas of attention for revision surgery include the agger nasi cell and superior uncinate process. In addition, a lateralized superior segment of the middle turbinate can cause iatrogenic frontal sinusitis. This can be addressed by either resecting the middle turbinate to its insertion along the skull base or by cutting the synechiae and medializing the middle turbinate with a stitch or a middle meatal spacer.

Packing and Stenting

- As long as there is at least 180° of intact frontal recess mucosa, stents are rarely needed in the frontal recess.

In extended frontal sinus procedures in which a drill is used to denude the mucosa and remove bone more than 180 around the frontal recess, stents can be employed to try to keep the recess open. However, there is not good evidence that they are better than local postoperative care, even in this situation. There are commercially available silicone stents, but we prefer using a thin silastic stent rolled into a tube and placed within the frontal recess, when for one reason or another, a decision to use a stent is made. These are easily removed in the clinic and can unfurl to cover the entire recess.

- Medializing the middle turbinate following surgery is often critical to the success of the procedure.

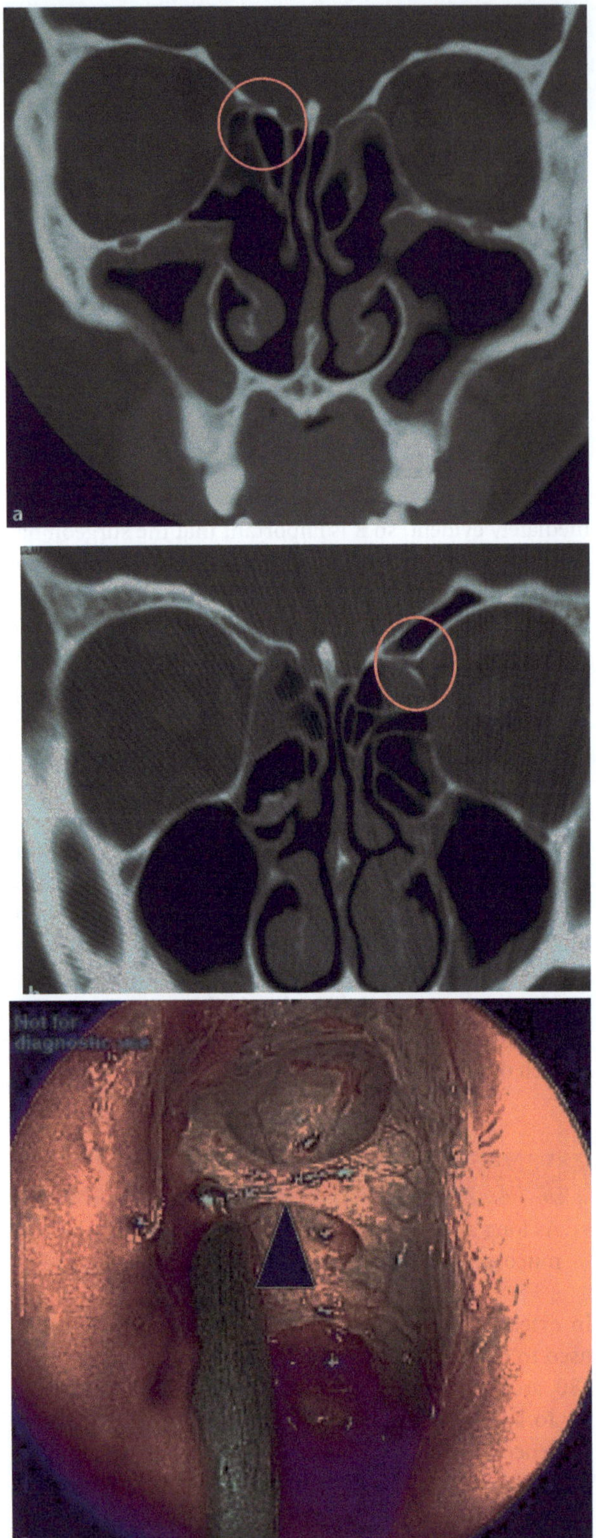

Fig. 10.7 Coronal CT scan views of an anterior ethmoid artery within the skull base (**a**) and traveling below the skull base (**b**). **c** An endoscopic view with a 30° endoscope. The *black arrowhead* is pointing to an anterior ethmoid artery below the skull base and without a bony mesentery

This allows easier postoperative access for debridements and helps prevent iatrogenic frontal recess obstruction from a lateralized middle turbinate. Often in revision cases, the horizontal portion of the basal lamellae has been removed, making the middle turbinate less stable. Medializing the middle turbinate against the septum can be done in a variety of methods. Scarring the medial surface of the middle turbinate and the opposing surface of the septum while placing a spacer in the middle meatus can create a controlled synechia, keeping the middle turbinate medialized (Fig. 10.8). Other techniques involve suturing both middle turbinates together through the septum.

Postoperative Care

- In the case of revision sinus surgery, postoperative care is often as important as the actual surgery itself.

Revision sinusotomies must be carefully and diligently examined following surgery. A failure to actively debride the recess and ostia, ensure its patency, and suction contaminated blood and mucus from the sinus is a recipe for restenosis and failure. To do this in a setting of an awake, often anxious patient, with topical analgesia alone makes this portion of the process very challenging, but can be aided by the careful application of topical ponticaine or even cocaine solution to the site. Where local debridements are necessary, 1% lidocaine with 1:100,000 epinephrine can be injected using a fine bent needle and a small syringe.

The timing of the first postoperative debridement varies with the individual surgeon's preference. Some debride on postoperative day one, while others wait for an additional 3–7 days. It is advantageous to have a full set of sinus instruments available in the clinic. This is coupled with angled suctions that are long and curved enough to reach into the frontal sinus and lateral and inferior regions of the maxillary sinus. Debridements should be aimed at clearing away fibrin debris and any loose bony fragments, while keeping trauma to the surrounding mucosa to a minimum.

While the mechanical care of revision antrostomies are important to prevent restenosis, medical management of the disease state is essential to long-term success. In a patient with significant polypoid edema, postoperative oral steroids can be used to keep the edema to a minimum. Intranasal steroids sprayed in the Moffit or head-down position, can help with delivery to the frontal recess. Postoperative antibiotics should also be given in an infectious setting, and antibiotics with good bone penetration should be used in patients with evidence of neo-osteogenesis. Other considerations in the management of these difficult patients includes local or oral antihis-

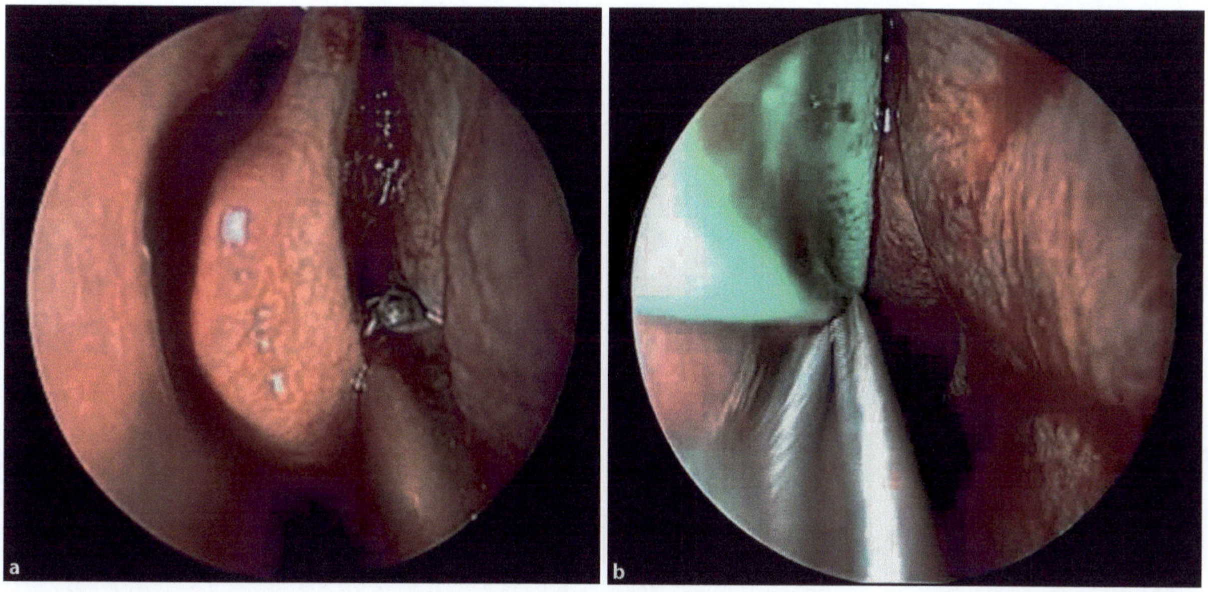

Fig. 10.8 Endoscopic views of creating a controlled synechiae between the right middle turbinate and nasal septum to prevent middle turbinate lateralization. The microdebrider is used to denude opposing surfaces of the middle turbinate and septum (**a**). A merocel sponge is then placed lateral to the middle turbinate and kept in place for 1–3 days (**b**)

tamines, antileukotriene medications, long-term irrigations, or an even a trial of itraconazole. In the latter situation, the patient's liver function tests should be evaluated prior to therapy and monitored during the treatment, and the patient should be aware of the off-label usage of this medication in this situation.

This routine of mechanical debridement and postoperative medication should be continued on a weekly basis until the mucosa of maxillary, ethmoids, and frontals are healed. The medical treatment is guided almost entirely by the endoscopic appearance of the cavity and the presence of residual, typically asymptomatic, disease. Once the cavity is secure, routine surveillance by nasal endoscopy should continue for the life of the patient.

Conclusion

Revision endoscopic sinus surgery remains a great challenge to all who practice sinus surgery. Surgical technique aside, the most important decisions are still made in the office. These entail assessing whether or not the patient is a good surgical candidate, identification of the patient's anatomy that is contributing to patient's symptoms and disease process, and the institution of aggressive adjuvant medical therapy.

References

1. Bowden MT, Church CA, Chiu AG, et al. (2004) Informed consent in functional endoscopic sinus surgery: the patient's perspective. Otolaryngol Head Neck Surg 131:126–132
2. Chandra RK, Schlosser R, Kennedy DW (2004) Use of the 70-degree diamond burr in the management of complicated frontal sinus disease. Laryngoscope 114:188–192
3. Glicklich RE, Metson R (1997) Effects of sinus surgery on quality of life. Otolaryngol Head Neck Surg 117:12–17
4. King JM, Caldarelli DD, Pigato JB (1994) A review of revision functional endoscopic sinus surgery. Laryngoscope 104:404–408
5. Senior BA, Kennedy DW, Tanabodee J, et al. (1998) Long-term results of functional endoscopic sinus surgery. Laryngoscope 108:151–157

Chapter 11

Septal and Turbinate Surgery in Revision Sinus Surgery

11

Joseph Raviv and Peter H. Hwang

Core Messages

- Septal deviation and turbinate variants can encroach on sinus drainage pathways and may benefit from correction in the revision surgical patient.
- Preoperative nasal endoscopy is critical to formulating a surgical plan regarding treatment of the septum and turbinates.
- Endoscopic septoplasty provides excellent visualization and facilitates dissection in cases of revision septoplasty.
- Surgical release of the lateralized middle turbinate may require adjunctive medialization techniques to prevent reformation of scarring.

Contents

Introduction

Functional endoscopic sinus surgery has a long-term success rate of approximately 90% for improving symptoms in patients with medically refractory chronic rhinosinusitis [10]. In the evaluation of patients with persistent postoperative disease, the paranasal sinuses are typically scrutinized for causative factors, but the closely related nasal septum and turbinates may often be overlooked. This chapter will discuss the role of the nasal septum and turbinates in chronic sinus disease and the specific treatment techniques available for successful outcomes in the revision surgical treatment of patients with chronic rhinosinusitis.

Anatomy

Septum

The nasal septum separates the two nasal cavities, provides structural support for the nose, influences airflow in the nasal cavity, and expresses olfactory neuroepithelium. The membranous septum connects the columella to the caudal margin of the quadrangular cartilage, which comprises the majority of the anterior septum. The posterior septum is bony, consisting of the perpendicular plate of the ethmoid bone posterosuperiorly and the vomer posteroinferiorly. Finally, the nasal, frontal, maxillary, and palatine bones each contribute nasal crests to the periphery of the septum. The cartilaginous and bony portions of the septum align during fetal development and fuse to form bony cartilaginous junctions. Displacement of the bony–cartilaginous interfaces results in deviations or deflections of the septum; this may occur congenitally as well as during periods of rapid facial growth, or consequent to external trauma.

Turbinates

The turbinates are intrinsic to the normal functioning of the nasal airway. They facilitate the filtering, warming, and humidification of inspired air. The middle and superior turbinates also participate in olfaction.

- In light of the functional nature of the turbinates, decision making in turbinate surgery requires a judicious consideration of the potential impact of surgical modification on nasal function.

The precursors of the nasal turbinates can be identified during the 8–10th week of fetal development as outgrowths from the lateral nasal wall [12]. These outgrowths, or ethmoturbinals, ultimately yield the middle and superior turbinates. The inferior turbinate is derived from the maxilloturbinal, a separate structure located inferior to the ethmoturbinals. Given its distinct embryonic derivation, the inferior turbinate is subject to fewer of the anatomic variations commonly seen in the middle and superior turbinates.

The three scroll-like turbinate bones divide the nasal lumen into meati. The inferior meatus is defined by the space between the inferior turbinate and the floor of the nose; the middle meatus by the space between the inferior and middle turbinates; and the superior meatus by the space between the middle and superior turbinates.

- The turbinate bones are encased by pseudostratified ciliated columnar respiratory epithelium, which contributes to mucociliary clearance of the nose. The inferior turbinate also possesses a vasoactive submucosal stroma that may hypertrophy and contribute to nasal obstruction.

Anatomic variations of turbinate structure are common, with pneumatization being the most commonly observed variant (Fig. 11.1). Concha bullosa of the middle turbinate is perhaps the most commonly encountered anatomic variant during surgery. A study reviewing 202 consecutive computed tomography (CT) scans found pneumatization of the vertical lamella of the middle turbinate in 46.2%, of the inferior or bulbous segment in 31.2%, and both the lamella and bulbous portion in 15.7% of cases [1]. Septal deviation and middle-turbinate concha bullosa often occur concurrently [11]. Nearly 80% of patients with a dominant concha bullosa have a concurrent deviated septum. There is also a strong association between unilateral concha bullosa and contralateral septal deviation. Pneu-

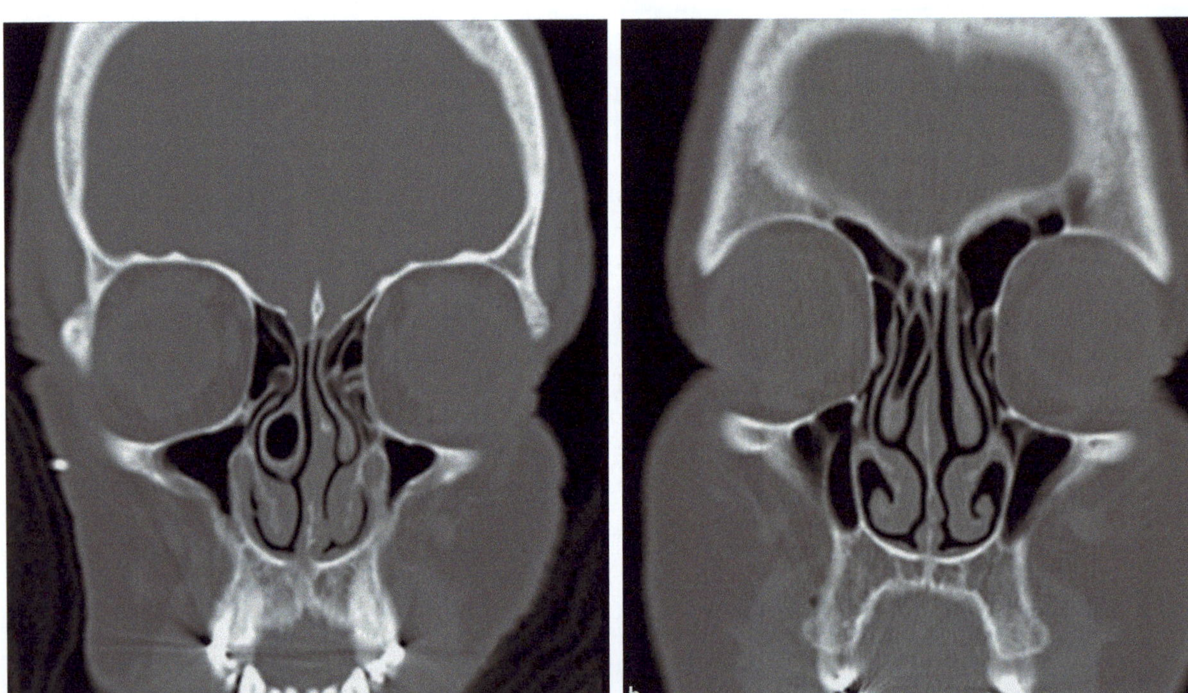

Fig. 11.1 Middle-turbinate pneumatization variants. **a** Pneumatization of the bulbous segment of the middle turbinate. **b** Pneumatization of the vertical lamella of the middle turbinate

matization of the superior turbinate is not uncommon [15, 17], and pneumatization of the inferior turbinate is a rare but acknowledged variant as well.

Association with Rhinosinusitis

- Variations in septal and turbinate anatomy may play a role not only in nasal obstruction, but also in the development of chronic sinus disease. This is believed to be due to both anatomic narrowing of the ostiomeatal complex (OMC) as well as to disruption of mucociliary function.

For example, septal deviation may displace the middle turbinate laterally, encroaching upon the maxillary ostium. Likewise, a pneumatized middle turbinate or superior turbinate may narrow the middle meatus or superior meatus, respectively [16]. Middle-turbinate concha bullosa has been associated with anterior ethmoid disease, while septal deviation has been associated with disease of the ostiomeatal complex, anterior ethmoid, and posterior ethmoid [2, 6].

In addition to contributing to anatomic narrowing of the OMC, septal deviation may also contribute to rhinosinusitis by impairing mucociliary clearance. Septal deviation has been associated with significantly longer mucociliary clearance times than in normal controls. Notably, normalization of mucociliary clearance has been observed after septoplasty [4, 13].

Preoperative Workup

Assessment of the revision surgical patient should include a historical review of previous septal or turbinate surgical procedures. Evidence of previous surgical treatment of the turbinates and/or septum should be correlated with findings on nasal endoscopy.

Diagnostic nasal endoscopy is an essential component of the evaluation of the revision surgical patient, and inspection of the turbinates and septum forms a key component of the endoscopy. The inferior turbinates should be examined before and after application of topical decongestant, in order to adequately assess the degree of soft tissue hypertrophy. Evidence of previous surgical treatment of the inferior turbinate can often be identified, including resection or out-fracture.

- If inspection of the inferior meatus reveals an accessory surgical antrostomy, the region should be carefully evaluated for possible recirculation around the inferior turbinate between the inferior meatal and middle meatal antrostomies.

The middle turbinate should be examined carefully for evidence of previous middle-turbinate resection or scarring to the lateral nasal wall. Several studies of patients requiring revision endoscopic sinus surgery found that the most common surgical alteration associated with recurrent sinus disease was partial middle turbinectomy resulting in middle meatal scarring and lateralization of the middle turbinate [4, 9].

- Lateralization and adhesions of the superior aspect of the middle turbinate may indicate underlying iatrogenic frontal sinus obstruction.

The superior turbinate and sphenoid ostia should be visualized as well if possible. Recirculation around the superior turbinate may occur if there is discontinuity between the surgical sphenoidotomy and the natural ostium of the sphenoid sinus. Finally, an endoscopic assessment of the nasal septum should be performed. Difficulty accessing the middle meatus during the office endoscopy indicates a strong likelihood that septoplasty would be beneficial.

Septoplasty is often a necessary complement to endoscopic sinus surgery for both intraoperative and postoperative access [3]. During surgery, endoscopic access to the middle meatus can be impaired by otherwise asymptomatic deflections of the septum. Postoperatively, examination and debridement of the sinus cavities can be more difficult if obstructive septal deflections are left uncorrected. In postsurgical failures, it is important to assess whether either lack of or incomplete correction of septal deviation contributed to the poor outcome. Evidence of prior septoplasty should be recognized prior to revision septal surgery and may be easier to assess endoscopically by palpation of the septum with a probe or suction as opposed to simple inspection.

Surgical Technique

Endoscopic Septoplasty

Please refer to Video 11.1. Traditional techniques for correction of septal deformity have relied on headlight illumination. The application of endoscopic techniques to septoplasty was initially described in 1992 [8], and offers several important advantages [5, 7] .

- Utilization of the endoscope allows excellent illumination and visualization, including enhanced identification of dissection planes, better assessment of posterior septal deflections, and earlier recognition of flap tears.

In addition, the endoscopic technique permits limited, minimally invasive approaches for isolated deviations by moving the incision to the immediate vicinity of an isolated septal deflection (Fig. 11.2).

- The ability to minimize mucosal elevation is a particular advantage in revision septoplasty, where adherent flaps from prior submucous resection may be difficult to dissect.

Furthermore, simultaneous endonasal endoscopic examination allows the surgeon to gauge the progress made toward achieving relief of nasal obstruction and adequate surgical exposure. Finally, the endoscopic approach provides an excellent teaching tool. Demonstration of surgical anatomy and technique on the video monitor provides an invaluable learning opportunity for students, residents, and surgical assistants.

The patient is positioned, prepared, and draped for septoplasty as is standard for endoscopic sinus surgery. Topical oxymetazoline is applied for decongestion and 1% lidocaine with 1:100,000 epinephrine injected subperichondrially.

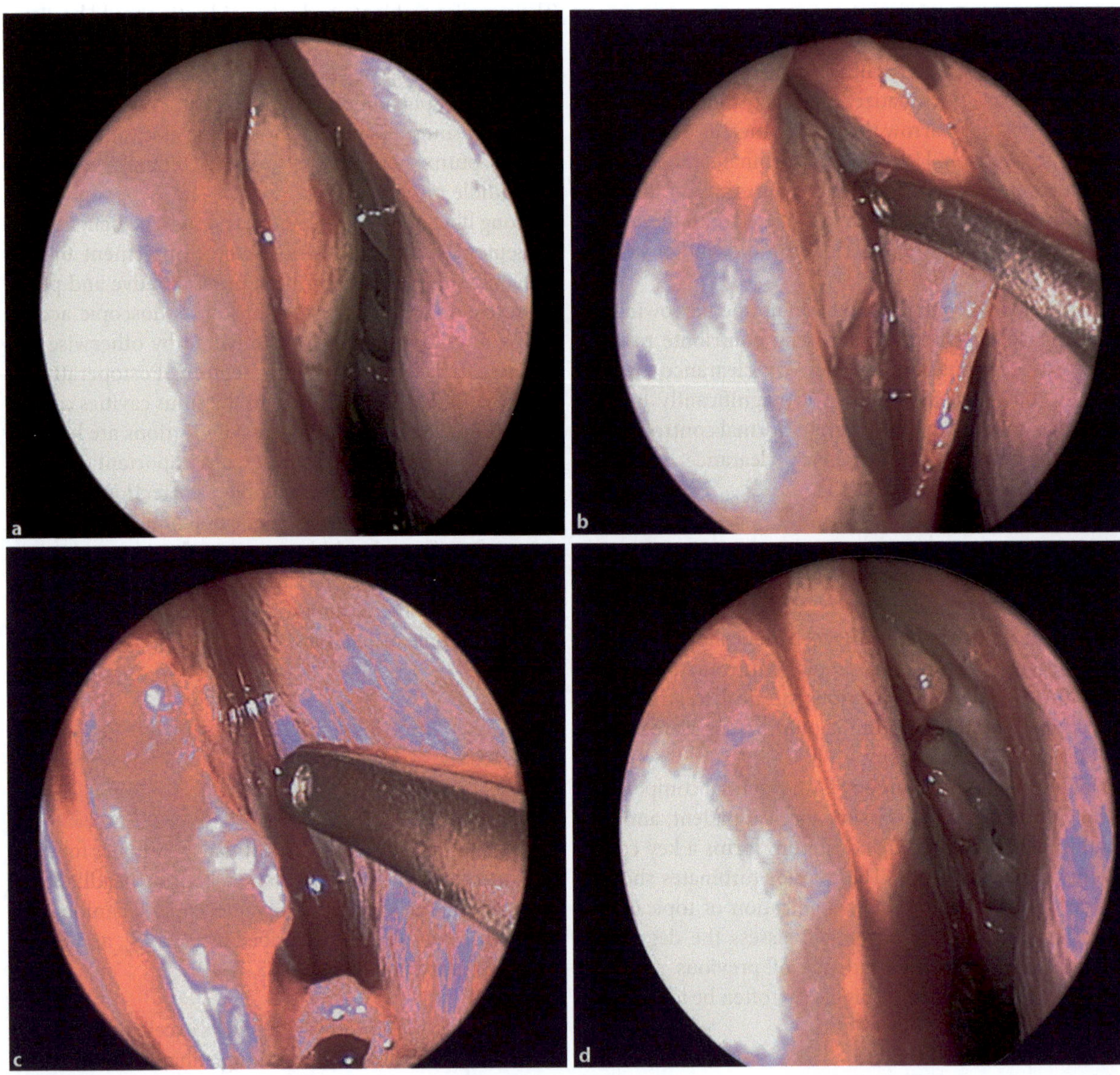

Fig. 11.2 Limited endoscopic septoplasty for isolated septal deflection. **a** Posteriorly placed incision just anterior to septal deviation. **b–c** Elevation of the mucoperichondrial flap and excision of the deviated cartilage and bone. **d** Reapposition of the mucosal flap and confirmation of adequacy of resection

Incision Design

- The incision is typically placed on the ipsilateral side of maximal deviation.
- For a broadly deviated septum, a standard hemi-transfixion incision is used.
- For more posterior isolated deformities or in revision septoplasty, a more posteriorly placed incision in the immediate vicinity of the deformity can be made with an angled scalpel blade.

Surgical Technique Principles

- Once the plane of dissection is established, the mucoperichondrial flaps are elevated with a suction Freer or Gorney elevator under direct endoscopic visualization.
- A scope irrigator can greatly enhance visualization while working beneath the septal flaps.
- After complete elevation of the ipsilateral septal flap, the septal cartilage is incised at the point of maximal deflection, and the contralateral flap elevated.
- Flap elevation is continued bilaterally until the complete extent of septal deformity has been dissected.
- The deviated septum is then excised using standard septoplasty instruments as well as endoscopic scissors, punches, or forceps.
- The adequacy of the septoplasty is confirmed by performing serial endoscopy of the nasal cavity.
- Closure involves reapposition of the septal flaps, followed by a running quilting stitch, which is placed endoscopically with a 4–0 plain gut suture on a Keith needle.
- When a hemi-transfixion incision has been made, the incision is closed under direct visualization with a 5–0 plain gut suture.
- When the incision has been placed posteriorly for limited septal work, no closure of the incision is required.
- No nasal packing is required.

The endoscopic septoplasty technique is also useful for removing isolated septal spurs. A longitudinal incision is made along the apex of the spur and mucosal flaps are then elevated above and below the spur to reveal the spur and allow its removal. The superior and inferior flaps can be then be reapproximated and the incision usually does not need to be closed with suture. This approach minimizes the degree of flap dissection and reduces the risk of flap perforation.

Inferior-Turbinate Reduction

Refractory chronic sinus disease is not typically due to inferior turbinate hypertrophy. However, symptoms of nasal obstruction are common among patients with significant sinonasal inflammation, and therefore inferior-turbinate reduction should be considered in the revision FESS candidate with turbinate hypertrophy and obstructive symptoms.

- The goal of inferior turbinate reduction is to provide a controlled reduction of the inferior turbinate soft tissue with maximal mucosal preservation.

Several different techniques are currently available for inferior turbinate soft-tissue reduction including laser, radiofrequency, and microdebrider submucous resection. The authors prefer the use of powered instrumentation for submucous resection of the inferior turbinates and believe that it offers several advantages.

Advantages of Microdebrider Inferior-Turbinate Reduction

- Microdebrider reduction is clinically efficacious while offering excellent mucosal preservation.
- The surgeon can sculpt targeted anatomic regions of the inferior turbinate that may not be as well approached with other techniques, including the superior–anterior and most inferior aspect of the turbinate.
- Finally, while thermal reduction techniques depend on the contracture of turbinate tissue that occurs over time as necrosed regions are replaced by fibroblasts, the results with microdebrider reduction are immediate.

The procedure can be performed in either the office or the operating room setting. A total of 1–2 ml of 1% lidocaine with 1:100,000 epinephrine solution is injected in the anterior aspect of the inferior turbinate. An incision at the anteriormost aspect of the inferior turbinate is made just behind the mucocutaneous border. The incision can be made with a number 15 scalpel or with a specially designed turbinate microdebrider blade with a built-in dissector (Medtronic, Jacksonville, Florida, USA). A submucoperiosteal flap is elevated along the anterior half of the inferior turbinate. The turbinate blade is then placed facing outward to reduce the soft tissue under endoscopic visualization via serial passes of the blade from posterior to anterior. The reduction in size of the inferior turbinate is usually recognized immediately as the procedure progresses. Out-fracture of the inferior turbinate using a Boies elevator is frequently performed concurrently as a complementary procedure. Hemostasis is typically achieved with topical epinephrine, and packing is very rarely required. The incision need not be closed.

Excision of Middle-Turbinate Concha Bullosa

- Surgical resection of a concha bullosa entails careful preservation of the medial lamella (which attaches to the skull base) and resection of only the lateral half of the turbinate (Fig. 11.3).

The extent of middle-turbinate pneumatization is evaluated on CT scans and allows the surgeon to anticipate points of safe entry into the lumen of the concha bullosa. Local anesthetic is injected as is routine for FESS, including the middle turbinate mucosa. The concha bullosa is then entered with sharp dissection using either a sickle knife or sharp Freer elevator. Because the lumen of the

11

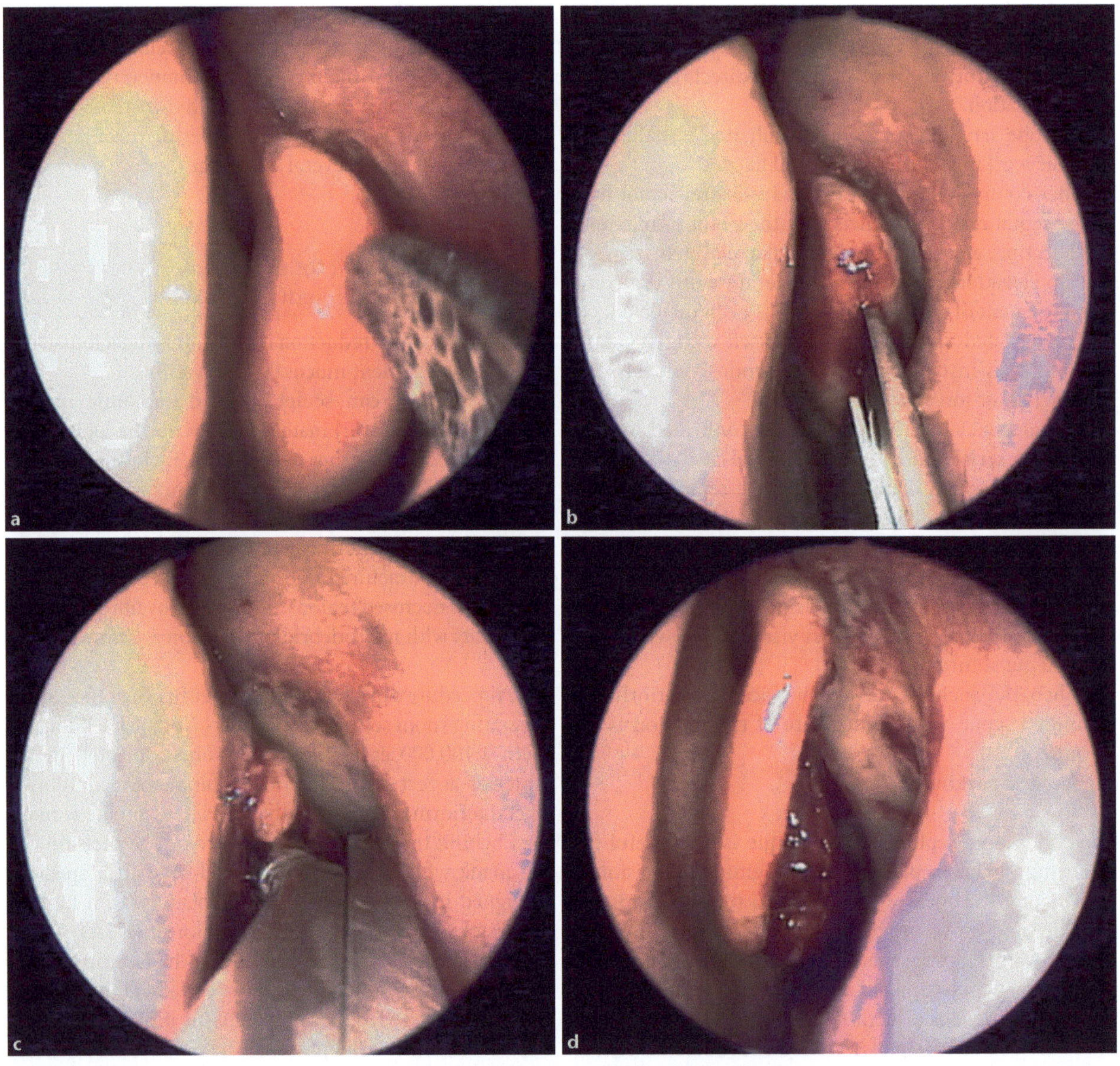

Fig. 11.3 Surgical resection of the concha bullosa. **a** The concha bullosa is entered sharply with a sickle knife. **b** The incision is extended superiorly and inferiorly with endoscopic scissors. **c** The lateral aspect of concha bullosa is resected with through-cutting forceps. **d** The medial lamella mucosa and attachment to the cribriform plate are preserved

concha bullosa is a functional ethmoid air cell, great care must be taken to enter the turbinate without disrupting the mucosal lining of the interior of the concha bullosa. Once proper entry is confirmed by endoscopic visualization, the incision is extended from superior to inferior with either endoscopic scissors or sickle knife, taking care to not destabilize the attachment of the medial lamella to the cribriform plate. Turbinate scissors and through-cutting forceps are then used to continue dissection posteriorly. Removal of the lateral lamella may be performed with a microdebrider or in a piecemeal fashion with through-cutting forceps. In certain cases, the pneumatized middle turbinate may be approached from the posterior free edge of the lateral lamella; dissection in these situations can proceed from posterior to anterior using a back biter forceps.

In the revision surgical approach to the partially resected concha bullosa, care should be taken to ensure that all areas of pneumatization have been addressed. Inadequate resection of the inferior bulbous portion of the middle turbinate can result in narrowing of the middle meatus, while incomplete resection of the pneumatized vertical lamella of the pneumatized turbinate can narrow the ethmoid cavity and frontal recess.

Lateralized Middle-Turbinate Release

Lateralization of the middle turbinate is a common finding in the post-FESS patient and may occur as a result of several factors. First, the turbinate may be attenuated and "floppy" due to over resection. Secondly, surgical trauma to the mucosal surface of the turbinate may predispose to the development of adhesions with the lateral nasal wall. Thirdly, inadequate postoperative debridement may allow early granulation to mature into adherent synechiae. Because middle-turbinate lateralization may collapse, scar, and narrow the sinus outflow tracts, surgical correction is often indicated in the revision FESS patient.

The patient is positioned, prepared, and draped as is standard for endoscopic sinus surgery. Topical oxymetazoline or epinephrine (1:1000) is applied preoperatively for decongestion. Intraoperative surgical navigation may be helpful during the initial diagnostic endoscopy, confirming the relationship of the middle-turbinate remnant to the medial orbital wall. The position of the skull base and cribriform plate should also be determined. Once these critical anatomic structures are delineated, safe infiltration of the middle-turbinate remnant and medial orbital wall with 1% lidocaine with 1:100,000 epinephrine solution is performed.

The initial step is a release of the scarred middle turbinate from the lateral nasal wall. The release is achieved through a vertically oriented incision between the turbinate remnant and the lateral nasal wall, parallel to the medial orbital wall. The synechiae can be divided with endoscopic scissors or a small through-cutting instrument, such as a pediatric Blakesley forceps (Fig. 11.4). Once the turbinate has been released from its lateral scarred position, the degree of previous middle-turbinate resection can be more fully assessed. When previous middle-turbinate resection has been limited, releasing the lateralized turbinate will reveal a near-normal appearing middle-turbinate remnant.

- The goal in cases with middle-turbinate lateralization is to allow the middle turbinate to heal in a medial position.

This can be achieved by placement of a middle meatal stent for approximately 7 days. Optional scarification of the middle turbinate to the nasal septum can be performed concurrently by abrading the apposing surfaces of the middle turbinate and adjacent septum; middle meatal stenting will bring these surfaces together to facilitate a favorable adhesion. Alternatively, suturing of the middle turbinate to the septum is an effective method of turbinate medialization. A simple dissolvable mattress suture (4–0 plain gut on a straight Keith needle) placed endoscopically will allow sufficient time for the medialized turbinate to heal without reforming adhesions to the lateral nasal wall.

If the middle-turbinate remnant is substantially truncated or ossified from prior resection, restoration of the turbinate to a medial position may not be possible. In such cases, selective resection of the lateralized portions of the turbinate may actually be necessary to relieve ethmoid or frontal obstruction.

Regardless of the surgical strategy employed, postoperative inspection and debridement of granulation is important to prevent early scar formation and relateralization.

Superior-Turbinate Resection

Although less common, revision surgery involving the superior turbinate can pose similar challenges to those posed by the middle turbinate. Just as the middle turbinate forms the medial border of the anterior ethmoid cavity, the superior turbinate defines the medial border of the posterior ethmoid cavity. As imprecise anterior ethmoid and frontal recess dissection can lead to destabilization and scarring of the middle turbinate, so too can posterior ethmoid and sphenoid surgery lead to superior-turbinate scarring and postsurgical failure.

When sphenoidotomy is performed through a transethmoidectomy approach, the inferior portion of the

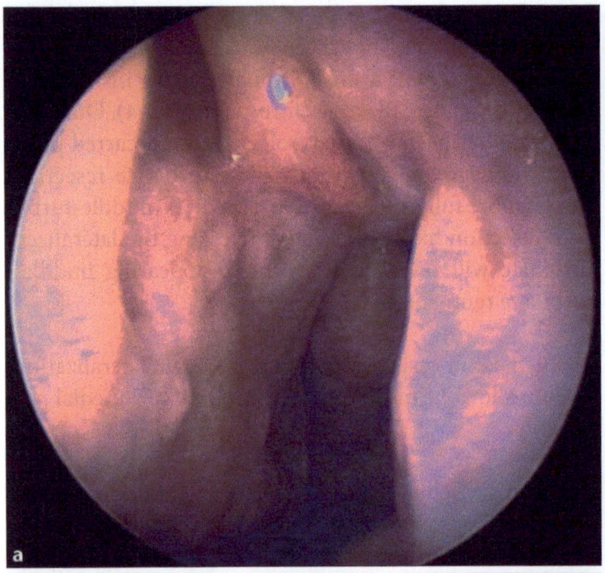

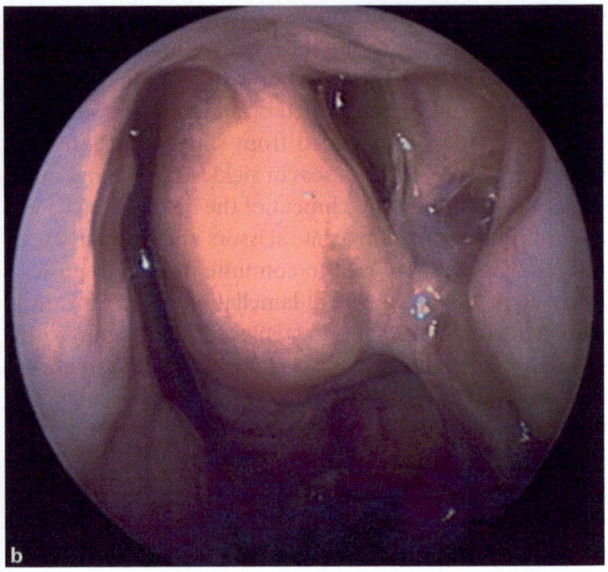

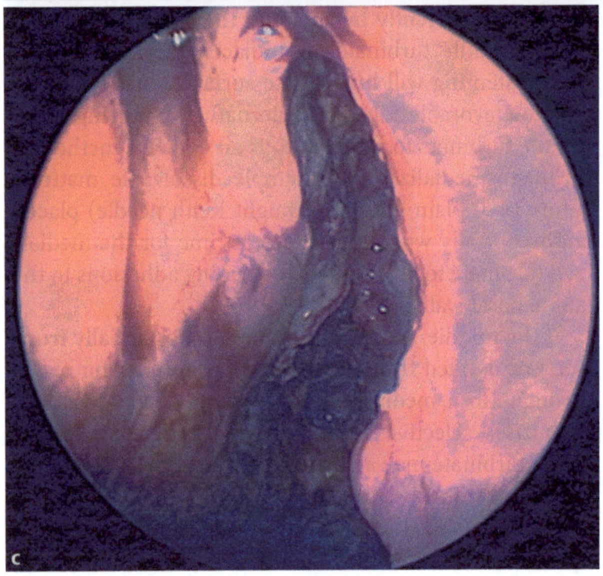

Fig. 11.4 Release of the lateralized middle turbinate. **a** Previous resection of the middle turbinate with lateralization and scarring to the lateral nasal wall. **b** Dense scar tissue between the middle-turbinate remnant and medial orbital wall. **c** Vertically oriented release of synechiae and medialization of the middle-turbinate remnant

superior turbinate is resected with a through-cutting instrument to expose the natural sphenoid ostium within the sphenoethmoid recess. Once identified, the sphenoid ostium is enlarged and the anterior wall of the sinus removed using through-cutting punches and forceps. In situations where the inferior portion of the superior turbinate is not resected cleanly, the remnant superior turbinate may form adhesions with adjacent tissue. The sphenoid outflow may then be compromised because either the natural ostium is obstructed or recirculation of mucous has developed around the superior turbinate between the natural ostium and surgical sphenoidotomy.

Surgical correction of a scarred superior turbinate is relatively straightforward. The first step is to identify and cannulate the natural ostium of the sphenoid sinus. At this point, resection of the scarred inferior aspect of the superior turbinate should be performed with a through-cutting forceps. The sphenoid ostium can then be enlarged and brought into continuity with the remainder of the surgical sphenoidotomy, as necessary.

- Conservative resection of the inferior third of the superior turbinate should not result in significant disturbance of the olfactory neuroepithelium.

Tips and Pearls to Avoid Complications

1. Palpate the septum carefully in revision septoplasty in order to anticipate the extent of prior submucous resection. Take extra caution in elevating the mucosal flaps over absent septal bone or

cartilage, or move the incision posteriorly to avoid dissecting in areas of prior surgery.
2. If possible, minimize dissection of the posterior third of the inferior turbinate during soft-tissue reduction. This area may carry feeding vessels from the sphenopalatine artery and may be more prone to postoperative bleeding.
3. Always confine concha bullosa excision to the lateral aspect of the turbinate. The medial turbinate carries the attachment to the skull base and should be left undisturbed.
4. Be aware of the presence of middle-turbinate lamellar cells, which can harbor disease and should be opened along with pneumatized portions of the bulbous middle turbinate.

References

1. Bolger WE, Butzin CA, Parson DS (1991) Paranasal sinus bony anatomic variations and mucosal abnormalities: CT analysis for endoscopic sinus surgery. Laryngoscope 101:56–64
2. Calhoun KH, Waggenspack GA, Simpson CB, et al (1991) CT evaluation of the paranasal sinuses in symptomatic and asymptomatic populations. Otolaryngol Head Neck Surg 104:480–483
3. Cantrell H (1997) Limited septoplasty for endoscopic sinus surgery. Otolaryngol Head Neck Surg 116:272–276
4. Chu CT, Lebowitz RA, Jacobs JB (1997) An analysis of sites of disease in revision endoscopic sinus surgery. Am J Rhinol 11:287–291
5. Chung BJ, Batra PS, Citardi MJ, et al (2007) Endoscopic septoplasty: revisitation of the technique, indications, and outcomes. Am J Rhinol 21:307–311
6. Elahi MM, Frenkiel S, Fageeh N (1997) Paraseptal structural changes and chronic sinus disease in relation to the deviated septum. J Otolaryngol 26:236–240
7. Hwang PH, McLaughlin RB, Lanza DC, et al (1999) Endoscopic septoplasty: indications, technique, and results. Otolaryngol Head Neck Surg 120:678–682
8. Lanza DC, Kennedy DW, Zinreich SJ (1991) Nasal endoscopy and its surgical application. In: Lee KJ (ed) Essential Otolaryngology: Head and Neck Surgery, 5th edn. Medical Examination, New York, pp. 373–387
9. Musy PY, Kountakis SE (2004) Anatomic findings in patients undergoing revision endoscopic sinus surgery. Am J Otolaryngol 25:418–422
10. Senior BA, Kennedy DW, et al (1998) Long-term results of functional endoscopic sinus surgery. Laryngoscope 108:151–157
11. Stallman JS, Lobo JN, Som PM (2004) The incidence of concha bullosa and its relationship to nasal septal deviation and paranasal sinus disease. Am J Neuroradiol 25:1613–1618
12. Stammberger H (1991) Functional Endoscopic Sinus Surgery. Decker, Philadelphia
13. Ulusoy B, Arbag H, Sari O, et al (2007) Evaluation of the effects of nasal septal deviation and its surgery on nasal mucociliary clearance in both nasal cavities. Am J Rhinol 21:180–183
14. Uslu H, Uslu C, Varoglu E, et al (2004) Effects of septoplasty and septal deviation on nasal mucociliary clearance. Int J Clin Pract 58:1108–1111
15. van Alyea OE (1939) Ethmoid labyrinth. Arch Otolaryngol 29:881–902
16. Yasan H, Dögru H, Baykal B, et al (2005) What is the relationship between chronic sinus disease and isolated nasal septal deviation? Otolaryngol Head Neck Surg 133:190–193
17. Zuckerkandl E (1882) Normale und pathologische Anatomie der Nasenhöhle und ihrer pneumatischen Anhänge. Wilhelm Braumüller, Wien

Chapter 12

Revision Endoscopic Surgery of the Ethmoid and Maxillary Sinus

12

Biana G. Lanson, Seth J. Kanowitz,
Richard A. Lebowitz, and Joseph B. Jacobs

Core Messages

- Revision FESS is substantially more complex than primary surgery due several factors.
- Etiologies for recalcitrant postsurgical chronic rhinosinusitis are classified broadly as environmental, host, or iatrogenic.
- In order to maximize the success rate of revision FESS the surgeon must be familiar with the evaluation, diagnosis, surgical anatomy, and management of these complex patients.

Contents

Introduction

Functional endoscopic sinus surgery (FESS) is indicated for the treatment of symptoms of chronic rhinosinusitis (CRS). Success rates after FESS have been reported as ranging from 74 to 97.5% [13, 14, 22], leaving 2.5–26% of patients still suffering from persistent symptoms and signs of chronic infectious and/or inflammatory sinus disease following surgery. As more and more primary FESS procedures are performed, the number of patients who are being evaluated for revision sinus surgery is also increasing. This chapter will help to educate the otolaryngologist about patients who present with failure of primary maxillary and ethmoid sinus surgery, whether due to inadequacy of the primary surgery or the recurrence of sinonasal mucosal disease resulting from underlying medical or immunologic conditions. The chapter will also provide a guideline for the diagnosis, management, and treatment of patients presenting with persistent symptoms of CRS after sinus surgery.

Causes for Surgical Failures

Causes of treatment failures following FESS include environmental factors, host systemic diseases, iatrogenic problems, and surgical deficiencies [6]. Taken as a whole these are thought to impair normal mucociliary clearance and cause postoperative surgical treatment failures. Environmental control is an important component in the medical management of patients with CRS; exposure to irritants and allergens should be minimized or eliminated whenever possible [6].

Similarly, host systemic diseases may cause excessive mucosal inflammation and result in further impairment of mucociliary clearance. These conditions include allergic diathesis [14], the recurrent sinonasal polyposis that can result from the inflammatory response seen in Churg Strauss Syndrome or Job's Syndrome, cystic fibrosis [19], granulomatous disease, neoplasia, and immotile ciliary syndrome [1]. Some authors propose that the presence of eosinophilic infiltration, as seen in both allergic and nonallergic rhinosinusitis, can be an important variant in predisposing a patient to the closure of a middle meatal antrostomy with subsequent persistence of inflammatory changes within the maxillary sinus [8, 10]. Similarly, in patients with sinonasal polyposis, a history of previous sinus surgery, asthma, or allergy predicted recurrence and need for revision surgery [23].

Iatrogenic causes of treatment failure can result from poor surgical technique (i.e., an improperly placed maxillary antrostomy), middle-turbinate resection with lateralization of the turbinate remnant, inadequate postoperative nasal debridement, or deficient postoperative medical management leading to a persistent infectious or inflammatory mucosal response. Furthermore, overaggressive removal of healthy mucosa resulting in bone exposure during primary FESS or, alternatively, failure to remove diseased bony ethmoid partitions may lead to significant scarring or an osteitic response.

A suggested important reason for surgical failure is a "missed ostium sequence" [21]:

- Inadequate surgical removal of the most anterior portion of the uncinate process blocks visibility of the most anterior fontanelle leading to failure to identify the natural maxillary ostium and incorporate it in the maxillary sinus antrostomy. An accessory maxillary ostium may be mistakenly enlarged resulting in persistent disease due to mucociliary flow being directed toward the obstructed natural outflow tract rather than toward the surgically created antrostomy.
- Surgical antrostomies that do not communicate with the natural ostia can also generate a "recirculation phenomenon" in which mucus is swept by the cilia out of the maxillary sinus via the natural ostium but then reenters the sinus though the improperly placed surgical antrostomy (Fig. 12.1) [21]. This may lead to persistence of maxillary sinus disease.

Surgical trauma to the nasal mucosa, associated with mucosal stripping and bone exposure, can often result in synechiae, fibrosis, regrowth of poorly ciliated epithelium, osteoneogenesis, and osteitis (Fig. 12.2), which have all been implicated as potential etiologies of surgical failure [21]. Bacterial invasion of exposed bone and the subsequent chronic inflammatory reaction are thought to potentiate the osteoneogenesis process. Inflammation within the bone is difficult to eradicate and can be a nidus for local production of additional inflammatory mediators causing persistent mucosal disease and inhibition of healing [6]. In addition, mucosal stripping and the creation of raw surfaces may result in postoperative lateralization of the middle turbinate and subsequent synechiae formation adhering the middle turbinate to the lateral nasal wall (Fig. 12.3). Secondary anatomic obstruction of the ostiomeatal pathways often results.

Ramadan reviewed 398 patients who did not have a medical history of immunodeficiency, systemic disorders, cystic fibrosis, or ciliary abnormality, but whose

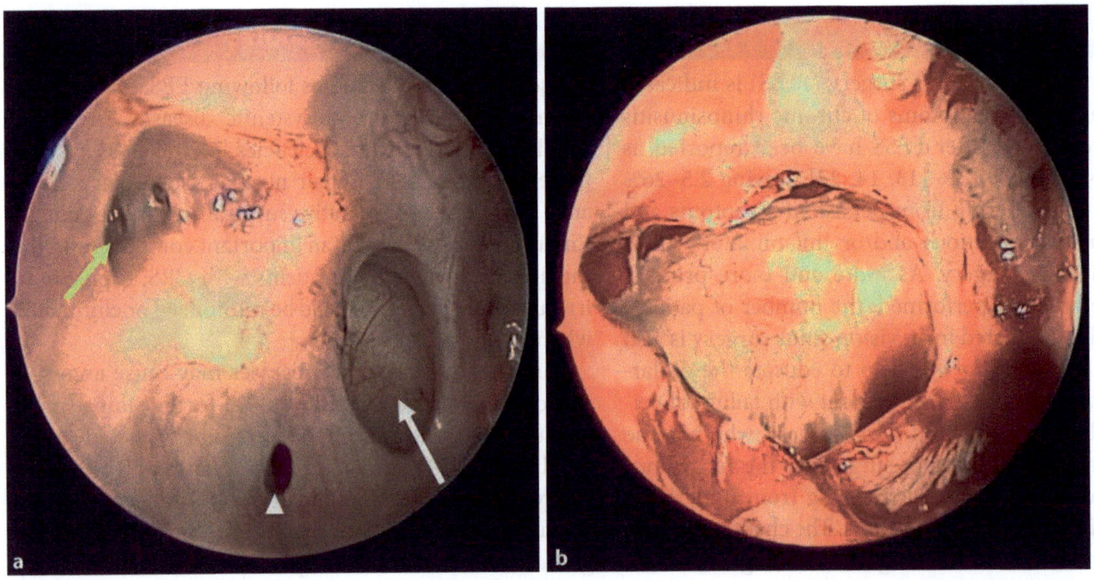

Fig. 12.1a,b Maxillary recirculation. **a** Endoscopic visualization (30 endoscope) of an improperly placed maxillary antrostomy. The natural maxillary sinus osier (*yellow arrow*) is not in continuity with the posterior maxillary antrostomy (*white arrow*) or accessory ostium (*white arrowhead*), as a result of either scar tissue formation or improper placement of the antrostomy in the posterior fontanelle during primary functional endoscopic sinus surgery (FESS). **b** After revision, the new maxillary antrostomy now includes the natural ostium, accessory ostium, and the antrostomy that had been created during primary FESS

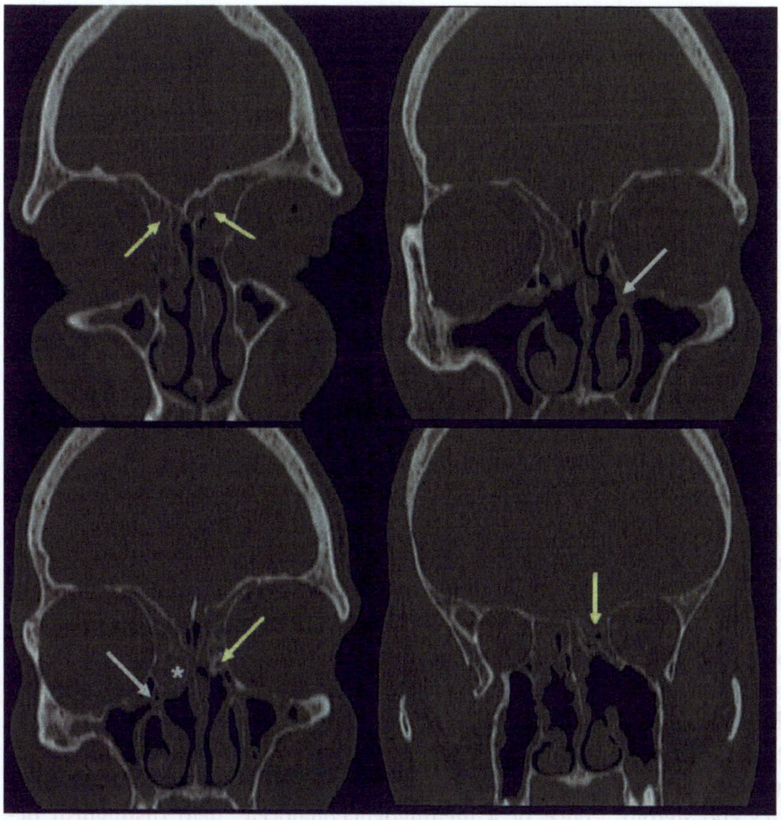

Fig. 12.2 Osteitis. Preoperative coronal computed tomography (CT) scan or the paranasal sinuses in a patient undergoing revision FESS. Areas of osteitic bone within the ethmoid cavity (*yellow arrows*), retained uncinate process (*white arrows*) leading to scarring of the maxillary antrostomy, and an undissected concha bullosa (*white asterisk*) have likely contributed to this patients primary FESS failure

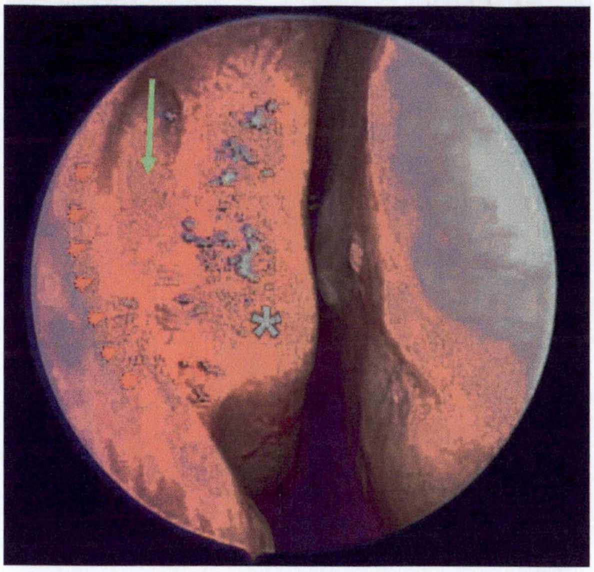

Fig. 12.3 Lateralized middle turbinate. Endoscopic visualization (0 endoscope) of a lateralized right middle turbinate (*asterisk*). A web of scar tissue (*yellow arrow*) has formed between the middle turbinate (*asterisk*) and the lateral nasal wall (*red arrowheads*), thus leading the lateralization of the middle turbinate and persistence of chronic rhinosinusitis after primary FESS

CRS symptoms persisted after their primary FESS procedure. Fifty-two of these patients required a revision FESS procedure. He found that the revision cases had a higher mean computed tomography (CT) score, according to the Lund-MacKay staging system, compared with non-revision cases. Fifty six percent of the revision cases had evidence of adhesions, and the most common cause of revision surgery was the presence of residual air cells and stenosis of sinus ostia [22] . Chambers et al. and Hinohira et al. noted that scarring in the middle meatus, residual ethmoid cells, and stenosis of the maxillary sinus ostium are the common causes for surgical failure [4, 12]. Chu et al. reported 153 patients requiring revision sinus surgery and found that the most common surgical alteration to be partial middle turbinectomy with resulting lateralization of the middle turbinate remnant and subsequent scarring of the middle meatus [5]. Thus, mucosal preservation during both primary and revision FESS is essential for a successful outcome. This can be achieved with use of through-cutting instruments and directed powered mucosal shaving techniques.

Incomplete surgery resulting in persistent symptoms following primary FESS may be due residual ethmoid air cells or the failure to address anatomic findings such as pneumatization of the middle turbinate (concha bullosa), deviation of the nasal septum, and the presence of infraorbital (Haller) cells [3, 20]. In a study by Musy and Kountakis, among 70 patients with primary surgical failure, 70% had a lateralized middle turbinate and 64% had an incomplete anterior ethmoidectomy [17]. A retained foreign body (e.g., infected dental implant in the maxillary cavity) can also cause persistent sinonasal infection and disease.

Preoperative Workup and Indications

Evaluation for revision sinus surgery begins with the patient's history, including a thorough review of the past medical history, as well as the physical exam. Potential environmental and host factor influences are carefully discussed. Close attention is paid to eliciting a history of immunodeficiency, cystic fibrosis, granulomatous and autoimmune disease, and genetic syndromes, such as Kartagener's syndrome and Churg Strauss Syndrome. The surgeon should also obtain original records and radiographs whenever possible. Prior surgical technique, perioperative medical therapy as well as a schedule of postoperative surgical debridements should to be reviewed. It is prudent to know whether a mucosal-preserving technique was used, appropriate antibiotics and steroid treatments prescribed, adequate and timely debridement procedures performed, and whether the patient had used sterile nasal saline irrigation and/or any other alternative therapies that may have complicated treatment [6].

Nasal endoscopic evaluation of the patient is also of utmost importance. The degree of inflammation and/or infection of the sinuses can be assessed. Moreover, most surgically created anatomic problems can be identified: retained uncinate process, scaring and synechiae formation, lateralized middle-turbinate remnants, improperly placed maxillary antrostomy, or residual infraorbital cells [6]. The mucosal findings are potentially reversible, especially if not associated with anatomic obstruction. The patient's symptoms can often be correlated with the endoscopic findings and therefore should be carefully documented. The revision surgeon should be convinced of the rhinologic origin of the patient's symptoms before planning surgery.

Preoperative identification and treatment of a resistant bacterial infection can aid in revision surgery. *Staphylococcus aureus*, methicillin-resistant *S. aureus*, and Gram-negative organisms, such as *Pseudomonas*, are the most common bacteria in patients presenting for revision surgery [2, 18]. Purulent secretions should be cultured and culture-directed antibiotics initiated prior to surgery. Therapy in patients suffering from allergic fungal sinusitis or eosinophilic mucin rhinosinusitis may include systemic and topical antifungals and steroids [9].

The majority of the patients are treated with topical steroid therapy as well as systemic antibiotic and steroid therapy as part of the initial medical management of their recurrent sinus disease. Many otolaryngologists advocate a short burst of high-dose oral steroids just prior to revision surgery, in order to reduce sinonasal mucosal edema and facilitate the delineation of anatomic structures. Preoperative steroids, 20–40 mg/day for 4–10 days can reduce polyp size, stabilize or reduce mucosal edema, and reduce intraoperative bleeding [6].

A recent CT scan of the paranasal sinuses is required after maximal medical therapy. In the case of revision maxillary and ethmoid sinus surgery, close attention should be paid to evaluation of the residual uncinate process, residual ethmoid cells and septae, supraorbital ethmoid cells, infraorbital ethmoid cells, and the presence of mucoceles. It is imperative to evaluate the skull base height (Keros I–III) and position of the lamina papyracea, as well as to check for evidence of previous breach of these boundaries. An example of a residual uncinate process seen on coronal CT of the sinuses is shown in Fig. 12.4.

Magnetic resonance imaging (MRI) can be a useful adjunct radiologic modality in the evaluation of patients with skull-base dehiscence, previous orbital injury, or in cases of sinonasal neoplasia. MRI can identify the presence of a meningoencephalocele, help distinguish between tumor, polyps, mucin, and secretions, and assess the integrity of the periorbita and dura.

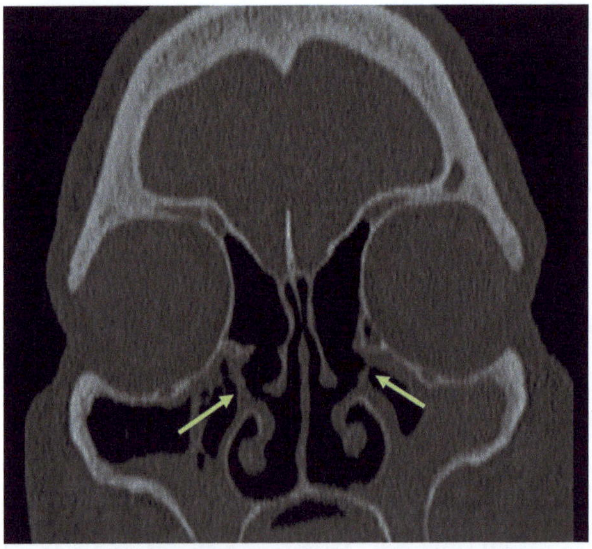

Fig. 12.4 Retained uncinate. Preoperative coronal CT scan of the paranasal sinuses in a patient undergoing bilateral revision endoscopic maxillary antrostomy. Fragments of retained uncinate process (*yellow arrows*) lead to scarring and eventual stenosis of the maxillary antrostomy bilaterally. As a result, the patient suffered from chronic maxillary rhinosinusitis after primary FESS

The use of intraoperative computer-assisted stereotactic surgical navigation has enhanced potential access with decreased morbidity to altered anatomic structures in complicated revision procedures [11]. Needless to say, the surgeon should still be vigilant about the identification of key anatomic structures and should not rely solely on the navigation system. Also, repeated visual confirmation of registration should be performed throughout the surgery.

Appropriate counseling of patients is also imperative once the decision has been made to proceed with surgery. Goals of surgery, increased risks of revision sinus surgery, patient expectations, need for long-term follow-up, postoperative debridement, and medical management should all be addressed.

Technique

General

Recent radiographic studies must be present in the operating room and the surgeon should reference these materials before and during the surgery. Correlation of CT images and intraoperative endoscopic findings can be especially helpful in revision surgery when the patient's sinonasal cavity lacks the usual anatomic landmarks. An attempt should also be made to identify the anterior ethmoid artery on the CT images as the normal bony covering may have been removed during previous surgery, thus making inadvertent injury more likely during revision procedures.

Before initiating surgery, decongestion and vasoconstriction of the sinonasal cavity may be achieved with topical oxymetazoline and injection of 1% xylocaine with 1:100,000 or 1:200,000 epinephrine. As in all surgical procedures, the surgeon is to work from "known" to "unknown." Both the maxillary and ethmoid cavities should be inspected with angled rigid endoscopes, and appropriate cultures obtained with suction traps. The primary landmarks in revision surgery are the middle turbinate/turbinate remnant, roof of the maxillary sinus, medial orbital wall, and skull base.

If the middle turbinate is scarred laterally and obstructing access to the ethmoid cavity it should be gently medialized. Synechiae and scarring should be released with a sharp sickle knife or through-cutting forceps, and all attempts should be made to preserve the mucosa [4].

- It is important to remember that when medializing the middle turbinate it may be thickened due to osteoneogenesis, thus making medialization more difficult and the risk of injury to the skull base greater.

When encountering osteitic bone, the bone should be debrided with curettes. In the case of diffuse osteitis, a high-speed suction irrigation, diamond-tipped drill can be utilized.

Revision Maxillary Sinus Surgery

- Key landmarks during maxillary sinus surgery include:
  1. Floor of the orbit.
  2. Lamina papyracea.
  3. Superior attachment of the inferior turbinate.
  4. Ascending process of the maxilla.

If the maxillary sinus roof (orbital floor) can be visualized through the previous maxillary antrostomy, the plane of the lamina papyracea can be established. The sinus should be visualized with angled telescopes. If the antrostomy is patent then it can be probed with a maxillary ostium seeker, making sure the angle of dissection is inferolateral and away from the orbit. The seeker can also be used to palpate the ascending process of the maxilla. A flexible fiberoptic endoscope can be helpful for visualization of the antrum via a small antrostomy.

If a retained uncinate process is visualized, it should be removed using a 90 Blakesley forceps, microdebrider, back-biting forceps, or down-biting forceps. Care must be taken to avoid injury to the nasolacrimal duct anteriorly. This region should be palpated with a maxillary ostium seeker prior to removal of any bony fragments. Remnants of the uncinate process can be gently medialized to help avoid damage to the nasolacrimal duct. If the natural maxillary ostium is obstructed, it can be enlarged using angled-through cutting forceps or Blakesley forceps. In the case of a maxillary antrostomy having been placed posteriorly, it should be brought into continuity with the natural ostium. This can be achieved by using through-cutting instruments to incise the soft tissue between the antrostomy and the natural ostia. It is helpful to remember that natural maxillary ostia are oblique – not in the same plane as the lateral nasal wall. Thus, visualization of the natural ostium with a 70 rigid endoscope is key to verify that it is in continuity with the newly created antrostomy.

- In cases of patients who suffer from failure of mucociliary transport, such as cystic fibrosis or Kartagener's syndrome, a large maxillary ostium is to be created that should encompass most of the medial wall of the maxillary sinus. This allows for copious nasal irrigation and drainage by gravity with appropriate head positioning.

In some cases a limited Caldwell-Luc approach for insertion of sinus instruments or endoscopes may be helpful to access disease located inferiorly or laterally within the maxillary sinus. The disease processes that may require such extended maneuvers include retained foreign bodies and fungal balls.

Finally, the maxillary sinus can have persistent disease from the infected secretions draining down from the frontal and ethmoid sinuses. Addressing the frontal/ethmoid disease is thus imperative in this situation.

Revision Ethmoid Sinus Surgery

Revision ethmoid sinus surgery seeks retained ethmoid cells, septae, and scarring that impairs mucociliary flow and clearance. In addition, foci of inflammatory mucosal disease and osteitis are identified and addressed. Care is taken to open residual air cells and their septae as well as to remove foci of inflammatory disease while sparing as much nasal mucosa as possible. The sphenoethmoid cell, the orbitoethmoid cell, and most anterior and superior ethmoid cells can be the most difficult and challenging cells to incorporate into the sinonasal cavity during revision ethmoid sinus surgery. When the bone has become markedly thickened from osteitis, part of the revision ethmoidectomy can be performed with a suction-irrigation drill [6].

As during primary FESS, it is imperative to identify the skull base, lamina papyracea, and sphenoid rostrum early during the surgical procedure. The preoperative CT scan is essential for the assessment of the integrity of the lamina papyracea and skull base, which may be thinned or eroded due to chronic disease or prior surgery. Some surgeons advocate finding the skull base in patients with extensive ethmoid disease or scarring by first entering the sphenoid sinus [7] and/or using image guidance to confirm its location.

If a bony skull-base defect is identified, MRI should be considered to determine whether a meningocele or encephalocele is present. Intrathecal injection of fluorescein may also be used to diagnose a meningocele and demonstrate a cerebrospinal fluid (CSF) leak.

Tips and Pearls to Avoid Complications

1. Recent radiographic studies must be present in the operating room and the surgeon should reference these materials before and during the surgery.
2. Key anatomic landmarks during revision maxillary sinus surgery include the floor of the orbit, lamina papyracea, superior attachment of the inferior turbinate, and ascending process of the maxilla.
3. Back-biting forceps, down-biting forceps, angled microdebrider, maxillary ostium seeker, and flexible fiberoptic endoscope are useful instruments when performing surgery in the previously operated maxillary sinus.
4. Key anatomic landmarks during revision ethmoid sinus surgery include the skull base, lamina papyracea, and face (rostrum) of the sphenoid.
5. The sphenoethmoid cell, the orbitoethmoid cell, and most anterior and superior ethmoid cells can be the most challenging and important cells for marsupialization into the sinonasal cavity during revision ethmoid sinus surgery.

Complications

Surgical complications of revision sinus surgery resonate those of primary sinus surgery. However, the revision surgeon should take special care in the surgical approach, as some of the normal anatomic landmarks may be absent or distorted by the previous surgery, and defects in the lamina and or skull base may be present.

Complications can be divided into local, orbital, skull base, and intracranial events [24]. Local events include bleeding and synechiae formation. Orbital complications include violation of the lamina papyracea, with orbital bleeding or injury to the medial rectus muscle, injury to the anterior ethmoid artery resulting in bleeding and/or orbital hematoma, and injury to the optic nerve. Skull-base injuries can manifest as an intraoperative or postoperative CSF leak and subsequent formation of a meningocele or encephalocele. Finally, intracranial injuries include subarachnoid hemorrhage, pseudoaneurysm, and extra-axial, parenchymal, or intravetricular hemorrhage. With the use of powered instrumentation, more severe complications can occur from inadvertent violation of the lamina or skull base.

Postoperative Care

- Aggressive medical therapy:
  1. Culture-directed antibiotics based on intraoperative microbiology specimen results.
  2. Systemic corticosteroids are often indicated. If eosinophil-predominant polyps and mucus point to an underlying allergic component, longer courses or frequent bursts may be indicated.
  3. Topical steroids. The physician should try to minimize oral steroid use and transition to a combination of topical and mechanical treatments as soon as the endoscopic exam findings allow.
  4. Sterile nasal saline irrigation.
  5. Management of underlying host and environmental factors, such as allergies.

- Meticulous postoperative debridement based upon endoscopic findings and close monitoring of the sinonasal mucosa.

- Close endoscopic follow-up with reevaluation of medical therapy based on exam findings:
  1. Endoscopic surveillance is an important tool in the postoperative care of revision sinus surgical patients.
  2. Medical therapy can be either tapered or reinitiated based on findings of mucosal inflammation, aeration, or secondary infection.

- Culture-directed antibiotic therapy for acute exacerbations of chronic rhinosinusitis.
- CT studies if the original symptoms persist or new symptoms occur that cannot be explained by endoscopic findings.

Outcomes

Moses et al. studied 90 revision FESS cases and reported a success rate of 67%. Extent of disease, history of polyps, allergy, previous traditional endonasal sinus surgery, male gender, chronic steroid use, and the presence of a deviated septum all appeared to adversely affect revision FESS outcome [16]. McMains and Kountakis studied 125 patients who underwent revision sinus surgery after failing both maximum medical therapy and prior sinus surgery for chronic rhinosinusitis. They followed their patients over a 3-year period and found an overall success rate of 92% when evaluating patient symptom scores, Sinonasal Outcome Test (SNOT-20), and nasal endoscopy scores. Patients with nasal polyposis were more apt to fail revision FESS than patients with other medical conditions [15]. We believe that close endoscopic monitoring of the patient's sinonasal cavities and timely treatment of early recurrent disease can help avoid repetitive surgeries.

References

1. Anand VK, Osguthorpe JD, Rice D (1997) Surgical management of adult rhinosinusitis. Otolaryngol Head Neck Surg 117:S50–S52
2. Bolger WE (1994) Gram negative sinusitis: an emerging clinical entity? Am J Rhinol 8:279–283
3. Bolinger WE, Woodruff WW, Parsons DS, et al. (1990) Maxillary sinus hypoplasia: classification and description of associated uncinate process hypoplasia. Otolaryngol Head Neck Surg 103:759–765
4. Chambers DW, Davis WE, Cook PR, et al. (1997) Long-term outcome analysis of functional endoscopic sinus surgery: correlation of symptoms with endoscopic examination findings and potential prognostic variables. Laryngoscope 107:504–510
5. Chu CT, Lebowitz RA, Jacobs JB (1997) An analysis of sites of disease in revision endoscopic sinus surgery. Am J Rhinol 11:287–291
6. Cohen NA, Kennedy DW(2006) Revision endoscopic sinus surgery. Otolaryngol Clin North Am 39:417–435
7. Cullen MM, Bolger WE (2001) Revision endoscopic sinus surgery for recurrent rhinosinusitis. In: Kennedy DW, Bolger WE, Zinreich SJ (eds) Diseases of the Sinuses. Diagnosis and Management. Decker, Hamilton, Ontario, Canada, pp 245–254
8. Davis WE, Templer JW, Lamear WR (1999) Middle meatus antrostomy: patency rates and risk factors. Otolaryngol Head Neck Surg 104:467–472
9. DeShazo RD, Chapin K, Swain RE (1997) Fungal sinusitis. N Engl J Med 337:254–259
10. Elwany S, Bassyouni M, Morad F (2002) Some risk factors fro refractory chronic sinusitis: an immunohistochemical and electron microscopic study. J Laryngol Otol 116:112–115
11. Fried MP, Moharir VM, Shin J, et al. (2002) Comparison of endoscopic sinus surgery with and without image guidance. Am J Rhinol 16:193–197
12. Hinohira Y, Yumoto E, Hyodo M, et al. (1995) Revision endoscopic sinus surgery – long-term follow up and operative findings. Nippon Jibiinkoka Gakkai Kaiho 98:1285–1290
13. Kennedy DW (1992) Prognostic factors, outcomes and staging in ethmoid sinus surgery. Laryngoscope 102:1–18
14. Levine HL (1990) Functional endoscopic sinus surgery: evaluation, surgery, and follow-up of 250 patients. Laryngoscope 100:79–84
15. McMains KC, Kountakis SE (2005) Revision functional endoscopic sinus surgery: objective and subjective surgical outcomes. Am J Rhinol 19:344–347
16. Moses RL, Cornetta A, Atkins JP Jr, et al. (1998) Revision endoscopic sinus surgery: the Thomas Jefferson University experience. Ear Nose Throat J 77:190, 193–195, 199–202
17. Musy PY, Kountakis SE (2004) Anatomic findings in patients undergoing revision endoscopic sinus surgery. Am J Otolaryngol 25:418–422
18. Nadel DM, Lanza DC, Kennedy DW (1998) Endoscopically guided cultures in chronic sinusitis. Am J Rhinol 12:233–241
19. Nishioka GJ, Cook PR, Davis WE, et al. (1994) Immunotherapy in patients undergoing functional endoscopic sinus surgery. Otolaryngol Head Neck Surg 110:406–412
20. Parsons DS, Nishioka GI (2001) Pediatric sinus surgery. In: Kennedy DW, Bolger WE, Zinreich SJ (2001) Diseases of the Sinuses: Diagnosis and Management. Decker, Hamilton, Ontario, pp 271–280

21. Parsons DS, Stivers FE, Talbot AR (1996) The missed ostium sequence and the surgical approach to revision functional endoscopic sinus surgery. Otolaryngol Clin North Am 29:169–183
22. Ramadan HH (1999) Surgical causes of failure in endoscopic sinus surgery. Laryngoscope 109:27–29
23. Wynn R, Har-El G (2004) Recurrence rates after endoscopic sinus surgery for massive sinus polyposis. Laryngoscope 114:811–813
24. Zeifer B (2002) Sinusitis: postoperative changes and surgical complications. Semin Ultrasound CT MR 23:475–491

Chapter 13

Revision Endoscopic Surgery of the Sphenoid Sinus

13

Richard R. Orlandi

Core Messages

- Revision sphenoid sinus surgery is usually most easily performed after a complete ethmoidectomy.
- The sphenoid sinus natural ostium can typically be found using the superior turbinate as a landmark, even in revision cases.
- Once a decision is made to enlarge the sphenoid sinus ostium, a maximally wide opening will minimize the risk of stenosis.
- Attempts at widening the natural ostium inferiorly and medially do not typically improve the chances of a patent ostium postoperatively and can lead to bleeding and unnecessary mucosal disruption.

Contents

Introduction

The need for revision of altered anatomic structures in the sphenoid region is not as common as in the ethmoid or frontal regions [5]. Nevertheless, even primary sphenoid sinus surgery challenges many sinus surgeons due to the proximity of the optic nerve and internal carotid artery. Landmarks in the posterior ethmoid sinus are few, making accurate identification of the natural ostium and verification of presence within the sphenoid sinus, not a posterior ethmoid cell, difficult. The alteration of the surgical field in revision sphenoid surgery serves to intensify these difficulties. While complications occur in 13% of sphenoidotomies overall and tend to be minor, the vast majority occur in revision cases [7].

Evaluation

Tips and Pearls

1. Sphenoid sinusitis following previous surgery is best evaluated both endoscopically and radiographically.
2. Many "revision sphenoidotomies" involve previously unopened sphenoid sinuses, where a posterior ethmoid cell was mistaken for the sphenoid sinus.
3. Thorough analysis of the cause of the previous failed sphenoidotomy minimizes the chances of it recurring.

Persistent or recurrent sphenoid disease may complicate up to 10% of primary sphenoidotomies [7]. Assessment of a previous sphenoidotomy can be achieved both radiographically and endoscopically. Because the anterior wall of the sphenoid sinus runs in the coronal plane, axial images are most helpful in assessing this structure. Review of coronal imaging may yield clues as to the cause of the sphenoidotomy failure, such as the presence of a sphenoethmoidal (Onodi) cell superior and lateral to the sphenoid sinus (Fig. 13.1).

Endoscopic evaluation of the sphenoid sinus is typically performed as part of a diagnostic nasal endoscopy in a patient who has undergone previous sinus surgery.

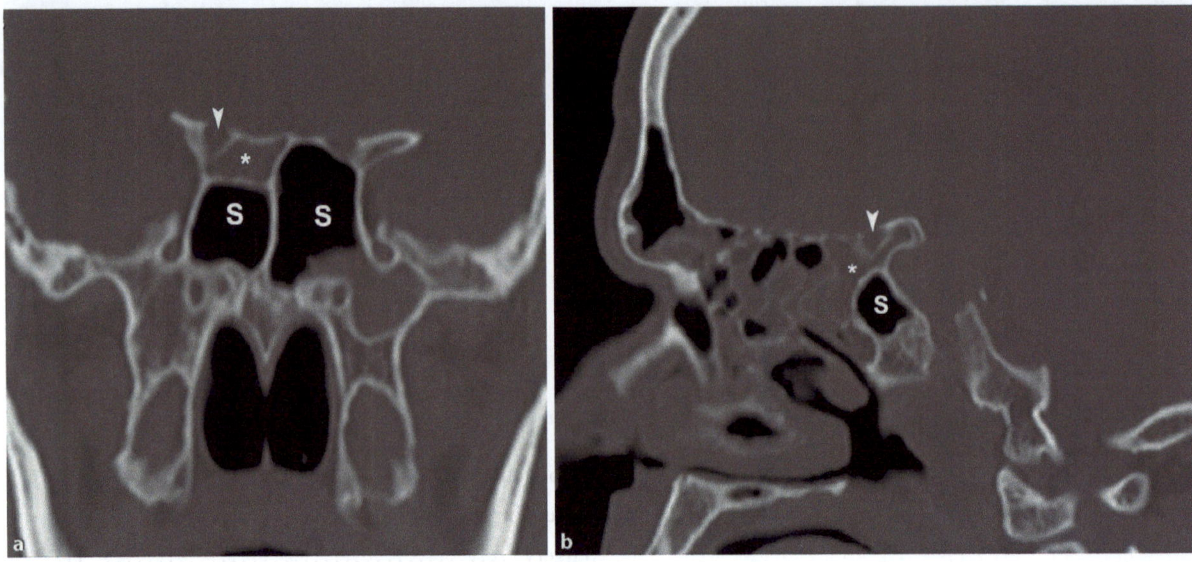

Fig. 13.1 Coronal (**a**) and sagittal (**b**) computed tomography (CT) scan of the sphenoid sinuses (*S*), demonstrating a right-sided sphenoethmoidal cell (*asterisk*). Note that the right optic nerve (*arrowhead*) runs in the lateral wall of the sphenoethmoidal cell, not the sphenoid sinus. In the sagittal image (**a**), the continuity of the sphenoethmoid cell with the remaining posterior ethmoid complex is clearly seen

13

Visualization of the surgical ostium of the sphenoid sinus is facilitated by using the middle and superior turbinates as reference landmarks. These two structures run in the same parasagittal plane and share a skull-base attachment, with the superior turbinate extending posteriorly and superiorly from the middle turbinate (Fig. 13.2) [6]. The superior turbinate forms a critical and nearly constant landmark for the sphenoid sinus [2]. Even patients who have undergone middle-turbinate resection will typically have a superior-turbinate remnant medially within the posterior ethmoid complex (Fig. 13.3).

The posterior ethmoid cavity should be assessed for persistent inflammation, which may contribute to continuing sphenoid rhinossinusitis. Scarring among residual posterior ethmoid partitions, particularly medially near the superior turbinate, indicates likely involvement of the sphenoid sinus drainage in the scarring. Occasionally purulence can be seen in the nasopharynx, descending vertically from the sphenoethmoidal recess (Fig. 13.4).

Planning for a revision sphenoidotomy begins with an analysis of why the previous surgical intervention failed. The first task in assessing patients with sphenoid sinus disease following previous sinus surgery is to determine whether the sphenoid sinus was indeed previously opened. During endoscopic sinus surgery, identification of the true sphenoid cavity can be challenging. Large posterior ethmoid cells and sphenoethmoidal (Onodi) cells can often be mistaken for the sphenoid sinus. In these cases, revision of the sphenoid sinus is not a true revision at all, but instead amounts to a primary sphenoidotomy via an operated posterior ethmoid sinus. Preoperative imaging can assist in determining if the sphenoid sinus was previously opened. The natural bone aperture of the sphenoid sinus ostium is typically only 3–4 mm in diameter so that a larger bone gap seen on imaging indicates a sphenoidotomy has likely been performed previously (Fig. 13.5). The natural ostium of the sphenoid sinus empties into the sphenoethmoidal recess, medial to the superior turbinate in all cases [4]. Openings in the sinus lateral to the superior turbinate indicate that the sinus has probably been previously opened surgically, but also that the opening probably did not include the natural ostium.

Other causes of failure can be seen on radiology as well as endoscopy. Previous sphenoidotomies may fail due to insufficient opening of the anterior sphenoid wall, excessive mucosal disruption with resulting scar contracture, and retained posterior ethmoid partitions and inflammation. Attention to these issues and learning from them reduces the chances of repeating them during revision surgery.

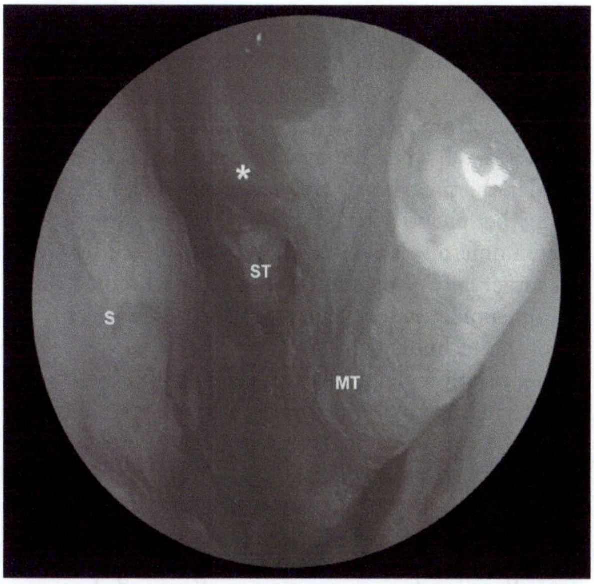

Fig. 13.2 Endoscopic view of the left middle (*MT*) and superior turbinates (*ST*) following a correction of a deviated nasal septum. The common skull base attachment of the turbinates (*asterisk*) is seen

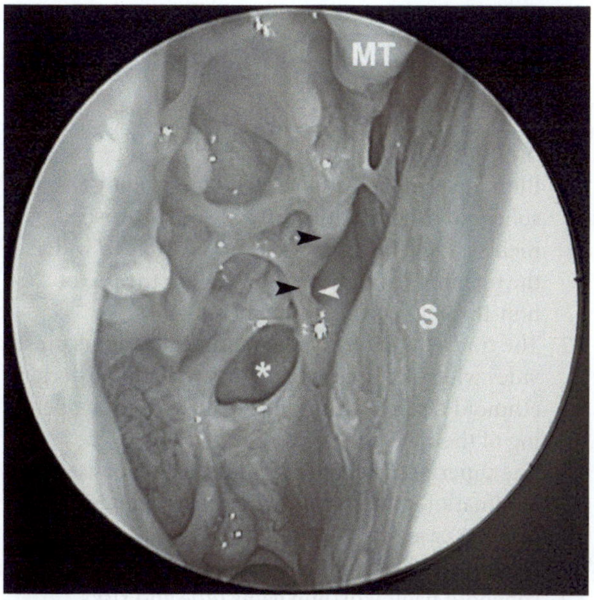

Fig. 13.3 Endoscopic view of the right ethmoid complex, demonstrating a partially resected middle turbinate and a superior turbinate remnant (*black arrowheads*). A posterior ethmoid cell (*asterisk*) is seen lateral to the superior turbinate remnant, and the sphenoid ostium (*white arrowhead*) is seen medial to it

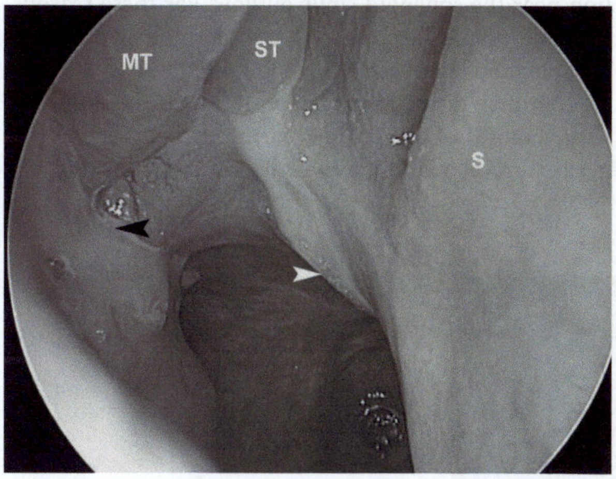

Fig. 13.4 Endoscopic view of the right nasopharynx. Purulence is seen emanating from the sphenoethmoidal recess (*white arrowhead*), between the superior turbinate and the septum. Purulence from the middle meatus (*black arrowhead*) is also seen, lateral to the middle turbinate

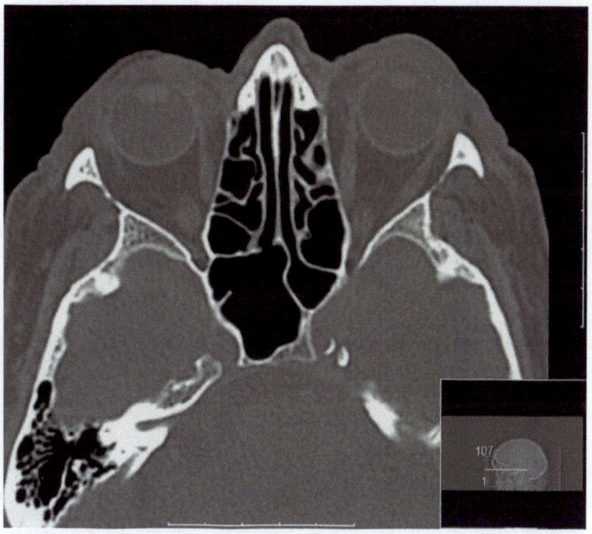

Fig. 13.5 Axial CT scan of the sphenoid and ethmoid sinuses. The sphenoid ostium opens medial to the superior turbinate (continuous with the more anterior middle turbinate at this level) and has about a 3-mm opening. The scale at the bottom of this figure is in centimeters

Surgery

Tips and Pearls

1. Blunt instruments can be useful for probing the sphenoid ostium, while through-cutting instruments should be used whenever possible to widen the opening. Thick bone may require the use of non-through-cutting instruments.
2. The transethmoid route to the sphenoid sinus provides wider access and addresses residual posterior ethmoid disease. This route facilitates a wide opening of the sphenoid sinus.
3. The superior turbinate provides a nearly constant landmark for the sphenoid natural ostium, even in revision cases.
4. Mucosal disruption medial and inferior to the sphenoid natural ostium gains little and risks circumferential stenosis.

Instrumentation for revision surgery of the sphenoid sinus is similar to that of primary sphenoidotomy (Fig. 13.6). Blunt instruments for probing can be helpful in safely identifying the previous surgical ostium, while forceps that cut close to the coronal plane assist in widening the ostium maximally. Through-cutting punches are much preferred over grasping instruments in order to maximally preserve mucosa and thus speed healing postoperatively. Occasionally the thick bone of the anterior sphenoid wall necessitates the use of Kerrison punches, but this is uncommon. In these rare cases, great care must be employed to avoid unnecessary mucosal loss. Powered cutting instruments should be used with great care, if at all, in the sphenoid region due to the potential for injury to the internal carotid artery and optic nerve. These structures, found in the lateral wall of the sphenoid sinus, lack a bone covering in a substantial number of patients. Cutting instruments that are designed to avoid injuring the lateral wall while removing the anterior wall are preferred in this area. Image guidance can be helpful in identifying the sphenoid sinus among posterior ethmoid cells where numerous landmarks have been altered by previous surgery. Revision surgery, posterior ethmoidectomy, and sphenoidotomy are all acceptable indications for the use of this technology [1].

Preoperative medical therapy should be directed at minimizing mucosal inflammation in order to diminish bleeding. Oxymetazoline spray is given just before surgery and is used throughout surgery on cotton pledgets to control hemorrhage. Injection of 1:100,000 epinephrine into the area of the sphenopalatine artery as it enters the nose significantly diminishes bleeding during sphenoidotomy [3, 9].

The route to the sphenoid sinus can be either transnasal – medial to the middle turbinate – or transethmoid – lateral to the middle turbinate. The transnasal route is more direct and does not require a total ethmoidectomy. However, the narrowness of the space between the middle turbinate and nasal septum typically requires fracture lateralization or resection of the middle turbinate. Leaving the posterior ethmoid cells intact also limits the extent to which the sphenoid sinus ostium can be widened laterally and potentially ignores a source of continued inflammation near the sphenoid sinus outflow. For these reasons, the author typically prefers the transethmoid approach to the sphenoid sinus, especially in revision cases.

Thorough dissection of the posterior ethmoid sinuses, with removal of all residual partitions between the superior turbinate and lamina papyracea, facilitates iden-

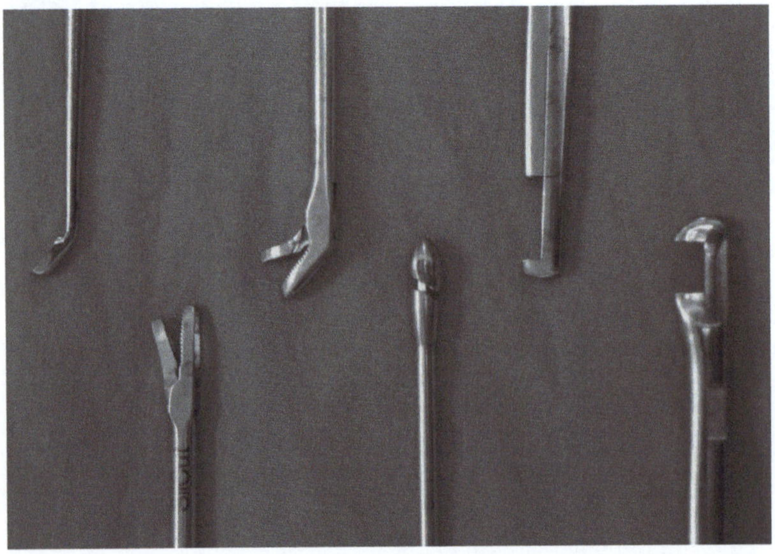

Fig. 13.6 Instruments useful for revision endoscopic sphenoid sinus surgery

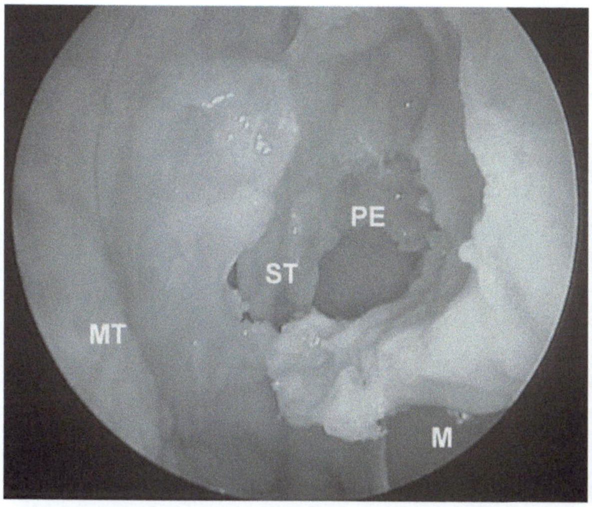

Fig. 13.7 Endoscopic view of the dissected left anterior and posterior ethmoid sinuses, using a 0 telescope placed lateral to the middle turbinate. The superior turbinate is seen directly posterior to the middle turbinate, in the medial portion of the posterior ethmoid sinuses (*PE*). The maxillary sinus (*M*) has also been opened. Adapted from Orlandi et al. [6]. Used with permission, OceanSide Publications

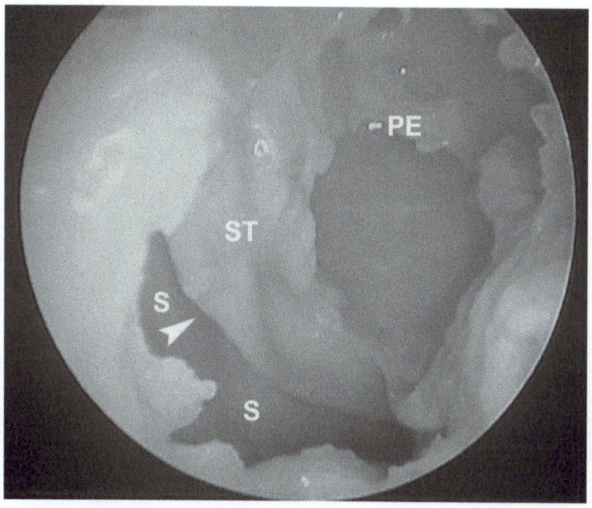

Fig. 13.8 Closer view of the superior turbinate, showing the sphenoethomidal recess (*arrowhead*) between the superior turbinate and the septum (*S*). Adapted from Orlandi et al. [6]. Used with permission, OceanSide Publications

tification and maximal opening of the sphenoid sinus. The superior turbinate is identified medially within the posterior ethmoid field, posterior to the middle turbinate (Figs. 13.7 and 13.8). This landmark reliably identifies the anterior wall of the sphenoid sinus and, if its inferior 3–4 mm are removed, facilitates identification of the sphenoid natural ostium (Fig. 13.9).

Some surgeons prefer to enter the sphenoid sinus medial to the superior turbinate (through the natural ostium), while others enter lateral to the superior turbinate [2, 6]. In revising the sphenoidotomy, the previous ostium should be sought and widened maximally. Cutting instruments are used to widen the opening laterally toward the lamina papyracea, and superiorly to the skull base. Palpating behind each partition prior to its removal reduces the risk of dissection beyond the limits of the sphenoid and posterior ethmoid sinuses. Maximal widening medially entails incorporating the sphenoid natural ostium while preserving the majority of the superior turbinate, thus reducing the risk of olfactory loss (Fig. 13.10) [8].

The vomer joins the pneumatized body of the sphenoid just medial to the sphenoid ostia. The thickness of the bone in this area precludes extension of the sphenoidotomy medial to the natural ostium with conventional instrumentation. Likewise, the clivus rapidly increases in thickness inferior to the sphenoid natural ostium, making inferior extension of the sphenoidotomy difficult. Wound contracture that takes place during the normal healing process tends to close circumferential defects, making it desirable to leave as much ostial mucosa intact while maximally widening the opening. For this reason only superior and lateral widening, with its inherent disruption of the ostial mucosa is recommended. Inferior and medial widening has nearly no advantage in typical cases and greatly increases the risk of stenosis or complete closure. Moreover, dissection inferior to the sphenoid ostium endangers bleeding from the septal branch of the sphenopalatine artery, which crosses the sphenoid anterior wall 2–3 mm below the ostium.

Postoperative Care and Outcomes

Tips and Pearls

1. Postoperative diagnostic endoscopy, possibly with debridement, is as important with revision sphenoid sinus surgery as it is following any endoscopic sinus procedure.
2. While outcome data for revision sinus surgery is lacking, patency rates appear to diminish over time, necessitating a sufficiently long follow-up to determine success.
3. Like any endoscopic sinus surgery, revision sphenoidotomy requires postoperative nasal endoscopy to debride crusting and retained secretions, and to guide medical therapy.

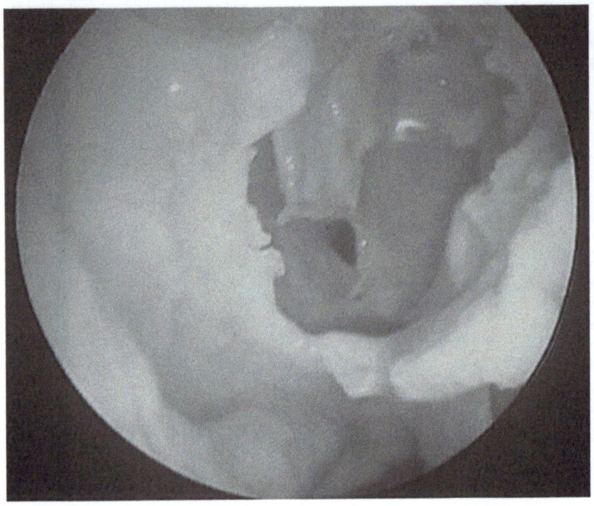

Fig. 13.9 The inferior portion of the superior turbinate has been sharply resected, showing the sphenoid ostium. Adapted from Orlandi et al. [6]. Used with permission, OceanSide Publications

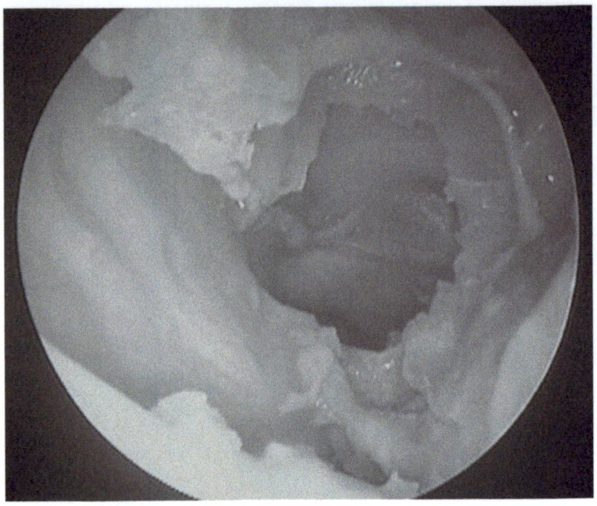

Fig. 13.10 The sphenoid anterior wall has been removed superior and lateral to the natural ostium. No dissection has taken place inferior or medial to the natural ostium and the superior turbinate remnant is intact. Adapted from Orlandi RR [6]. Used with permission, OceanSide Publications

Removal of crusts within the sphenoid opening, either with saline irrigation or debridement (or both), is essential to remove accumulated fibrin and other debris. These items can act as a scaffold for matrix deposition within the wound, with eventual scarring and stenosis. They can also impede secretion transport out of the sinus, favoring bacterial colonization and perpetuating inflammation. Postoperative medical therapy is aimed at reducing this inflammation and is managed according to the endoscopic appearance of the sphenoid and posterior ethmoid sinuses at each visit.

Outcome data for revision sphenoid sinus surgery is generally lacking. It is essential in evaluating patient success that sufficiently long follow-up be performed. As for the frontal sinus, the patency of the sphenoid sinus ostium can diminish over time. One study evaluated 74 patients following endoscopic sphenoidotomy and found 100% sphenoid patency at 1 month postoperatively. The patency rate decreased to 82% over the ensuing follow-up period, which ranged from 6 months to nearly 6 years [7].

Conclusion

Revision endoscopic surgery of the sphenoid sinus is challenging due to its anatomic relationships. The superior turbinate forms a reliable landmark in endoscopic sphenoid sinus surgery, even in revision cases. The ability to widen the sphenoid ostium is confined medially and inferiorly by thick bone. Once mucosal disruption of the sphenoid ostium has taken place, a maximally wide opening is encouraged in order to minimize the risk of postoperative stenosis due to wound contracture. The risk of complications appears to be higher in revision versus primary sphenoid sinus surgery, and a sufficiently long endoscopic follow-up period is necessary to ensure the patency of the surgical ostium.

References

1. AAO-HNS policy on intra-operative use of computer-aided surgery (2005) [cited 2007]. Available from: http://www.entlink.net/practice/rules/imageguiding.cfm
2. Bolger WE, Keyes AS, Lanza DC (1999) Use of the superior meatus and superior turbinate in the endoscopic approach to the sphenoid sinus. Otolaryngol Head Neck Surg 120:308–313
3. Douglas R, Wormald PJ (2006) Pterygopalatine fossa infiltration through the greater palatine foramen: where to bend the needle. Laryngoscope 116:1255–1257
4. Millar DA, Orlandi RR (2006) The sphenoid sinus natural ostium is consistently medial to the superior turbinate Am J Rhinol 20:180–181

5. Musy PY, Kountakis SE (2004) Anatomic findings in patients undergoing revision endoscopic sinus surgery Am J Otolaryngol 25:418–422
6. Orlandi RR, Lanza DC, Bolger WE, et al. (1999) The forgotten turbinate: the role of the superior turbinate in endoscopic sinus surgery Am J Rhinol 13:251–259
7. Rosen FS, Sinha UK, Rice DH (1999) Endoscopic surgical management of sphenoid sinus disease Laryngoscope 109:1601–1606
8. Say P, Leopold D, Cochran G, et al. (2004) Resection of the inferior superior turbinate: does it affect olfactory ability or contain olfactory neuronal tissue? Am J Rhinol 18:157–160
9. Wormald PJ, Athanasiadis T, Rees G, et al. (2005) An evaluation of effect of pterygopalatine fossa injection with local anesthetic and adrenalin in the control of nasal bleeding during endoscopic sinus surgery Am J Rhinol 19:288–292

Chapter 14

Endoscopic and Microscopic Revision Frontal Sinus Surgery

14

Ulrike Bockmühl and Wolfgang Draf

Core Messages

- There must be a reasonable correlation between a patient's complaints and radiologic findings.
- High-resolution computed tomography and magnetic resonance imaging are the most valid imaging modalities.
- Revision surgery is most often necessary due to incomplete removal of obstructing agger nasi cells, superior attachment of the ethmoid bulla or uncinate process (incomplete anterior ethmoidectomy), lateralization of middle-turbinate remnants, neo-osteogenesis of the frontal recess, and polypoid mucosa obscuring the recess.
- Endonasal revision frontal sinus surgery requires detailed anatomical knowledge.
- In the majority of patients revision can be managed successfully via the endonasal route by performing Draf's type I–III drainages.
- In aspirin triad, patients with severe polyposis, Draf's type III drainage is indicated as the first revision procedure.
- Contraindications for endonasal frontal sinus revision surgery are anterior–posterior dimension less than 0.5 cm, inadequate surgical training, and lack of proper instrumentation.
- The external osteoplastic, mostly obliterative frontal sinus operation must be part of the armamentarium of the experienced sinus surgeon for the resolution of exceptionally difficult frontal sinus problems.

Contents

Introduction

Chronic frontal sinusitis is a disease that continues to pose a significant challenge to surgeons despite considerable advances in instrumentation and surgical techniques [4, 5, 11, 31, 33]. Primary endoscopic or microscopic sinus surgery can often result in scarring of the frontal recess, especially when there is an incomplete removal of obstructing agger nasi cells, superior attachment of the ethmoid bulla, or uncinate process [3, 5]. Failure to recognize frontal recess cells and supraorbital ethmoid cells can mislead the surgeon into believing the frontal recess has been opened. Other common causes of failure of primary surgery, including lateralization of middle-turbinate remnants, neo-osteogenesis of the frontal recess, and polypoid mucosa obscuring the recess, all contribute to the difficulty and danger of revision surgery [4]. Historically, surgeons treating recurrent or persistent frontal sinus disease advocated either reestablishing drainage from an intranasal approach, reestablishing drainage from an external approach, or obliteration of the sinus. Since the introduction of endoscopic technology to manage paranasal sinus diseases, interest in reestablishing drainage from an intranasal approach has flourished and several endoscopic techniques, many bearing a resemblance to procedures developed by Draf [6], have been described. These include:

1. Anterior ethmoidectomy without alteration of the frontal ostium itself (i.e., drainage type I according to Draf) [6].
2. Endoscopic frontal sinusotomy according to Stammberger and Posawetz, characterized as "uncapping the egg" [32].
3. Enlargement of the frontal ostium medially until the middle turbinate (i.e., drainage type IIa according to Draf) [6].
4. Removal of the entire frontal floor on one side until the nasal septum in front of the olfactory fossa (i.e., drainage type IIb according to Draf) [6].
5. Median drainage of frontal sinuses removing both frontal sinus floors, upper nasal septum, and septum (septa, if several) sinuum frontalium (i.e., drainage type III according to Draf or endoscopic modified Lothrop procedure) [6, 13].

In general, the first two procedures are indicated in primary surgery, techniques 3 and 4 mainly in revision cases, and Draf's type III drainage and the modified Lothrop procedure are most often performed as rescue surgery. Using maximal medical therapy, a stepwise progression from less to more invasive procedures, and an aggressive postoperative regimen of debridement, excellent results can be achieved treating this difficult clinical problem.

14

Indications for revision surgery:

- Persistent chronic frontal rhinossinusitis as failure of appropriate medical therapy and/or previous surgery due to polypoid mucosa obscuring the recess.
- Persistent chronic frontal sinusitis due to anatomical particularities after previous surgery (e.g., persistent agger nasi cells, superior attached ethmoid bulla or uncinate process, lateralization of the middle turbinate, and neo-osteogenesis of the frontal recess).
- Patients with aspirin triad (i.e., polyposis, aspirin intolerance, and bronchial asthma).
- Frontal sinus mucoceles.
- Primary or recurrent tumors (i.e., inverted papilloma, osteoma, ossifying fibroma, and malignancies).

Contraindications:

- Narrow anterior–posterior (AP) dimension of the frontal sinus floor, hypoplastic frontal sinus.
- Failure of adequate endonasal type III drainage.
- Patients with aspirin triad and condition after several endonasal revision procedures.
- Inexperience of the surgeon.
- Unavailability of proper instrumentation.

Preoperative Workup

The decision for revision surgery is not easy to make for either the patient or the surgeon. If the patient complains about persistent or recurrent symptoms like frontal headache, reduced smelling or nasal obstruction, endoscopy of the nose is indicated first followed by magnetic resonance imaging (MRI) verification and, in case of likelihood for revision surgery, computed tomography (CT) scans should be performed. CT images should be scanned in the axial direction with a maximum of 0.65-mm sections, and from there, coronal as well as sagittal views should be reconstructed. The most common sign of persistent or recurrent disease is mucosal thickening within the frontal recess and/or sinus.

- Anatomic evaluation of the frontal sinus region with CT scans is key to the feasibility and safety of endoscopic or microscopic revision frontal sinus surgery.

CT scans should reveal the number and location of frontal recess air cells, as well as barriers that have to be removed to reach the internal frontal sinus ostium [10, 39].

The coronal CT views are excellent to determine the following structures:

- Remaining agger nasi cells or neo-osteogenesis of the frontal recess (Fig. 14.1).
- Superior uncinate process.
- Depth of the olfactory fossa.
- Anterior ethmoid artery.
- Bulla frontalis (cell above the agger nasi with expansion into the frontal sinus; Fig. 14.1b).
- Supraorbital ethmoid cells

Sagittal and axial CT views are important to determine the following structures:

- AP dimension of the frontal recess (Figs. 14.2 and 14.3).
- Frontal recess.
- Supraorbital ethmoid cells.
- Bulla frontalis (cell above the agger nasi with expansion into the frontal sinus).
- Interseptal frontal sinus cell.

The important anatomic AP dimension is the distance from the nasal bones at the root of the nose to the anterior skull base [12, 14, 19, 36]. This dimension includes the AP thickness of the nasal beak and the distance from the beak to the anterior skull base. Recently, it was determined that an accessible dimension of at least 5 mm is required to allow safe removal of the nasal beak and frontal sinus floor [10]. An accessible dimension less than 5 mm would preclude the patient's candidacy for endo-

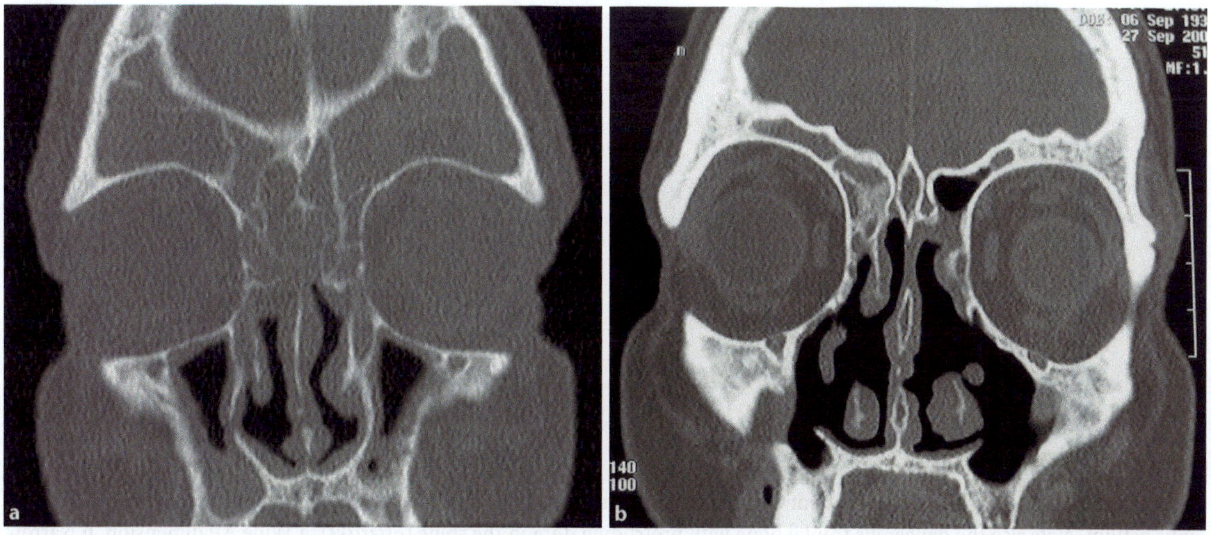

Fig. 14.1 **a** Coronal computed tomography (CT) view showing a recurrent chronic pansinusitis including the frontals sinuses. Above the agger nasi cells left after previous operation there are cells with expansion into the frontal sinus (bullae frontales). **b** Coronal CT scan showing neo-osteogenesis of the right frontal recess

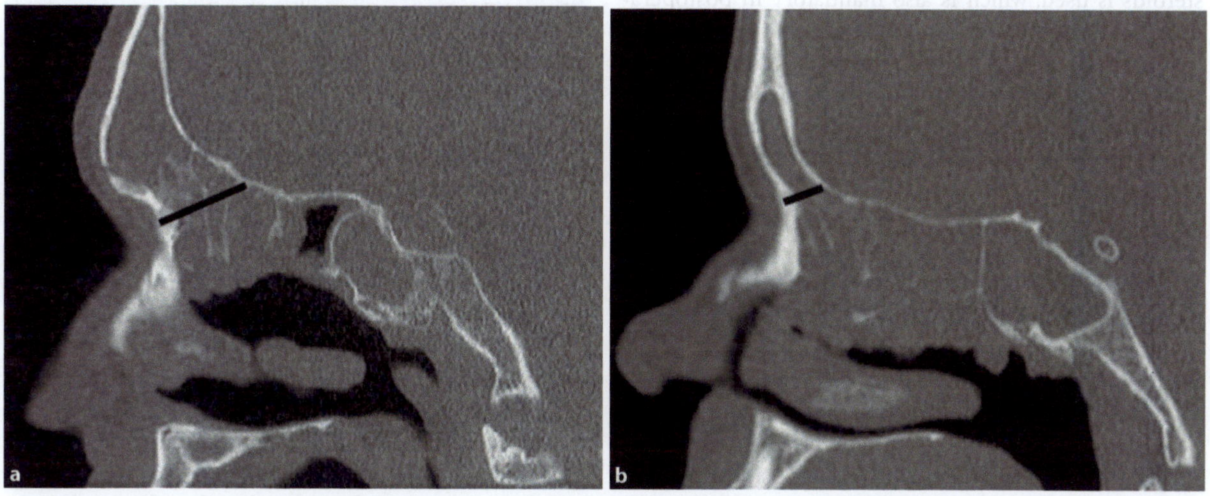

Fig. 14.2 Sagittal CT views showing persistent chronic sinusitis after incomplete ethmoidectomy, and demonstrating different anterior to posterior (AP) dimensions of the frontal recess (*black bar*). **a** Wide AP dimension. **b** Narrow AP dimension

nasal frontal sinus surgery. Furthermore, it is of utmost importance to analyze the images for dangerous anatomical findings like skull-base and lamina papyracea defects or a very deep cribriform plate. Recognizing the so-called dangerous frontal bone decreases the danger of creating a dural defect when removing an incomplete frontal sinus septum (Fig. 14.3a).

Whenever possible the updated images should be compared with the previous ones. However, there must be a reasonable correlation between patients' complaints and radiologic findings (i.e., it should not be forgotten that the surgeon operates patients and not CTs or MRIs). In case of headaches, neurological consultation is sometimes important, particularly if the patient reports about migraine in the family.

- Prior to surgery, the patient's underlying condition causing frontal sinus disease should be optimized medically.

Therefore, a selective combination of nasal irrigations, antibiotics, leukotriene antagonists, topical, and/or oral

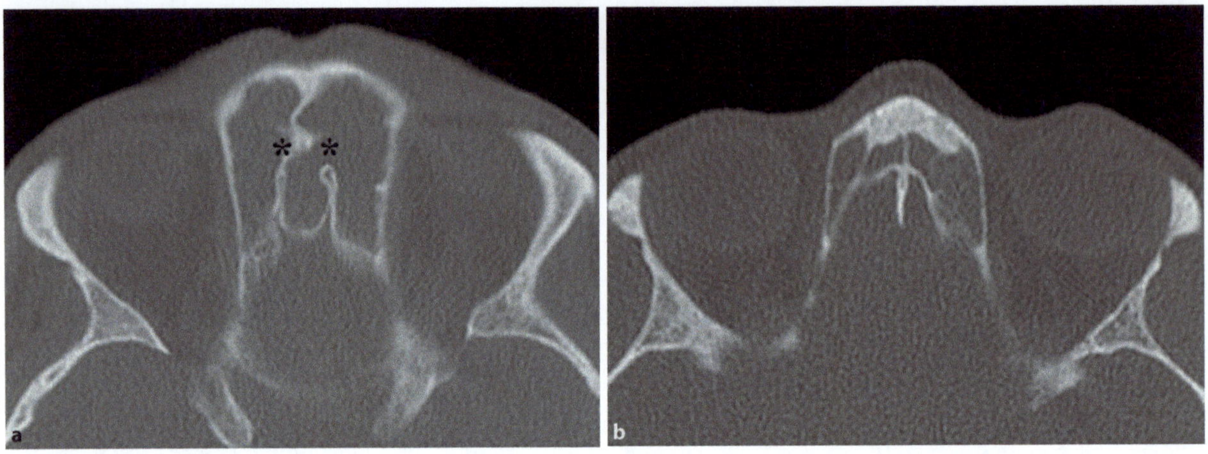

Fig. 14.3 Axial CT views showing persistent chronic frontal sinusitis, and demonstrating different AP dimensions of the frontal sinus ostium. Note also the dangerous frontal bone with protruding dura in the spine (*asterisks*). **a** Wide AP dimension. **b** Narrow AP dimension

steroids is used, which is also mandatory in postoperative care to prevent restenosis, leading to another disease recurrence. This is especially important for patients with more aggressive disease (i.e., aspirin triad patients). In preparation for surgery, these patients regularly take 50 mg prednisone per day for the 10 immediately preoperative days.

Surgical Technique

Once revision surgery is indicated, careful individual planning is essential to decide whether the endonasal technique is still suitable or an external procedure should be preferred. In case of endonasal revision frontal sinus surgery, in our hands a stepwise progression from less (Draf's type I or IIa/b drainages) to more invasive procedures (Draf's type III drainage) has stood the test of time [6, 8, 9, 14, 18, 36]. For the Draf III drainage to be successful, special surgical equipment is necessary: 45° angled endoscope with irrigation and suction, angled instruments, suction irrigation drills (between 35° and 70°), and computer image guidance is often helpful.

General anesthesia is required for revision frontal sinus surgery. In addition, topical decongestion helps to provide a dry field. The nasal cavities are first decongested using topical xylometazoline, and then the septum and the lateral nasal wall at the agger nasi are injected with up to 12 ml of 1% lidocaine and 1:200,000 epinephrine solution. The extent and type of local decongestant applied depends on the medical condition of each individual patient.

Type I Drainage According to Draf

In general, prior to surgery on the frontal recess and sinus, at least an anterior, but better a complete ethmoidectomy has to be performed. It is important to remove all agger nasi cells. To minimize the risk of complications it is essential to visualize the attachment of the middle turbinate medially, the lamina papyracea laterally, and the anterior skull base with the anterior ethmoid artery superiorly. It should be kept in mind that in revision surgery the anatomy is significantly distorted and landmarks such as the middle turbinate may be partially resected, making them unreliable for anatomic localization. However, it should be remembered that the skull base is usually most easily identified in the posterior ethmoid or sphenoid sinus, where it is horizontal and the ethmoid cells are larger. Care always needs to be taken at the ethmoid roof near the anterior ethmoid artery and toward the attachment of the middle turbinate, as the skull base is thinnest in this area. Therefore, one should stay close and parallel to the lamina papyracea, opening one or two supraorbital ethmoid cells that are located anterior to the vessel. Once the frontal recess has been clearly identified, adjacent bony partitions can be fractured and teased out, which is as important as the preservation of mucosa. This opening corresponds to a simple drainage or type I drainage according to Draf (Fig. 14.4). An alternative when the middle turbinate has been retracted laterally due to previous surgery and is obstructing the frontal sinus drainage, is the so-called "frontal sinus rescue procedure" by Kuhn et al. [20].

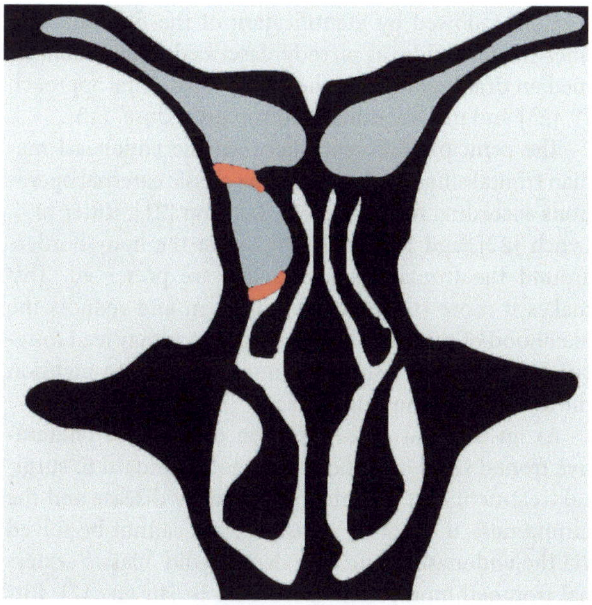

Fig. 14.4 Schematic illustration of a type I drainage according to Draf. The structures marked in *red* are those that have to be resected

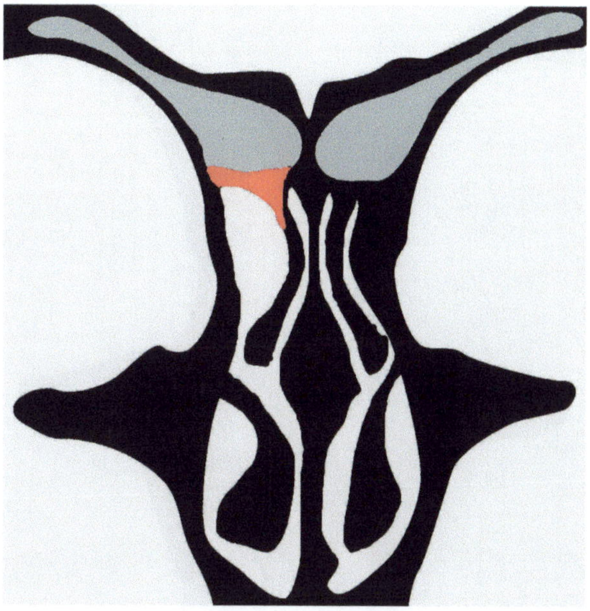

Fig. 14.5 Schematic illustration of a type II drainage according to Draf. The structures marked in *red* are those that have to be resected

Type II Drainage According to Draf

Type II drainage according to Draf (Fig. 14.5) is an extended drainage procedure that is achieved by resecting the floor of the frontal sinus between the lamina papyracea and the middle turbinate (type IIa) or the nasal septum (type IIb) anterior the ventral margin of the olfactory fossa either with the punch, curette, or with angled forceps [36]. Hosemann et al. [14, 15] showed in a detailed anatomical study that the maximum diameter of a neo-ostium of the frontal sinus (type IIa), which could be gained using a spoon or a curette, was 11 mm, with an average of 5.6 mm. If one needs to achieve a larger drainage opening like type IIb, one has to use a drill because of the increasing thickness of the bone going more medially toward the nasal septum. Care is needed to ensure that the frontal sinus opening is left bordered by bone on all sides and that the mucosa is preserved at least on one part of the circumference. In case one feels the type IIa drainage opening is too small with regard to the underlying pathology, it is better to perform the type IIb drainage. The wide approach to the ethmoid is obtained by exposing the lacrimal bone and reducing it as well as parts of the agger nasi and part of the frontal process of the maxilla until the lamina papyracea is clearly visible.

Type III Drainage According to Draf

Type III drainage according to Draf (Fig. 14.6) is a median drainage procedure that involves removal of the upper part of the nasal septum and the lower part of the frontal sinus septum or septa, if there is more than one, in addition to the type IIb drainage of both frontal sinuses (Fig. 14.7). To achieve the maximum possible opening of the frontal sinus it is very helpful to identify the first olfactory fibers on both sides: the middle turbinate is exposed and cut, millimeter by millimeter, from anterior to posterior along its origin at the skull base. After about 10–15 mm one will see the first olfactory fiber coming out of a little bony hole. Finally, the so-called "frontal T" [7] results (Fig. 14.8). Its long crus is represented by the posterior border of the perpendicular ethmoid lamina resection, the shorter wings on both sides are provided by the posterior margins of the frontal sinus floor resection. This provides an excellent landmark for the anterior border of the olfactory fossa on both sides, which allows the completion of frontal sinus floor resection close to the first olfactory fiber. In difficult revision cases one can begin the type III drainage primarily from two starting points, either from the lateral side, as already described, or from medially. The primary lateral approach is recommended if the previous ethmoidectomy was incomplete and the middle turbinate is still present as a landmark.

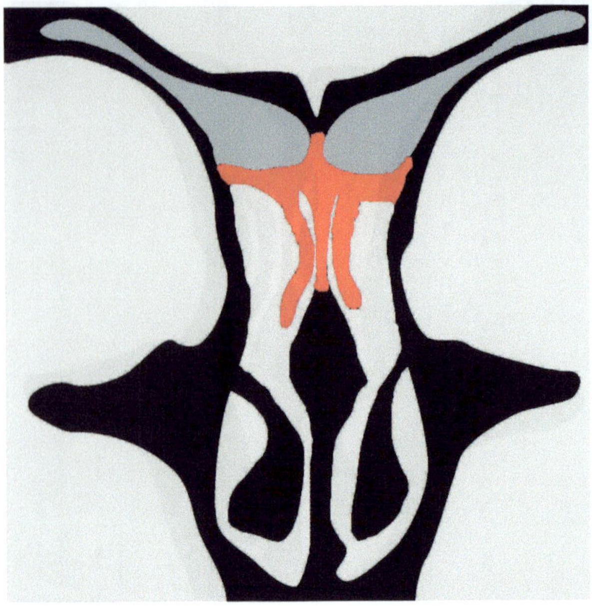

Fig. 14.6 Schematic illustration of a type III drainage according to Draf. The structures marked in *red* are those that have to be resected

One should adopt the primary medial approach if the ethmoid has been cleared and/or if the middle turbinate is absent. The primary medial approach begins with the partial resection of the perpendicular plate of the nasal septum, followed by identification of the first olfactory fiber on each side, as already described. The endonasal median drainage corresponds with nasofrontal approach IV [23] and the "modified Lothrop procedure" [13].

The principle difference between the endonasal median frontal sinus drainage and the classic external operations according to Jansen [17], Lothrop [21], Ritter [27], Lynch [22], and Howarth [16] is that the bony borders around the frontal sinus drainage are preserved. This makes it more stable in the long term and reduces the likelihood of reclosure by scarring, which may lead to recurrent frontal sinusitis or a mucocele, not to mention the avoidance of an external scar.

As an external procedure, the osteoplastic obliterative frontal sinus operation is the gold standard in surgical treatment of a chronic inflammatory disease and the ultima ratio if a frontal sinus problem cannot be solved via the endonasal route. The decades-old "classic" external frontoethmoidectomy according to Jansen [17], Ritter [27], Lynch [22], or Howarth [16], achieved via an infraeyebrow incision, has to be judged as "obsolete" since the frequency of postoperative mucoceles increases with the duration of postoperative follow up, to 40% and more. The strategy of the osteoplastic obliterative operation is to remove very meticulously all mucosa of the frontal sinuses using a microscope and endoscope as visual aids. The naked eye is not sufficient! Ear cartilage and fascia are used to create a reliable barrier between the nose and ethmoid on one side and the frontal sinus on the other. Then the frontal sinuses have to be filled with freshly harvested

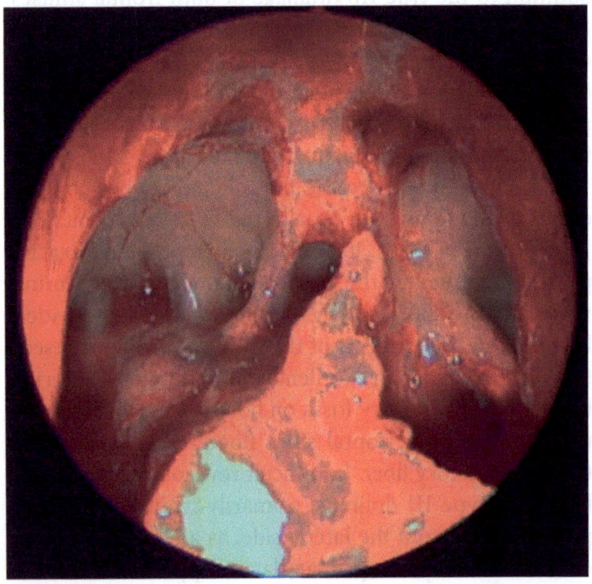

Fig. 14.7 Intraoperative condition after opening the frontal sinuses in the way of a type III drainage according to Draf (median drainage)

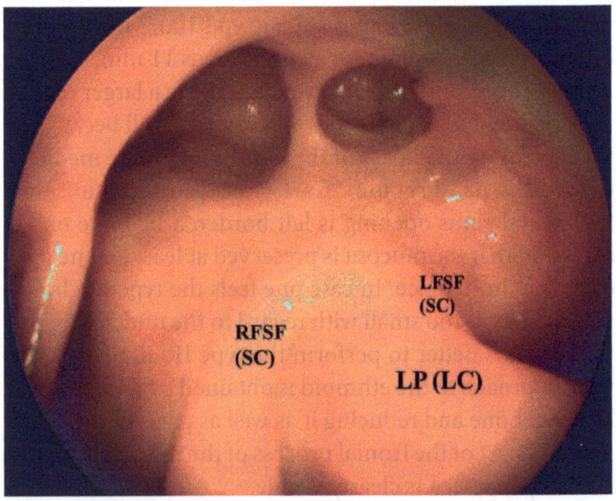

Fig. 14.8 Schematic illustration of the "frontal T" according to Draf. *LC* long crus, *LFSF* left frontal sinus floor, *LP* lamina perpendicularis, *RFSF* right frontal sinus floor, *SC* short crus

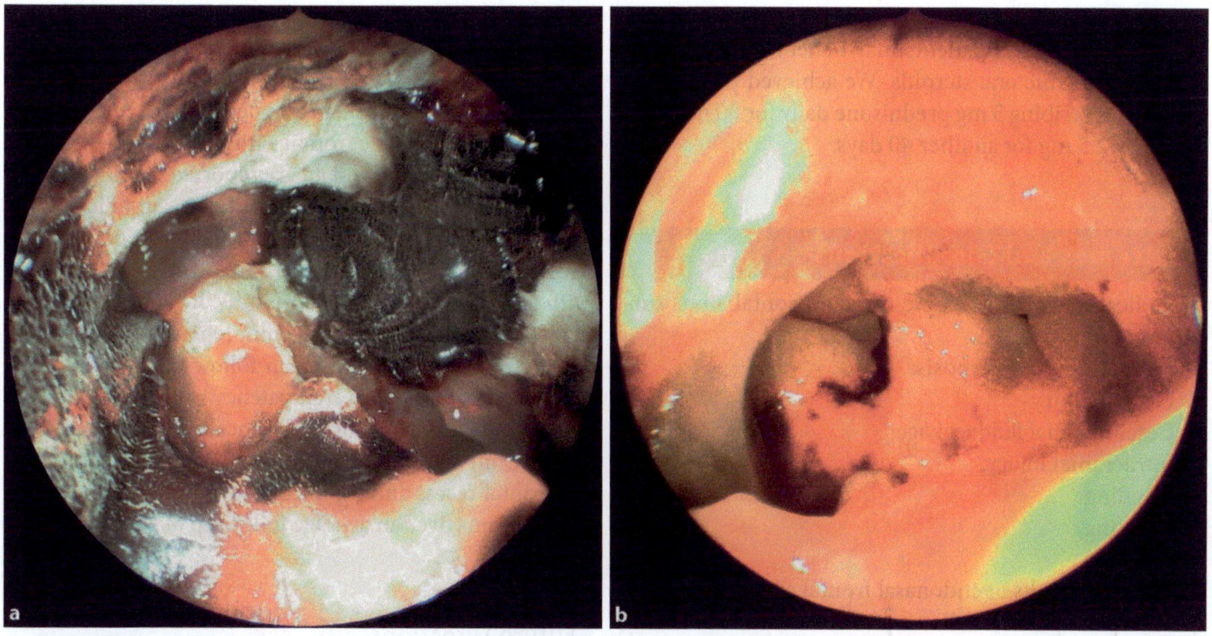

Fig. 14.9 Conditions around the 7th postoperative day showing differences in wound healing. **a** Severe crusting. **b** Mild crusting with swollen mucosa

autogenic fat in smaller cubes. By this method the frontal sinuses are excluded from the paranasal sinus system [2]. In experienced hands the rate of postoperative mucocele does not exceed 10% [34].

Postoperative Care

Rubber finger stalls are used as nasal packages that will be left in place for 5 days in type III drainage and 3 days in type II drainages. Some authors advocated the use of soft, flexible silicone stents in cases of a frontal sinus neo-ostium less than 5 mm in diameter, since more rigid silicone tubes have not given satisfying results [26, 28, 37, 38]. So far, the techniques using soft silicone drainage devices have not shown promising results in long-term observations.

All patients with type III drainage are placed on postoperative antibiotics (our preferred choice is clarithromycin) for at least 5 days. After removing the packing, patients are instructed to perform nasal saline irrigations twice daily until healing is complete. The degree of crusting can be very different (Fig. 14.9). In general, leaving rubber finger stalls for longer reduces crusting because faster re-epithelization is stimulated, like in a moistened chamber. In addition, all patients receive an intranasal steroid spray, and they are requested to use it for at least 3 months. Endoscopic debridement is performed in the office setting 1 and 2 weeks after surgery and is repeated every 2 weeks thereafter until the crusting disappears. We achieve better results and less painful postoperative treatment by being less aggressive and removing only mobile crusts. Figure 14.10 shows an optimal postoperative result.

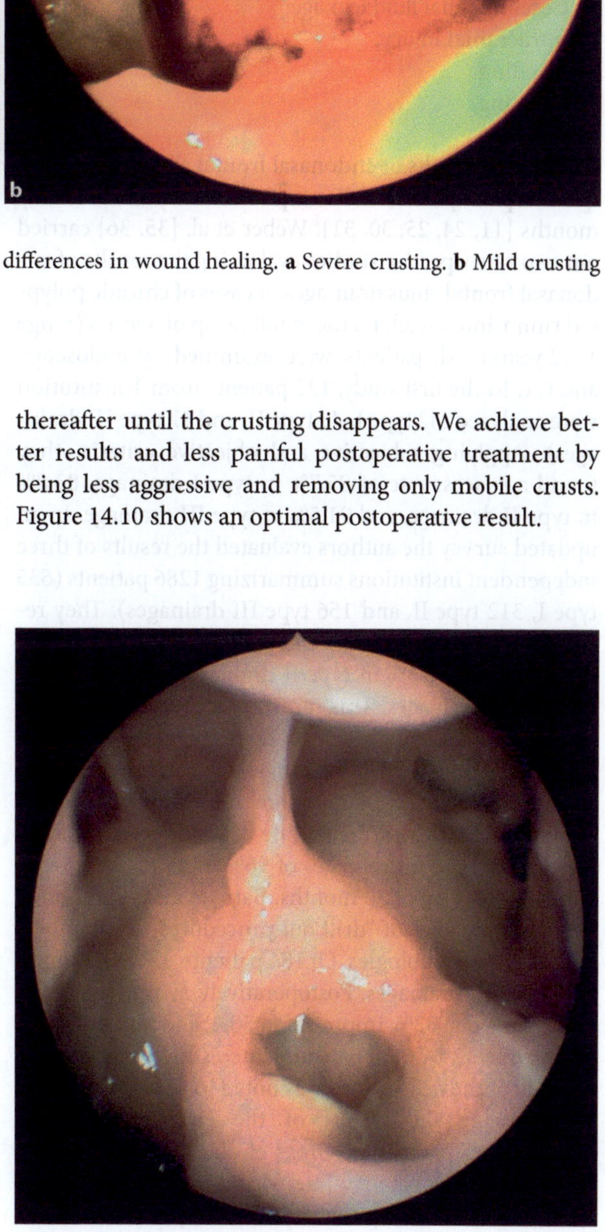

Fig. 14.10 Optimal result after type III drainage according to Draf (3 years postoperatively)

Patients with hyperplastic sinusitis and nasal polyposis, and aspirin triad patients may benefit from tapering doses of systemic oral steroids. We achieved positive effects by prescribing 5 mg prednisone daily for 30 days followed by 2.5 mg for another 40 days.

Outcomes and Complications

Complications of endoscopic revision frontal sinus surgery:

- Frontal ostium restenosis.
- Orbital injury.
- Cerebrospinal fluid leakage.
- Intracranial injury.
- Bleeding.
- Crusting.

Judging the results of endonasal frontal sinus surgery requires a postoperative follow up of several years, not only months [11, 24, 25, 30, 31]. Weber et al. [35, 36] carried out two retrospective studies evaluating the results of endonasal frontal sinus drainages in cases of chronic polypoid rhinosinusitis after a mean follow up of 5 years (range 1–12 years). All patients were examined by endoscopy and CT. In the first study, 132 patients from 1 institution were analyzed (42 type I, 43 type II, and 47 type III drainages). Applying subjective and objective criteria, they found a success rate of 85.7% in type I drainage, 83.8% in type II drainage, and 91.5% in type III drainage. In an updated survey the authors evaluated the results of three independent institutions summarizing 1286 patients (635 type I, 312 type II, and 156 type III drainages). They reported a primary patency rate of 85.2–99.3% in type I drainages, 79–93.3% in type II drainages, and 91.5–95% in type III drainages. This means that despite the choice of prognostically unfavorable cases, type III drainages appeared to show the best results, although this was not statistically significant among the three groups. Recently, Eviatar et al. [9] described a rate of ventilated frontal sinuses after type II drainages of 96% in 25 patients, with a mean follow up of 30 months. Batra et al. [1] presented surgical outcomes of "drill out procedures" for complex frontal sinus pathologies. Of 186 patients, 13.4% required type II or III drainages. Postoperatively, symptomatology was resolved in 32%, improved in 56%, and remained unchanged in 12% of the patients. Interestingly, endoscopic patency of the neo-ostium was noted in 92%.

Reviewing the results of the endoscopic modified Lothrop procedure, Gross et al. [13] found a 95% frontal drainage patency rate with a mean follow up of 12 months, but as experience with the procedure accumulated and patients were followed for longer periods of time, the overall patency success rate was reduced. Schlosser et al. [29] followed 44 patients for an average of 40 months. Of these, 9 (20%) patients required revision modified Lothrop surgery and 8 (18%) eventually needed an osteoplastic frontal sinus operation with obliteration. Almost similar data are reported by Shirazi et al. [30], who analyzed 97 patients with a mean follow up of 18 months; 23% required revision surgery. In contrast, Wormald et al. [40] indicated a 93% primary patency rate with a mean follow up of 22 months. Recently, Friedman et al. [11] published the most comprehensive study evaluating 152 patients with a mean follow up of 72 months, and showing a 71.1% overall patency rate.

Regardless of the surgical procedure among 67 patients, Chiu and Vaughan [5] found 86.6% to have a patent frontal recess and significant subjective improvement in symptoms over an average follow up of 32 months.

Future Directions

Endonasal revision surgery of the frontal sinus remains a great challenge to all surgeons regardless of their experience. It requires proper training and special instruments. However, recurrent or persistent frontal sinus disease after surgery can be addressed with endoscopic or microscopic techniques with a high success rate and low complication rate. These techniques offer several advantages over frontal sinus obliteration and should be in every rhinologist's armamentarium for use in the appropriate clinical situation. Only long-term follow up can determine whether the current endoscopic or microscopic methods will result in consistently permanently favorable results. Despite the progress in surgery, it remains the task to identify the underlying mechanisms causing chronic rhinosinusitis or triad and to develop appropriate medication to cure the disease.

Tips and Pearls

1. Sagittally reconstructed CT scans, especially indicating the AP dimension, are required to assess patient's candidacy for an endonasal revision procedure.
2. For anatomical orientation it is important to determine the presence of remaining agger nasi cells, the superior uncinate process, anterior ethmoid artery, bulla frontalis and supraorbital ethmoid cells, and the depth of the olfactory fossa.
3. When drilling, care has to be taken to preserve the mucosa on the lateral and posterior wall of the frontal recess in order to prevent complications and postoperative stenosis.

4. A large resection of the upper nasal septum is required to provide adequate drainage of the frontal sinuses, and to avoid restenosis.
5. Pre- and postoperative medical management support wound healing, and regular surveillance should be carried out to assure surgical outcome and prevent disease recurrence.

References

1. Batra PS, Cannady SB, Lanza DC (2007) Surgical outcomes of drillout procedures for complex frontal sinus pathology. Laryngoscope 117:927–931
2. Bockmühl U (2005) Osteoplastic frontal sinusotomy and reconstruction of frontal defects. In: Kountakis S, Senior B, Draf W (eds) The Frontal Sinus. Springer, Berlin Heidelberg New York, pp 281–289
3. Bradley DT, Kountakis SE (2004) The role of agger nasi air cells in patients requiring revision endoscopic frontal sinus surgery. Otolaryngol Head Neck Surg 131:525–527
4. Chandra RK, Palmer JN, Tangsujarittham T, Kennedy DW (2004) Factors associated with failure of frontal sinusotomy in the early follow-up period. Otolaryngol Head Neck Surg 131:514–518
5. Chiu AG, Vaughan WC (2004) Revision endoscopic frontal sinus surgery with surgical navigation. Otolaryngol Head Neck Surg 130:312–318
6. Draf W (1991) Endonasal micro-endoscopic frontal sinus surgery. The Fulda concept. Oper Tech Otolaryngol Head Neck Surg 2:134–240
7. Draf W (2005) Endonasal frontal sinus drainage type I-III according to Draf. In: Kountakis S, Senior B, Draf W (eds) The Frontal Sinus. Springer, Berlin Heidelberg New York, pp 219-232
8. Draf W, Weber R, Keerl R, Constantinidis J, Schick B, Saha A (2000) Endonasal and external micro-endoscopic surgery of the frontal sinus. In: Stamm A, Fraf W (eds) Micro-endoscopic Surgery of the Paranasal Sinuses and the Skull Base. Springer, Berlin, Heidelberg, New York, pp 257–278
9. Eviatar E, Katzenell U, Segal S, Shlamkovitch N, Kalmovich LM, Kessler A, Vaiman M (2006) The endoscopic Draf II frontal sinusotomy: non-navigated approach. Rhinology 44:108–113
10. Farhat FT, Figueroa RE, Kountakis SE (2005) Anatomic measurements for the endoscopic modified Lothrop procedure. Am J Rhinol 19:293–296
11. Friedman M, Bliznikas D, Vidyasagar R, Joseph NJ, Landsberg R (2006) Long-term results after endoscopic sinus surgery involving frontal recess dissection. Laryngoscope 116:573–579
12. Gross CW, Schlosser RJ (2001) The modified Lothrop procedure: lessons learned. Laryngoscope 111:1302–1305
13. Gross WE, Gross CW, Becker D, Moore D, Phillips D (1995) Modified transnasal endoscopic Lothrop procedure as an alternative to frontal sinus obliteration. Otolaryngol Head Neck Surg 113:427–434
14. Hosemann W, Gross R, Goede U, Kuehnel T (2001) Clinical anatomy of the nasal process of the frontal bone (spina nasalis interna). Otolaryngol Head Neck Surg 125:60–65
15. Hosemann W, Kuhnel T, Held P, Wagner W, Felderhoff A (1997) Endonasal frontal sinusotomy in surgical management of chronic sinusitis: a critical evaluation. Am J Rhinol 11:1–9
16. Howarth WG (1921) Operations on the frontal sinus. J Laryngol Otol 36:417–421
17. Jansen A (1894) Zur Eröffnung der Nebenhöhlen der Nase bei chronischer Eiterung. Arch Laryng Rhinol (Berl) 1:135–157
18. Kennedy DW, Senior BA (1997) Endoscopic sinus surgery. A review. Otolaryngol Clin North Am 30:313–330
19. Kountakis S (2005) Endoscopic modified Lothrop procedure. In: Kountakis S, Senior B, Draf W (eds) The Frontal Sinus. Springer, Berlin Heidelberg New York, pp 233–241
20. Kuhn FA, Javer AR, Nagpal K, Citardi MJ (2000) The frontal sinus rescue procedure: early experience and three-year follow-up. Am J Rhinol 14:211–216
21. Lothrop HA (1914) Frontal sinus suppuration. Ann Surg 29:175–215
22. Lynch RC (1921) The technique of a radical frontal sinus operation which has given me the best results. Laryngoscope 31:1–5
23. May M (1991) Frontal sinus surgery: endonasal endoscopic osteoplasty rather than external osteoplasty. Oper Tech Otolaryngol Head Neck Surg 2:247–256
24. Neel HB 3rd, McDonald TJ, Facer GW (1987) Modified Lynch procedure for chronic frontal sinus diseases: rationale, technique, and long-term results. Laryngoscope 97:1274–1279
25. Orlandi RR, Kennedy DW (2001) Revision endoscopic frontal sinus surgery. Otolaryngol Clin North Am 34:77–90
26. Rains BM 3rd (2001) Frontal sinus stenting. Otolaryngol Clin North Am 34:101–110
27. Ritter G (1906) Eine neue Methode zur Erhaltung der vorderen Stirnhöhlenwand bei Radikaloperationen chronischer Stirnhöhleneiterungen. Dtsch Med Wschr 19:905–907
28. Schaefer SD, Close LG (1990) Endoscopic management of frontal sinus disease. Laryngoscope 100:155–160
29. Schlosser RJ, Zachmann G, Harrison S, Gross CW (2002) The endoscopic modified Lothrop: long-term follow-up on 44 patients. Am J Rhinol 16:103–108

30. Shirazi MA, Silver AL, Stankiewicz JA (2007) Surgical outcomes following the endoscopic modified Lothrop procedure. Laryngoscope 117:765–769
31. Sonnenburg RE, Senior BA (2004) Revision endoscopic frontal sinus surgery. Curr Opin Otolaryngol Head Neck Surg 12:49–52
32. Stammberger H, Posawetz W (1990) Functional endoscopic sinus surgery. Concept, indications and results of the Messerklinger technique. Eur Arch Otorhinolaryngol 247:63–76
33. Tran KN, Beule AG, Singal D, Wormald PJ (2007) Frontal ostium restenosis after the endoscopic modified Lothrop procedure. Laryngoscope 117:1457–1462
34. Weber R, Draf W, Keerl R, Kahle G, Schinzel S, Thomann S, Lawson W (2000) Osteoplastic frontal sinus surgery with fat obliteration: technique and long-term results using magnetic resonance imaging in 82 operations. Laryngoscope 110:1037–1044
35. Weber R, Draf W, Keerl R, Schick B, Saha A (1997) Endonasal microendoscopic pansinus operation in chronic sinusitis. II. Results and complications. Am J Otolaryngol 18:247–253
36. Weber R, Draf W, Kratzsch B, Hosemann W, Schaefer SD (2001) Modern concepts of frontal sinus surgery. Laryngoscope 111:137–146
37. Weber R, Hochapfel F, Draf W (2000) Packing and stents in endonasal surgery. Rhinology 38:49–62
38. Weber R, Mai R, Hosemann W, Draf W, Toffel P (2000) The success of 6-month stenting in endonasal frontal sinus surgery. Ear Nose Throat J 79:930–932, 934, 937–938
39. Wormald PJ (2003) Salvage frontal sinus surgery: the endoscopic modified Lothrop procedure. Laryngoscope 113:276–283
40. Wormald PJ, Ananda A, Nair S (2003) Modified endoscopic Lothrop as a salvage for the failed osteoplastic flap with obliteration. Laryngoscope 113:1988–1992

Chapter 15

Revision Endoscopic Frontal Sinus Surgery

15

Patricia A. Maeso, Subinoy Das, and Stilianos E. Kountakis

Core Messages

- Revision endoscopic frontal sinus surgery is a challenging procedure that should be undertaken only by the experienced sinus surgeon.
- Evaluation and understanding of the frontonasal outflow tract in the setting of previously surgically altered anatomy is essential.
- Choice of procedure for the revision frontal sinus surgery depends not only on careful preoperative evaluation of available computed tomography radiography, but also on the underlying pathology.
- Careful postoperative debridement and monitoring is essential for the success of any revision frontal sinus operation.

Contents

Introduction

Revision endoscopic frontal sinus surgery remains one of the greatest challenges facing the skilled endoscopic surgeon. Primary endoscopic sinus surgery has a long-term success rate greater than 90%; therefore, patients requiring revision frontal sinus surgery represent a subset of patients with advanced or poorly controlled disease. To increase the chance of success, the endoscopic surgeon should reevaluate the underlying cause of the patient's symptoms. If they are attributable to frontal sinus pathology, then a thorough evaluation should be performed as to the cause underlying failure of the previous operation. The patient's surgical anatomy should be properly reevaluated and the surgeon should be prepared for altered and unusual findings, such as missing and/or distorted landmarks, missing bone, prolapsed orbital contents, encephaloceles, and tumors. A proper revision procedure should be selected and performed by an endoscopic surgeon skilled in this approach, using advanced technology such as computerized image guidance and advanced frontal sinus instrumentation when appropriate. Finally, medical management directed at the patient's underlying pathophysiology, meticulous postoperative debridement, and comprehensive patient education will improve the likelihood of success in this often difficult to manage subset of sinus patients.

Patient Selection/Preoperative Evaluation

Prior to consideration for any revision endoscopic procedure, a thorough reevaluation should be carried out for each patient by performing a comprehensive history and physical examination with angled rigid and/or flexible endoscopy. Initially, a reevaluation should be made as to whether a patient's signs and symptoms are attributable to chronic frontal sinusitis.

Tips and Pearls

1. Primary complaints of headache, while more common with frontal sinusitis, are poor predictors of surgically amenable sinus disease.
2. Evaluation for migraines and other causes of headaches by a qualified neurologist should be pursued with a very low threshold for patients with headache and absent rhinosinusitis symptoms.

Similarly, evaluation for allergic, rheumatologic, psychiatric, and other causes of a patient's symptomatology should always be considered. A review of previous records including previous radiology and pathology reports should be performed whenever possible and will be helpful in ascertaining the true nature of the patient's disease.

Chronic mucosal diseases such as aspirin-induced asthma (Samter's triad), cystic fibrosis, ciliary dysmotility, allergic fungal rhinosinusitis, chronic eosinophilic hyperplastic sinusitis, and others increase the likelihood that the patient's symptoms are attributable to recurrent frontal sinusitis. A comprehensive physical examination will allow the sinus surgeon to detect possible systemic manifestations of an underlying disease that may reveal the true diagnosis for a patient. Angled rigid sinonasal endoscopy and flexible endoscopy (often performed consecutively) are helpful in evaluating the frontal sinus outflow tract and may alert the sinus surgeon to subtle mucosal disease and iatrogenic findings. Photodocumentation of endoscopic findings should be utilized whenever possible.

15

Repeat radiographic imaging is essential for analyzing the diseased frontal sinus. High-resolution computed tomography (CT) analyzed in the coronal, axial, and sagittal planes will allow the surgeon to gain an understanding of the altered three-dimensional anatomy of the frontal sinus and frontal sinus outflow tract. Postoperative films should be compared to preoperative films whenever possible. Magnetic resonance imaging should be supplemented when necessary, as it allows the surgeon to gain a better understanding of the soft-tissue anatomy of a previously operated frontal sinus. This includes distinguishing mucoceles versus encephaloceles, identifying defects in the lamina with periorbital fat herniation, and alerting the sinus surgeon to possible tumors such as inverting papillomas and other rare benign and malignant sinus and skull-base tumors.

Preoperative Assessment/Planning

If the patient's disease is attributable to chronic frontal sinus pathology, then a thorough analysis for the failure of previous frontal sinus surgery should be performed. Broadly, causes for frontal sinus disease in the setting of previous frontal sinus surgery can represent lack of optimal medical management, persistent disease due to incomplete surgery, iatrogenic disease, and recurrent disease following a successful procedure.

Prior to consideration of any repeat surgical procedure, the rhinologist should ascertain the previous medical management of the patient's disease and, in particular, their compliance to these regimens. Nasal saline irrigations, culture-directed oral and intranasal antimicrobial drugs, intranasal steroid sprays and irrigations, mucolytics, and oral anti-inflammatory agents such as leukotriene inhibitors and oral steroids have all been used with varying efficacy in controlling chronic frontal rhinosinusitis. Often, patients with poor outcomes following initial surgery have a poor history of compliance to medical regimens. Time spent in the office educating patients on the necessity and proper techniques of medical management may obviate the need for further operations.

- The best likelihood of success with a repeat operation is in the setting of persistent disease due to a previous incomplete or inadequate surgery.

The quality of previous surgery in the setting of persistent disease varies significantly, with some patients having minimal prior frontal recess surgery being performed and some patients having extensive frontal recess surgery, with the critical obstruction of the frontal sinus still remaining. Reviewing CT scans in multiple planes is very helpful, and sagittal reconstructions are now available on most image-guidance workstations and advanced image viewers.

- The most common causes of persistent frontal sinus obstruction are obstruction from a remnant agger nasi cell and a medially displaced superior remnant of the uncinate process (Fig. 15.1).

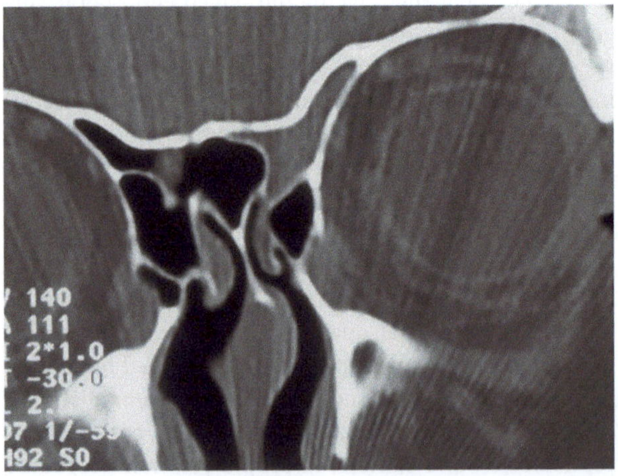

Fig. 15.1 Agger nasi obstructing the frontal sinus outflow tract

Often, a remnant cap of an ethmoid bulla (mistaken to be the true frontonasal outflow tract) is the cause of persistent frontal sinus outflow obstruction. This is particularly common when angled endoscopes were not used in prior surgeries, as a 45 and often only a 70 endoscope allow visualization of the roof of the frontal sinus.

Tips and Pearls

Common causes of persistent frontal sinus disease:

1. Remnant Agger nasi.
2. Remnant cap of ethmoid bulla.
3. Retained frontal cells.
4. Retained supraorbital ethmoid cells.
5. Persistent polyps.
6. Iatrogenic scarring of the frontal recess and ostium.

Other causes of persistent disease include retained frontal cells, retained supraorbital ethmoid cells, and persistent polyps. These persistent entities may critically obstruct the frontonasal outflow tract and be missed during initial surgeries.

While patients with persistent anatomical obstruction often have excellent outcomes with revision surgical techniques, patients with iatrogenic causes of chronic frontal rhinosinusitis are often the most difficult to cure. Furthermore, iatrogenic scarring and neo-osteogenesis can unfortunately convert a patient with previously mild to moderate symptoms into one with crippling disease. As a result, iatrogenic frontal sinus disease is best avoided by using sound and meticulous technique when performing primary frontal sinus operations.

Commonly, iatrogenic disease is the result of cicatricial scarring from circumferential stripping of the frontal recess mucosa. In addition, mucosal stripping can also lead to neo-osteogenesis, which leads to the deposition of inflamed and hardened bone in the frontal recess, which can be very difficult to remove. Often, a drill is required to remove neo-osteogenesis, and leads to the further risk of greater fibrin deposition, neo-osteogenesis, and eventually restenosis.

Another common cause of iatrogenic disease is frontal sinus mucocele formation. This can be the result of previous frontal sinus procedures such as frontal sinus obliteration with incomplete removal of frontal sinus mucosa, or other less aggressive forms of frontal sinus surgery. Frontal sinus mucoceles can occur several years to decades after previous surgery. They often lead to erosion of the anterior and/or posterior table of the frontal sinus and should be suspected particularly if the patient has had a long asymptomatic interval between symptoms.

- Recurrent frontal sinus disease is most commonly a result of mucosal edema in the frontal recess outflow tract and represents a flare-up of the patient's underlying mucosal pathology.

Often, recurrent frontal disease responds to topical medical therapy appropriately delivered to the frontal sinus. Also, limited surgery such as a frontal sinus polypectomy or removal of a few remnant cells is often all that is needed to surgically address recurrent frontal sinus disease. The surgeon should pay close attention to the underlying remnant anatomy to see if anatomical variations make the patient prone to recurrences and could be surgically ameliorated. On the other hand, the risk of creating iatrogenic injury and scarring is often higher with revision frontal sinus surgery, and prudence is warranted.

Relevant Anatomy

In particular, the surgeon should look for radiographic evidence of iatrogenic causes of frontal sinusitis including an absent middle turbinate, or a scarred or lateralized middle turbinate or turbinate remnant. Evidence of a residual superior uncinate or remaining anterior ethmoid/frontal cells may reveal evidence for previous inadequate surgery (Fig. 15.2). Given the likelihood of distorted anatomy, the sinus surgeon should have a clear three-dimensional understanding of the anatomy of the patient's individual frontal recess prior to commencing with surgery. The skull base and the lamina should be carefully evaluated for any potential dehiscence that may be the result of prior surgery, and intraoperatively, suspicious areas should be considered dehiscent unless bone is palpated or confirmed with accurate image guidance. In revision frontal sinus cases, the surgeon should look for the following common causes of pathology:

1. A partially amputated middle turbinate or lateralization of the entire middle turbinate (due to complete resection of the basal lamella) causing obstruction of frontal sinus outflow.
2. Scarring of the superior uncinate to the middle turbinate medial to the frontal sinus outflow tract.
3. Scarring, circumferential stenosis, and/or osteoneogenesis in the frontal ostium area.
4. A remnant ethmoid bulla cap mistakenly considered the frontal recess.
5. Agger nasi or frontal cells left undissected, and/or recurrence of polyposis in the frontal outflow system [3].

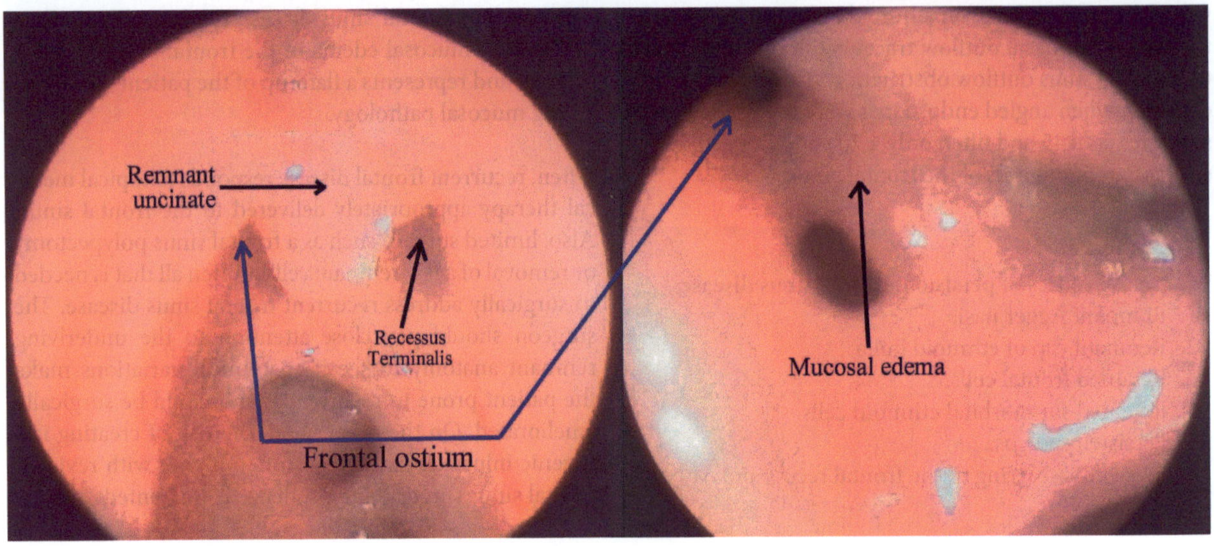

Fig. 15.2 The recessus terminalis is a blind pouch formed by the superior attachment of the uncinate process, as it attaches to lamina papyracea. It can frequently be mistaken for the frontal sinus. The frontal sinus ostium will usually be found posterior and medial to this location

Operative Techniques

Tips and Pearls

1. The mucosa of the lateral frontal recess should not be disturbed since this helps restore frontal sinus function.
2. Frontal sinus obliteration is now utilized infrequently.
3. The "above and below" technique addresses lateral or cephalad frontal sinus lesions and type II or IV frontal cells, which cannot be reached endoscopically.
4. When using the "above and below" technique, oval-shaped trephinations increase working space while minimizing the chance for cosmetic deformity.

Surgery for frontal sinus disease should follow an organized progression from least aggressive to most aggressive. There are multiple procedures from which to choose; however, endoscopic procedures should be at the forefront of the thought process when considering frontal sinus surgery. Frontal sinus obliterations should be performed only rarely with the advent of improved frontal sinus instruments and technology.

The endoscopic frontal recess drainage procedure or Draf I procedure is a complete anterior ethmoidectomy with drainage of the frontal recess without manipulation of the frontal sinus outflow tract [7]. It is often used as first-line surgery for management of frontal sinus disease since it carries minimal risk for scarring of the frontal recess; however, it has little role in revision frontal sinus surgery.

Endoscopic Frontal Sinusotomy

Endoscopic frontal sinusotomy involves enlargement of the frontal sinus outflow tract. This extended drainage procedure has been classified into Draf IIA, which corresponds to removing anterior ethmoidal cells that protrude into and/or obstruct the frontal recess (Fig. 15.3). The goal of this procedure is to create an opening of at least 5 mm into the frontal sinus between the middle turbinate medially and the lamina papyracea laterally by removing bony partitions, while sparing frontal recess mucosa. In the presence of a narrow frontal recess, removal of an intersinus septal cell or a Draf IIB procedure may be performed. A Draf IIB involves resection of the frontal sinus floor between the lamina papyracea and the nasal septum (Fig. 15.4). In revision cases, an incomplete previous frontal sinusotomy may be addressed by carefully identifying the true frontonasal outflow tract and removing any obstructing frontal, ethmoid, or agger nasi cells. When the middle turbinates have been resected and the remnant has lateralized and scarred across the frontal sinus outflow tract, the frontal sinus rescue procedure or revision frontal sinusotomy with mucoperiosteal flap

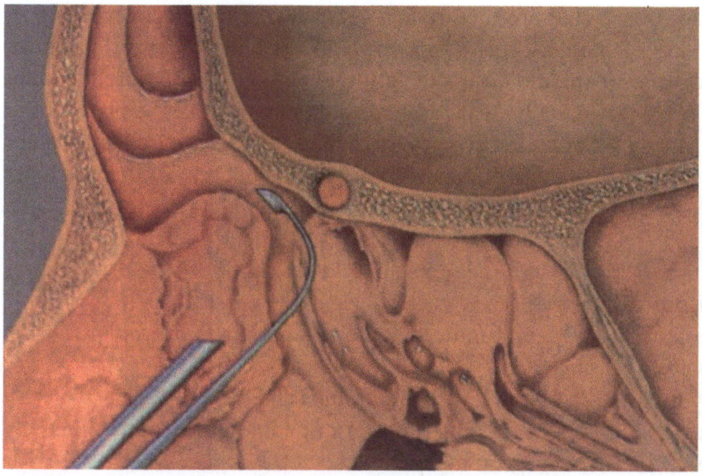

Fig. 15.3 Representative image of a Draf IIA procedure or frontal sinusotomy where ethmoidal cells protrude into frontal recess and removal is necessary via "uncapping the egg"

advancement is used to remove any bony and soft-tissue obstruction caused by the destabilized middle-turbinate remnant [1].

External Frontal Sinus Trephination with Endoscopic Frontal Sinus Surgery: the "Above and Below Technique"

Endoscopic approaches to the frontal sinus are usually favored; however, there are some circumstances where the simple trephine along with an endoscopic approach or the "above and below technique" can facilitate the surgery and obviate the need for a more aggressive approach to the frontal sinus. Indications for this procedure are ever expanding since it is minimally invasive and cosmetically appealing, yet allows the surgeon to reach areas that are not available via endonasal techniques. Among the indications for the procedure, the most common remain lateral or cephalad frontal sinus lesions, type II or IV frontal cells, which cannot be addressed endoscopically, tumors or inflammatory lesions involving the frontal sinus, frontal sinus trauma, and distorted anatomy of the frontal recess (Fig. 15.5). When performing the trephination, the position of the frontal sinus can be confirmed by utilizing a properly registered and accurate image-guidance system. If image guidance is not available, then the position of the frontal sinus is confirmed on preoperative CT in relation to the supraorbital rim or via a six-foot Caldwell radiograph that can be cut to be used as a template in order to adequately outline the frontal sinus. The endoscopic portion of the surgery should be completed first. After this is done, an incision is made through the medial eyebrow at the level of the supraorbital rim without shaving this region. Once the incision is done, a 4 mm drill bit may be utilized to enter the sinus at the previously confirmed location. The trephine may be enlarged up to 6–8 mm to accommodate instruments as well as the endoscope [6]. Oval-shaped trephinations increase working space while minimizing the chance for cosmetic deformity. Having both the endonasal and external exposure gives the surgeon the advantage of better visualization and improved instrumentation in the area of the frontal sinus, and allows for superior based irrigation of the frontal sinus, which can be very helpful in identifying the frontal recess outflow tract with distorted anatomy as well as in assessing the final opening to the frontal recess after the frontal sinusotomy is completed. The operation is done so that both aspects of the procedure are complimentary (Video 15.1). For example, visualization can be performed endonasally while instrumentation can be done through the trephination, and vice versa. The above

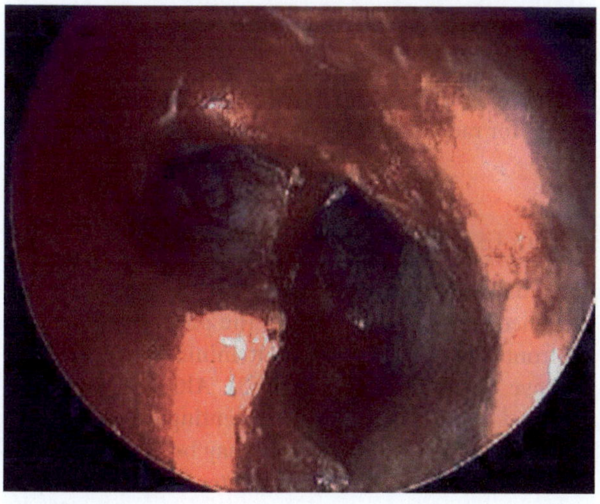

Fig. 15.4 Postoperative view of a Draf IIB procedure

and below approach should be part of any sinus surgeon's repertoire as it has many applications given its ease of performance, safety profile, and minimal cosmetic disfigurement.

Endoscopic Modified Lothrop or Draf III Procedure

This procedure, also known as the Draf type III procedure, can be utilized as an alternative to osteoplastic flap frontal surgery. The procedure has the surgical objective of creating a large nasofrontal communication by utilizing a totally intranasal approach and avoiding an external incision, while preserving the frontal sinus mucosa [2].

The indications for the endoscopic modified Lothrop procedure include [8]:

1. Failed prior endoscopic sinus surgery techniques.
2. Significant neo-osteogenesis in the frontal recess and frontal ostium.
3. Frontal recess adhesions.
4. Disease processes that have resulted in the loss of the posterior wall or floor of the frontal sinus.
5. Failed previous osteoplastic flap with obliteration and mucocele formation.
6. Tumor removal from the frontal sinus.

15

The procedure involves identifying the true frontal ostia, which can be difficult, and often is facilitated by the use of computer-aided image guidance, a wire probe, and/or an external minitrephination approach with the use of saline/fluorescein. The superior uncinate and frontal recess cells are then resected. Drilling is then performed in an anterior direction through the anterior insertion of the middle turbinate until the nasal beak is removed and the nasal bone is reached, and laterally until the plane of the lamina papyracea is reached. A superior 2×2 cm septectomy is then performed at the junction of the quadrangular cartilage and perpendicular plate of ethmoid bone. The contralateral frontal sinus floor is then drilled away through the septectomy defect until the opposite lamina papyracea is reached (Fig. 15.6; Video 15.2).

Contraindications to the modified Lothrop procedure include:

1. Hypoplastic frontal sinus and frontal recess.
2. Narrow anteroposterior depth of the frontal sinus.
3. Surgeon inexperience.
4. Lack of proper instrumentation [4].

The modified endoscopic Lothrop is a valuable endonasal approach that should be readily available and always entertained for those patients who are candidates for more aggressive frontal sinus surgery (Fig. 15.7).

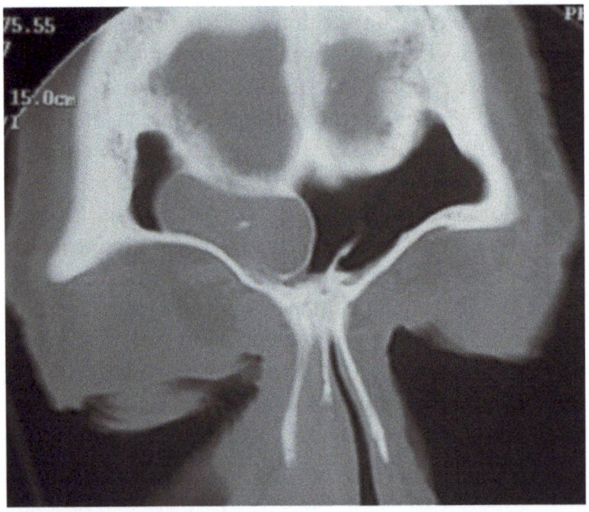

Fig. 15.5 Computed tomography scan: coronal image of a type IV frontal sinus cell

Osteoplastic Flap and External Approaches

The osteoplastic flap has been described historically as the definitive procedure for the treatment of recalcitrant frontal sinusitis and frontal sinus disease not amenable to endoscopic approaches [5]. Relative indications to this external approach include chronic frontal sinusitis refractory to endoscopic surgery, mucopyocele, severe trauma with fractures involving the drainage pathways, and after resection of large frontal tumors near the frontal recess. Other external approaches have also been described for the management of frontal sinus disease, but have mostly fallen out of favor.

- Endoscopic procedures not only have the absence of any external scars, but they also help maintain the physiologic ventilation of the sinuses, which is important for radiologic and clinical follow up.

Frontal Sinus Stenting

The indications and benefits of frontal sinus stenting has remained a controversial issue. The purpose of stenting the frontal sinus outflow tract is to minimize stenosis and improve mucosalization (Video 3). Although there are no standardized indications for stenting, there are several situations in which stenting may be considered: (1) the frontal sinus neo-ostium diameter is less than 5 mm, (2) there is extensive or circumferential exposure of bone

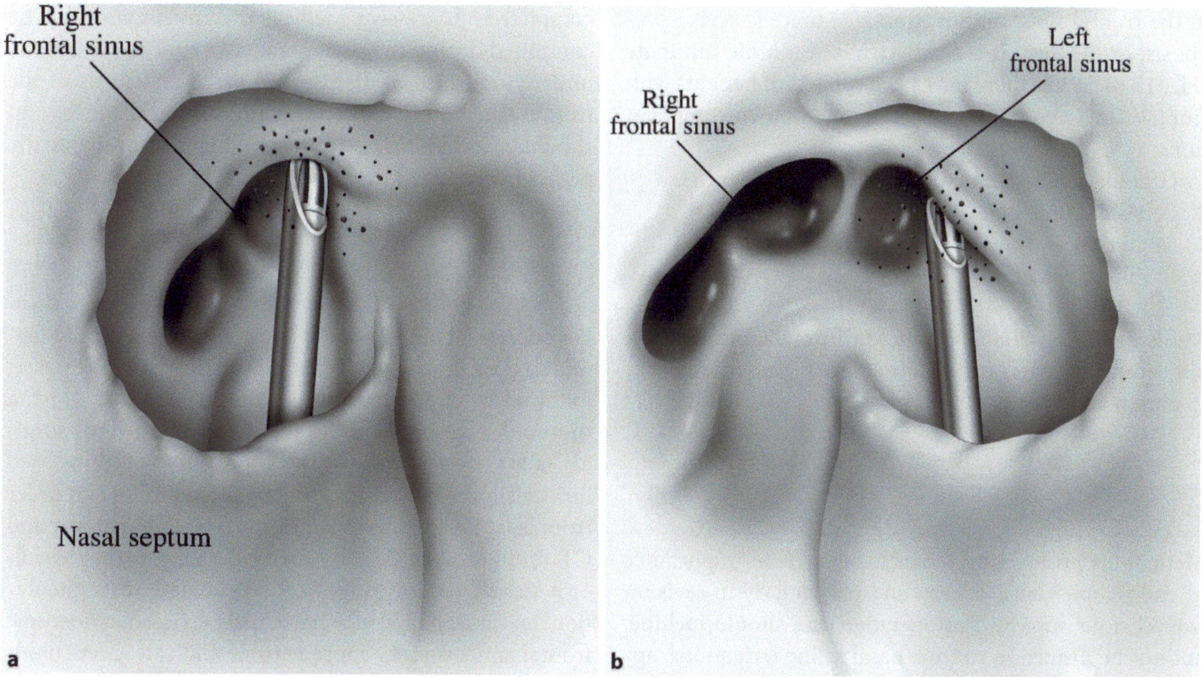

Fig. 15.6 Drilling through the nasal beak to remove the opposite frontal sinus floor and complete the modified Lothrop procedure. **a** Drilling through the midline. **b** Completion of the drilling toward the opposite frontal sinus modified Lothrop procedure

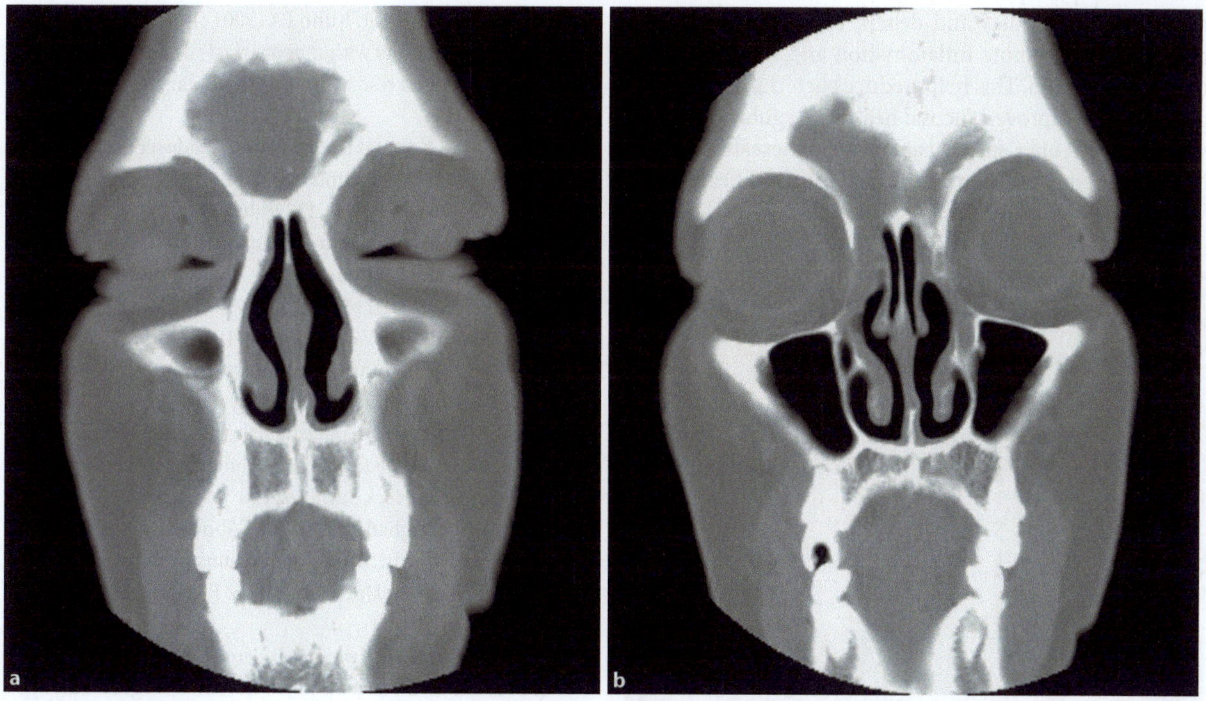

Fig. 15.7 Persistent frontal disease and frontal recess scar formation after multiple sinus surgeries, necessitating more aggressive revision frontal surgery (endoscopic modified Lothrop procedure)

in the frontal sinus outflow tract, (3) there is severe polyposis, or (4) there is a flail, lateralized middle turbinate (Fig. 15.8). While there have been reports of benefits with frontal sinus stenting, there are several known complications:

1. Granulation tissue formation around the stent.
2. Persistent crusting.
3. Migration.
4. Biofilm formation.

Stents maybe a valuable adjunct in frontal sinus surgery, but careful selection and follow up are necessary in order to obtain good results.

Postoperative Care

Meticulous postoperative care is of extreme importance in endoscopic sinus surgery, and particularly in revision frontal sinus surgery. Postoperative care should include, but not be limited to routine nasal saline irrigations, appropriate antibiotic therapy as deemed necessary, as well as topical and systemic agents that control inflammation.

- Endoscopic debridement of the frontal recess is an integral part of good postoperative care.

Meticulous postoperative debridement will allow the removal of any crusts and debris, retained mucus, and blood, which promote inflammation and scarring in the neofrontal ostium. This helps reduce bacterial and/or fungal load and improve mucosal healing. Regular follow up within 1 week after surgery and closely thereafter should be performed in order to ensure that mucosal healing has completed. Aggressive medical therapy should also be continued during the perioperative period to control the underlying mucosal disease and avoid restenosis of the frontal sinus outflow tract. Finally, long-term follow up should be individualized for each patient according to the pathophysiology of his or her frontal sinus disease.

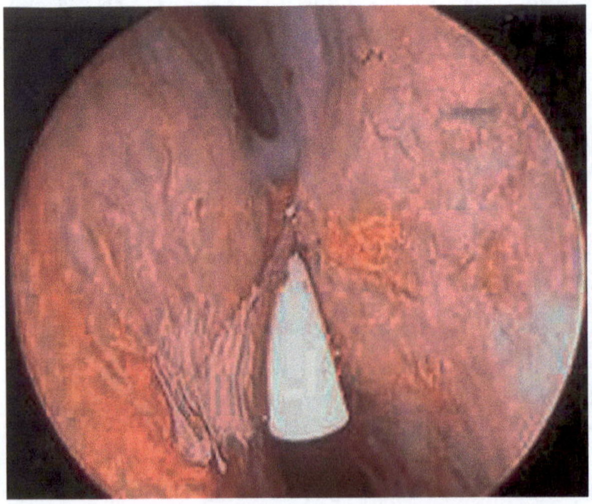

Fig. 15.8 Postoperative view of a frontal sinus stent in place

Conclusions

For successful outcomes the revision surgeon should first undertake a thorough reevaluation of the patient's disease, followed by efforts to optimize medical therapy. Next, a thorough investigation into the causes of previous surgical failure should ensue. The choice of procedure used for revision frontal sinus surgery should follow an order from least invasive to most, dictated by the anatomy and CT findings as well as by the underlying pathophysiology. Advancements in optical technology, instrumentation, and image guidance have made revision endoscopic frontal sinus surgery more feasible and safe. Meticulous postoperative care and adherence to individualized medical regimens will lead to greater success in the care of this difficult subset of patients.

References

1. Citardi JM, Javer AR, Kuhn FA (2001) Revision endoscopic frontal sinusotomy with mucoperiosteal flap advancement: the frontal sinus rescue procedure. Otolaryngol Clin N Am 34:123–132
2. Farhat FT, Kountakis SE (2004) Endoscopic modified Lothrop. Oper Tech Otolaryngol Head Neck Surg 15:4–7
3. Friedman M, Bliznikas D, Vidyasagar R, Landsberg R, (2004) Frontal sinus surgery: update of clinical anatomy and surgical techniques. Oper Tech Otolaryngol Head Neck Surg 15:23–31
4. Gross CW, Gross WE, Becker D (1995) Modified transnasal endoscopic Lothrop procedure: frontal drillout. Oper Tech Otolaryngol Head Neck Surg 6:193–200
5. Jacobs JB (2000) Osteoplastic flap with obliteration: is this an ideal procedure for chronic frontal sinusitis? Arch Otolaryngol Head Neck Surg 126:100
6. Patel AM, Vaughan WC (2005) "Above and Below" FESS: simple trephine with endoscopic sinus surgery. In: Kountakis SE, Senior BA, Draf W (eds) The Frontal Sinus. Springer, Berlin, pp 191–199
7. Weber R, Draf W, Kratzsch B, Hosemann W, Schaefer SD (2001) Modern concepts of frontal sinus surgery. Laryngoscope 111:137–146
8. Wormald PJ (2003) Salvage frontal sinus surgery: the modified Lothrop procedure. Laryngoscope 113:275–283

Chapter 16

Postoperative Medical Management 16

Dennis F. Chang, David B. Conley, and Robert C. Kern

Core Messages

- A common and frustrating dilemma associated with sinus surgery is scarring between the middle turbinate and lateral nasal wall.
- The most common adverse event associated with the procedure is failure to alleviate the initial presenting complaints.
- After sinus surgery, mucociliary function of the paranasal sinuses is inhibited for 6–12 weeks.
- Most sinus surgeons feel that aggressive debridement of the postsurgical sinus cavity is critical for success.
- Postoperative debridement may decrease the rate of adhesions and synechiae.
- Postoperative nasal saline irrigations reduce crusting and edema and improve nasal obstruction.
- Intranasal corticosteroids play an integral role in the postoperative management of the surgically treated sinus cavities.
- Because of the multiple side effects of long-term oral steroid use, short oral steroid bursts should be used judiciously, with nasal topical therapy being the preferred treatment.
- In cases of extensive nasal polyps, an ideal solution would involve delivering a large amount of steroid to the diseased sinuses while minimizing systemic absorption.
- Culture-directed antibiotic therapy is necessary for infectious exacerbations of chronic sinus disease, especially after sinus surgery.

Contents

Introduction

Functional endoscopic sinus surgery (FESS) is one of the most commonly performed operations by otolaryngologists. The popularity and success of this procedure has been attributed in part to excellent improvement in patient symptoms both in the short term as well as long term postoperative period [33]. Although much has been written about the rare, devastating complications of FESS – cerebrospinal fluid leak and blindness – the most common adverse event associated with the procedure remains failure to alleviate the initial presenting complaints. Meticulous postoperative care and maximal medical management are widely believed to be crucial to obtaining optimal results. In many respects, the techniques and methods employed after the operation to maintain healthy and open sinus cavities may be as important as the initial surgery itself.

Multiple obstacles can present themselves in the postoperative patient, but a common and frustrating dilemma is scarring between the middle turbinate and lateral nasal wall. This phenomenon often leads to partial or complete obstruction of the ostiomeatal complex with recurrence of symptomatology. After FESS, mucociliary function of the paranasal sinuses is inhibited for 6–12 weeks [16]. Debris composed of fibrin, blood clots, crusts, and viscous secretions tend to accumulate during this time period and the patient is then particularly vulnerable to discomfort, perioperative infection, and postoperative formation of synechiae. Numerous protocols and techniques have been formulated to deal with these challenges and optimize postoperative healing. The decision as to what constitutes the "best" management philosophy is often controversial. This chapter will cover the following major points: postoperative debridement, pros, cons, timing, frequency, nasal saline irrigation and lavage, steroids, oral, topical, and nebulized antibiotic therapy, and allergic fungal sinusitis (AFS).

The various methods and packing used to prevent lateralization of the middle turbinate are beyond the scope of this chapter and will be covered in detail elsewhere in this volume.

Postoperative Debridement

The role of postoperative debridement and the exact timing and frequency of debridement are not standardized. The management philosophies are based mainly on empiric data with a dearth of prospective, double-blinded, randomized, controlled studies addressing this topic. Most sinus surgeons feel that aggressive debridement of the postsurgical sinus cavity is critical for success. The rationale underlying debridement is that if debris composed of crusts, blood clots, bone chips, and fibrin are allowed to accumulate, there will be a tendency for increased adhesions and synechiae formation with resultant scar and recurrent rhinosinusitis. Ancillary arguments for debridement include more rapid relief of nasal congestion and fewer postoperative infections [3]. A minority of surgeons consider debridement unnecessary, opting instead to prevent postoperative adhesions by placing packing in the middle meatus.

- A major disadvantage to regular and routine aggressive debridements is the increased bleeding and pain associated with both injection of local anesthetic and the instrumentation of the sensitive postoperative nasal cavity.

Debridement also can be time-consuming in the edematous and inflamed surgical cavity and can potentially cause additional mucosal damage that delays wound healing.

The literature on this topic has been somewhat conflicted and controversial. A study by Nissen et al. [23] looked at 17 patients and compared symptom scores, healing, and adhesion rates between debrided and nondebrided sides in the same patient over a 3-month period of time. Although there was no statistical significance shown, the numbers of patients enrolled and the short follow-up period are more consistent with a pilot study and only limited conclusions can be drawn. Ryan et al. [30] analyzed 120 patients in a retrospective review. His group found that despite minimal postoperative follow up with an average of only 2.8 visits and 1 debridement, 78% of patients reported either significant improvement in symptoms or outright cure at 18 months follow up. Postoperative antibiotic therapy and topical nasal corticosteroids were both used routinely and the authors suggest that these are more critical in the absence of regular postoperative debridements. Probably the best study to date on the topic, however, included 60 patients in a randomized, partially blinded, controlled, prospective trial [3]. Debrided patients had significantly less crusting in the sinus cavities as well as significantly less postoperative adhesion formation compared to those who had saline irrigation alone. The procedure did induce more postoperative pain but there was no difference in bleeding. The study concluded that increased adhesions from increased crusts and debris may increase the need for revision sinus surgery, and that debridements should be undertaken to prevent this as much as possible.

- The current weight of evidence supports debridement to remove crusts, bone chips, and fibrin as a method to prevent adhesions and synechiae in adult patients following FESS.

An interesting perspective can be gained by looking at the pediatric FESS population and the role that debridement plays in postoperative management. Pediatric patients have a limited tolerance for office endoscopy and debridement, traditionally mandating a return to the operating room under general anesthesia for second-look and cleansing of the sinus cavities 2–4 weeks after the primary operation. Over time, this management has been challenged with several groups contending in prospective studies that postoperative improvement in nasal obstruction, drainage, and chronic cough was identical in pediatric patients with and without any postoperative debridement [21, 22]. Pediatric patients undergoing revision surgery and those suffering from cystic fibrosis were excluded from these trials. Since the extent of sinus surgery, and possibly the disease itself, may be different from the adult population, any conclusions based on data from the pediatric FESS literature cannot be readily extrapolated.

The timing and frequency of debridements is also a matter of contention. Kuhnel et al. [19] noted that avulsion of epithelium occurred in 23% of patients when debrided in the 1st week and advised the first postoperative manipulation be delayed until the 2nd week after surgery. Bugten et al. performed debridements at 6 and 12 days and found that crusts and adhesions were significantly reduced [3]. A third debridement was reserved for patients with infections or recalcitrant crusting. Some surgeons advocate aggressive debridements daily in the 1st week of surgery or weekly over 6–8 weeks until healing is complete, although patient comfort is significantly impacted and these regimens have fallen somewhat out of favor.

- A recent position statement by the American Rhinologic Society maintains that four postoperative debridements in a 6-week period for routine FESS patients is reasonable and six debridements in the complex patient is fair.

- However, treatment ultimately must be tailored to each individual patient and disease case.

Nasal Saline Irrigation and Lavage

The effectiveness of daily saline irrigation of the sinuses and nares in the treatment of chronic rhinosinusitis as well as allergic and nonallergic rhinitis is well established. Postoperatively, nasal saline remains a crucial component in maintaining clean, moist, well-aerated sinus cavities. Crusting is significantly reduced and nasal obstruction and edema are improved. The exact manner, technique, and volume of delivery will vary from institution to institution at the preference of both the surgeon and the patient, but there appears to be a consensus that saline lavage is both recommended and necessary in the post-FESS patient.

Nasal saline irrigation protocol:

1. During postoperative days 1–7, patients are discouraged from irrigating the nose vigorously as the surgical site is still fresh and sore. They are encouraged to begin gently instilling commercially prepared normal saline spray in their nares twice daily.
2. After the first postoperative visit and debridement, they are given an instruction sheet that teaches them how to mix their own saline solution.
3. They are taught to adjust both the amount of salt and the temperature of the solution to optimize comfort.
4. Noniodized salt should be used as iodine may irritate the nose.
5. Patients are informed of the various devices for irrigation including bottles designed for irrigation or a similar-sized bulb syringe.
6. They are taught to lean over, breathe through their mouth, and passively irrigate one naris and then another without snorting in the saline solution.
7. Saline lavage should be done at least twice a day and separately from any other concurrent nasal steroid spray.
8. This regimen is continued for at least 3–6 months while the sinus cavities complete healing.

The postoperative course, the presence of polyps, the incidence of perioperative infections, and other factors will then determine whether antibiotics and steroids are added to the saline solution. The only randomized single-blinded trial to look at saline lavage in the postoperative patient compared mechanical lavage with pressurized saline to chemical lavage with saline impregnated with an antiseptic and a mucolytic [24]. Ultimately there was no difference in efficacy between the two groups, although there was a trend toward significance with the chemical lavage group causing less crusting.

A commercially available oily mixture made of nasal emollient derived from pine and eucalyptus has proven especially effective in relieving patients of excessive nasal crusting after sinus surgery. This problem is minimized by preserving the turbinates during surgery; however, some aspect of crusting is usually unavoidable. In some cases, the middle turbinates have completely degenerated into polypoid form and preservation is impractical.

Corticosteroids

Intranasal corticosteroids have long been a part of preoperative maximal medical therapy, having minimal systemic absorption and mild, local side effects. The continued use of intranasal corticosteroids postoperatively is justified primarily for two reasons. First, the continued anti-inflammatory effect of the steroid may be increased in efficacy since there should theoretically be greater delivery to the more open postoperative sinus cavity. The removal of the uncinate process, the medialization of the middle turbinate, and the exposed skull base mucosa from a complete ethmoidectomy are all anatomic factors that facilitate greater distribution of topical medications to the sinus mucosa. Second, in the case of nasal polyps, disease recurrence is common and the persistent daily use of intranasal corticosteroids is widely believed to reduce the rate of recurrence. Rowe-Jones et al. [29] studied 72 patients over a 5-year period in a prospective, randomized, placebo-controlled, and double-blinded manner. A statistically significant improvement was demonstrated not only in patient subjective symptoms, but also in endoscopic edema and polyp scores and total nasal volume. The placebo group also required more oral steroid tapers, and of the 12 patients who failed the study due to excessive requirements for oral steroid tapers, 10 were from the placebo group. Older studies using flunisolide and beclomethasone have also shown improvement in the prevention of nasal polyp recurrence at 1 year and 2.5 years [11, 18]. A more recent paper by Desrosiers' group demonstrated an interesting effect of postoperative intranasal steroid use [8]. In a prospective observational study of 157 patients, intranasal corticosteroid use was associated with lower rates of bacterial recovery, especially for revision FESS patients. This phenomenon may be partially explained by the high rate of colonization of post-FESS patients with *Staphylococcus aureus* and the potentially anti-inflammatory and proinnate immune actions of intranasal corticosteroids, which could result in improved

S. aureus clearance from the sinuses. [31] While corticosteroids are known to suppress inflammation, it has only recently become clear that they enhance the innate immune defenses of airway epithelium.

- Postoperative corticosteroids appear to not only suppress inflammation, but also reduce the rate of bacterial colonization.

Conflicting literature arguing against the beneficial effects of topical steroids can also be cited, however. Dijkstra et al. [10] followed 162 patients in a prospective, double-blinded, placebo-controlled, randomized study focused on fluticasone and found no significant difference in recurrence rates of either chronic rhinosinusitis or nasal polyps 1 year after sinus surgery. Another paper evaluating Beconase nasal spray and olfaction recovery in post-nasal polypectomy patients also revealed no difference [13]. These results represent a minority point of view.

Oral glucocorticoids are also a mainstay of therapy for both allergic rhinitis, chronic rhinosinusitis with and without nasal polyposis, and postoperative mucosal edema [20]. They are also frequently given both perioperatively to decrease inflammation and operative bleeding as well as together with antibiotics for acute sinusitis and exacerbations of chronic sinusitis. In the postoperative period, oral steroid bursts with either prednisone or methylprednisolone can be crucial in slowing or preventing nasal polyp recurrence. Unfortunately, the list of side effects for chronic oral steroid use is potentially problematic.

16

The side effects of chronic oral steroid use include:

1. Immunosuppression.
2. Exacerbation of diabetes or unmasking of latent diabetes.
3. Precipitation into diabetic ketoacidosis.
4. Osteoporosis.
5. Peptic ulcer disease.
6. Hypertension.
7. Psychological effects such as depression and psychosis.
8. Muscle wasting.
9. Cataracts.
10. Impaired wound healing.
11. Avascular joint necrosis.
12. Facial changes ("buffalo hump" and "steroid facies").

Consequently, even short oral steroid bursts should be used judiciously, with nasal topical therapy being the preferred treatment.

In the setting of polyps in particular, intranasal corticosteroids alone are frequently insufficient to control postoperative mucosal disease. A more ideal solution would involve delivering a large amount of steroid to the diseased sinuses while minimizing systemic absorption. This philosophy is similar to the use of ototopical antibiotic drops delivered in very high local concentrations to the external ear canal and middle ear space. Various attempts to achieve the same effect in the sinuses have been made. Budesonide respules, which are traditionally used for asthma treatment, have been adapted for sinusitis. Respules are dissolved in saline solution and used to irrigate the postoperative sinus regularly for at least 6–8 weeks. While there have been anecdotal tales of success, no prospective randomized, controlled trial in the literature has been performed to study this.

Recently, a retrospective review by DelGaudio et al. [6] studied a variety of topical steroid drops formulated for ophthalmic and otologic use and their effect on sinus ostia stenosis in the postoperative period of revision FESS patients. The solutions include dexamethasone ophthalmic (0.1%), prednisolone ophthalmic (1%), and ciprofloxacin-dexamethasone otic (0.3/0.1%) drops. They found that of 67 sides treated, 64% were patent, 14.9% were stable, and 20.9% failed. There was only one complication secondary to lowered morning cortisol levels, which necessitated discontinuation of the drops. Mean follow up was 4.8 months. An interesting perspective was put forth as a possible explanation for the occasional ineffectiveness of intranasal corticosteroids. Conventional nasal steroid sprays are often deposited in the anterior nasal cavity. With topical steroid drops, patients were instructed to extend the head at a 45 angle and turned slightly to the side of drop application for 5 min. This variation of the Mygind technique was shown to improve delivery of medication versus sprays [17]. The paper advocates, based on previous work by Citardi and Kuhn [5], that anatomic position is critical for the delivery of steroid to the targeted frontal recess.

- The route of topical steroid delivery (spray, drops or irrigation) may play a significant role in the efficacy of these therapies.

Antibiotic Therapy

Antibiotics therapy is a key component of the management of acute and chronic rhinosinusitis and their role in the preoperative setting has been studied extensively and documented in the literature.

Many studies have reported the presence of typical upper respiratory tract organisms in acute and chronic rhinosinusitis. *Streptococcus pneumoniae, Hemophilus influenzae*, and *Moraxella catarrhalis* remain the top three bacteria implicated in uncomplicated acute rhinosinusitis [27]. The microbiology of chronic rhinosinusitis particularly in the postoperative setting is more complicated. While *S. aureus*, anaerobes, and Gram-negative organisms have always been recognized as more significant contributors in chronic versus acute disease, their presence in the postoperative patient is increased. Bhattacharyya et al. [2] demonstrated that *Strep. pneumoniae*, *H. influenzae*, and *M. catarrhalis* combined, only made up 10.8% of over 290 cultures taken from post-FESS sinus cavities. Of special interest, *S. aureus* and coagulase-negative staphylococcus represented the number one and number two most cultured organism, and together represented nearly 30% of all organisms. *Pseudomonas aeruginosa* was third at 7.2%. Fungal organisms were cultured in only 1.7% of the specimens.

- *S. aureus* frequently colonizes chronic rhinosinusitis and postoperative patients and may play a role in the progression of mucosal inflammation.

S. aureus is widely believed to be a significant pathogen in the etiology of chronic rhinosinusitis and its presence in the operated sinus cavity is a cause for concern. Recent reviews illustrate a convincing argument for staphylococcal superantigens and their nonspecific activation of local T-cell receptors as a factor in the development of chronic rhinosinusitis with nasal polyposis [32, 36]. Another striking finding is the relatively high prevalence of *Pseudomonas* bacteria in the postoperative setting; these bacteria have a very strong propensity for developing multidrug resistance.

Antibiotic resistance is an emerging problem in all fields of medicine and post-FESS patients have often received multiple long-term courses before undergoing surgery. Consequently, it should come as no surprise that these patients often present with infections by multidrug resistance bacteria that are difficult to eradicate. The study by Bhattacharyya makes a strong argument for culture directed antibiotic therapy in the postoperative setting and points out that a good FESS should provide much improved access to at least the maxillary antrum and ethmoid cavity for representative specimens [2].

The issue of resistance coupled with possible systemic side effects from protracted use of oral antibiotics has led to an increased interest in the topical delivery of antibiotics. As nasal saline irrigation was already a well-established regimen used by patients, a natural extension was the addition of both corticosteroids and antibiotics to the wash. The philosophy was to increase delivery of antibiotic to the affected sinus cavities while decreasing systemic absorption. The prevalence of *Staphylococcus* and *Pseudomonas* in the postoperative patient made the addition of two types of antibiotics especially attractive. For staphylococcal coverage, mucopirocin is added to saline rinses; gentamycin and tobramycin represent the most popular antibiotics mixed into saline for pseudomonal coverage.

One criticism of using saline to deliver antibiotics centers on the concentration of the antibiotic in the solution. While it offers an improvement over oral ingestion alone, the presence of large amounts of saline significantly dilutes whatever antibiotic is mixed and ultimately decreases the concentration delivered to the sinus cavities. A more suitable alternative would appear to be the delivery of a small volume of solution by means of a nebulizer. Initial trials by Vaughan et al. [34] and Desrosiers et al. [7] demonstrated safety as well as improvement in infection clearance rates, nasal symptomatology, and quality of life surveys. Vaughan's study was an uncontrolled pilot study, which not only showed a longer disease-free interval (17 weeks versus 7 weeks) for the nebulized antibiotic treatment group, but also decreased facial pain and postnasal drip [34].

- A randomized controlled study on intranasal antibiotic use by Desrosiers' group showed that there was symptomatic improvement, but comparison between a nebulized saline control group and the nebulized tobramycin group revealed no significant differences [7].

The paper concluded that large-particle nebulized aerosol therapy in and of itself may offer a safe and effective management alternative, but was unable to show any additional benefit of tobramycin [7].

Recent research has placed new emphasis on biofilm formation and the role that it plays in recalcitrant chronic rhinosinusitis, especially in the operated patient. Previous work had demonstrated the increased prevalence of *Staphylococcus* and *Pseudomonas* species in the post-FESS patient and various theories had been advanced as to why infections in this patient population were so difficult to clear [2]. Both *Staphylococcus* and *Pseudomonas* are known biofilm producers and it is now thought that bacterial biofilms help to explain the decreased efficacy of oral antibiotics, since the minimal inhibitory concentration (MIC) of antibiotics delivered in oral form is simply inadequate to affect bacteria in biofilms. An impractical solution would simply be to increase the MIC of various antibiotics, as studies have shown that high MICs are capable of overcoming biofilm resistance [15]. As high concentrations are difficult to attain in serum due to systemic toxicity, the focus is placed on topical antibiotics, which may achieve concentrations high enough to penetrate biofilms and eradicate bacteria but with negligible systemic absorption. Preliminary work by Desrosiers et al. [9] recently demonstrated the capacity of supra-MIC levels of moxifloxacin to kill bacteria in biofilms in vitro. An elegant animal model for both inducing chronic rhinosinusitis and then studying the effects of various topical medications on the maxillary sinus through a surgically implanted irrigating catheter has recently been published [4]. Irrigation with saline alone demonstrates no significant difference from untreated animals with regard to the degree of inflammation of sinus mucosa and underlying bone, and no changes in the amount of purulence could be found. Further work will concentrate on the effects of topical antibiotics and steroids in the rabbit model and future clinical trials to establish safety profiles, dosages, and regimens will also be needed.

Allergic Fungal Sinusitis

AFS represents a special subgroup of chronic rhinosinusitis whose treatment is especially challenging [1]. Even with intranasal corticosteroids and multiple courses of systemic steroids, disease recidivism requiring revision FESS is common. Part of the difficulty in elucidating optimal medical therapy for AFS is the fact that the etiology of this disease remains unclear. Complete eradication of fungus from the sinus cavities with both surgical and medical therapy would appear to be a reasonable goal. Unfortunately, the extreme toxicity of systemic antifungal therapy has limited its use in patients with AFS.

The usefulness of postoperative immunotherapy in AFS was highlighted by Folker et al. [14]. Results demonstrated improved mucosal staging, improved sinusitis-specific quality of life, and decreased reliance on both systemic and topical nasal corticosteroids. The study was not blinded and the decision was made not to withhold fungal immunotherapy from any patients with AFS who desired it. As such, the control group was selected retrospectively. Future work would focus on a true parallel prospective, controlled study with blinding. This work suggests the importance that atopy to fungal antigens plays in the etiology of AFS.

Practical management of AFS consists of surgical removal of polyps and reestablishment of sinus aeration with complete removal of fungal mucin. Medical management is then aggressively employed to prevent reobstruction of the ostia via polyps or edema. If the polypoid disease progresses to the point of obstruction, then the cycle of fungal mucin reaccumulation and polyp formation typically requires revision surgery. Aggressive medical and topical therapy is usually required to maintain postoperative AFS patients.

Ponikau et al. [25] suggested that a fungal-mediated process may be the primary etiologic agent not just in AFS, but in all forms of chronic rhinosinusitis. Initially, treatment with topical antifungal medications such as amphotericin B was advocated with some studies showing positive results [26, 28]. These were nonblinded and uncontrolled observational studies. A recent paper by Weschta et al. [35], which examined topical amphotericin B therapy in 60 patients in a prospective, controlled, double-blinded trial. found no difference in any of the parameters studied. Furthermore, a larger, more recent, randomized multi-institutional trial failed to show any efficacy with the use of amphotericin nasal rinses [12].

- The efficacy of topical antifungal medications for any form of chronic rhinosinusitis is currently unproven.

Conclusion

The management of chronic rhinosinusitis can be challenging. While surgical therapy is often required, the postoperative medical management of the disease is believed to be critical for optimal outcome. Postoperative debridement, steroids, saline lavages, antibiotics, topical and nebulized therapy, and the special challenges presented by AFS have been discussed in detail. Many of these issues remain controversial and further research is needed to clarify their role in the treatment of chronic rhinosinusitis.

References

1. Bent JP, Kuhn FA (1994) Diagnosis of allergic fungal sinusitis. Otolaryngol Head Neck Surg 111:580–587
2. Bhattacharyya N, Kepnes LJ (1999) The microbiology of recurrent rhinosinusitis after endoscopic sinus surgery. Arch Otolaryngol Head Neck Surg 125:1117–1120
3. Bugten V, Nordgard S, Steinsvag S (2006) The effects of debridement after endoscopic sinus surgery. Laryngoscope 116:2037–2043
4. Chiu AG, Antunes MB, Feldman M, Cohen NA (2007) An animal model for the study of topical medications in sinusitis. Am J Rhinol 21:5–9
5. Citardi MJ, Kuhn FA (1998) Endoscopically guided frontal sinus beclomethasone instillation for refractory frontal sinus/recess mucosal edema and polyposis. Am J Rhinol 12:179–182
6. DelGaudio JM, Wise SK (2006) Topical steroid drops for the treatment of sinus ostia stenosis in the postoperative period. Am J Rhinol 20:563–567
7. Desrosiers M, Salas-Prato M (2001) Treatment of chronic rhinosinusitis refractory to other treatments with topical antibiotic therapy delivered by means of a large-particle nebulizer: results of a controlled trial. Otolaryngol Head Neck Surg 125:265–269
8. Desrosiers M, Abdolmohsen H, Frenkiel S, Kilty S, Marsan J, Witterick I, Wright E (2007) Intranasal corticosteroid use is associated with lower rates of bacterial recovery in chronic rhinosinusitis. Otolaryngol Head Neck Surg 136:605–609

9. Desrosiers M, Bendouah Z, Barbeau J (2007) Effectiveness of topical antibiotics on *Staphylococcus aureus* biofilm in vitro. Am J Rhinol 21:149–153
10. Dijkstra MD, Ebbens FA, Poublon ML, Fokkens WJ (2004) Fluticasone propionate aqueous nasal spray does not influence the recurrence rate of chronic rhinosinusitis and nasal polyps 1 year after functional endoscopic sinus surgery. Clin Exp Allergy 34:1395–1400
11. Dingsor G, Kramer J, Olsholt R, Soderstrom T (1985) Flunisolide nasal spray 0.025% in the prophylactic treatment of nasal polyposis after polypectomy. A randomized, double-blind, parallel, placebo controlled study. Rhinology 23:49–58
12. Ebbens FA, Scadding GK, Badia L, Hellings PW, Jorissen M, Mullol J, Cardesin A, Bachert C, van Zele TP, Dijkgraaf MG, Lund V, Fokkens WJ (2006) Amphotericin B nasal lavages: not a solution for patients with chronic rhinosinusitis. J Allergy Clin Immunol 118:1149–1156
13. El Naggar M, Kale S, Aldren C, Martin F (1995) Effect of Beconase nasal spray on olfactory function in post-nasal polypectomy patients: a prospective controlled trial. J Laryngol Otol 109:941–944
14. Folker RJ, Marple BF, Mabry RL, Mabry CS (1998) Treatment of allergic fungal sinusitis: a comparison trial of postoperative immunotherapy with specific fungal antigens. Laryngoscope 108:1623–1627
15. Ghannoum M, O'Toole GA (2004) Biofilm antimicrobial resistance. In: Ghannoum M, O'Toole GA (eds) Microbial Biofilms. ASM, Washington DC, pp 250–268
16. Gross CW, Gross WE (1994) Post-operative care for functional endoscopic sinus surgery. Ear Nose Throat J 73:476–479
17. Hardy JG, Lee SW, Wilson CG (1985) Intranasal drug delivery by sprays and drops. J Pharm Pharmacol 37:294–297
18. Karlsson G, Rundcrantz H (1982) A randomized trial of intranasal beclomethasone dipropionate after polypectomy. Rhinology 20:144–148
19. Kuhnel T, Houseman W, Wagner W, Fayed K (1996) How traumatizing is mechanical mucuous membrane care after interventions in paranasal sinuses? A histological immunohistochemical study. Laryngorhinootologie 75:575–579
20. Mabry R (1987) Corticosteroids in rhinology. In: Goldman JL, Blaugrund SM, Shugar JMA (eds) The Principles and Practice of Rhinology. John Wiley, New York, pp 847–853
21. Mierzwinski J, Krzysztof D, Piotr L, Olijewski J, Piziewicz A, Burduk K (2006) Functional endoscopic sinus surgery in children – our experience. Otolaryngol Pol 60:517–520
22. Mitchell RB, Pereira KD, Younis RT, Lazar H (1997) Pediatric functional endoscopic sinus surgery: is a second look necessary? Laryngoscope 107:1267–1269
23. Nilssen EL, Wardrop P, El-Hakim H, White PS, Gardiner Q, Ogston S (2002) A randomized control trial of post-operative care following endoscopic sinus surgery: debridement versus no debridement. J Laryngol Otol 116:108–111
24. Pigret D, Jankowski R (1996) Management of post-ethmoidectomy crust formation: randomized single-blind clinical trial comparing pressurized seawater versus antiseptic/mucolytic saline. Rhinology 34:38–40
25. Ponikau JU, Sherris DA, Kern EB, Homburger HA, Frigas E, Gaffey TA, Roberts GD (1999) The diagnosis and incidence of allergic fungal sinusitis. Mayo Clin Proc 74:877–884
26. Ponikau JU, Sherris DA, Kita H, Kern EB (2002) Intranasal antifungal treatment in 51 patients with CRS. J Allergy Clin Immunol 110:862–866
27. Ramadan HH (1995) What is the bacteriology of chronic sinusitis in adults? Am J Otolaryngol 16:303–306
28. Ricchetti A, Landis BN, Maffioli A, Giger R, Zeng C, Lacroix J (2002) Effect of anti-fungal nasal lavage with amphotericin B on nasal polyposis. J Laryngol Otol 116:261–263
29. Rowe-Jones JM, Medcalf M, Durham SR, Richards DH, MacKay I (2005) Functional endoscopic sinus surgery: 5 year follow up and results of a prospective, randomized, stratified, double-blind, placebo controlled study of postoperative fluticasone propionate aqueous nasal spray. Rhinology 43:2–10
30. Ryan RM, Whittet HB, Norval C, Marks NJ (1996) Minimal follow-up after functional endoscopic sinus surgery. Does it affect outcome? Rhinology 34:44–45
31. Schleimer RP (2004) Glucocorticoids suppress inflammation but spare innate immune responses. Proc Am Thorac Soc 1:222–230
32. Seiberling KA, Grammer LC, Kern RC (2005) Chronic rhinosinusitis and superantigens. Otolaryngol Clin North Am 38:1215–1236
33. Senior BA, Kennedy DW, Tanabodee J, Kroger H, Hassab M, Lanza D (1998) Long-term results of functional endoscopic sinus surgery. Laryngoscope 108:151–157
34. Vaughan WC, Carvalho G (2002) Use of nebulized antibiotics for acute infections in chronic sinusitis. Otolaryngol Head Neck Surg 127:558–568
35. Weschta M, Rimek D, Formanek M, Polzehl D, Podbielski A, Riechelmann H (2004) Topical antifungal treatment of chronic rhinosinusitis with nasal polyps: a randomized, double-blind clinical trial. J Allergy Clin Immunol 113:1122–1128
36. Zhang N, Gevaert P, van Zele T, Perez-Novo C, Patou J, Holtappels G, van Cauwenberge P, Bachert C (2005) An update on the impact of *Staphylococcus aureus* enterotoxins in chronic rhinosinusitis with nasal polyposis. Rhinology 43:162–168

Chapter 17

Evaluation and Treatment of Recurrent Nasal Polyposis

Frederick C. Roediger and Andrew N. Goldberg

17

Core Messages

- Nasal polyposis is the defining feature of a more severe subset of chronic rhinosinusitis.
- Patients with primary or recurrent disease should be evaluated for associated disorders such as asthma, allergic fungal rhinosinusitis, aspirin sensitivity, cystic fibrosis, immunoglobulin subclass deficiency, and primary ciliary dyskinesia.
- Oral and intranasal corticosteroids are the cornerstone of medical therapy for patients with chronic rhinosinusitis with nasal polyposis.
- Patients with medically refractory chronic rhinosinusitis with nasal polyposis or allergic fungal rhinosinusitis are surgical candidates.
- Intensive perioperative medical management and selective use of powered instrumentation facilitate safe and effective surgery.
- Close surveillance, early detection of recurrent polyposis, and tailored medical therapy are required to decrease the need for revision surgery and increase the interval between surgeries in refractory cases.

Contents

Introduction

Nasal polyposis (NP) is a clinical and pathological manifestation of chronic inflammation in the paranasal sinuses. Population-based surveys have shown a prevalence of 2–4% in the general population, while autopsy studies suggest a much higher rate of preclinical lesions [25, 35, 42].

In the past, the literature referred to NP as a clinical entity distinct from chronic rhinosinusitis (CRS). Today, NP is recognized as the defining feature of a more severe and treatment-refractory subset of rhinosinusitis, CRS with nasal polyposis (CRSwNP) [40]. Patients with CRSwNP demonstrate decreased disease-specific quality of life (QOL) and greater extent of disease on computed tomography (CT) scans than their nonpolypoid counterparts [14]. CRSwNP patients also commonly have symptoms that persist despite maximal medical therapy, and improve less after surgery than patients with CRS without nasal polyposis (CRSsNP) [14, 29]. Despite ongoing research, the pathogenesis of NP remains elusive.

- The majority (>80%) of polyps appear to be the product of eosinophilic inflammation, characterized by subepithelial caps of eosinophils, pseudocyst formation with deposition of albumin, and elevated levels of the inflammatory mediators interleukin-5 and eotaxin [6].

Others, such as those associated with ciliary dysmotility, are neutrophil-rich, yet may appear identical on clinical examination [58]. The reason for these findings is still unknown. Theories explaining polyp formation, regardless of the inciting event, are numerous and include loss of autonomic innervation, dysregulation of water and ion transporters, and chronic vascular changes leading to congestion and exudation [6, 42].

Since NP may be the presenting manifestation of several conditions, such as allergic fungal rhinosinusitis (AFRS) and cystic fibrosis (CF), specialized testing and referrals should be arranged if an underlying disorder is suspected. Those patients with disease refractory to maximal medical therapy are considered for surgical intervention. Well-designed and sometimes intensive medical regimens are essential in both the immediate perioperative period and the long-term for successful management.

Evaluation

Besides querying symptoms of CRS [10], a treatment history should be carefully elicited. Prior medical regimens should be assessed for adequacy of dose, duration, patient adherence, and medication interactions. A history of complications of oral steroid use, such as worsening hypertension, poor diabetic control, psychological disturbances, or osteoporosis, is worrisome, since systemic corticosteroids play a central role in the treatment of recurrent disease. Early identification of non-steroid-responsive NP can minimize risks in patients who may not derive a benefit from corticosteroids.

Past surgical history, including complications and perioperative medical care, is explored to gauge the severity, extent, and laterality of the disease. Prior operative reports should be scrutinized, noting that although sinus surgery has evolved from simple polypectomy under local anesthesia in the pre-endoscopic era to formal FESS today, a wide range of prior procedures are possible.

- Reports of visual disturbance, watery nasal discharge (particularly unilateral), meningitis, excessive bleeding, epiphora, and facial numbness may indicate involvement of critical structures related to previous surgery or complications of severe polyposis.

A comprehensive head and neck examination, including an assessment of the cranial nerves with attention to trigeminal nerve function and extraocular movements, should be performed. Further ophthalmic evaluation may identify unilateral visual acuity loss, proptosis, or epiphora. The nose is examined externally for weakened cartilaginous support or widening from bony expansion from nasal polyps or neoplasm. Anterior rhinoscopy pre- and postapplication of a topical decongestant is then used to assess nasal cavity patency, mucosal health, septal position, and inferior turbinate size and response to vasoconstriction.

Nasal endoscopy is an essential component of the rhinologic exam in patients with recurrent polyposis. The procedure can define the extent and character of NP, detect subtle mucosal changes in the sinus cavities, and examination of the fovea ethmoidalis, cribriform region, and sphenoid may reveal pulsation related to dehiscence of the skull base or carotid. In addition, movement of nasal contents during ballottement of the eye during office endoscopy can signify dehiscence of the orbital wall. Treatment planning, postoperative care, and surveillance all depend heavily on the findings during nasal endoscopy.

A contemporary CT scan of the paranasal sinuses with fine cuts should be carefully analyzed for the extent of disease, skull-base and orbital integrity, nasolacrimal ducts, middle turbinates, and remaining surgical landmarks. Hallmarks of specific diagnoses, such as an expansile lesion with central serpiginous calcifications in AFRS or the dense bone associated with chronic infection, should be noted. MRI of the paranasal sinuses with gadolinium enhancement may also be indicated, for example to identify encephalocele or meningocele when skull-base dehiscence is detected on CT.

Serum total immunoglobulin E (IgE) levels are helpful in patients with concurrent asthma, since IgE levels correlate with airway hyperresponsiveness [56, 62]. However, the exact role of IgE in predicting the severity of CRS continues to be debated, with a correlation between serum total IgE level and mucosal disease on CT scan demonstrated in some studies [7] but not others [52]. No significant change in IgE is seen 1 year after sinus surgery in patients reporting improvement in symptoms, indicating that IgE levels are not a sensitive barometer for changes in CRS [34]. In contrast, peripheral eosinophilia has been shown to correlate with the degree of nasal polyposis [32] as well as disease severity on CT scan [7, 32, 52]. For those patients progressing to sinus surgery, an elevated mucosal eosinophil level (>5 cells per high-power field) indicates more severe disease [32].

Specialized testing for associated disorders, as outlined in Table 17.1, should be considered on a case by case basis.

Although recurrent nasal polyposis most likely indicates a diagnosis of CRSwNP alone, several associated disorders must be considered during history-taking (Table 17.1).

Inhalant Allergy

Allergic rhinitis (AR) is present in 15–20% of the general population [42]. However, although both atopy and NP

Table 17.1 Disorders associated with nasal polyposis

Disorder	Age of onset	Laterality	Associated findings	Confirmatory studies
Allergic rhinitis (AR)	Bimodal peaks in early school and early adult years	Bilateral	• Pale, edematous inferior turbinates • Transverse nasal crease • Dark, edematous infraorbital skin • Mouth breathing	• Allergy skin testing or radio-allergosorbent test (RAST)
Asthma	May develop at any age, but most (75%) diagnosed before age 7 years	Bilateral	• Episodic wheeze, cough, and difficulty breathing triggered by exercise, cold air, or allergens • Personal/family history of atopy	• Pulmonary function tests (PFTs) demonstrating variable expiratory airflow obstruction
Allergic fungal rhinosinusitis (AFRS)	Adolescents and young adults (mean age 22 years)	Often unilateral, may be bilateral	• Unilateral thick, dark rhinorrhea • AR, asthma (> 50%) • Facial/ocular dysmorphia	• Elevated serum IgE • Type I hypersensitivity by history, skin testing, or RAST • Characteristic computed tomography scan • Eosinophilic mucus • Positive fungal stain of sinus contents
Aspirin sensitivity	Third to fourth decade	Bilateral	• Wheezing, rhinorrhea, nasal congestion, tearing, and/or facial flushing 30–120 min after ingestion of aspirin or nonsteroidal anti-inflammatory drugs	• Serial monitoring of PFTs after aspirin challenge • Concurrent rise in urinary leukotrienes
Cystic fibrosis (CF)	Most (> 90%) identified by age 8 years	Bilateral	• Recurrent respiratory infections • Failure to thrive • Steatorrhea	• Elevated sweat chloride (> 60 mEq/l) on two or more occasions (95% sensitive) • Molecular testing for 20–30 most common mutations (> 90% sensitive)
Immunoglobulin subclass deficiency	Adolescents and young adults	Bilateral	• Recurrent sinopulmonary infections with common bacterial pathogens • Osteomyelitis, meningitis, diarrhea, skin infections	• Complete blood count with differential • Total IgG, IgA, complement (CH50), and individual IgG subclass levels
Primary ciliary dyskinesia (PCD)	Children	Bilateral	• Recurrent respiratory infections, bronchiectasis • Situs inversus • Infertility in men, decreased fertility in women	• Endoscopic sinonasal mucosal biopsy with electron microscopy
Young's syndrome	Onset in early childhood	Bilateral	• Infertility secondary to obstructive azoospermia • Less sinopulmonary infections as an adult	• Normal CF and PCD testing
Antrochoanal polyp	Young adults (mean age 27 years)	Unilateral	• Unilateral nasal obstruction, rhinorrhea, protrusion into the superior oropharynx	• Surgical excision and pathological examination to exclude inverted papilloma and AFRS

occur in subsets of patients with CRS, a direct or causal relationship between inhalant allergies and NP has yet to be proven.

- Positive skin tests occur in a similar percentage of patients with and without nasal polyps [6].

Less than 5% of patients with inhalant allergies have NP, similar to the general population [42], and the prevalence of NP is actually higher in nonallergic rhinitis than the corresponding allergic form [58].

Asthma

The frequencies of NP in allergic and intrinsic asthma are approximately 5% and 13%, respectively [58]. NP occurs most frequently in nonatopic asthma patients over age 40 years with severe, steroid-dependent disease [58]. Treating sinus disease in asthmatics is an important component of their care; a reduction of total annual oral prednisone and antibiotic use in patients with concurrent asthma has been well documented after FESS [47, 57, 64].

Allergic Fungal Rhinosinusitis

AFRS is thought to represent a type I hypersensitivity reaction to noninvasive fungus. Nearly all AFRS patients have NP [55]. Most AFRS patients present with a history of progressive nasal obstruction, anosmia, and dark nasal discharge predominantly affecting one side. The characteristic CT scan findings include opacification of multiple ipsilateral sinuses containing areas of hyperattenuation from calcification and products of fungal metabolism (iron, magnesium, manganese) and expanding borders caused by mass effect of debris and dense polyposis [5, 11]. Bony erosion with skull-base or orbital involvement leading to proptosis occurs in roughly half of patients [23]. Recent work suggests that AFRS is a subset of eosinophilic mucin chronic rhinosinusitis [21, 48]. Despite thorough surgical debridement and intensive medical therapy, AFRS frequently recurs and requires reoperation [33].

Aspirin Sensitivity

Aspirin sensitivity (AS) is a clinical syndrome in which patients typically develop refractory CRS and asthma in the third to fourth decade of life, with acute respiratory exacerbations precipitated by aspirin or nonsteroidal anti-inflammatory drugs, and is associated with NP 36% of the time [58]. These patients generally have worse respiratory disease than non-AS asthmatics [20]. The triad of aspirin sensitivity, asthma, and NP is termed Samter's triad, or aspirin-exacerbated respiratory disease.

Cystic Fibrosis

- CF should be considered in the workup of any child with NP.

Most patients with CF present with either recurrent respiratory infections or manifestations of pancreatic insufficiency, such as failure to thrive or steatorrhea [54]. Most develop CRS, with approximately 20% of affected patients demonstrating NP on nasal endoscopy and >90% having pan-opacification of the sinuses on CT [58, 70].

Immunoglobulin Subclass Deficiency

Deficiency of one or more of the immunoglobulin G (IgG) subclasses occurs in up to 20% of the general population, yet most individuals are asymptomatic [46]. Some present in adolescence and early adulthood with CRSwNP and recurrent pulmonary infections. Testing reveals normal or near-normal total serum IgG with one or more subclass levels greater than two standard deviations below the age-adjusted mean [26]. Early diagnosis and immunoglobulin replacement can reduce the frequency and severity of infections and increase life expectancy.

Primary Ciliary Dyskinesia

This autosomal recessive disease is characterized by recurrent childhood respiratory infections and CRSwNP secondary to ciliary immotility [1]. Fifty percent of cases are associated with situs inversus [44]. The triad of bronchiectasis (after repeated pulmonary infections), CRS, and situs inversus is termed Kartagener's syndrome [2]. Patients with PCD generally have a normal lifespan and have a lower rate of decline of lung function than patients with CF, so they are more likely to present undiagnosed as a young adult with NP [44].

Young's Syndrome

This disorder is characterized by azoospermia, NP, and recurrent sinopulmonary infections [24]. Patients have normal sweat chloride values and pancreatic function, unlike those with CF, and motile cilia, distinguishing them from patients with PCD.

Unilateral Recurrent Nasal Polyps

- Patients with unilateral recurrent nasal polyps should be closely scrutinized for inverted papilloma and neoplasm.

Past pathology slides can be requested and examined. AFRS and antrochoanal polyp can also present with unilateral disease.

Medical Treatment

- Oral corticosteroids are used frequently in the treatment of severe, recurrent nasal polyps.

Their efficacy has been noted anecdotally for decades and continues to be documented in the literature [36, 65]. One small, randomized clinical trial addressed the short-term effects of systemic steroids [4]. This study showed that patients with severe NP had significant improvements in general QOL after a 2-week prednisone burst and taper compared to a control group with similar disease that received no treatment [4]. The same investigators also showed improvements in nasal symptoms, polyp size, and nasal patency at 2 weeks with this medical regimen [9]. Chronic oral steroid use may be necessary in some patients, particularly those with concomitant pulmonary disease. Effort should be made to reduce oral steroid levels to the lowest possible to control disease with the goal of a regimen of every-other-day steroid dosing to minimize adrenal suppression. Patients requiring more than three courses of systemic corticosteroids can be considered for functional endoscopic sinus surgery (FESS) [13, 45]. Using this guideline, on average 10–30% of patients with CRSwNP undergoing close observation and intensive medical treatment for 1 year will progress to need surgery [13, 45].

- Intranasal corticosteroids have an exceedingly low systemic bioavailability [3] and should be used in the long-term to safely suppress inflammation.

Intensive medical treatment of NP with the strategy of a combination of short-course systemic and long-term topical corticosteroids is the most common approach today and its efficacy continues to be documented [13, 28, 37, 50, 61].

Oral antibiotics are used widely in the medical management of recurrent CRSwNP. Coverage should include both aerobic and anaerobic bacteria and should be culture-directed if possible [43]. In the absence of cultures, suitable empiric broad-spectrum antibiotics include penicillin derivatives with a beta-lactamase inhibitor (amoxicillin/clavulanate), fluoroquinolones (levofloxacin), or macrolides (erythromycin). The macrolides have received much attention for their anti-inflammatory and immunomodulatory effects and the potential for inducing polyp regression when courses longer than 4 weeks are prescribed [38]. For example, an 8- to 12-week course of clarithromycin in patients with CRSwNP was shown to significantly decrease interleukin-8 levels in nasal lavage and reduce polyp size in 40% of cases [69]. Clinical improvement manifests as decreased nasal secretions, postnasal drip, and nasal obstruction [38].

Topical application of antibiotics in irrigation solutions is a common practice despite little data on their use in NP patients [66]. One study, in which one-third of patients had NP, showed successful treatment of drug-resistant bacterial exacerbations with mupirocin irrigations [59]. Despite one small study of patients with CRSwNP showing improvements in objective CT findings and endoscopic scores with the use of topical amphotericin B [51], larger studies of CRS patients in which the majority (80–100%) had NP have shown no benefit to this therapy [19, 67].

Leukotriene blockade provides a benefit in patients with asthma, especially those with AS, improving lung function and decreasing medication use and exacerbations [16]. Identification of increased leukotriene release in the nasal cavities of patients with NP and observations that NP was reduced in Samter's triad patients treated with leukotriene inhibitors led to the hypothesis that CRSwNP patients would benefit from similar treatment.

- Leukotriene blockade may benefit patients with nasal polyps.

A recent clinical trial using the cysteinyl leukotriene receptor antagonist zafirlukast and the 5-lipoxygenase inhibitor zileuton in patients with NP showed significant improvements in sinonasal symptom scores and reductions in the degree of polyposis and oral steroid use with leukotriene blockade [49].

Aspirin desensitization should be offered to all patients with Samter's triad. This therapy requires several days of inpatient treatment with continuous daily aspirin ingestion until the desensitized state is achieved [60]. Maintenance with daily aspirin, typically 650 mg of enteric-coated aspirin twice daily, can reduce the number of asthma exacerbations and hospitalizations per year, limit the need for sinus surgery, and reduce antibiotic and corticosteroid use [63].

Adjunctive measures in the treatment of CRSwNP include nasal saline rinses, smoking cessation, and addressing atopy. Normal saline applied to the nasal cavities three times a day has been shown to decrease sinonasal symptoms and endoscopically observed mucosal edema and secretions, and increase QOL in patients with CRS refractory to medical and surgical therapy [15]. Smoking cessation is highly recommended since a history of tobacco use portends a prolonged course with increased recurrence rates [30]. Treatment of inhalant allergies is important in the overall care of the patient with CRSwNP and may help alleviate certain nasal symptoms such as rhinorrhea or pruritis. Immunotherapy (IT) is unlikely to have a significant direct effect on the degree of nasal polyposis in CRSwNP, but postoperative IT with specific fungal antigens is highly effective in improving QOL and endoscopic findings and decreasing steroid use in patients with AFRS [8, 22].

Patient Selection for Surgical Treatment

In a comparison of medical and surgical therapy, Blomqvist et al. treated patients with CRSwNP with a 10-day burst and taper of oral prednisolone and a concurrent month of topical budesonide, then randomized the subjects to have FESS on either the right or left side [12]. One year after surgery, patients reported a greater improvement on the surgical side compared to the medically treated side in terms of nasal obstruction, nasal secretions, and sinus pressure, yet only 25% pursued FESS on the medical side when it was offered [12].

While this intriguing study appears to show an advantage for surgery, in general only patients with CRSwNP refractory to maximal medical therapy are considered candidates for surgical treatment. The basis for this practice is a randomized, controlled clinical trial comparing medical and surgical therapy for CRS, showing improvements in subjective symptoms, QOL, and endoscopic score at 6 and 12 months in both treatment groups with no statistical difference between the two arms of the study [53]. Roughly 40% of participants had CRSwNP and subset analysis demonstrated the same findings.

- A course of maximal medical therapy, ideally including a macrolide or another appropriate antibiotic, oral and/or topical corticosteroids, and nasal saline irrigations, is recommended for all CRS patients prior to considering sinus surgery.

The one notable exception to these guidelines is AFRS, since surgery to remove the offending agent is the primary treatment modality. Also, in patients with persistently refractory disease, it may be reasonable to discuss the role of scheduling FESS at given intervals, when symptom severity peaks.

Perioperative Medical Care

It has long been recognized that medical therapy in the immediate postoperative period is critical to the success of surgery for NP. Two placebo-controlled clinical trials of budesonide [27] and flunisolide [17] after polypectomy emerged in the early 1980s, showing greater symptom improvement, delayed recurrence, and greater interval between surgeries for the treatment groups compared to placebo.

Current methods include the use of burst and taper oral corticosteroids started the week preceding surgery. Evidence to support this approach is now emerging and supports prior anecdotal descriptions of less inflammation, reduced polyp size, and improved technical ease during surgery with the use of perioperative systemic corticosteroids [68]. The taper is continued for at least 2 weeks after surgery and adjusted according to nasal endoscopic findings during postoperative examination and debridement. Patients with allergic fungal sinusitis may benefit from a slower taper of oral steroids lasting >6 weeks. Broad-spectrum antibiotics are given during the same 3-week period surrounding the surgery. Topical corticosteroids are continued for long-term maintenance.

Surgical Technique

Surgery concentrates on complete removal of nasal polyps and bony septations, particularly in the ethmoid sinus, and includes wide openings in the maxillary, sphenoid, and frontal regions, if they are involved. The use of Kerrison rongeurs for removal of thick bony partitions and otherwise diseased bone is helpful when osteitic changes and osteoneogenesis have taken place. Thickened mucosa without polyps is not typically removed, as the regenerated mucosa demonstrates less effective ciliary regrowth and a reduction in mucous gland density.

The use of image guidance is helpful in surgery for recurrent NP because landmarks are frequently distorted or obscured by the disease or absent after prior intervention.

Powered instrumentation greatly facilitates surgery on recurrent CRSwNP, allowing the removal of polyps rapidly and effectively with reduced bleeding. Continuous suction is available when using a microdebrider without switching instruments.

Safe use of the microdebrider requires strict adherence to several principles:

1. The tip should be visualized at all times, especially when cutting. The teeth of the microdebrider, even when not spinning, can abrade mucosa during passage of the instrument in and out of the nasal cavity.

2. Prior to engaging tissue at any phase of the surgery, the suction port should be opened by tapping the foot pedal and spinning the blade a fraction of a turn. In general, only tissue that moves freely into the open suction is removed.
3. The cutting face of the tip should be aimed away from important structures.
4. There must be constant assessment of the field and decisions made regarding which mucosa to preserve. The tip should be pointed away from mucosa that is to be spared.

The microdebrider plays a more prominent role and provides a greater advantage in the polyp-debulking steps of the surgery than during the refined components, such as identification of the skull base and treatment of sphenoid and frontal sinus disease. However, when used judiciously, the instrument is useful in delicate work and special angulated blades are available. Powered instrumentation helps achieve the primary surgical goal of removing disease from its origin in the maxillary and ethmoid sinuses. The creation of well-aerated, accessible cavities facilitates office-based endoscopic surveillance and delivery of topical medications in the postoperative and maintenance phases of treatment.

Intraoperative specimen sent for aerobic, anaerobic, and fungal culture as well as pathologic analysis of thick secretions and debris can aid in directing antibiotics at offending organisms. Pathologic analysis of debris removed from the sinuses as well as analysis of tissue specimen can identify fungal elements, eosinophilic infiltration, and tissue invasion that may guide postoperative care and provide valuable prognostic information.

At the conclusion of surgery, techniques that reduce synechiae formation, such as middle-turbinate medialization, can be employed to optimize results. It is likely that future dressings will incorporate pharmacotherapy, such as steroid deposition, to reduce inflammation and avoid the systemic effects of oral steroid therapy.

Surgical Outcomes

Historically, higher recurrence rates after FESS have been observed in patients with CRSwNP compared to those with CRSsNP [18, 29], and a recent study documented that patients with CRSwNP experience less improvement symptomatically after FESS and a higher rate of requiring revision surgery (10% versus 0.8%) than CRSsNP patients [14]. Furthermore, NP is also associated with failure of revision FESS [31, 39, 41]. For these reasons, more vigilant surveillance and adjustments to medical therapy are required in patients with CRSwNP than in those without polyposis to prevent recidivism.

Future Directions

The pathophysiology of recurrent NP, like that of its parent disease, CRS, remains enigmatic. Current investigations into the various molecular mechanisms of the underlying inflammatory response as well as the etiologic agents will hopefully identify new therapeutic targets. While surgical therapy remains an option for medically refractory disease, more refined medical treatments should further reduce the need for systemic corticosteroids and improve the overall care of patients with NP.

Tips and Pearls

1. Always consider cystic fibrosis in the workup of children with NP.
2. Suspect AFRS, inverted papilloma, or an underlying malignancy in patients with unilateral NP.
3. Combine antibiotics such as macrolides, oral and topical corticosteroids, and adjunctive measures such as nasal saline to administer maximal medical therapy.
4. Always use systemic corticosteroids perioperatively to improve the surgical field and make refined, thorough, and safe surgery possible.
5. Be wary of reducing the postoperative oral steroid taper too quickly and allowing regrowth of polyps in the surgical healing phase.
6. Regular surveillance is required to improve long-term outcomes and determine the timing of treatment intervention.

References

1. Afzelius BA (2004) Cilia-related diseases. J Pathol 204:470–477
2. Afzelius BA, Stenram U (2006) Prevalence and genetics of immotile-cilia syndrome and left-handedness. Int J Dev Biol 50:571–573
3. Allen A, Down G, Newland A, Reynard K, Rousell V, Salmon E, Scott R (2007) Absolute bioavailability of intranasal fluticasone furoate in healthy subjects. Clin Ther 29:1415–1420
4. Alobid I, Benitez P, Pujols L, Maldonado M, Bernal-Sprekelsen M, Morello A, Picado C, Mullol J (2006) Severe nasal polyposis and its impact on quality of life. The effect of a short course of oral steroids followed by long-term intranasal steroid treatment. Rhinology 44:8–13
5. Aribandi M, McCoy VA, Bazan C 3rd (2007) Imaging features of invasive and noninvasive fungal sinusitis: a review. Radiographics 27:1283–1296
6. Bachert C, Gevaert P, Holtappels G, Cuvelier C, van Cauwenberge P (2000) Nasal polyposis: from cytokines to growth. Am J Rhinol 14:279–290

7. Baroody FM, Suh SH, Naclerio RM (1997) Total IgE serum levels correlate with sinus mucosal thickness on computerized tomography scans. J Allergy Clin Immunol 100:563–568
8. Bassichis BA, Marple BF, Mabry RL, Newcomer MT, Schwade ND (2001) Use of immunotherapy in previously treated patients with allergic fungal sinusitis. Otolaryngol Head Neck Surg 125:487–490
9. Benitez P, Alobid I, de Haro J, Berenguer J, Bernal-Sprekelsen M, Pujols L, Picado C, Mullol J (2006) A short course of oral prednisone followed by intranasal budesonide is an effective treatment of severe nasal polyps. Laryngoscope 116:770–775
10. Benninger MS, Ferguson BJ, Hadley JA, Hamilos DL, Jacobs M, Kennedy DW, Lanza DC, Marple BF, Osguthorpe JD, Stankiewicz JA, Anon J, Denneny J, Emanuel I, Levine H (2003) Adult chronic rhinosinusitis: definitions, diagnosis, epidemiology, and pathophysiology. Otolaryngol Head Neck Surg 129:S1–S32
11. Bent JP 3rd, Kuhn FA (1994) Diagnosis of allergic fungal sinusitis. Otolaryngol Head Neck Surg 111:580–588
12. Blomqvist EH, Lundblad L, Anggard A, Haraldsson PO, Stjarne P (2001) A randomized controlled study evaluating medical treatment versus surgical treatment in addition to medical treatment of nasal polyposis. J Allergy Clin Immunol 107:224–228
13. Bonfils P, Nores JM, Halimi P, Avan P (2003) Corticosteroid treatment in nasal polyposis with a three-year follow-up period. Laryngoscope 113:683–687
14. Deal RT, Kountakis SE (2004) Significance of nasal polyps in chronic rhinosinusitis: symptoms and surgical outcomes. Laryngoscope 114:1932–1935
15. Desrosiers MY, Salas-Prato M (2001) Treatment of chronic rhinosinusitis refractory to other treatments with topical antibiotic therapy delivered by means of a large-particle nebulizer: results of a controlled trial. Otolaryngol Head Neck Surg 125:265–269
16. Drazen JM, Israel E, O'Byrne PM (1999) Treatment of asthma with drugs modifying the leukotriene pathway. N Engl J Med 340:197–206
17. Drettner B, Ebbesen A, Nilsson M (1982) Prophylactive treatment with flunisolide after polypectomy. Rhinology 20:149–158
18. Dursun E, Korkmaz H, Eryilmaz A, Bayiz U, Sertkaya D, Samim E (2003) Clinical predictors of long-term success after endoscopic sinus surgery. Otolaryngol Head Neck Surg 129:526–531
19. Ebbens FA, Scadding GK, Badia L, Hellings PW, Jorissen M, Mullol J, Cardesin A, Bachert C, van Zele TP, Dijkgraaf MG, Lund V, Fokkens WJ (2006) Amphotericin B nasal lavages: not a solution for patients with chronic rhinosinusitis. J Allergy Clin Immunol 118:1149–1156
20. Fahrenholz JM (2003) Natural history and clinical features of aspirin-exacerbated respiratory disease. Clin Rev Allergy Immunol 24:113–124
21. Ferguson BJ (2000) Eosinophilic mucin rhinosinusitis: a distinct clinicopathological entity. Laryngoscope 110:799–813
22. Folker RJ, Marple BF, Mabry RL, Mabry CS (1998) Treatment of allergic fungal sinusitis: a comparison trial of post-operative immunotherapy with specific fungal antigens. Laryngoscope 108:1623–1627
23. Ghegan MD, Lee FS, Schlosser RJ (2006) Incidence of skull base and orbital erosion in allergic fungal rhinosinusitis (AFRS) and non-AFRS. Otolaryngol Head Neck Surg 134:592–555
24. Handelsman DJ, Conway AJ, Boylan LM, Turtle JR (1984) Young's syndrome. Obstructive azoospermia and chronic sinopulmonary infections. N Engl J Med 310:3–9
25. Hedman J, Kaprio J, Poussa T, Nieminen MM (1999) Prevalence of asthma, aspirin intolerance, nasal polyposis and chronic obstructive pulmonary disease in a population-based study. Int J Epidemiol 28:717–722
26. Herrod HG (1993) Clinical significance of IgG subclasses. Curr Opin Pediatr 5:696–699
27. Karlsson G, Rundcrantz H (1982) A randomized trial of intranasal beclomethasone dipropionate after polypectomy. Rhinology 20:144–148
28. Keith P, Nieminen J, Hollingworth K, Dolovich J (2000) Efficacy and tolerability of fluticasone propionate nasal drops 400 microgram once daily compared with placebo for the treatment of bilateral polyposis in adults. Clin Exp Allergy 30:1460–1468
29. Kennedy DW (1992) Prognostic factors, outcomes and staging in ethmoid sinus surgery. Laryngoscope 102:1–18
30. Kennedy DW, Wright ED, Goldberg AN (2000) Objective and subjective outcomes in surgery for chronic sinusitis. Laryngoscope 110:29–31
31. King JM, Caldarelli DD, Pigato JB (1994) A review of revision functional endoscopic sinus surgery. Laryngoscope 104:404–408
32. Kountakis SE, Arango P, Bradley D, Wade ZK, Borish L (2004) Molecular and cellular staging for the severity of chronic rhinosinusitis. Laryngoscope 114:1895–1905
33. Kuhn FA, Javer AR (2000) Allergic fungal sinusitis: a four-year follow-up. Am J Rhinol 14:149–156
34. Lal D, Baroody FM, Weitzel EK, deTineo M, Naclerio RM (2006) Total IgE levels do not change 1 year after endoscopic sinus surgery in patients with chronic rhinosinusitis. Int Arch Allergy Immunol 139:146–148
35. Larsen PL, Tos M (2004) Origin of nasal polyps: an endoscopic autopsy study. Laryngoscope 114:710–719
36. Lildholdt T, Fogstrup J, Gammelgaard N, Kortholm B, Ulsoe C (1988) Surgical versus medical treatment of nasal polyps. Acta Otolaryngol 105:140–143

37. Lund VJ, Flood J, Sykes AP, Richards DH (1998) Effect of fluticasone in severe polyposis. Arch Otolaryngol Head Neck Surg 124:513–518
38. Majima Y (2004) Clinical implications of the immunomodulatory effects of macrolides on sinusitis. Am J Med 117:S20–25S
39. McMains KC, Kountakis SE (2005) Revision functional endoscopic sinus surgery: objective and subjective surgical outcomes. Am J Rhinol 19:344–347
40. Meltzer EO, Hamilos DL, Hadley JA, Lanza DC, Marple BF, Nicklas RA, Bachert C, Baraniuk J, Baroody FM, Benninger MS, Brook I, Chowdhury BA, Druce HM, Durham S, Ferguson B, Gwaltney JM Jr, Kaliner M, Kennedy DW, Lund V, Naclerio R, Pawankar R, Piccirillo JF, Rohane P, Simon R, Slavin RG, Togias A, Wald ER, Zinreich SJ; American Academy of Allergy, Asthma and Immunology; American Academy of Otolaryngic Allergy; American Academy of Otolaryngology-Head and Neck Surgery; American College of Allergy, Asthma and Immunology; American Rhinologic Society (2004) Rhinosinusitis: establishing definitions for clinical research and patient care. Otolaryngol Head Neck Surg 131:S1–S62
41. Moses RL, Cornetta A, Atkins JP Jr, Roth M, Rosen MR, Keane WM (1998) Revision endoscopic sinus surgery: the Thomas Jefferson University experience. Ear Nose Throat J 77:190, 193–5, 199–202
42. Mygind N, Dahl R, Bachert C (2000) Nasal polyposis, eosinophil dominated inflammation, and allergy. Thorax 55: S79–S83
43. Nadel DM, Lanza DC, Kennedy DW (1998) Endoscopically guided cultures in chronic sinusitis. Am J Rhinol 12:233–241
44. Noone PG, Leigh MW, Sannuti A, Minnix SL, Carson JL, Hazucha M, Zariwala MA, Knowles MR (2004) Primary ciliary dyskinesia: diagnostic and phenotypic features. Am J Respir Crit Care Med 169:459–467
45. Nores JM, Avan P, Bonfils P (2003) Medical management of nasal polyposis: a study in a series of 152 consecutive patients. Rhinology 41:97–102
46. Ochs, HD, Stiehm, ER, Winkelstein, JA, Cunningham-Rundles C, Durandy A, Lederman HM, Notarangelo LD, Rawlings DJ, Roifman CM (2004) Antibody deficiencies. In: Stiehm ER, Ochs HD, Winkelstein JA (eds) Immunologic Disorders in Infants and Children (5th edn). Elsevier, Philadelphia, pp 356–426
47. Palmer JN, Conley DB, Dong RG, Ditto AM, Yarnold PR, Kern RC (2001) Efficacy of endoscopic sinus surgery in the management of patients with asthma and chronic sinusitis. Am J Rhinol 15:49–53
48. Pant H, Kette FE, Smith WB, Macardle PJ, Wormald PJ (2006) Eosinophilic mucus chronic rhinosinusitis: clinical subgroups or a homogeneous pathogenic entity? Laryngoscope 116:1241–1247
49. Parnes SM, Chuma AV (2000) Acute effects of antileukotrienes on sinonasal polyposis and sinusitis. Ear Nose Throat J 79:18–20, 24–5
50. Penttila M, Poulsen P, Hollingworth K, Holmstrom M (2000) Dose-related efficacy and tolerability of fluticasone propionate nasal drops 400 microg once daily and twice daily in the treatment of bilateral nasal polyposis: a placebo-controlled randomized study in adult patients. Clin Exp Allergy 30:94–102
51. Ponikau JU, Sherris DA, Weaver A, Kita H (2005) Treatment of chronic rhinosinusitis with intranasal amphotericin B: a randomized, placebo-controlled, double-blind pilot trial. J Allergy Clin Immunol 115:125–131
52. Poznanovic SA, Kingdom TT (2007) Total IgE levels and peripheral eosinophilia: correlation with mucosal disease based on computed tomographic imaging of the paranasal sinus. Arch Otolaryngol Head Neck Surg 133:701–704
53. Ragab SM, Lund VJ, Scadding G (2004) Evaluation of the medical and surgical treatment of chronic rhinosinusitis: a prospective, randomised, controlled trial. Laryngoscope 114:923–930
54. Ratjen F, Doring G (2003) Cystic fibrosis. Lancet 361:681–689
55. Ryan MW, Marple BF (2007) Allergic fungal rhinosinusitis: diagnosis and management. Curr Opin Otolaryngol Head Neck Surg 15:18–22
56. Sears MR, Burrows B, Flannery EM, Herbison GP, Hewitt CJ, Holdaway MD (1991) Relation between airway responsiveness and serum IgE in children with asthma and in apparently normal children. N Engl J Med 325:1067–1071
57. Senior BA, Kennedy DW, Tanabodee J, Kroger H, Hassab M, Lanza DC (1999) Long-term impact of functional endoscopic sinus surgery on asthma. Otolaryngol Head Neck Surg 121:66–68
58. Settipane GA (1987) Nasal polyps: epidemiology, pathology, immunology, and treatment. Am J Rhinol 1:119–126
59. Solares CA, Batra PS, Hall GS, Citardi MJ (2006) Treatment of chronic rhinosinusitis exacerbations due to methicillin-resistant *Staphylococcus aureus* with mupirocin irrigations. Am J Otolaryngol 27:161–165
60. Stevenson DD (2003) Aspirin desensitization in patients with AERD. Clin Rev Allergy Immunol 24:159–168
61. Subramanian HN, Schechtman KB, Hamilos DL (2002) A retrospective analysis of treatment outcomes and time to relapse after intensive medical treatment for chronic sinusitis. Am J Rhinol 16:303–312
62. Sunyer J, Anto JM, Sabria J, Roca J, Morell F, Rodriguez-Roisin R, Rodrigo MJ (1995) Relationship between serum IgE and airway responsiveness in adults with asthma. J Allergy Clin Immunol 95:699–706
63. Sweet JM, Stevenson DD, Simon RA, Mathison DA (1990) Long-term effects of aspirin desensitization – treatment for aspirin-sensitive rhinosinusitis-asthma. J Allergy Clin Immunol 85:59–65

64. Uri N, Cohen-Kerem R, Barzilai G, Greenberg E, Doweck I, Weiler-Ravell D (2002) Functional endoscopic sinus surgery in the treatment of massive polyposis in asthmatic patients. J Laryngol Otol 116:185–189
65. Van Camp C, Clement PA (1994) Results of oral steroid treatment in nasal polyposis. Rhinology 32:5–9
66. Vining EM (2006) Evolution of medical management of chronic rhinosinusitis. Ann Otol Rhinol Laryngol Suppl 196:54–60
67. Weschta M, Rimek D, Formanek M, Polzehl D, Podbielski A, Riechelmann H (2004) Topical antifungal treatment of chronic rhinosinusitis with nasal polyps: a randomized, double-blind clinical trial. J Allergy Clin Immunol 113:1122–1128
68. Wright ED, Agrawal S (2007) Impact of perioperative systemic steroids on surgical outcomes in patients with chronic rhinosinusitis with polyposis: evaluation with the novel Perioperative Sinus Endoscopy (POSE) scoring system. Laryngoscope 117:1–28
69. Yamada T, Fujieda S, Mori S, Yamamoto H, Saito H (2000) Macrolide treatment decreased the size of nasal polyps and IL-8 levels in nasal lavage. Am J Rhinol 14:143–148
70. Yung MW, Gould J, Upton GJ (2002) Nasal polyposis in children with cystic fibrosis: a long-term follow-up study. Ann Otol Rhinol Laryngol 111:1081–1086

Chapter 18

Revision Surgery for Allergic Fungal Rhinosinusitis

18

Subinoy Das, Patricia A. Maeso, and Stilianos E. Kountakis

Core Messages

- Recurrent disease is common in allergic fungal rhinosinusitis (AFR) and close follow-up is necessary.
- Both optimal medical and surgical therapy are needed for the adequate treatment of AFRS to minimize recurrence.
- Care should be taken to avoid dural resection to prevent future intracranial dissemination of disease.
- Image-guided surgery is useful for revision surgery for AFRS in the face of altered anatomical landmarks.
- Recurrence after treatment of AFRS is common.

Contents

Introduction

Over the past 30 years, there has been an increasing understanding of role fungi in chronic rhinosinusitis. Allergic fungal rhinosinusitis (AFRS) is now believed to be an inflammatory reaction mounted by an immunocompetent host to environmental fungi, most commonly of the dematiaceous species.

The diagnostic criteria for AFRS are as follows:

1. Gel and Coombs type I (IgE-mediated) hypersensitivity to fungus, as confirmed either by history, serology, or examination.
2. Nasal polyposis.
3. Characteristic radiographic findings such as hyperattenuation and bony expansion with or without erosion.
4. Eosinophilic mucin without fungal invasion into sinus tissue.
5. Positive fungal stain of sinus contents removed at the time of surgery.

AFRS affects approximated 5–10% of patients affected by chronic rhinosinusitis. Most cases reported are located in temperate regions of relatively high humidity. AFS is most common among adolescents and young adults, with a similar male to female ratio. Over thirty fungal species have been identified as a cause for AFRS, with *Bipolaris*, *Curvilaria*, and *Aspergillus* species being the most common subtypes. Revision surgery for AFRS is common, with up to 80% of patients developing recurrent disease. Close lifetime follow-up is mandatory for patients with AFRS.

Clinical Presentation

AFRS unfortunately tends to be recurrent and resistant to even the most aggressive and compliant medical treatment, with numerous surgical procedures over the course of a patient's life being the rule rather than the exception. Recurrence can be detected early in the form of mucosal edema, or later with frank polyps and fungal debris. Reasons for recurrence include inadequate initial debridement, irregular follow-up, and not cleaning the postoperative cavities appropriately, and of course the nature of the disease. Appropriate follow-up allows the identification of recurrent disease at an earlier stage, thus making it more amenable to medical therapy.

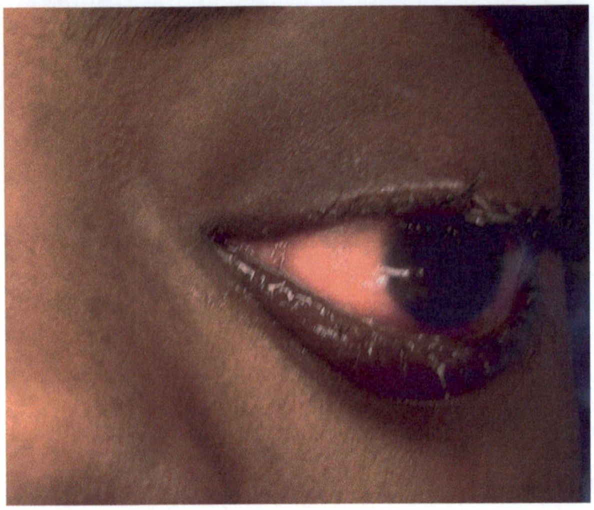

Fig. 18.1 Orbital proptosis secondary to allergic fungal rhinosinusitis (AFRS)

- Recurrent symptoms of anosmia and nasal obstruction may signal the onset of recurrence.

Recurrent facial remodeling and/or orbital proptosis are typically rare in patients educated about their disease who maintain regular follow-up appointments, but are obviously warning signs of severe disease that may need further surgical intervention (Fig. 18.1).

Imaging

Radiologic evaluation of the paranasal sinuses of patients with recurrent AFRS may reveal mild findings of recurrent polyposis or opacification of residual sinus cells, or may reveal severe findings similar to the characteristic findings used to diagnose AFRS (Fig. 18.2). Computed tomography (CT) is typically the first line of imaging chosen for patients with a history of AFRS, and careful comparison with preoperative images is required. Often, with removal of the tenacious allergic mucin, bone remodeling occurs over time to restore the natural contours of facial anatomy. Areas that are not remodeling and opacified, particularly in the lateral frontal sinuses, may signify persistent or recurrent disease. Magnetic resonance imaging findings are also sensitive for fungal debris, with hypointense signaling in T1-weighted images, central signal voids in T2-weighted images, and increased peripheral T1/T2 enhancement along the sinus walls as specific indicators for AFRS (Fig. 18.3) [3].

Medical Treatment

Therapy for recurrent AFRS is varied due to the multifactorial etiology of the disease. After complete surgical extirpation of all fungal debris, intranasal corticosteroid treatment and nasal saline irrigations are the first line of therapy for the long-term treatment of AFRS. Intranasal steroid irrigations have several advantages:

1. Their potent anti-inflammatory and immunomodulatory effects can reverse early polypoid degeneration and inflammatory damage to sinus mucosa.
2. They dilute and wash away inciting fungal antigens.
3. They lead to greater delivery of steroids to the sinus mucosa with less systemic absorption compared to oral steroids, leading to a much greater safety profile.

18

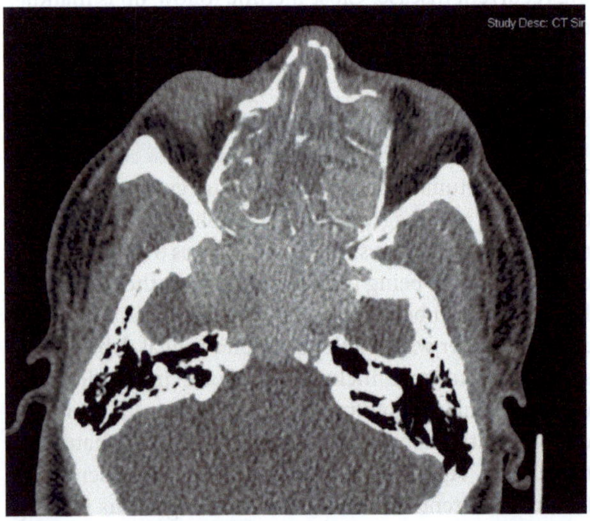

Fig. 18.2 Axial computed tomography (CT) scan with characteristic findings of AFRS

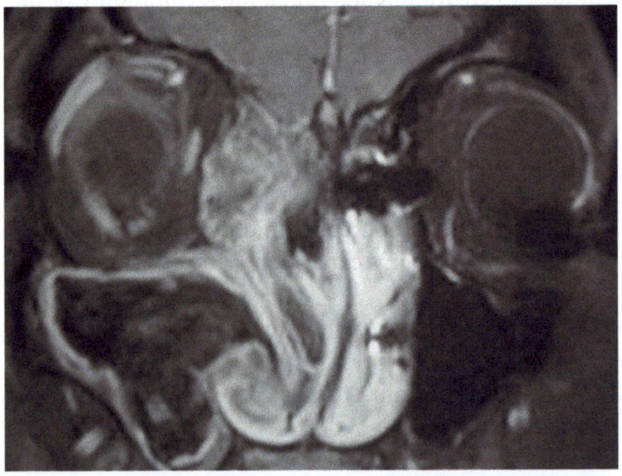

Fig. 18.3 Magnetic resonance imaging of a patient with AFRS

Intranasal steroid irrigations do cause low levels of systemic absorption, and should be used with caution in patients sensitive to chronic steroid medication. However, confirmation of the patient's use of this medication and compliance with this regimen is recommended before pursuing revision surgery in most cases. Oral steroids are effective in reversing the inflammatory cycle that causes recurrent disease in AFRS. However, chronic oral steroid use is associated with a significant side effect profile, and therefore should be used with caution.

Leukotriene inhibitors may also be beneficial in the prevention of AFRS recurrence. These drugs are active in blocking the formation and/or action of leukotrienes in the inflammatory cascade of AFRS, and have a more favorable side-effect profile compared to oral steroid therapy; however, supportive data is lacking.

Immunotherapy has also been used as an adjunct to AFRS therapy. Studies have suggested that AFRS recurrence diminishes markedly in patients who are place in an immunotherapy regimen [2]. In addition, the role of topical antifungals in the treatment of AFRS has been explored. Controversy exists regarding their use as AFRS is now known to be an inflammatory disease; systemic antifungals have historically been not effective in reversing the inflammation and are associated with severe systemic side effects. Recently, daily topical antifungals have been used in an effort to minimize recurrence of AFRS, but supportive data is pending.

Revision Surgery

Once obvious allergic mucin and polyps are identified that are not responding to adequate medical therapy, revision surgery is necessary.

Tips and Pearls

1. The goals of revision surgery are to extirpate fungal debris and inflammatory mucin and polyps completely from the nasal cavities, as well as to improve access to nasal cavities for future office surveillance and postoperative irrigations.
2. Revision surgery should be staged and/or aborted if visualization is poor during the operation, the surgeon becomes disoriented, or if blood loss or anesthetic risk becomes too great.
3. Staging the procedure when necessary permits the sinus surgeon to reorient himself within the surgical field and procure additional imaging if necessary.
4. Utmost importance should be given to preventing dural injury and/or cerebrospinal fluid leak during the procedure. Intradural contamination can lead to devastating consequences and vastly increase the difficulty of future operations.

As with any revision sinus surgery case, the patient who undergoes revision surgery for AFS should undergo a complete reassessment of their condition. This is especially important in the case of the patient who was previously operated on by another surgeon. Specific attention should be given to the postsurgical scans, which should ideally consist of coronal, axial, and sagittal imaging, and be formatted to be available to image-guidance systems.

All of the following aspects should be comprehensively evaluated by studying all CT images [1]:

1. The entire skull base is evaluated for slope, height, erosions, asymmetry, and neo-osteogenesis.
2. The medial orbital wall is examined for integrity, residual uncinate process, position, and erosion.
3. The ethmoid vessels are located and their relationship to the skull base needs to be examined.
4. The posterior ethmoid sinuses are evaluated for their vertical height, the presence of an Onodi cell, and neo-osteogenesis.
5. The maxillary sinuses are evaluated for Haller cells and accessory ostia.
6. The sphenoid sinuses are evaluated for the position of the intersinus septum location and appreciation of a bony dehiscence of the carotid artery and optic nerve.
7. The frontal recess and sinuses are evaluated for the presence of agger nasi and supraorbital pneumatization, frontal sinus drainage, and anteroposterior diameter of the frontal sinus.
8. The presence or absence of the middle turbinate, uncinate process, septal defects, and other distortions should be fully evaluated.

In the face of the altered anatomical landmarks as well as any skull-base or orbital erosion that may be encountered in AFRS and in revision sinus surgery, the use of computer-aided image guidance is recommended for revision surgery for AFRS.

It is important to understand that while normal anatomical landmarks may be altered in revision surgery for AFRS secondary to the disease process itself or because of the primary surgery, there are certain constant anatomical landmarks that may provide a guide during revision sinus surgery:

1. The junction of the medial and superior maxillary walls indicate the sagittal plane of the lamina papyracea.
2. The axial plane at the level of the superior maxillary wall (orbital floor) approximates the location of sphenoid ostium.
3. The distance from the anterior nasal spine to the posterior maxillary wall approximates the location of the sphenoid rostrum.
4. Once at the sphenoid, the lowest height of the skull base can be identified and careful dissection through the ethmoid sinuses in a posterior-to-anterior fashion can be done safely.

It is also important to note that the middle turbinate may not always be identifiable in revision sinus surgery cases. Dissection should be kept as lateral as possible near the medial orbital wall in order to avoid dissecting near the middle turbinate insertion to the skull base. This area is particularly susceptible to dural violation. Finally, dissection in the area of the frontal recess should be done with great care. Given the distorted anatomy, the anterior ethmoidal artery may lie completely out of its bony covering and may be prone to injury. Good visualization of both the skull base and medial orbital wall is paramount to dissection in this area.

Allergic mucin and polyps will be encountered in patients who undergo revision surgery for AFRS. The sinuses may be packed with the fungal debris and cavities will be expanded by both the debris and the sinuses (Fig. 18.4). The sinus surgeon should take advantage of this common feature of the disease when performing revision surgery. Using powered instrumentation, the polyps can be carefully followed. Slow careful removal of the polyps will lead to the sinus ostium and subsequently to the affected sinus.

- The slow expansile nature of AFRS can enlarge natural sinus openings; therefore, even if fungal mucin resides in areas that are typically difficult to approach, the expansile tendency enlarges the natural outflow tracts, enabling greater access to the sinus cavity (Fig. 18.5).

Thick allergic mucin will be encountered inside the sinuses and possibly in the nasal cavity itself (Video 18.1). Careful removal of all the allergic mucin is very important for the success of the surgery. However, it is well known that removal of all of the allergic mucin can be very challenging. Being patient and using suction and blunt curetting instruments along with normal saline irrigation help in the removal of this tenacious material (Video 18.1). Once this material is removed, improved access to the paranasal sinuses in the face of altered anatomical landmarks is obtained.

18

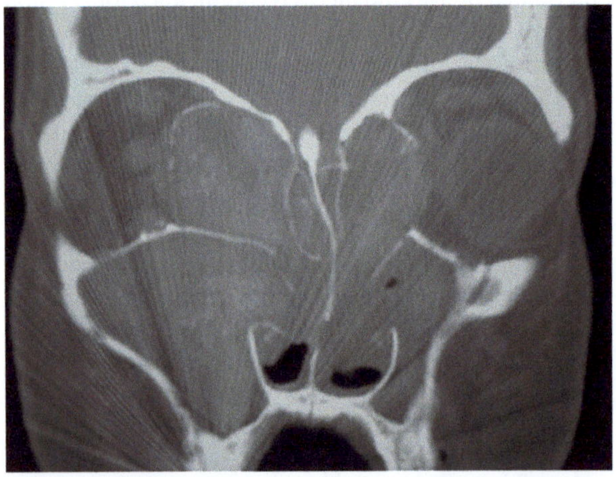

Fig. 18.4 Coronal CT showing expanded sinus cavities

Complications

The incidence of surgical complications is increased in revision sinus surgery cases. As for any revision sinus surgery case, the most severe complications related to revision surgery for AFRS are intraorbital and intracranial injuries. The most series quote such serious complications occurring in one out of every 200 cases [1]. Serious vascular injuries should also be considered in the case of revision surgery for AFRS. Among the minor complications that may be encountered are: scarring, bleeding, infection, epiphora, synechiae formation, mucocele, and disease persistence or recurrence with the need for further surgery. All of these potential complications need to be preoperatively discussed at length with the patient and they should be part of the informed consent.

Open Approaches

Open approaches can serve as a valuable adjunct to endoscopic approaches in revision AFRS cases. External frontal sinus trephination combined with endoscopic frontal sinusotomy ("the above and below technique") can be very valuable for extirpating frontal sinus disease, particularly with significant disease in the lateral frontal sinus or type IV frontal cells.

- When thick fungal debris is located in the remote regions of the frontal sinus, above and below techniques assist in their safe and complete removal.

The Caldwell-Luc approach is typically unnecessary due to the advent of curved microdebriders and malleable instruments. Osteoplastic flap with frontal sinus obliteration is now performed uncommonly. AFRS typically dilates the natural ostia of individual sinuses and the frontal recess, so if frontal debris can be extirpated, the frontal sinus typically regains normal function with plentiful access to medical irrigations. As with all operations, surgeons should not expect that any particular operation will serve as the definitive procedure for this highly recalcitrant disease.

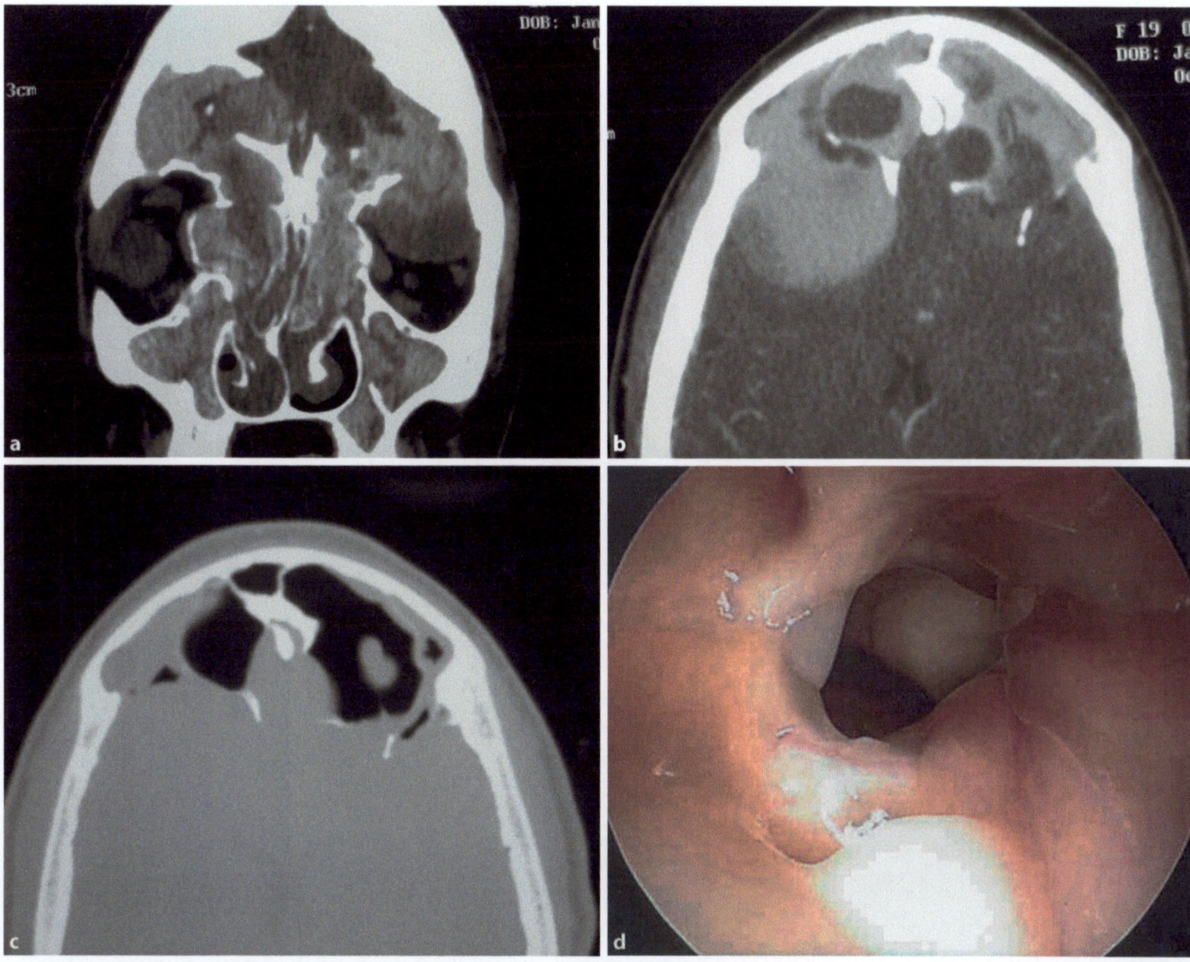

Fig. 18.5 **a** Coronal CT with extensive frontal and superior orbital wall erosion. Widened frontal recess and ostia. **b** Axial CT with extensive erosion of the posterior plate of the frontal sinus. **c** Postoperative axial CT after endoscopic frontal surgery and removal of fungal debris. **d** Postoperative endoscopic view of the widened frontal ostium

Conclusions

It is important to consider that any one particular surgery may not suffice in the treatment of this aggressive disease. Medical therapy should be maximized prior to pursuing any revision surgery and should be directed at modulating the immune response to fungus. Surgery serves to eliminate the fungal debris present in the sinus cavities as well as to provide access for postoperative debridement and irrigations. Further harm during revision surgery should be conscientiously avoided. Revision surgery for AFRS is common; however, by following standard anatomical landmarks and by staging the procedure when needed, it can be performed safely with few complications.

References

1. Govindaraj S, Antunes M, Kennedy DW (2007) Revision sinus surgery. In: Kountakis SE, Onerci M (eds) Rhinologic and Sleep Apnea Surgical Techniques. Springer, Germany, pp 199–210
2. Mabry RL, Marple BF, Folker RJ, Mabry CS (1998) Immunotherapy for allergic fungal sinusitis: three years experience. Otolaryngol Head Neck Surg 119:648–651
3. Manning SC, Merkel M, Kriesel K, et al. (1997) Computed tomography and magnetic resonance diagnosis of allergic fungal sinusitis. Laryngoscope 107:170–176

Chapter 19

Revision Endoscopic Surgery for Benign Sinonasal Tumors

19

Michael J. Sillers and Yvonne Chan

Core Messages

- While benign tumors can be safely and completely removed from the paranasal sinuses using endoscopic techniques, there is a generally infrequent but not negligible rate of recurrence.
- Long-term follow up with endoscopic and appropriate imaging surveillance is critical in recognizing early tumor recurrence.
- A high index of suspicion should be employed when there is a change in the endoscopic examination.
- Multimodality imaging is essential when there may be multiple sites of tumor recurrence.
- Intraoperative frozen section analysis is a vital step in assuring complete tumor removal at the time of revision surgery.

Contents

Introduction

Benign tumors of the nasal cavity and paranasal sinuses have been successfully removed utilizing transnasal endoscopic approaches for over the last two decades. With increased experience and skill, improved instrument design, and computer-aided surgery, an endoscopic approach has become the default choice for most rhinologic surgeons for the surgical management of sinonasal benign neoplastic diseases. Whether utilizing traditional open approaches or transnasal endoscopic techniques, there is an infrequent but not negligible rate of recurrent and residual tumor, which creates a unique clinical situation that deserves special discussion.

When performing revision surgery, the following questions should be answered:

1. Why did the previous surgery fail?
2. Was the nature/extent of disease underappreciated (Figs. 19.1 and 19.2)?
3. Were certain anatomic or imaging signs not recognized preoperatively?
4. Was intraoperative frozen section analysis utilized?
5. Were appropriate surgical techniques employed?

The answers to these questions will shed light on the reasons for failure and help assure success during subsequent surgery.

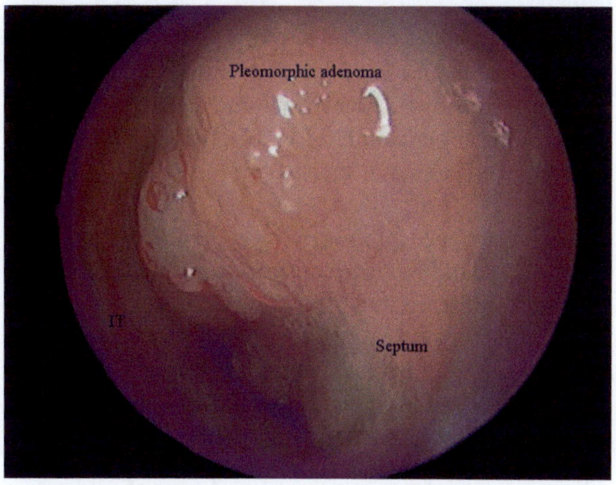

Fig. 19.1 Endoscopic view of recurrent pleomorphic adenoma of the nasal septum. The lesion was initially removed during a septoplasty at an outside facility. *IT* Inferior turbinate

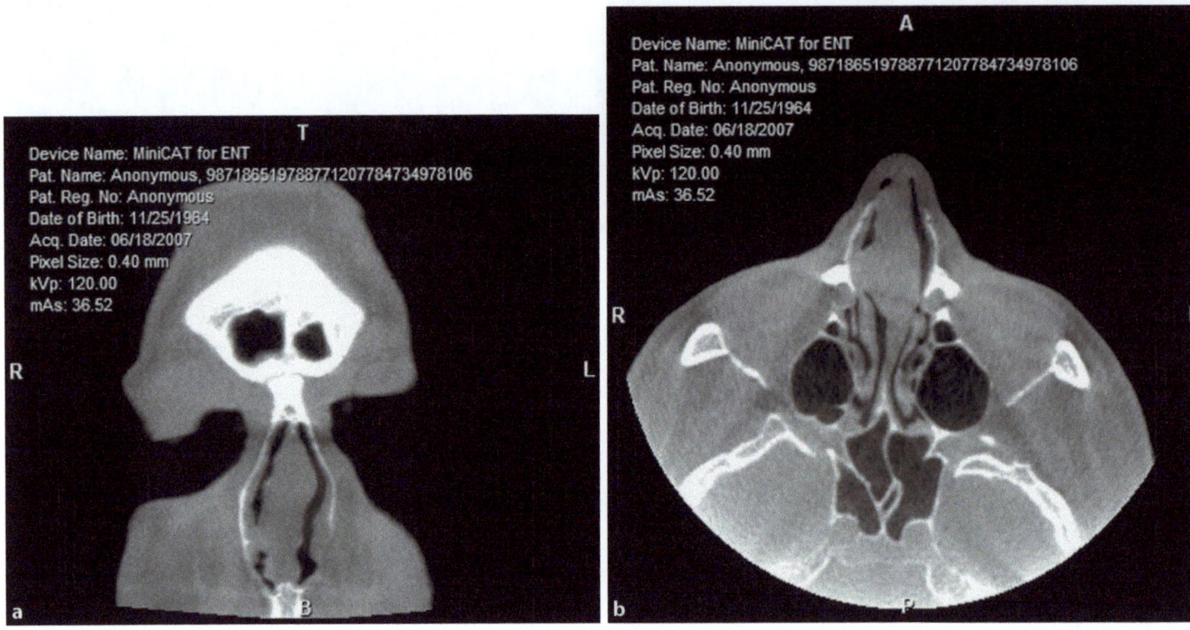

Fig. 19.2 Coronal (**a**) and axial (**b**) computed tomography (CT) scans of recurrent pleomorphic adenoma of the nasal septum. The lesion was isolated to the nasal septum

While most benign tumors encountered in the nasal cavity and paranasal sinuses do not have malignant potential, the most commonly encountered one, inverted papilloma, is reported to undergo malignant degeneration in 5–15% of patients, with a working risk of 10% [6, 12]. For this reason, revision surgery for inverted papilloma will be discussed in detail, while other less commonly encountered tumors will be mentioned in more general terms.

Inverted Papilloma

Inverted papilloma is specifically the most commonly encountered Schneiderian papilloma and in general the most commonly encountered benign neoplasm of the nasal cavity and paranasal sinuses.

- The recurrence of inverted papilloma ranges from 0 to 78% and has been related to surgical approach, extent of disease, and prior surgery.

When comparing open vs. endoscopic resection, recurrence rates for endoscopic approaches are favorable, and in some recent series, lower. Most of these studies, including one of the most recent, are retrospective reviews and meta-analyses [7]. However, as with most disease processes, the extent of disease is the single most important factor impacting recurrence. Lee et al. found the recurrence rate in their series of reoperations for inverted papilloma to be 27.3% with Krouse stage III tumors, while lower stages did not recur [5]. Sautter et al. also found that extent of disease was the most important variable and that the surgical approach did not impact recurrence [10].

Preoperative Workup

When patients undergo surgery for inverted papilloma, regular endoscopic surveillance should be performed (Figs. 19.3 and 19.4). At times, early recurrent or residual disease can be identified and treated by simple excision in the office setting. Care should be taken to properly document the suspected site and the specimen sent to pathology. When there is suspicion for more advanced disease, radiographic evaluation should be performed to assist in determining the stage of disease. Computed tomography (CT) and magnetic resonance imaging (MRI) are both helpful in identifying the extent of disease and allow a preoperative staging of the patient's recurrent disease. CT scan will also serve to demonstrate bony erosion or invasion into the skull base or the orbit. In patients with recurrent disease, there may be multiple distinct sites of neoplasia and a pure "stage" may not be determined. Prior surgery may also lead to postobstructive changes with mucocele formation, which cannot always be distinguished by CT alone. MRI is helpful in further distinguishing the nature of CT opacification (i.e., inspissated mucous vs. soft tissue). In addition to preoperative planning, this also has implications for prognosis (Figs. 19.5 and 19.6).

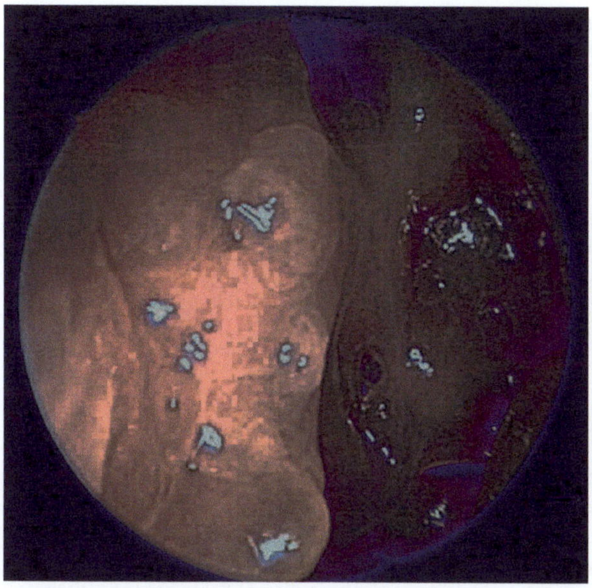

Fig. 19.3 Endoscopic view of recurrent inverted papilloma on the right lamina papyracea

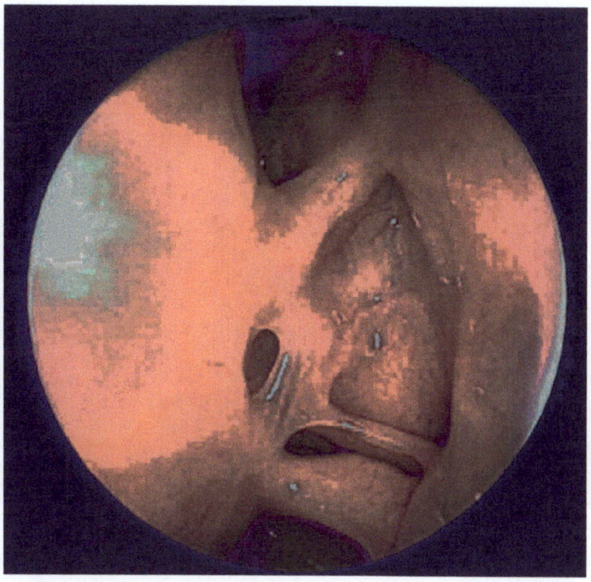

Fig. 19.4 Endoscopic inspection of the right lamina papyracea 2 years postresection of recurrent inverted papilloma

- Areas of hyperostosis/osteoneogenesis on CT should be identified as this has been shown to highly correlate with site of origin of inverted papilloma (Fig. 19.7b) [4, 14].

Comparison with CT imaging taken prior to the initial surgical procedure, if available, will be helpful in this setting as new areas of hyperostosis may be the result of prior surgery and not necessarily recurrent tumor origin. When CTs are obtained, a surgical navigation protocol should be employed so that this technology can be utilized during the revision surgical procedure.

Currently, there are several staging systems for inverted papilloma, with that proposed by Krouse used most commonly (Table 19.1) [8]. Citardi et al. have proposed a new classification that eliminates malignancy, which was included in the Krouse system (Table 19.2) [1]. Regardless

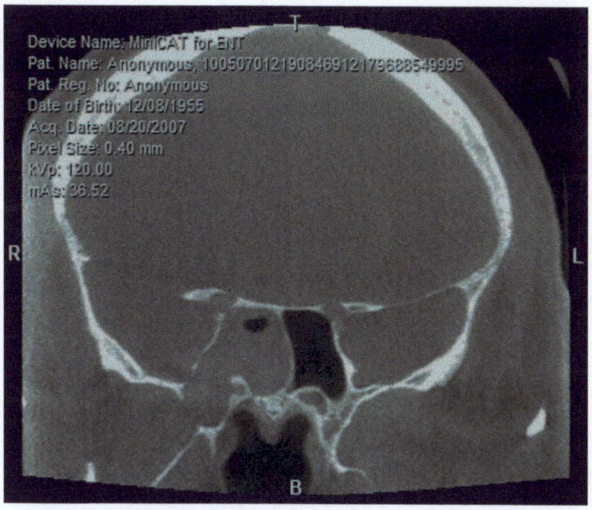

Fig. 19.5 Coronal CT showing opacified sphenoid sinus with extensive pterygoid recess pneumatization in a patient with posterior ethmoid sinus inverted papilloma

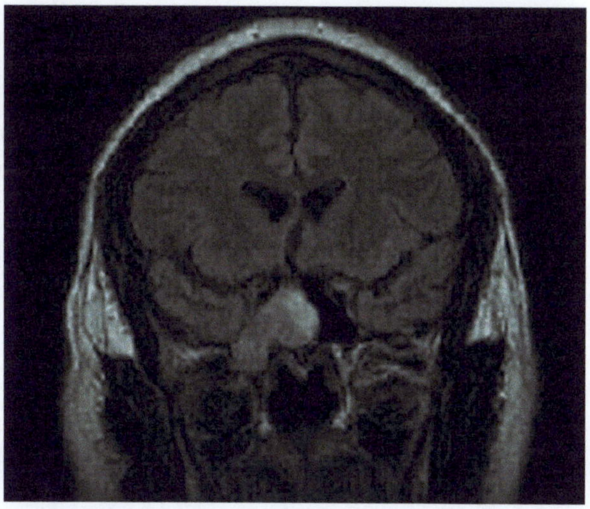

Fig. 19.6 T1-weighted coronal magnetic resonance image showing intermediate signal intensity in the sphenoid sinus

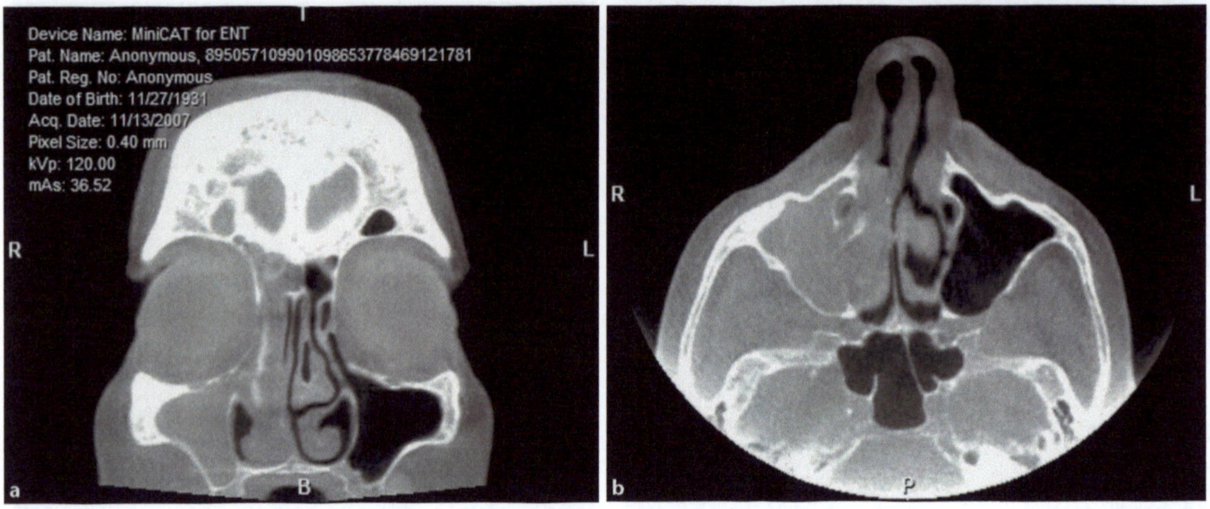

Fig. 19.7 Coronal (**a**) axial (**b**) CT demonstrating hyperostosis of the uncinate process suggesting site of origin of tumor

of the system chosen, the most effective approach is to assimilate the endoscopic and imaging data in order to counsel the patient as to the appropriate choice of procedure as well as prognosis on an individual basis.

Once the preoperative stage and the extent of disease have been determined, a plan for revision surgery should be made. Patients are instructed to discontinue medications that would lead to unnecessary bleeding at the time of surgery. Decreased visualization related to a bloody field can lead to increased risk for complications and incomplete surgery resulting in residual/recurrent disease. It is important to ask specifically about the use of nonprescription medications (nonsteroidal anti-inflammatory drugs, aspirin, vitamin E) and herbal products (green tea, *Ginkgo biloba*), which are not often disclosed but can lead to troublesome bleeding. Discontinuation of prescription anticoagulants is best managed after discussion with the prescribing physician regarding the risks of medical complications associated with their cessation.

Commonly encountered risks of endoscopic sinus surgery should be discussed with each patient. Specific risks related to the extent of proposed surgery should be further disclosed. For example, removal of a recurrent osteoma along the ethmoid roof may require/involve removing a

Table 19.1 Krouse staging system for inverted papilloma [8]

T1	Confined to the nasal cavity
T2	Ostiomeatal complex region, ethmoid, or medial maxillary involvement (with or without nasal cavity involvement)
T3	Any wall of the maxillary sinus but medial, frontal sinus, or sphenoid with or without T2 criteria
T4	Any extrasinus involvement or malignancy

Table 19.2 Citardi staging system for inverted papilloma [1]

Group A	Confined to the nasal cavity, ethmoid sinuses, or medial maxillary wall
Group B	Involvement of any maxillary wall (other than the medial maxillary wall), frontal, or sphenoid sinus
Group C	Extension beyond the paranasal sinuses

portion of the ethmoid roof, resulting in an anticipated cerebrospinal fluid leak and its attendant repair.

- Depending on the location of the surgery (hospital vs. ambulatory surgery center), special arrangements may need to be made to ensure that intraoperative frozen section analysis is available as an integral part of the revised surgical procedure.

Surgical Technique

Once the patient is brought to surgery, maximal decongestion of the nasal mucosa is started in the preoperative holding area by applying topical decongestants. In the operating room, the choice of general anesthetic agents is important. Wormald et al. have proposed total intravenous anesthesia as a method by which the peripheral vasodilatation associated with certain inhalation agents is avoided. The importance of controlling the heart rate in addition to blood pressure is emphasized in this technique [13]. Once appropriately anesthetized, local infiltration of vasoconstrictors is carried out along the lateral nasal wall and in the region of the sphenopalatine artery, either transnasally or transpalatally via the greater palatine foramen. Finally, topical vasoconstrictors are applied to the nasal mucosa using cotton pledgets. While these steps may be time consuming, they will lead to improved hemostasis, which makes the surgical procedure much less problematic.

As an initial step, secretions and crusts are removed from the operative site. Suspicious areas should be sampled and sent to the pathologist for frozen section analysis (Fig. 19.8). Care must be taken to document these sites as there may be multiple separate foci of tumor that needs to be addressed. En bloc resection is preferred but not always possible in revision surgery. All gross tumor must be removed along with surrounding, normal-appearing tissue to assure complete resection. The permanent specimen should be clearly marked for orientation. Intraoperative frozen section analysis of surgical margins is important and will help dictate further resection.

- In general with benign disease, natural barriers such as the lamina papyracea and dura should not be removed unless there is obvious tumor involvement.

Areas of hyperostosis should be carefully reduced with a diamond bur on the microdebrider. Computer-aided surgery is helpful in these instances in gauging progress (Fig. 19.9). Depending on the location and extent of disease, the operating surgeon should be comfortable with advanced endoscopic techniques, such as the endoscopic modified Lothrop procedure and the transmaxillary/

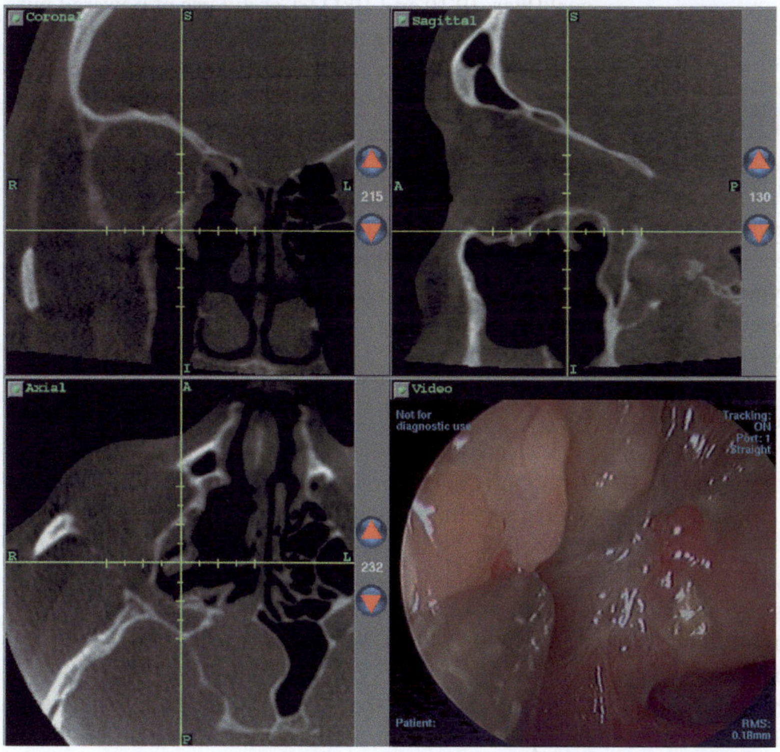

Fig. 19.8 Intraoperative view of the right posterior ethmoid sinus with recurrent inverted papilloma

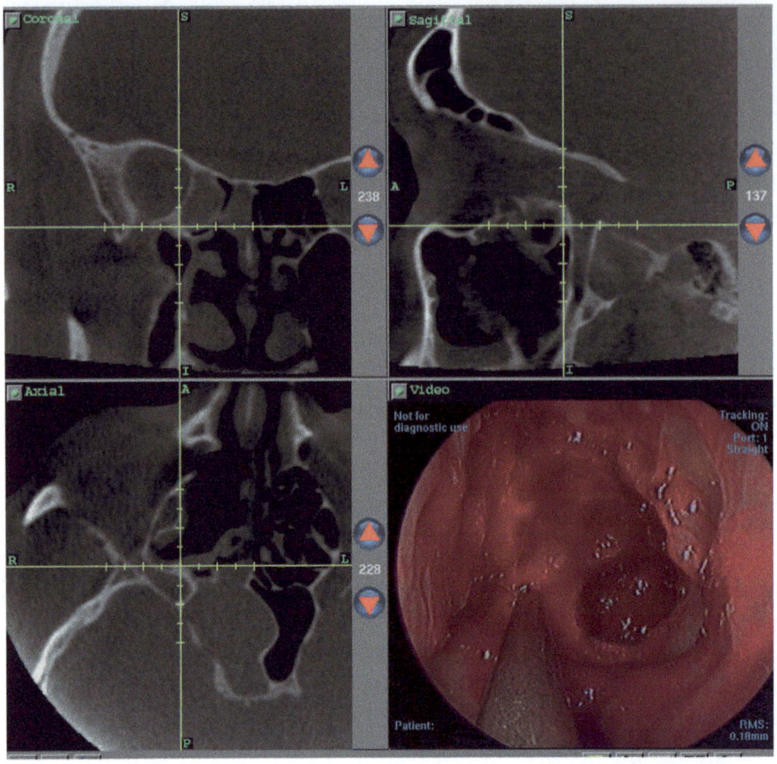

Fig. 19.9 Intraoperative view after tumor resection and reduction of the hyperostotic region with a diamond bur

transpterygoid approach to an extensively pneumatized sphenoid sinus. Hemostasis is achieved in the surgeon's preferred fashion and nasal packing is placed as indicated.

Other Benign Neoplasms

Fibro-osseous Lesions

Osteoma, ossifying fibroma, and fibrous dysplasia constitute the range of fibro-osseous lesions affecting the paranasal sinuses. It is generally agreed that symptomatic lesions should be removed and complete resection is likely with osteoma and ossifying fibroma. However, complete removal is rarely achievable with fibrous dysplasia as it usually develops along existing bony planes.

- Sacrifice of vital structures is not appropriate when treating benign neoplasia.

Tumor recurrence of osteoma and ossifying fibroma is related to incomplete resection. At times the operating surgeon may elect to leave a "shell" of tumor along the skull base or lamina papyracea during primary surgery to avoid the risk of intracranial or intraorbital injury associated with complete tumor removal. The indications for revision surgery are no different than for primary surgery. Removal of symptomatic recurrent lesions is appropriate and complete tumor removal should be the goal (Figs. 19.10 and 19.11). Careful use of powered burs is helpful in reducing the overall bulk of these lesions. As with primary surgery, identifying a cleavage plane is helpful in separating the base of the lesion from the surrounding site of attachment. The use of a curette or osteotome enables the surgeon to safely remove the tumor while avoiding injury to underlying structures. The potential for orbital and intracranial complications should be discussed in advance with the patient, including intraoperative plans for repair and their impact on recovery should they occur.

Angiofibroma

Angiofibroma is relatively uncommon and recurrence, as with other tumors, is often related to the extent of disease at the time of initial surgery.

- Angiofibroma skull-base invasion was associated with recurrence in 27.5% of patients [3].

Herman et al. urged that all patients, including those with asymptomatic tumor remnants, be followed closely with

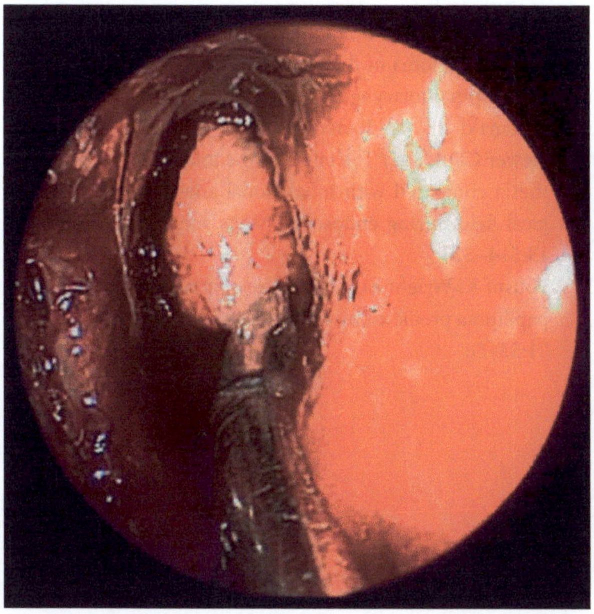

Fig. 19.10 Intraoperative view of recurrent left frontal sinus osteoma

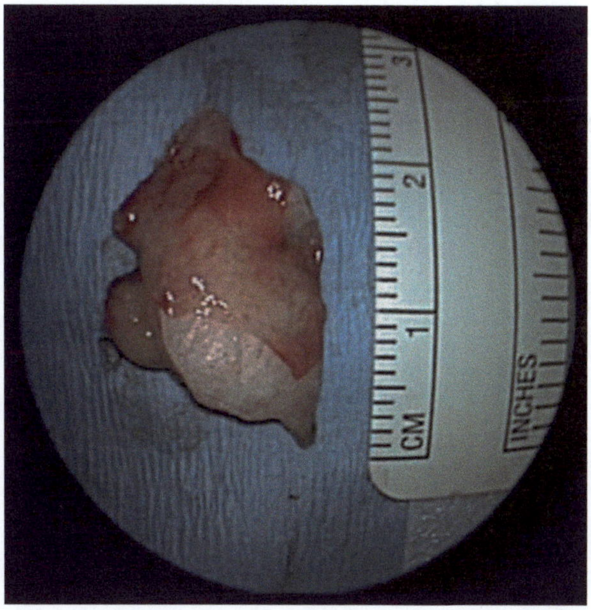

Fig. 19.11 Intraoperative view of osteoma specimen as it was resected

serial CT [3]. Some small remnants may involute, while those that become symptomatic can be treated with radiation therapy or revision surgery. Scholtz et al. found as low as 15% recurrence in 14 patients over an 11-year period [11]. Seven patients underwent a transnasal endoscopic approach, which they conclude to be appropriate in patients with lesions that involve the nasopharynx, nasal cavity, paranasal sinuses, and pterygopalatine fossa. Preoperative arteriography with embolization has been shown to reduce intraoperative blood loss [2, 9].

Conclusion

Benign tumors presenting in the nasal cavity and paranasal sinuses can be safely and successfully removed using transnasal endoscopic techniques. Success has also been achieved when tumors have extended beyond the confines of the nasal cavity and paranasal sinuses. The single most important factor in tumor recurrence is the extent of disease at initial presentation. Patients should be followed closely long term to enable early detection of recurrent disease. Questionable findings on endoscopic surveillance should be viewed with a high index of suspicion and appropriate biopsy and/or imaging studies obtained. Depending on the extent of tumor and the skills of the operating surgeon, endoscopic techniques once again can be safely used to address recurrent disease.

References

1. Cannady SB, Batra PS, Sautter NB, Roh HJ, Citardi MJ (2007) New staging system for sinonasal inverted papilloma in the endoscopic era. Laryngoscope 117:1283–1287
2. Economou TS, Abemayor E, Ward PH (1998) Juvenile nasopharyngeal angiofibroma: an update of the UCLA experience, 1960–1985. Laryngoscope 98:170–175
3. Herman P, Lot G, Chapot R, Salvan D, Huy PI (1999) Long term follow-up of nasopharyngeal angiofibromas: analysis of recurrences. Laryngoscope 109:140–147
4. Lee DK, Chung SK, Dhong HJ, Kim HY, Kim HJ, Bok KH (2007) Focal hyperostosis on CT of sinonasal inverted papilloma as a predictor of tumor origin. AJNR Am J Neuroradiol 28:618–621
5. Lee TJ, Huang SF, Lee LA, Huang CC (2004) Endoscopic surgery for recurrent inverted papilloma. Laryngoscope 114:106–112
6. Lesperance MM, Esclamdo RM (1995) Squamous cell carcinoma arising in inverted papilloma. Laryngoscope 105:178–183
7. Mirza S, Bradley PJ, Acharya A, Stacey M, Jones NS (2007) Sinonasal inverted papillomas: recurrence, and synchronous and metachronous malignancy. J Laryngol Otol 121: 857–864
8. Krouse JH (2000) Development of a staging system for inverted papilloma. Laryngoscope 110:965–968

9. Onerci TM, Yücel OT, Oğretmenoğlu O (2003) Endoscopic surgery in treatment of juvenile nasopharyngeal angiofibroma. Int J Pediatr Otorhinolaryngol 67:1219–1225
10. Sautter NB, Cannady SB, Citardi MJ, Roh HJ, Batra PS (2007) Comparison of open versus endoscopic resection of inverted papilloma. Am J Rhinol 21:320–323
11. Scholtz A, Appenroth E, Kammen-olly K, Scholtz LU, Thumfart WF (2001) Juvenile nasopharyngeal angiofibroma: management and therapy. Laryngoscope 111:681–687
12. von Buchwald C, Bradley PJ. Risks of malignancy in inverted papilloma of the nose and paranasal sinuses (2007) Curr Opin Otolaryngol Head Neck Surg 15(2):95–98
13. Wormald PJ, van Renen G, Perks J, Jones JA, Langton-Hewer CD (2005) The effect of the total intravenous anesthesia compared with inhalational anesthesia on the surgical field during endoscopic sinus surgery. Am J Rhinol 19:514–520
14. Yousuf K, Wright ED (2007) Site of attachment of inverted papilloma predicted by CT findings of osteitis. Am J Rhinol 21:32–36

Chapter 20

Recurrent Cerebrospinal Fluid Leaks and Meningoencephaloceles

20

Sarah K. Wise, Richard J. Harvey, and Rodney J. Schlosser

Core Messages

- Endoscopic repair of cerebrospinal fluid (CSF) leaks and meningoencephaloceles is largely successful, with rates of skull-base defect closure greater than 90%.
- Certain factors may increase the potential for recurrence of CSF leak or meningoencephalocele. Identification of such factors in the preoperative period allows the surgeon to alter treatment protocols accordingly.
- Diagnosis of recurrent CSF leaks and meningoencephaloceles often incorporates preoperative and intraoperative techniques. A combination of laboratory testing, radiologic imaging, and special procedures may be required to accurately diagnose the site of a skull-base defect.
- Surgical techniques for endoscopic repair of recurrent CSF leaks and meningoencephaloceles vary by the site and size of the skull-base defect, as well as surgeon experience. Certain types of recurrent CSF leaks and meningoencephaloceles may require additional perioperative measures for increased repair success.

Contents

Introduction

In 1926, Dandy reported the first successful intracranial repair of a cranial defect in a patient with pneumocephalus [9]. Extracranial repair of a skull-base defect and cerebrospinal fluid (CSF) leak via naso-orbital incision was subsequently reported in 1948 by Dohlman [10]. The first report of endonasal endoscopic skull-base defect repair occurred in a case of iatrogenic skull-base injury and was published by Wigand in 1981 [53]. Following this, Mattox and Kennedy described the techniques for endoscopic repair of CSF leaks in detail and expanded the indications to skull-base defects caused by craniofacial trauma and meningoencephaloceles [24].

In present times, success rates for closure of skull-base defects by endoscopic techniques remain greater than 90% in most series [6, 8, 15, 17–19, 21–24, 26, 29, 56], as compared to traditional open skull-base defect repair via craniotomy, with success rates reported in the range of 60–80% [1, 16, 34]. In addition, endoscopic transnasal approaches for CSF leak repair circumvent the morbidities of intracranial approaches, which include anosmia, cerebral edema, seizures, and memory deficits [25]. The exceptional visualization provided by rigid endoscopes reduced morbidity over craniotomy, and higher success rates as compared to open approaches has made endoscopic repair of CSF leaks and meningoencephaloceles the preferred approach [15, 18, 24].

As surgeons develop increased comfort with endoscopic skull-base repair techniques, more challenging cases are being undertaken. Endoscopic surgeons are increasingly involved in addressing pathology along the skull base and beyond the skull base, often in conjunction with their neurosurgical colleagues. In addition, revision skull-base defect repair is frequently performed endoscopically following failure of primary endoscopic or open procedures. In each case, the endoscopic surgeon should be aware of factors that could lead to failure of skull-base defect repair. By identifying factors that may contribute to failure, surgeons can employ adjunctive perioperative and intraoperative measures that may improve the success of their repair.

Indications for Transnasal Endoscopic Repair of CSF Leaks and Meningoencephaloceles

1. Active CSF leak.
2. Pneumocephalus.
3. Skull-base defect with a history of meningitis.
4. Meningoencephalocele with active CSF leak or history of meningitis.
5. Skull-base defect created during endoscopic sinus surgery or skull-base surgery.
6. Skull-base defect accessible by transnasal endoscopic techniques.

Contraindications for Transnasal Endoscopic Repair of CSF Leaks and Meningoencephaloceles

1. Medical issues that render a patient unfit for surgery or general anesthesia.
2. Skull-base defect not accessible by transnasal endoscopic means.
3. Untreated tumor in the area of the skull-base defect. In this case, the tumor should be treated prior to definitive repair of the skull-base defect.
4. Surgeon discomfort or inexperience with endoscopic repair techniques.
5. Equipment or instrumentation unavailable.
6. Active meningitis (relative contraindication).

Preoperative Workup

Diagnosis of CSF Leak – Laboratory

Whether a patient presents with a primary or recurrent CSF leak, confirmation of true CSF rhinorrhea should be made. Studies used in the past, such as fluid analysis for glucose, protein, and electrolytes are no longer encouraged due to high false-positive and false-negative rates. Currently, β2-transferrin testing is advocated due to its high sensitivity and specificity for the detection of CSF [45]. β2-transferrin is found only in the CSF, ocular vitreous humor, and perilymph [45]. While false-positives may occur, these cases are rare, arising in patients with chronic liver disease, genetic variations of the transferrin gene, and inborn errors of glycoprotein metabolism [36, 47]. Analysis for β2-transferrin requires only 0.17 ml of rhinorrhea fluid, and results may be obtained in less than 3 h with immunofixation electrophoresis techniques [33].

- Diagnosis of CSF rhinorrhea by β2-transferrin is the most sensitive, specific, and readily available laboratory technique currently available.

A second protein, β-trace protein, may also be analyzed to detect CSF in rhinorrhea fluid. β-trace protein is an enzyme also known as prostaglandin D synthase, which is produced in the leptomeninges and choroid plexus and subsequently secreted into the CSF [52]. Although β-trace protein is found in fluids throughout the body, its concentration is much higher in the CSF [27], and detection of this protein is also highly sensitive and specific for CSF [3].

Diagnosis of CSF Leak – Radiology

Following confirmation of CSF rhinorrhea by laboratory testing, radiologic evaluation is undertaken to identify the site of the skull-base defect. In cases of recurrent CSF leak, the surgeon should evaluate carefully all areas of the skull base on imaging studies. Certain patients, such as those with traumatic or spontaneous CSF leaks, often have multiple skull-base defects, which may or may not be actively leaking CSF [38]. In addition, patients who have undergone previous skull-base repair may present at a later date with CSF leak from a separate anatomic location [54].

Computed tomography (CT) scan is generally the initial study by which to assess the bony anatomy of the skull base. CT scans are typically acquired in a thin slice (less than 1.5 mm) axial protocol, with coronal and sagittal images created by reformatting the axial data set (Fig. 20.1).

Evaluation of images in a bone-window algorithm provides the most accurate assessment of skull-base integrity. The roof of the ethmoid and sphenoid sinuses is best viewed in the coronal plane, while the posterior table of the frontal sinus is visualized in the axial or sagittal plane. Finally, the integrity of the sella and clivus may also be assessed in the sagittal plane.

- Once diagnosis of CSF rhinorrhea is confirmed by laboratory testing, the integrity of the skull base should be assessed radiographically. This evaluation typically begins with a fine-cut axial CT scan, with triplanar image reformations viewed in bone-window algorithm.

When multiple bony skull-base defects are visualized on fine-cut CT scan or additional information is needed to accurately identify the site of active CSF leak, a CT cisternogram may be obtained by giving intrathecal contrast at the time of the CT scan. The nasal cavity and paranasal sinuses are then evaluated for pooling of contrast material (Fig. 20.2). Since the patient must be actively leaking CSF during the study for the best results, this test has sensitivities ranging from 48 to 96% [48]. Low-flow or intermittent CSF leaks have a decreased chance of being detected on a CT cisternogram. Although valuable information may be obtained from a CT cisternogram, this procedure is invasive and carries the risks of lumbar puncture and intrathecal contrast.

When evaluation of soft tissue along the skull base is necessary, such as in cases of suspected recurrent meningoencephalocele or skull-base tumor, magnetic resonance imaging (MRI) is frequently added to the diagnostic algorithm. Patients with spontaneous CSF leaks have a high rate of meningoencephalocele formation [6, 32, 38] and present with multiple simultaneous meningoencephaloceles in 31% of cases [38]. In such cases, MRI is valuable in determining the presence of meningoencephalocele and the contents of meningoencephalic sacs (Fig. 20.3). In patients with previous treatment for skull-base tumor, MRI may assist in the assessment of possible recurrence prior to attempting closure of a skull-base defect.

Magnetic resonance cisternography is an additional technique by which to localize CSF leaks, which has a reported sensitivity of 85–92% and 100% specificity [46]. The MRI protocol involves a fast spin-echo with fat suppression and image reversal [46], which demonstrates CSF as black against surrounding tissues, which have diminished intensity.

Finally, radionuclide cisternograms may be performed. This technique involves placement of pledgets at specific sites within the nasal cavity (cribriform recess, middle meatus, and sphenoethmoid recess), followed by lumbar

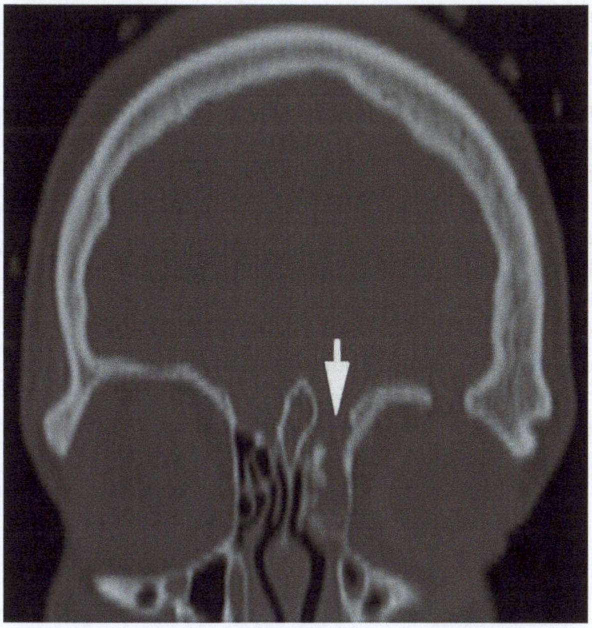

Fig. 20.1 Coronal computed tomography (CT) scan in a bone window algorithm, reconstructed from fine-cut axial data set. A left ethmoid roof defect (*arrow*) is visible following head trauma

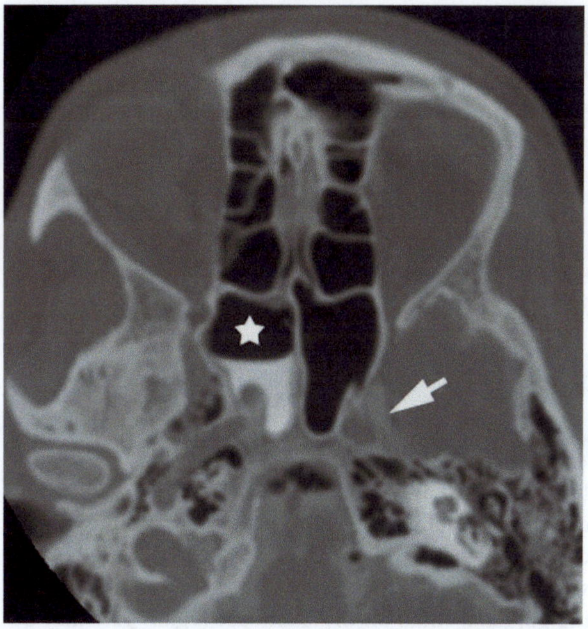

Fig. 20.2 Axial CT cisternogram image in a patient with a spontaneous cerebrospinal fluid (CSF) leak. Contrast enhancement is seen in the intracranial CSF spaces (*arrow*). In addition, contrast-enhanced CSF is present in the right sphenoid sinus (*star*)

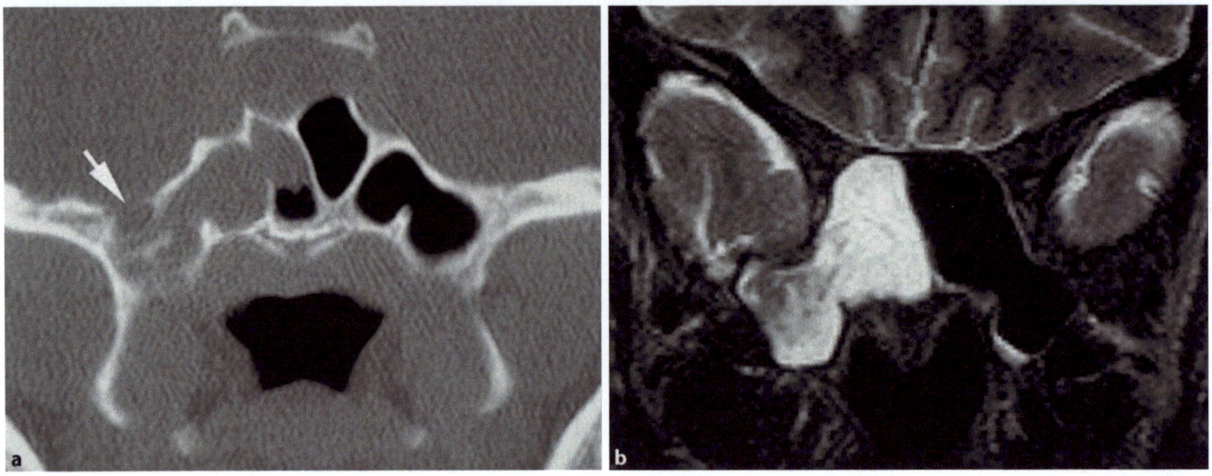

Fig. 20.3 **a** Coronal CT scan of a patient with a spontaneous CSF leak. A skull-base defect is noted in the lateral recess of the right sphenoid sinus (*arrow*). The exact etiology of the sphenoid sinus opacification cannot be determined by CT scan alone. **b** T2-weighted magnetic resonance imaging (MRI) scan of the same patient revealing a large meningoencephalocele protruding into the right sphenoid sinus

puncture and injection of intrathecal tracer [41]. Radioactivity is subsequently measured on the pledgets after a period of hours. In comparison to other localization techniques, the sensitivity of radionuclide cisternogram is low (62–76%), with a 33% false-positive rate [12, 16, 48]. However, for low-volume or intermittent CSF leaks, pledgets may be left in the nasal cavity for days to allow for detection of the leak, dependent on the half-life of the tracer used [13].

- Following the assessment of skull-base integrity by fine-cut CT scan, further testing to localize the site of the CSF leak (CT cisternogram, magnetic resonance cisternogram, radionuclide cisternogram) or to assess soft tissue along the skull base (MRI) may be necessary, depending on the individual case.

Perioperative Adjuncts

Lumbar Drains

Lumbar drains are often used as an adjunct in the repair of CSF leaks and meningoencephaloceles, although their use is somewhat controversial. A lumbar drain can assist in decreasing intracranial CSF pressure and alleviating potential strain on the skull-base repair. This may be helpful in cases of elevated intracranial pressure, such as in trauma patients with cerebral edema, cases of hydrocephalus, or spontaneous CSF leaks [43, 44]. In addition, the lumbar drain catheter can provide a conduit for injection of intrathecal fluorescein, as described below. Lumbar drains, however, have been associated with numerous complications, including the development or worsening of pneumocephalus, headache, nausea and vomiting, radicular pain, meningitis, vocal cord paralysis, and cerebral herniation [7, 11, 20, 37, 50, 51].

When the decision is made to use a lumbar drain, the surgeon should ensure that instructions for operating and monitoring the drain are clear and care of the drain is diligent. In a protocol to prevent the worsening of pneumocephalus with lumbar drains, Chan et al. advocate a passive gravity-dependent drainage system and avoidance of overdrainage [7]. Our protocol is similar, specifying the pressure above which CSF should be drained. This avoids the potential for intracranial "negative" pressures and the development of pneumocephalus, which can be life-threatening. The timing of lumbar drain removal varies depending on surgeon experience and preference, as well as patient-related factors, but in most cases, lumbar drains are removed 2–3 days postoperatively.

- Lumbar drains are a useful adjunct to CSF leak repair in certain cases. The surgeon should be mindful of potential complications associated with lumbar drains, however, and ensure that close monitoring and diligent care of the drain is available.

Intrathecal Fluorescein

Many surgeons use intrathecal fluorescein as an additional measure to localize the site of a skull-base defect intraoperatively. In this instance, injection of fluorescein is often performed at the time of lumbar drain insertion in the operating room. Intrathecal fluorescein is not approved by the United States Food and Drug Administration, and complications such as seizures, extremity weakness, and opisthotonus have been reported [30, 35]. These complications are rare, however, and may be related to high concentration, suboccipital injection, or rapid intrathecal injection [35, 55].

When using intrathecal fluorescein, our protocol involves the slow (over 10 min) intrathecal injection of 0.1 ml of 10% sodium fluorescein diluted in 10 ml of CSF. At the completion of the intrathecal fluorescein injection, the lumbar drain is clamped and the patient is placed into the Trendelenburg position to allow the fluorescein to collect along the skull base. Upon exposure of the skull base intraoperatively, fluorescein is often visible with routine endoscopic lighting. However, visualization of fluorescein may be enhanced with a blue light filter, if necessary.

Although it may be argued that intrathecal fluorescein is not necessary for every CSF leak repair, the challenge of repairing recurrent CSF leaks and meningoencephaloceles may necessitate adjunctive measures such as intrathecal fluorescein. In patients who have undergone previous repair of CSF leaks and meningoencephaloceles, recurrence may be due to failure of repair at the primary site. However, the surgeon should also be mindful that patients may present with new skull-base defects at anatomic sites remote from the original repair. This is especially true in cases of trauma and spontaneous CSF leaks, where multiple bony skull-base defects may be present (Fig. 20.4, Video 20.1) [38]. In such cases, the entire skull base may require intraoperative evaluation, and clear CSF can be difficult to detect. Intrathecal fluorescein provides an additional tool for intraoperative evaluation of the skull base and detection of the skull-base defect in need of repair.

Image-Guided Computer Navigation Systems

Image-guidance systems are commonly used in advanced endoscopic surgery and skull-base surgery. These systems may assist the surgeon intraoperatively in localizing skull-base defects and defining their dimensions. A series of endoscopic nasal CSF leak closures with and without the use of an image-guidance system was reported in 2005 by Tabaee et al. [49]. Although a statistically significant benefit in the success of CSF leak closure was not found with the use of image guidance [49], other authors have reported an increase in surgeon confidence with the use of image-guidance systems [2, 28]. In cases of revision CSF leak and meningoencephalocele repair, image-guidance systems may provide an added benefit of precisely localizing the dimensions of a bony skull-base defect in a previously operated and scarred field.

An additional tool available with image-guided surgery systems is the availability of image fusion. With this tool, images obtained by different modalities, such as CT and magnetic resonance, may be fused on a computer workstation to allow visualization of both the bone and soft-tissue components of the skull-base defect. This can be helpful in assessing meningoencephaloceles and bony skull-base defects with surrounding soft tissue and scar, such as in the case of recurrent CSF leaks.

- Intraoperative adjuncts for the localization of skull-base defects include intrathecal fluorescein and image-guided navigation systems.

Surgical Techniques

Specific techniques for the endoscopic repair of CSF leaks and meningoencephaloceles continue to evolve. While changes in technique will continue to occur over time, some basic principles are presented here. Surgery is generally performed with the patient under general anesthesia and in the supine position. In patients with known skull-base defects, positive-pressure ventilation with the bag-mask apparatus is avoided during anesthesia induction in order to decrease the risk of pneumocephalus [41, 42]. Once the patient is intubated, a lumbar drain may be inserted if the surgeon prefers, and the patient may be placed in the Trendelenburg position to increase the chance of identifying clear drainage or fluorescein from the skull base. If a lumbar drain is inserted, the drain is typically clamped during the early portions of the procedure to keep CSF pressure high and allow for better detection of the site of CSF leak. The nasal cavities are then decongested topically, and perioperative intravenous antibiotics with intrathecal penetration are administered. Under endoscopic visualization, intranasal structures are injected with local anesthesia according to surgeon preference.

The site of the skull-base defect is then identified, utilizing the principles and techniques of endoscopic sinus surgery. Depending on the specific site of the skull-base defect, the extent of sinus dissection will vary. However, in general, the skull-base defect should be adequately exposed to allow for visualization of the entire defect. This often requires some combination of uncinectomy, maxillary antrostomy, ethmoidectomy, sphenoidotomy, and frontal sinusotomy, depending on the location of the defect. For defects in the lateral recess of the sphenoid sinus, Bolger has described the endoscopic transpterygoid approach, which provides improved access to this difficult area over traditional transseptal and transethmoid approaches [4]. In addition, while this chapter focuses on endoscopic repair of skull-base defects, it should be kept in mind that

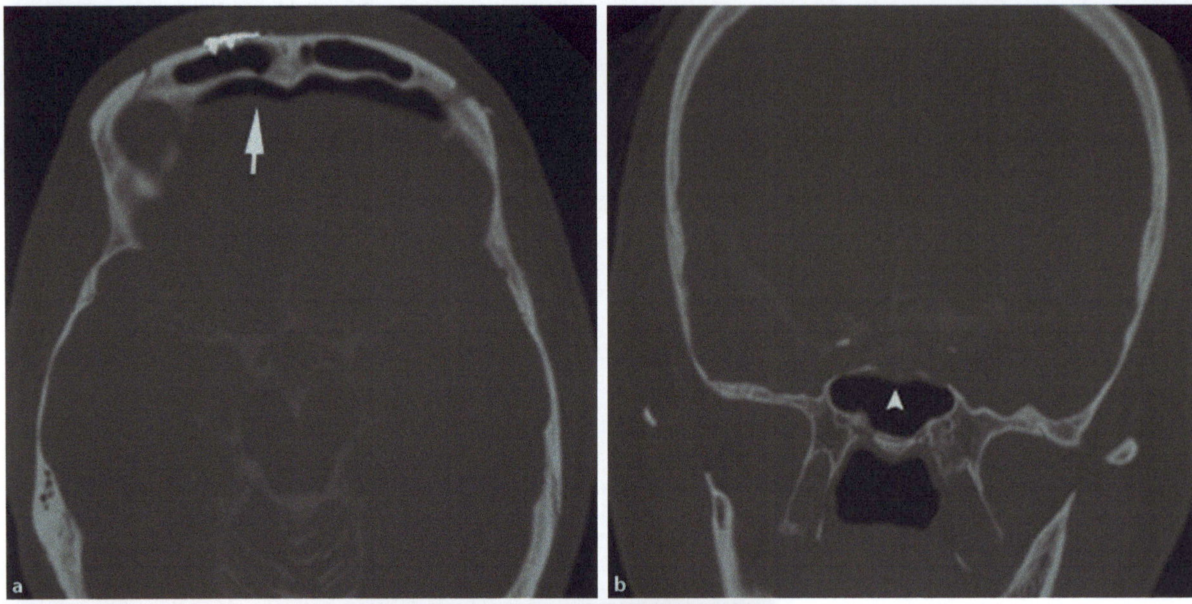

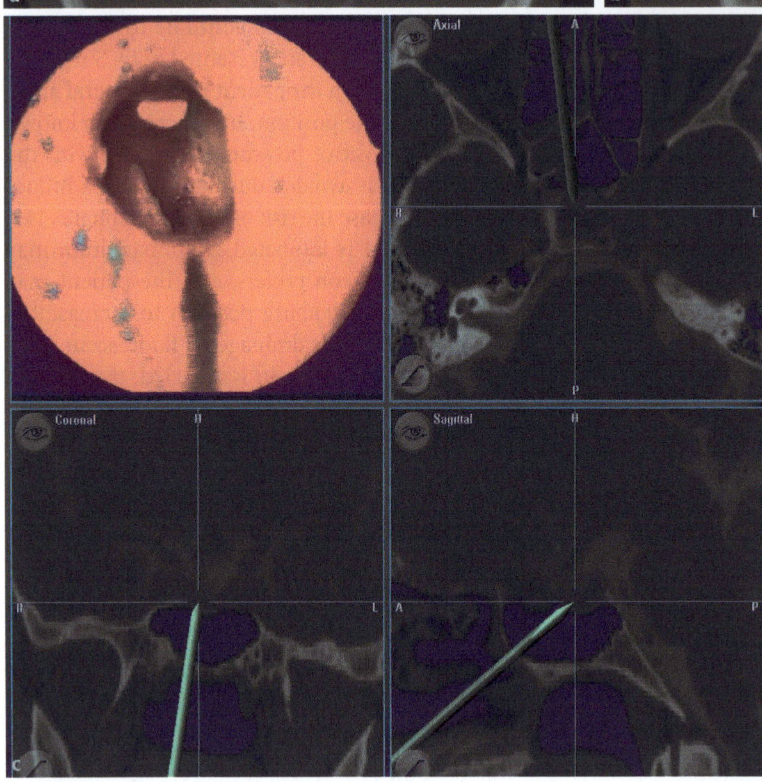

Fig. 20.4a–c Patient status post traumatic brain injury, craniotomy, and frontal sinus fracture repair referred for evaluation of persistent pneumocephalus 2 months after the initial injury. **a** A small bony defect is visualized in the right frontal sinus posterior table with adjacent pneumocephalus (*arrow*). **b** A second bony defect is noted in the sphenoid roof (*arrowhead*). CT cisternogram contrast is also seen along the sphenoid defect, but no contrast is pooling in the sphenoid sinus. **c** Intrathecal fluorescein highlights a small meningocele identified intraoperatively along the sphenoid roof. Image-guidance pointer rests on the sella, with the meningocele anterior

most of the principles described may also be applied to combined open/endoscopic approaches, as well as purely open approaches via an osteoplastic flap. The specific location of the defect and surgeon comfort and experience will dictate which approach is necessary to provide adequate exposure and visualization of the defect.

As in endoscopic sinus surgery for inflammatory disease, dissection is often facilitated by the use of angled endoscopes and giraffe instruments along the anterior ethmoid roof and in the frontal recess (Fig. 20.5). Angled endoscopes are also helpful in the lateral recess of the sphenoid sinus, where visualization can be difficult. During surgical dissection and exposure of skull-base defects, frontal and sphenoid sinusotomies should also be considered to prevent mucocele formation and allow for adequate assessment of ostia patency in the postoperative period.

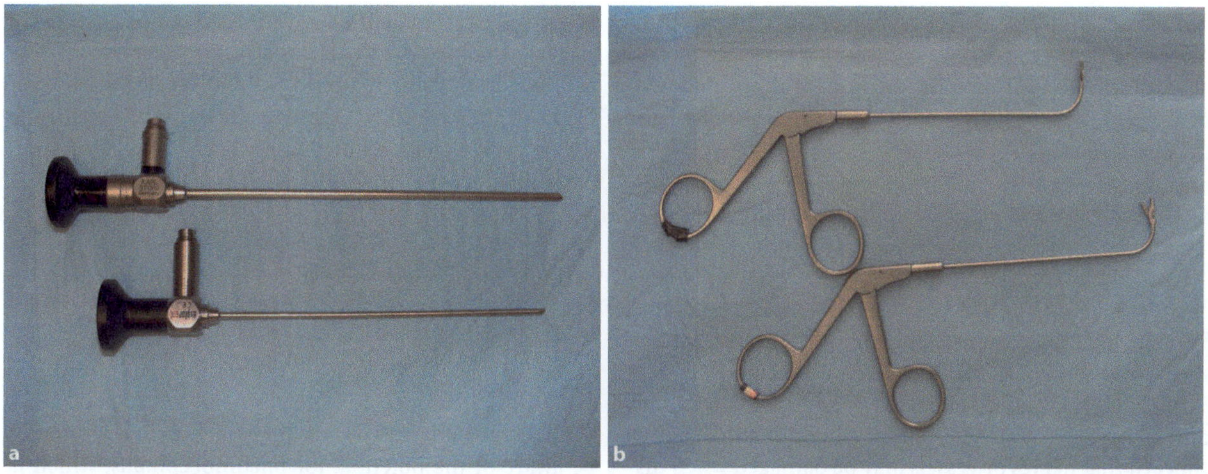

Fig. 20.5 **a** Angled rigid nasal endoscopes improve visualization of the frontal sinus/recess and lateral sphenoid recess for skull-base defect repair. **b** Giraffe angled instruments allow frontal sinus/recess manipulation

- Dissection of the paranasal sinuses surrounding the skull-base defect should be thorough. This allows for adequate visualization and access of instrumentation to perform the repair.

Once the skull-base defect is identified and exposed, the bone of the defect is denuded of surrounding mucosa for several millimeters (Fig. 20.6, Video 20.2). This prevents secretion of mucus from any mucosa underlying the graft, which may cause the graft to separate from its recipient bed [41, 42]. At this time, any meningoencephaloceles that are present at the site of skull-base defect are reduced to an intracranial position with bipolar cautery. This completes preparation of the recipient bed at the site of the skull-base defect. At this time, if an active CSF leak is present, CSF pressure may be diverted away from the

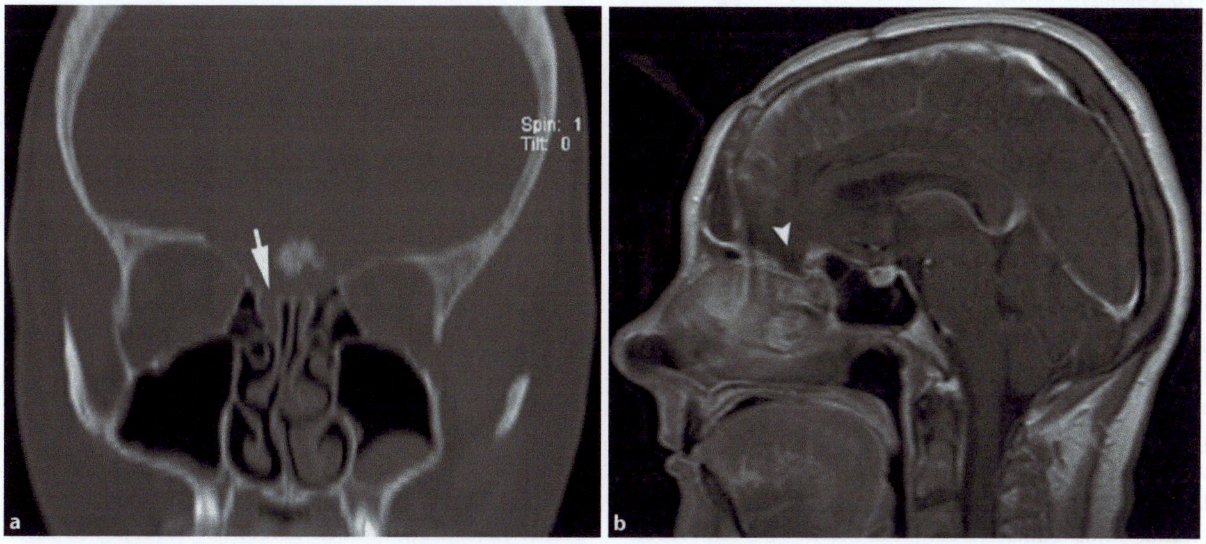

Fig. 20.6a,b Patient with recurrent CSF rhinorrhea following craniotomy for resection of olfactory meningioma. **a** Skull-base defect with likely meningocele identified in posterior ethmoid roof (*arrow*) on coronal CT scan in the bone window algorithm. **b** Presence of a posterior ethmoid meningocele (*arrowhead*) confirmed on sagittal MRI images. Video 20.2 shows endoscopic reduction of this meningocele and repair of the skull-base defect

site of the skull-base defect by taking the patient out of the Trendelenburg position and placing him/her in a 30 head-up position. If present, the lumbar drain may also be opened to drain approximately 5–10 ml per hour for the remainder of the procedure.

- Careful removal of mucosa surrounding the bony skull-base defect prevents the secretion of mucus, which may separate the graft from the recipient bed.

Specific techniques for repair will vary based on the site, size, and etiology of the defect. For small (less than 3 mm) defects, simple soft-tissue overlay grafts will typically close the defect successfully. In addition, if there is concern that nerves or vessels may be damaged when dissecting the dura away from the skull base, overlay grafting is recommended [15]. For larger defects, multilayer repairs are advocated. Repair layers may consist of soft tissue only, or a structural layer of bone may be added for support of very large defects or defects in patients with increased intracranial pressure [41, 42].

Various grafting materials have been used, and graft choice will depend on surgeon comfort and preference. Free bone graft choices include septal bone, turbinate bone, and mastoid bone. Free cartilage grafts may also be used. Autologous septal and turbinate mucosa, temporalis fascia, and abdominal fat have also been used, as have alloplastic collagen, and cadaveric dermis, fascia, and pericardium [42]. One may also consider intranasal vascularized pedicle grafts in patients with large defects or in patients with significant scarring, history of skull-base radiation therapy, or decreased blood supply to the recipient bed. Tissue adhesives may be applied following graft placement, if desired.

Whenever possible, placement of a soft-tissue or bone underlay graft in the epidural space, followed by a soft-tissue overlay graft intranasally, should be considered. A few caveats should be kept in mind, however. First, mucosal grafts should not be placed in an intracranial underlay position due to the risk of intracranial infection and mucocele [42]. Secondly, in patients with spontaneous CSF leaks and increased intracranial pressure, the entire skull base is often attenuated [42]. Significant manipulation of the skull base in these patients may lead to fracture and creation of larger defects. Finally, when placing grafts, the surgeon should remain aware of surrounding sinus ostia and avoid iatrogenic ostia obstruction during graft placement. When working near the frontal sinus outflow tract, short-term (1 week) insertion of a soft silastic stent may be useful in preventing iatrogenic obstruction during placement of the graft and packing material.

Once the graft materials are in place, the nose is packed to support the graft. Packing should begin with absorbable materials against the graft, followed by nonabsorbable materials if desired. Placement of absorbable materials in proximity to the graft allows any nonabsorbable materials to be removed without risking disruption of the graft. Absorbable materials will dissolve naturally over a period of approximately 6 weeks.

Potential Complications

Intracranial Complications

Pneumocephalus

With a known defect in the skull base, the surgeon should be aware of the potential for pneumocephalus, which is reported to carry a 25% risk of meningitis and 16% mortality [31]. Positive pressure from the external environment, such as sneezing, vomiting, continuous positive airway pressure respiratory devices, and application of bag-mask apparatus during general anesthesia induction can force air intracranially, leading to tension pneumocephalus. Patients should be alerted to this potential and instructed accordingly prior to their surgery. In addition, intubation protocols that avoid positive pressure during anesthesia induction are advisable [41, 42].

Intracranial Hemorrhage

When working along the skull base with a meningoencephalocele or skull-base tumor, vessels present in the mass often track intracranially. Traction forces on such masses may lead to rupture of the vessels in the intracranial cavity, leading to dangerous hemorrhage [41, 42]. Bipolar cautery for reduction of meningoencephaloceles and excision of skull-base tumors is typically advocated to safely cauterize these vessels without avulsing them [18].

Creation of New Skull-Base Defects

During the course of preoperative planning for endoscopic skull-base defect repair, the surgeon will carefully assess the skull base for the site of possible defects. As in preparation for endoscopic sinus surgery, sites of potential new complications involving the skull base should also be evaluated, such as asymmetry of the skull base, low-lying skull base, or tall middle-turbinate lateral lamellae. Awareness of such anatomic variants will alert the surgeon to possible sites for creation of new skull-base defects. This is especially important in the case of recurrent CSF leak or meningoencephalocele, given the altered anatomy and likely scarring from previous repairs.

Ocular Complications

Ocular complications are generally rare in endoscopic sinus surgery, and the same is true for endoscopic skull-base defect repair. However, the principles that guide the endoscopic surgeon during both types of procedure remain the same. Assessment of the patient's anatomy on preoperative CT scan will alert the surgeon to any anatomic variants and the position and integrity of the lamina papyracea, optic nerve, and optic nerve bony canal. As many skull-base defects are located in the sphenoid sinus, the surgeon should be keenly aware of the location of the optic nerve and cavernous sinus when working in this area.

Frontal and Sphenoid Ostium Stenosis

In the course of repairing skull-base defects, multiple layers of grafts and packing material are often required to ensure adequate repair. Depending on the site of skull-base defect, the ostia of the frontal or sphenoid sinus may be in the vicinity of the repair if the defect is located in the anterior ethmoid roof or frontal recess. In such cases, application of sufficient packing material may be difficult while maintaining the patency of the sinus ostia. Our typical protocol in such cases is to adequately open the sinus ostia during the course of the repair, leaving as much mucosa intact around the ostium as possible. The repair is then completed in the routine fashion. Upon completion of repairs near the frontal recess, we consider placement of a soft T-shaped silastic stent for 5–7 days. This stent can then be gently removed in the clinic without disturbing the graft or packing material and may increase the chances of maintaining frontal patency long term. In addition, during the course of postoperative care, a probe or very light suction may be carefully passed into the ostium to ensure its patency while avoiding disturbance of the graft site.

Tips and Pearls for Avoiding Complications

1. Carefully evaluate preoperative imaging for anatomic variants of the orbit and skull base, as well as integrity of the carotid canal and optic nerve canal.
2. Avoid the application of positive pressure to decrease the risk of pneumocephalus.
3. In order to reduce the chance of intracranial hemorrhage from torn vessels, use bipolar cautery along the skull base to reduce meningoencephaloceles and resect tumors.
4. For repairs near the frontal sinus ostium, identify and enlarge the ostium intraoperatively, meticulously preserving surrounding mucosa. Postoperatively, gently probe or suction the frontal sinus to ensure its patency while avoiding disturbance of the skull-base graft.

Factors Contributing to Failure in Skull-Base Repair

Factors leading to failure of skull-base defect repair have not been evaluated comprehensively. However, certain factors may alert the surgeon to potential failure and deserve mention. Most frequently, the presence of increased intracranial pressure is cited as placing patients at risk for failure [29, 56]. Various authors have described a clinical association between spontaneous CSF leaks, increased intracranial pressure, obesity, and empty sella syndrome [20, 38–40, 43]. Entities such as spontaneous CSF leaks and meningoencephaloceles, traumatic brain injury, and hydrocephalus may place patients at increased risk of skull-base repair failure due to the concomitant increased intracranial pressure. Often, perioperative adjuncts such as lumbar drains and diuretics, as well as placement of underlay bone grafts are advocated in such patients to decrease their propensity for failure.

Lindstrom et al. [20] also note increased failure rate for skull-base defects located in the lateral sphenoid recess, citing the technical difficulty of visualization and repair in this region. Another surgical factor that may make skull-base repair challenging is large skull-base defect size, especially following significant trauma or extirpation of skull-base tumors [20, 54].

A recent series at our institution designed to assess factors differentiating patients undergoing primary skull-base defect repair as compared to those undergoing revision repair identified several additional factors thought to play a role in skull-base defect repair failure [54]. These included failure to precisely localize the skull-base defect during the initial surgery (Video 20.3) and identification of a new skull-base defect at an anatomic location remote from the original repair. Factors that may influence wound healing were also present in higher percentages in revision patients, such as prior skull-base surgery, prior radiation therapy to the skull base, intracranial infection, and history of a skull-base neoplasm (excluding pituitary neoplasms). This highlights the importance of fully assessing each patient's clinical picture to ensure that surgical factors as well as patient-related factors are taken into account to provide the best possible repair circumstances.

Postoperative Care

While postoperative care and office debridement is integral to good surgical outcomes in endoscopic sinus surgery for inflammatory disease, office debridement is generally minimal in the setting of endoscopic transnasal CSF leak and meningocele repair. Postoperative protocols will vary depending on the operating surgeon and the individual case. However, some of our general principles following endoscopic CSF leak repair are discussed.

At the time of hospital discharge, patients are instructed to avoid heavy lifting and strenuous activity for approximately 6 weeks. We also recommend stool softeners and laxatives as necessary to avoid straining. In patients with spontaneous CSF leaks and increased intracranial pressure, we add diuretic therapy to decrease CSF production and alleviate stress on the repair site. Acetazolamide decreases CSF production by as much as 48% [5], and a mean reduction in intracranial pressure by 10 cmH_2O has been shown with the institution of acetazolamide postoperatively [44].

During surgery, the nose is typically packed with both absorbable and nonabsorbable packing after placement of graft material over the skull-base defect. In general, nonabsorbable packs are removed 5–7 days postoperatively. At that time, we briefly evaluate the nasal cavity with an endoscope to ensure that there is no obvious recurrence of CSF leak in the early postoperative period, but no significant debridement is performed. Over the next 6 weeks, the patient is endoscopically evaluated approximately every 2–3 weeks, and minimal debridements are performed with care not to disturb the graft site. For defects in the anterior ethmoid and frontal recess, the area of the frontal sinus ostium may be carefully probed or debrided to ensure that the frontal sinus remains patent. As previously discussed, any frontal recess stents are generally removed within 1 week. At 6 weeks postoperatively, the majority of the absorbable packing has dissolved and the graft site is usually visible. During the postoperative course, the patient does not perform any nasal irrigation, as nasal drainage following irrigations may often be mistaken for recurrence of CSF leak.

Outcomes

20

With success rates for endoscopic repair of CSF leaks and meningoencephaloceles greater than 90% in most series [6, 8, 15, 17–19, 21–24, 26, 29, 56], transnasal endoscopic repair of skull-base defects has become a preferred approach. However, recurrent CSF leaks and meningoencephaloceles may put forward challenges not present in primary cases. In a recent series at our institution, endoscopic primary skull-base defect repairs were compared to revision repairs. While the success rate for the overall group was high (93%), patients undergoing revision repair had a lower rate of successful closure (85%) than patients undergoing primary repair (97%) [54].

Patients with recurrent CSF leaks and meningoencephaloceles should be carefully assessed for factors that may contribute to failure of their repair. Such factors include spontaneous CSF leaks and meningoencephaloceles with increased intracranial pressure [14, 29], location of a skull-base defect in the lateral sphenoid sinus [20], and a large skull-base defect [20]. Other factors that may play a role in predisposing patients to recurrent CSF leaks and meningoencephaloceles include failure to accurately localize the skull-base defect, development of new skull-base defects, history of prior skull-base surgery or craniotomy, history of skull-base radiation, intracranial infections, and skull-base neoplasm (other than pituitary neoplasms) [54]. It is important to recognize these surgical factors and patient-related factors in order to adequately plan for surgery and for the care of the patient in the perioperative period.

References

1. Aarabi B, Leibrock LG (1992) Neurosurgical approaches to cerebrospinal fluid rhinorrhea. Ear Nose Throat J 71:300–305
2. Anon JB (1998) Computer-aided endoscopic sinus surgery. Laryngoscope 108:949–961
3. Arrer E, Meco C, Oberascher G (2002) Beta trace protein as a marker for cerebrospinal fluid rhinorrhea. Clin Chem 48:939–941
4. Bolger WE (2005) Endoscopic transpterygoid approach to the lateral sphenoid recess: surgical approach and clinical experience. Otolaryngol Head Neck Surg 133:20–26
5. Carrion E, Hertzog JH, Medlock MD (2001) Use of acetazolamide to decrease cerebrospinal fluid production in chronically ventilated patients with ventriculoperitoneal shunts. Arch Dis Child 84:68–71
6. Casiano RR, Jassir D (1999) Endoscopic cerebrospinal fluid rhinorrhea repair: is lumbar drain necessary? Otolaryngol Head Neck Surg 121:745–750
7. Chan E, Meiteles L (2007) Otogenic tension pneumocephalus caused by therapeutic lumbar CSF drainage for posttraumatic hydrocephalus: a case report. ENT Ear Nose Throat 86:391–393
8. Chin GY, Rice DH (2003) Transnasal endoscopic closure of cerebrospinal fluid leaks. Laryngoscope 113:136–138
9. Dandy WE (1926) Pneumocephalus: intracranial pneumatocele or aerocele. Arch Surg 12:949–982
10. Dohlman G (1948) Spontaneous cerebrospinal rhinorrhoea: case operated by rhinologic methods. Acta Otol Suppl 67:20–23
11. Dowd G, Molony T, Voorhies R (1998) Spontaneous otogenic pneumocephalus: case report and review of the literature. J Neurosurg 89:1036–1039
12. Eljammel MS, Pidgeon CN, Toland J (1994) MRI cisternography and localization of CSF fistulae. Br J Neurosurg 8:433–437

13. Flynn BM, Butler SP, Quinn RJ (1987) Radionuclide cisternography in the diagnosis and management of cerebrospinal fluid leaks: the test of choice. Med J Aust 146:82–84
14. Gendeh BS, Mazita A, Selladural BM, et al. (2005) Endonasal endoscopic repair of anterior skull base fistulas: the Kuala Lumpur experience. J Laryngol Otol 119:866–874
15. Hegazy HM, Carrau RL, Snyderman CH, et al. (2000) Transnasal endoscopic repair of cerebrospinal fluid rhinorrhea: a meta-analysis. Laryngoscope 110:1166–1172
16. Hubbard JL, McDonald TJ, Pearson BW, et al. (1985) Spontaneous cerebrospinal fluid rhinorrhea: evolving concepts in diagnosis and surgical management based on the Mayo Clinic experience from 1970 through 1981. Neurosurgery 16:314–321
17. Kirtane MV, Gauitham K, Upadhyaya SR (2005) Endoscopic CSF rhinorrhea closure: our experience in 267 cases. Otolaryngol Head Neck Surg 132:208–212
18. Lanza DC, O'Brien DA, Kennedy DW (1996) Endoscopic repair of cerebrospinal fluid fistulae and encephaloceles. Laryngoscope 106:1119–1125
19. Lee TJ, Huang CC, Chauang CC, et al. (2004) Transnasal endoscopic repair of cerebrospinal fluid rhinorrhea and skull base defect: ten-year experience. Laryngoscope 114:1475–1481
20. Lindstrom DR, Toohill RJ, Loerhl TA, et al. (2004) Management of cerebrospinal fluid rhinorrhea: the Medical College of Wisconsin experience. Laryngoscope 114:969–974
21. Locatelli D, Rampa F, Acchiardi I, et al. (2006) Endoscopic endonasal approaches for repair of cerebrospinal fluid leaks: nine year experience. Neurosurgery 58:ONS246–257
22. Lopatin AS, Kapitanov DN, Potapov AA (2003) Endonasal endoscopic repair of spontaneous cerebrospinal fluid leaks. Arch Otolaryngol Head Neck Surg 129:859–863
23. Marshall AH, Jones NS, Robertson IJA (1999) An algorithm for the management of CSF rhinorrhoea illustrated by 36 cases. Rhinology 37:182–185
24. Mattox DE, Kennedy DW (1990) Endoscopic management of CSF leaks and cephaloceles. Laryngoscope 100:857–862
25. McCormack B, Cooper PR, Persky M, et al. (1990) Extracranial repair of cerebrospinal fluid fistulas: techniques and results in 37 patients. Neurosurgery 27:412–417
26. McMains KC, Gross CW, Kountakis SE (2004) Endoscopic management of cerebrospinal fluid rhinorrhea. Laryngoscope 114:1833–1837
27. Melegos DN, Diamandis EP, Oda H, et al. (1996) Immunofluorometric assay of prostaglandin D synthase in human tissue extracts and fluids. Clin Chem 42:1984–1991
28. Metson RB, Cosenza MJ, Cunningham MJ, et al. (2000) Physician experience with an optical based image guided system for sinus surgery. Laryngoscope 110:972–976
29. Mirza S, Tahaper A, McClelland L, et al. (2005) Sinonasal cerebrospinal fluid leaks: management of 97 patients over 10 years. Laryngoscope 115:1774–1777
30. Moseley JI, Carton CA, Stern WE (1978) Spectrum of complications in the use of intrathecal fluorescein. J Neurosurg 48:765–767
31. Noth J (1971) On the importance of intracranial air. Brit J Surg 58:826–829
32. Ommaya AK, DiChiro G, Baldwin M, et al. (1968) Nontraumatic cerebrospinal fluid rhinorrhea. J Neurol Neurosurg Psychiatry 31:214–215
33. Papadea C, Schlosser RJ (2005) Rapid method for beta-2 transferrin in cerebrospinal fluid leakage using an automated immunofixation electrophoresis system. Clin Chem 51:464–470
34. Park JL, Strelzow VV, Friedman WH (1983) Current management of cerebrospinal fluid rhinorrhea. Laryngoscope 93:1294–1300
35. Rainer K, Rainer W, Wolfgang D, et al. (2004) Use of sodium fluorescein solution for detection of cerebrospinal fluid fistulas: an analysis of 420 administrations and reported complications in Europe and the United States. Laryngoscope 114:266–272
36. Roelandse FWC, Van de Zwart AZJ, Didden JH (1998) Detection of CSF leakage by isoelectric focusing on polyacrylamide gel, direct immunofixation of transferrin and silver staining. Clin Chem 44:351–353
37. Roland PS, Marple BF, Meyerhoff WL, et al. (1992) Complications of lumbar spinal fluid drainage. Otolaryngol Head Neck Surg 107:564–569
38. Schlosser RJ, Bolger WE (2002) Management of multiple spontaneous nasal meningoencephaloceles. Laryngoscope 112:980–985
39. Schlosser RJ, Bolger WE (2003) Significance of empty sella in cerebrospinal fluid leaks. Otolaryngol Head Neck Surg 128:32–38
40. Schlosser RJ, Bolger WE (2003) Spontaneous nasal cerebrospinal fluid leaks and empty sella syndrome: a clinical association. Am J Rhinol 17:91–96
41. Schlosser RJ, Bolger WE (2004) Nasal cerebrospinal fluid leaks: critical review and surgical considerations. Laryngoscope 114:255–265
42. Schlosser RJ, Bolger WE (2006) Endoscopic management of cerebrospinal fluid rhinorrhea. Otolaryngol Clin North Am 39:523–538
43. Schlosser RJ, Wilensky EM, Grady MS, et al. (2003) Elevated intracranial pressure in spontaneous CSF leaks. Am J Rhinol 17:191–195
44. Schlosser RJ, Wilensky EM, Grady MS, et al. (2004) Cerebrospinal fluid pressure monitoring after repair of cerebrospinal fluid leaks. Otolaryngol Head Neck Surg 130:443–448
45. Sibler H (1978) The normal cerebrospinal fluid proteins identified by means of thin-layer isoelectric focusing and crossed immunoelectrofocusing. J Neurol Sci 36:273–288

46. Sillers MJ, Morgan E, El Gammal T (1997) Magnetic resonance cisternography and thin coronal computerized tomography in the evaluation of cerebrospinal fluid rhinorrhea. Am J Rhinol 11:387–392
47. Skedros DG, Cass SP, Hirsch BE, et al. (1993) Sources of error in use of beta-2 transferrin analysis for diagnosing perilymphatic and cerebral spinal fluid leaks. Otolaryngol Head Neck Surg 109:861–864
48. Stone JA, Castillo M, Neelon B, et al. (1999) Evaluation of CSF leaks: high resolution CT compared with contrast-enhanced CT and radionuclide cisternography. AJNR Am J Neuroradiol 20:706–712
49. Tabaee A, Kassenoff TL, Kacker A, et al. (2005) The efficacy of computer assisted surgery in the endoscopic management of cerebrospinal fluid rhinorrhea. Otolaryngol Head Neck Surg 133:936–943
50. Ugarriza L, Cabedudo J, Lorenzana L, et al. (2001) Delayed pneumocephalus in shunted patients: report of three cases and review of the literature. Br J Neurosurg 15:161–167
51. Villarejo F, Carceller F, Alvarez C, et al. (1998) Pneumocephalus after shunting for hydrocephalus. Childs Nerv Syst 14:333–337
52. Watanabe K, Urade Y, Mader M, (1994) Identification of beta-trace protein as prostaglandin D synthase. Biochem Biophys Res Commun 203:1110–1116
53. Wigand ME (1981) Transnasal ethmoidectomy under endoscopic control. Rhinology 19:7–15
54. Wise SK, Harvey RJ, Neal JG, et al. (2007) Factors contributing to failure in skull base defect repair. Presented at the fall meeting of the American Rhinologic Society, September 5, Washington DC
55. Wolf G, Greistorfer K, Stammberger H (1997) Endoscopic detection of cerebrospinal fluid fistulas with a fluorescence technique: report of experience with over 925 cases. Laryngorhinootologie 76:588–594
56. Zweig JL, Carrau RL, Celin SE, et al. (2000) Endoscopic repair of cerebrospinal fluid leaks to the sinonasal tract: predictors of success. Otolaryngol Head Neck Surg 123:195–201

Chapter 21

Delayed Complications Following Sinus Trauma

21

David M. Poetker and Timothy L. Smith

Core Messages

- The most common complication following sinus trauma is sinusitis, usually resulting from edema, blood, retained bone or soft-tissue fragments, or foreign bodies.
- Craniofacial trauma accounts for approximately 28% of mucoceles.
- Mucoceles can present decades after the inciting trauma, so life-long follow up is indicated.
- Foreign bodies of the paranasal sinuses are associated with trauma in 70% of cases, and most commonly involve the maxillary sinus. Thorough and complete debridement in the acute setting is essential to prevent long-term complications.
- Paranasal sinus epidermoids have been reported to occur following traumatic implantation of squamous mucosa.
- Management of paranasal sinus epidermoids involves ventilation of the affected sinuses with long-term endoscopic follow up.
- Traumatic aneurysms of the internal carotid artery can present as an isolated sinus mass.

Contents

Introduction

Maxillofacial trauma is a common occurrence and has been well studied in the literature. Given the anatomical relationships, the paranasal sinuses are often involved in this trauma. Interestingly, relatively little has been written in the literature addressing the various complications of sinus trauma, and their respective management. Of the reports on sinus trauma, more attention has been paid to management of the acute complications rather than long-term or delayed complications. Management of such things as reduction of the bony fractures, removal of foreign bodies, and management of cerebrospinal fluid (CSF) leaks have all been described. In this chapter, we attempt to review the common, and some of the not-so-common delayed complications seen following the initial management of sinus trauma.

Rhinosinusitis

Acute complications associated with trauma include:

1. Sinus wall fractures.
2. Bleeding.
3. Sinus foreign bodies.
4. CSF leaks.

Each of these should be managed in the acute setting. However, if they are not appropriately managed, they can lead to delayed complications. The most common complication following sinus trauma is rhinosinusitis. Rhinosinusitis can result from edema and blood, retained bone or soft-tissue fragments, or foreign bodies. These can obstruct the outflow tract of the sinus and/or disrupt the mucociliary function of the mucous membrane. Either can lead to mucous retention in the sinus and ultimately chronic rhinosinusitis. This has been well described in the case of frontal sinus fractures that obstruct the outflow tract [11, 14]. Often, at the time of the acute injury, the blood and edema associated with the fracture make it very difficult to identify which frontal sinus fractures will result in obstruction of the outflow tract. Occasionally, a computed tomography (CT) scan obtained in a sagittal plane will help identify damage to the outflow tract. Smith and colleagues have discussed the option of medical treatment and observation of frontal sinus disease following the reduction of fractures of the anterior table of the frontal sinus, and any naso-orbitoethmoid fractures [14]. If this fails to resolve the sinus disease, a repeat of the medical management is recommended.

- Only if the second round of medical management fails do Smith et al. recommend endoscopic sinus surgery addressing the frontal sinus outflow tract [14].

This can be done through a Draf II procedure (extended endoscopic frontal sinusotomy), or a Draf III procedure (an endoscopic modified Lothrop procedure) [14]. These endonasal approaches can be augmented with a frontal sinus trephination. This allows for an additional access point for instrumentation and visualization. An osteoplastic flap may be considered in the case of a failed endonasal approach or a particularly recalcitrant case of frontal rhinossinusitis.

Post-traumatic rhinosinusitis involving the paranasal sinuses must be managed using the same principles as non-trauma-related rhinosinusitis. Initial medical management using broad-spectrum antibiotics with good sinus penetration, along with a corticosteroid to decrease outflow tract edema is recommended. Surgically, the sinus ostia must be opened, facilitating proper mucociliary function and sinus drainage. In a study reporting on maxillary sinus evaluation following trauma, the authors report that 9 of the 15 patients (60%) with maxillary sinus fractures report delayed complaints related to rhinosinusitis [16]. Six of the 9 patients required medications for the sinusitis. Follow-up CT scans of the sinuses performed between 9 and 47 months post-trauma (mean 19.8 months) showed diminished maxillary sinus volume in the traumatized sinus, mucosal thickening, and bone defects; 3 patients had their maxillary sinuses filled with soft tissue [16]. Since the focus of the article was not management, no mention was made of how these patients were treated, or the outcomes following treatment.

Mucoceles

A mucocele is an expanded, mucous-filled paranasal sinus that is most commonly found in the frontal sinus [5, 10]. Chronic rhinosinusitis and allergic sinonasal disease are the most common causes of paranasal sinus mucoceles [10]. Craniofacial trauma is the reported cause in approximately 28% of mucoceles [9]. Maxillary sinus mucoceles are said to account for up to 10% of all mucoceles, and are less commonly associated with trauma when compared to frontal mucoceles [2, 10]. Primary, or true mucoceles, occur when the outflow tract of the sinus is blocked, either due to trauma or inflammation. Secondary mucoceles occur when fractures result in mucosal entrapment and subsequent retention cyst formation [3, 15].

Patients present with a variety of signs and symptoms when suffering from a mucocele. These can range from severe headache to facial/sinus pressure, facial/sinus pain, vision complaints such as diplopia, and even obvious facial deformities. It is not uncommon to see bony erosion and remodeling of the sinus walls in the case of a mucocele. In the frontal sinus, this remodeling can extend anteriorly or posteriorly through the anterior and posterior tables, respectively. It can also extend inferiorly into the orbit leading to increased pressure on the globe, proptosis, and diplopia. This bony remodeling and erosion has been associated with the production of bone-resorbing factors produced by the lining of the mucoceles [15]. It is also believed that the intramucocele pressure is transmitted to the surrounding sinus bones, thus causing them to remodel. This remodeling often leads to gross changes in the shape of the sinus wall, and thinning of that wall. In the maxillary sinus, bone remodeling and erosion can lead to lateral nasal wall displacement, bulging of the hard palate, and even displacement of the maxillary alveolar dentition [2].

As mentioned, mucoceles can present years, and even decades from trauma.

- The average time between trauma and surgical confirmation of a mucocele has been reported at 7.5 years [15].

Koudstaal and his colleagues reported a series of three mucoceles following maxillofacial trauma. The longest delay in presentation in their series was 35 years [9]. For this, they advocate lifelong follow up for patients who have suffered sinus trauma. Although these are rare, they must be kept in the differential for patients presenting with a history of trauma.

Infection of the mucocele leads to formation of a mucopyocele. This infection can lead to rapid enlargement of the mucocele with increased risks of extrasinus complications.

- Pathogens associated with mucopyoceles are often common sinus pathogens associated with acute and chronic rhinosinusitis [15].

These rapid expansions of the mucocele increase the risk of intracranial complications [5]. Cultrera and colleagues report a patient who developed meningitis from a frontal sinus mucocele that had eroded through the posterior table of the frontal sinus, and through the dura. The patient was 9 years out from craniofacial trauma [5].

- Management of mucoceles and mucopyoceles due to maxillofacial trauma observes the same tenets of those due to inflammatory mucosal disease.

The mucocele must be opened, and the cavity drained. Although some authors still recommend complete evacuation of the cystic cavity with complete removal of the respiratory mucosa, most otolaryngologists would argue against that [15]. By opening the mucocele and allowing for drainage, mucociliary clearance may be re-established. Often times, the bony remodeling will return to a near-normal state, responding to the external pressures on the sinus once the intramucocele pressure has been relieved.

Foreign Bodies

As discussed, sinus foreign bodies can be identified in many acute trauma settings. Foreign bodies such as glass, bone fragments, gravel, and even teeth have been reported [1, 17].

- Sinus foreign bodies reportedly occur more than half of the time in the maxillary sinus, and are associated with trauma in 70% [17].

With the use of CT as the gold standard in the diagnostic imaging of maxillofacial trauma, it seems unlikely that foreign bodies are not discovered upon the initial radiographic evaluation. However, there are reports of facial fractures being treated many years ago, before the routine use of these imaging modalities, so retained foreign body should remain on the differential. In addition, it is quite possible to misinterpret the CT findings with the usual compliment of blood and edema in the sinuses in the acute setting.

Alessandro and colleagues at the University of Rome reported a case of a 26-year-old male who presented with a 14-month history of recurrent headaches and swelling of the left upper lid region. His history was significant for a severe motor vehicle collision (MVC) 2 years prior to evaluation. During that collision, he had suffered a left fronto-orbital fracture with a laceration over the left eyelid [1]. A CT scan demonstrated a foreign body lodged subcutaneously that extended into the anterior table of the frontal sinus. The sinus demonstrated mucosal thickening in the area of the foreign body. Upon surgical debridement, it was found to be a fragment of an ink pen [1]. Long-term follow up reportedly demonstrated resolution of the patient's symptoms.

Another report described a woman who suffered extensive facial fractures following an MVC [8]. These included Le Fort I, II, and III fractures, a midline palatal fracture, and a mandible fracture. A mold of her palate was made using a synthetic material made up of polyacrylic acid and polyethylmethacrylate. She underwent an open reduction of her fractures, and the palate and mandible fractures were addressed with a gunning splint. The woman recovered well from her injuries; however, she began having ipsilateral maxillary sinus complaints as soon as 1 year following the repair. She underwent several courses of antibiotics, and even a sinus washout. Although these helped, they did not solve the problem. Imaging demonstrated a right maxillary sinus opacification. Twenty-nine years after her trauma, she underwent resection of a mass from that maxillary sinus. Pathology reports described chronic inflammation with dense fibrosis, spicules of bone, and foreign material. The authors hypothesized that a small amount of the palate mold was introduced into the maxillary sinus, and the chronic sinus issues she suffered was from the sinus foreign body [8].

Silent Sinus Syndrome

There have been two reports to date of orbital floor fractures causing a silent sinus syndrome with delayed enophthalmos and hypoglobus (Fig. 21.1) [6,13]. In the first case, a 50-year-old male was struck in the face with a tree branch, suffering a minimally displaced orbital floor fracture. His ocular motility was normal, as was his vision,

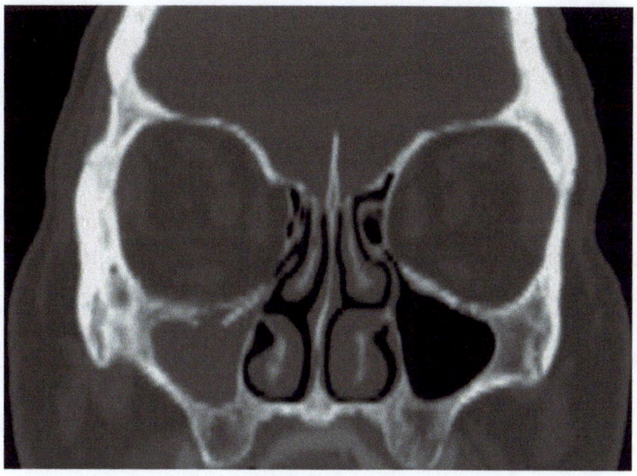

Fig. 21.1 A coronal computed tomography (CT) of the paranasal sinuses demonstrating an opacified right maxillary sinus. This patient sustained a right orbital blow out fracture 20 years prior to evaluation. She was initially referred to an ophthalmologist for contralateral proptosis. Note the right orbital floor prosthesis and the inferior displacement of the right orbital floor. Also note the lateralization of the ipsilateral uncinate process

so the fracture was managed conservatively. At 2 months post-trauma, he returned to the clinic for a 2-week progressive enophthalmos with diplopia. A CT of the orbits and sinuses revealed a completely opacified ipsilateral maxillary sinus with a severely depressed orbital floor. He was taken to surgery for maxillary antrostomy and orbital floor reconstruction. He was found to have obstruction of the natural maxillary ostium from herniated orbital contents. His symptoms resolved postoperatively [6]. The second case was of a 27-year-old man who was assaulted [13]. A CT scan demonstrated a minimally displaced left zygomaticomaxillary fracture and a moderately displaced orbital floor fracture, with an air-fluid level in the ipsilateral maxillary sinus. The patient was managed conservatively because he had no functional deficit. Six months after his trauma, he re-presented with vertical diplopia, limited vertical gaze, enophthalmos, and hypoglobus. A repeat CT scan revealed left inferior orbital expansion and a left maxillary sinus contracture with complete opacification. The patient underwent maxillary antrostomy with orbital floor reconstruction. At the time of surgery, thick, opaque mucous was cleared from the sinus, with bony fragments found obstructing the maxillary ostium. The patient had resolution of his diplopia. He was observed for an additional 4 months with no recurrence of his visual disturbances [13]. The two groups hypothesized that the mechanism of action was similar to that believed to cause silent sinus syndrome, where bone or herniated orbital contents led to obstruction of the ostium. This obstruction led to hypoventilation of the sinus, which in turn led to mucosal absorption of the oxygen and a negative pressure within the sinus. This negative pressure collapsed the sinus, pulling the orbital floor inferiorly. The authors advocate management directed at reestablishing the aeration of the sinus in these cases [13].

Paranasal Sinus Epidermoids

21

There are approximately two dozen reports of paranasal sinus epidermoids, or cholesteatomas, in the literature over the past 100 years [3,7].

- The most common locations of paranasal sinus epidermoids is the frontal sinus, but have also been reported in the ethmoid and maxillary sinuses [3].

Etiologic causes of epidermoid sinus tumors:

1. Congenital – they can theoretically be due to:
   a. Migration of squamous epithelium.
   b. Traumatic implantation.
   c. Metaplasia of the native respiratory mucosa.
2. Acquired – usually felt to be due to:
   a. Traumatic implantation.
   b. Metaplasia [3].

Patients often experience chronic pain, pressure, chronic infection, and disfigurement due to expansion and erosion caused from the epidermoid [3]. In addition, it is felt that these can degenerate into a carcinoma if not adequately addressed [7].

- Treatment of epidermoid lesions includes marsupialization and exteriorization of the cyst, as well as complete excision of the cyst lining [3].

Chandra and Palmer recently reported a series of three patients with paranasal sinus epidermoids. One patient had extension of a petrous apex epidermoid; however, the remaining two patients both had histories of craniofacial trauma, supporting the theory of traumatic implantation of the squamous mucosa. One woman had an epidermoid of the pterygopalatine space that expanded anteriorly, causing the posterior wall of the maxillary sinus to bulge anteriorly. The epidermoid was widely marsupialized through the posterior wall, using a maxillary antrostomy. She remained free of disease for 30 months at last follow-up [3].

The second patient was a young woman who developed an expanding mass of the left supraorbital ethmoid. Initially it was felt to be a mucocele; however, upon entering into the sinus, keratinaceous debris was encountered. She too underwent a wide marsupialization into the frontal sinus. As of 14 months postdebridement, she was without evidence of disease [3]. The authors acknowledge that more aggressive management such as an osteoplastic flap for frontal or ethmoid lesions is possible. They point out that the goal of their surgery was to ventilate the sinuses with functional mucociliary clearance. They also point out that wide marsupialization without complete excision of the cyst lining requires long-term endoscopic follow up with regular debridements [3].

Traumatic Aneurysms

Approximately one half of all intracranial traumatic aneurysms involve the internal carotid artery [12]. Of those, 60% occur in the cavernous portion of the internal carotid artery. They result from injury to all three layers of the artery, and often times are detected in the setting of fractures of the walls of the sphenoid sinus [12,18]. Interestingly, the initial angiograms performed will commonly show no aneurysm (Fig. 21.2); however, the patients may present with delayed epistaxis or an isolated sphenoid or ethmoid mass [12]. A clinical triad of craniofacial trauma, monocular blindness, and epistaxis should result in a high index of suspicion for a traumatic aneurysm. This severe epistaxis can occur anywhere from a few days to more than 6 months out from the trauma [12]. It has been recommended that an angiogram be performed in

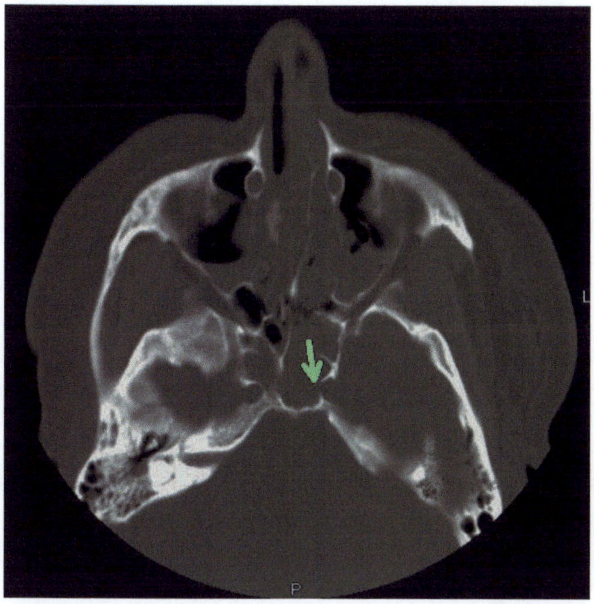

Fig. 21.2 An axial CT of the head demonstrating a fracture of the left lateral wall of the sphenoid sinus in a patient following a motor vehicle crash (*arrow*). An initial angiogram was negative for an aneurysm; however she remains at risk for development of a traumatic aneurysm

patients who have CT evidence of a sphenoid sinus or carotid canal fractures [18].

- Immediate angiograms should be performed in the fracture patients who have massive epistaxis.

Those without epistaxis should have an angiogram performed 2–3 weeks after the trauma. In patients without CT evidence of sphenoid sinus fractures, an angiogram should be performed if they demonstrate a delayed subarachnoid hemorrhage, unexplained neurological deterioration, or cranial nerve palsy. A repeat angiogram should be performed for patients with repeated epistaxis even if the initial angiogram was negative [18].

Ramos and colleagues present a patient who was evaluated for episodic dizziness and progressive visual complaints over an 8-year period. His past medical history was significant for severe craniofacial trauma 12 years prior to presentation. Imaging studies showed a mass in the sphenoid sinus, with the carotid arteries producing a normal signal in the region of the cavernous sinus bilaterally. The CT scan demonstrated erosion of the superior wall of the sphenoid. Initial biopsy attempts were nondiagnostic, so an endoscopic examination was performed. A well-encapsulated mass was identified, and profuse bleeding occurred when the mass was pierced. An angiogram demonstrated a very large aneurysm from the cavernous portion of the right internal carotid artery. This was successfully embolized, and ultimately the patient did well [12].

Cerebrospinal Fluid Leak

Cerebrospinal fluid leaks can occur in both the acute and delayed settings following craniofacial and sinus trauma. The delayed CSF leaks have been reported to occur months after the initial trauma [4]. Management of these delayed leaks is similar to that for a leak following an acute injury, or of a spontaneous CSF leak. This is outlined more extensively elsewhere in this text.

Conclusion

As discussed, there is a paucity of information in the literature about long-term or delayed complications from sinus trauma. Even with a remote trauma history, complicating factors may arise. One must be aware of these potential pitfalls in order to prepare adequately for their diagnosis and management.

References

1. Alessandro A, Sassano P, Mustazza MC, et al. (2006) Complex-type penetrating injuries of craniomaxillofacial region. J Craniofac Surg 17:442–446
2. Billing KJ, Davis G, Selva D, et al. (2004) Post-traumatic maxillary sinus mucocele. Ophthalmic Surg Lasers Imaging 35:152–155
3. Chandra RK, Palmer JN (2006) Epidermoids of the paranasal sinuses and beyond: endoscopic management. Am J Rhinol 20:441–444
4. Chen K, Chen C, Mardini S, et al. (2006) Frontal sinus fractures: a treatment algorithm and assessment of outcomes based on 78 clinical cases. Plast Reconstr Surg 118:457–468
5. Cultrera F, Giuffrida M, Mancuso P (2006) Delayed posttraumatic frontal sinus mucopyocoele presenting with meningitis. J Craniomaxillofac Surg 34:502–504
6. Gagnon MR, Yeatts RP, Williams Z, et al. (2004) Delayed enophthalmos following a minimally displaced orbital floor fracture. Ophthal Plast Reconstr Surg 20:241–243
7. Hartman JM, Stankiewicz JA (1991) Cholesteatoma of the paranasal sinuses: case report review of the literature. Ear Nose Throat J 70:719–725
8. Kirkpatrick WNA, Cook C, Joshi N, et al. (2003) Complications of the orbital floor and maxillary sinus 30 years after Coe-Pak misplacement in the management of pan-facial fractures. Orbit 22:55–61

9. Koudstaal MJ, Van der Wal KGH, Bijvoet HWC, et al. (2004) Post-trauma mucocele formation in the frontal sinus; a rationale for follow up. Int J Oral Maxillofac Surg 33:751–754
10. Marks SC, Latoni JD, Mathog RH (1997) Mucoceles of the maxillary sinus. Otolaryngol Head Neck Surg 117:18–21
11. Poetker DM, Smith TL (2006) Endoscopic treatment of the frontal sinus outflow tract in frontal sinus trauma. Oper Tech Otolaryngol Head Neck Surg 17:66–72
12. Ramos A, Tobio R, Ley E, et al. (1996) Traumatic aneurysm of the internal carotid artery: a late finding presenting as a mass in the sphenoid sinus. Am J Neuroradiol 17:222–225
13. Ross JJ, Kersten RC (2005) Late enophthalmos mimicking silent sinus syndrome secondary to orbital trauma. J Craniofac Surg 16:840–843
14. Smith TL, Jan JK, Loehrl TA, et al. (2002) Endoscopic management of the frontal recess in frontal sinus fractures: a shift in the paradigm? Laryngoscope 112:784–790
15. Smoot EC III, Bowen DG, Lappert P, et al. (1995) Delayed development of an ectopic frontal sinus mucocele after pediatric cranial trauma. J Craniofac Surg 6:327–331
16. Top H, Aygit C, Sarikaya A, et al. (2004) Evaluation of maxillary sinus after treatment of midfacial fractures. J Oral Maxillofac Surg 62:1229–1236
17. Tung T, Chen Y, Santamaria E, et al. (1998) Dislocation of anatomic structures into the maxillary sinus after craniofacial trauma. Plast Reconstr Surg 101:1904–1908
18. Uzan M, Cantasdemir M, Seckin MS, et al. (1998) Traumatic intracranial carotid tree aneurysms. Neurosurgery 43:1314–1320

Chapter 22

Recurrent Mucoceles

Benjamin Bleier, James N. Palmer, and Bradford A. Woodworth

22

Core Messages

- Management of recurrent mucoceles has shifted from open surgical resection toward more conservative, endoscopic marsupialization techniques.
- Recurrent mucocele formation may result from incomplete marsupialization of the primary lesion or unfavorable scarring of a sinus ostium or free mucosal edge.
- Mucoceles that violate the boundaries of the sinonasal cavity are at higher risk for recurrence due to the increased complexity of complete marsupialization by strictly endoscopic techniques.
- Infected mucoceles (mucopyoceles) can rapidly expand and increase the incidence of local complications.
- Computed tomography is absolutely required for evaluation and preoperative management, and magnetic resonance imaging is highly recommended if the primary lesion demonstrates skull-base erosion or frank intracranial extension.
- The overall goal of revision mucocele surgery includes complete adjacent sinusotomy followed by wide-field marsupialization of the cyst wall to minimize the risk of scarring and entrapment of residual secretory mucosa.
- Extended frontal sinus procedures, such as the Draf III (endoscopic modified Lothrop) procedure, are often necessary for recurrent frontal sinus mucoceles to increase the chances of success.
- Partial (modified) endoscopic medial maxillectomy is recommended for recurrent maxillary sinus mucoceles.
- Sphenoid mucoceles are addressed via a transnasal/transseptal or transethmoid approach.
- Endoscopic drainage appears to be an effective technique with little morbidity in the proper hands. However, open approaches are still necessary in select cases.

Contents

Introduction

Sinonasal mucoceles are indolent, expansile cysts that contain mucus and are lined with functional respiratory epithelium. These benign lesions may be locally destructive due to chronic expansion with reactive bone remodeling and may become secondarily infected, resulting in a mucopyocele. Classically, recurrent lesions were felt to require complete surgical resection, often with obliteration of the involved sinus cavities. With the advent of endoscopic surgical techniques and newer imaging modalities over the past 30 years, management of recurrent mucoceles has shifted toward more conservative marsupialization techniques.

Epidemiology

Mucoceles most commonly present between the ages of 40 and 60 years and have no discernable sex predilection [1]. Those presenting in children are usually idiopathic, although some authors advocate cystic fibrosis screening in any child found to have a mucocele [5, 7]. Paranasal sinus mucoceles occur most frequently in the frontal sinus [11]. Several large case series have reported incidences of 60–90% in the frontal sinus and 8–30% within the ethmoid sinus. Mucoceles of the maxillary and sphenoid sinus are rare, although some authors report an incidence of up to 5% and 10%, respectively [1, 9, 13].

Pathophysiology

The current paradigm for management of mucoceles and their recurrences derives from a more complete understanding of the pathophysiology of this disease. Studies by Lund et al. [14] demonstrated that the mucocele lining is composed of functional respiratory mucosa, namely ciliated pseudostratified columnar epithelium.

- Primary and recurrent mucocele development can be extrapolated to an event resulting in retained mucus with a concomitant loss of a normal outflow tract.

One proposed mechanism of primary mucocele formation implicates the cystic degeneration of a seromucinous gland with formation of a retention cyst [2]. Sinus outflow obstruction resulting from intranasal neoplasm or iatrogenic causes may also contribute to mucocele formation. One series reported a 9.3% incidence of frontal sinus mucocele following osteoplastic flap [8]. Recurrent mucocele formation may result from incomplete marsupialization of the primary lesion or unfavorable scarring of a sinus ostium or free mucosal edge. Other etiologic factors include a history of chronic sinusitis, allergic rhinitis, and previous maxillofacial trauma.

- Once formed, mucoceles may affect bony remodeling via an inflammatory cascade focused at the bone–mucocele interface.

Inflammatory mediators including interleukin (IL)-1 and IL-2 as well as fibroblast-derived prostaglandin E2 and collagenase act to promote bone resorption, which in conjunction with the mass effect of the lesion itself, can result in local bony destruction and displacement of adjacent soft tissue structures [14–16].

Local complications arise from chronic cyst wall expansion that may result in intraorbital extension with globe displacement or skull-base erosion. The incidence of intracranial extension has been reported as high as 55%, half of which had a larger intracranial than sinus component [9]. Lesions that violate the boundaries of the sinonasal cavity tend to be at higher risk for recurrence secondary to the increased complexity of complete marsupialization by strictly endoscopic techniques [18].

Bacterial invasion of the cyst can also occur, resulting in a mucopyocele. This may lead to rapid expansion of the lesion with a resultant increased incidence of local complications. Common culture isolates from these lesions include *Staphylococcus aureus*, alpha-hemolytic *Streptococci*, *Haemophilus influenzae*, *Pseudomonas aeruginosa*, and anaerobes including *Propionibacterium acnes*, *Prevotella*, and *Fusobacterium* [3, 5].

- Common etiologies of paranasal sinus mucoceles include:
  1. Chronic rhinosinusitis.
  2. Prior sinus surgery (external or endoscopic).
  3. Maxillofacial trauma.
  4. Allergy.
  5. Neoplasm.
  6. Idiopathic.

Presentation

Presenting symptoms of a recurrent mucocele are often referable to its location and include congestion, headache, rhinorrhea, and pressure. Diplopia, eye pain, decreased visual acuity, epiphora, and proptosis may be present with significant intraorbital involvement. In some cases of recurrent disease, prior loss of bony orbital architecture may result in profound exophthalmos, leading to exposure keratopathy and central retinal block [6]. Frontal mucoceles may also present with a forehead mass secondary to erosion of the anterior table. Conversely, patients with full-thickness posterior table erosion may present with a cerebrospinal fluid leak or meningitis.

Preoperative Workup

The evaluation of a patient with a suspected recurrent mucocele relies primarily on history and physical exam coupled with radiographic evaluation. If the prior marsupialization included sinusotomy with skull-base clearance, a portion of the cyst wall may be readily apparent on nasal endoscopy. While plain films have been utilized in the past to assess paranasal sinus disease, computed tomography (CT) has become the modality of choice to evaluate these lesions. Mucoceles appear as well-circumscribed cysts with homogenous mucoid contents whose attenuation increases with chronicity of the lesion secondary to increasing protein content (10–40 Hounsfield Units). High-resolution images in both axial and coronal planes provide valuable information regarding the integrity of surrounding bony structural elements and help to plan surgical intervention.

Magnetic resonance imaging (MRI) is also useful when attempting to differentiate between mucocele and other sinonasal soft tissue lesions, and is highly recommended if the primary lesion demonstrates skull-base erosion or frank intracranial extension. Mucoceles will be low intensity on T1-weighted and gadolinium-enhanced images, while appearing high intensity on T2-weighted imaging [13].

- Imaging the characteristics of mucoceles:
  1. Computed Tomography.
     a. Non-contrast enhanced.
     b. Well circumscribed with homogenous mucoid content.
        i. New lesions 10–18 Hounsfield Units.
        ii. Chronic Lesions 20–40 Hounsfield Units.
     c. Contrast enhanced.
     d. Rim enhancement.
  2. Magnetic resonance imaging.
     a. T1-weighted sequence – dark.
     b. T2-weighted sequence – bright.
     c. Gadolinium enhanced – does not enhance.

Several systems have been devised that classify mucoceles according to the site and degree of local invasion. Intracranial extent is a critical element in most systems as it predicts surgical complexity and potential need for skull-base repair or sinus obliteration at the time of surgery.

- Classification of paranasal sinus mucoceles [4]:
  1. Type 1 – anterior without intracranial extension.
  2. Type 2 – anterior with intracranial extension.
  3. Type 3 – posterior midline without intracranial extension.
  4. Type 4 – posterior with intracranial extension.

- As part of the preoperative evaluation the surgeon should do the following:
  1. Perform a complete history and physical examination including nasal endoscopy.
  2. Obtain a high-resolution CT with axial and coronal cuts. The use of image guidance for recurrent lesions is advocated.
  3. Carefully review CT with specific attention to site of involvement, the presence of bony erosion, and the degree of intraorbital and/or intracranial extension.
  4. Obtain an MRI with any significant intracranial involvement in primary or recurrent lesions or concern over sinonasal neoplasm.

Surgical Technique

Traditionally, open surgical resection, rather than marsupialization, was the gold standard treatment for primary or recurrent sinonasal mucoceles. Techniques such as the Lynch-Howarth frontoethmoidectomy or osteoplastic flap with subsequent sinus obliteration were associated with significant morbidity and cosmetic deformity as well as a relatively high recurrence rate [17]. As early as 1921 it was recognized that marsupialization was a rational alternative to these more radical approaches. This concept has been supported by subsequent studies demonstrating essentially normal mucociliary transport mechanisms within previously marsupialized cavities [10]. With the introduction of nasal endoscopes, microsurgical instruments, and image-guided surgical navigation, endoscopic transnasal marsupialization has become the treatment of choice and obviated the need for external incisions in the vast majority of cases.

Surgical management of recurrent lesions is largely dictated by the location, amount of residual bony partitions, and degree of local extension noted on preoperative CT.

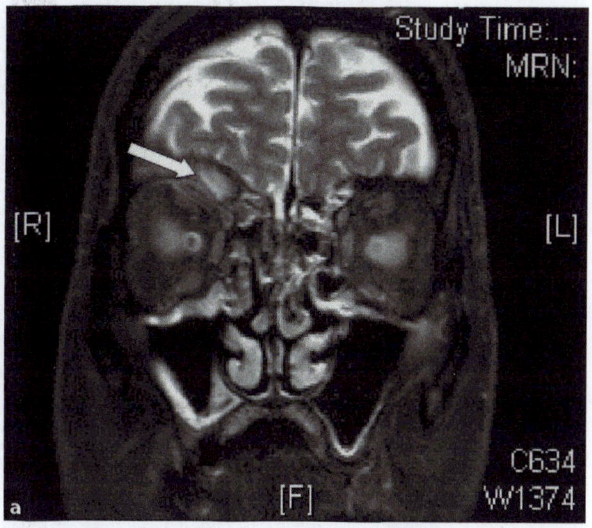

Fig. 22.1 Supraorbital ethmoid sinus mucocele. A patient with a history of right frontal mucocele drained at an outside institution presented with proptosis and eye pain. T2-weighted coronal magnetic resonance imaging scan reveals a right supraorbital ethmoid mucocele (*white arrow*) that probably developed secondary to inadequate drainage and iatrogenic scarring of the supraorbital outflow tract. **a** Intraoperative triplanar imaging and endoscopic view following drilling with a 70 diamond burr. **b** Intraoperative computed tomography (CT) scan and real-time updating of image-guidance was performed to confirm that the mucocele was completely marsupialized (**c**) **b–c** *see next page*

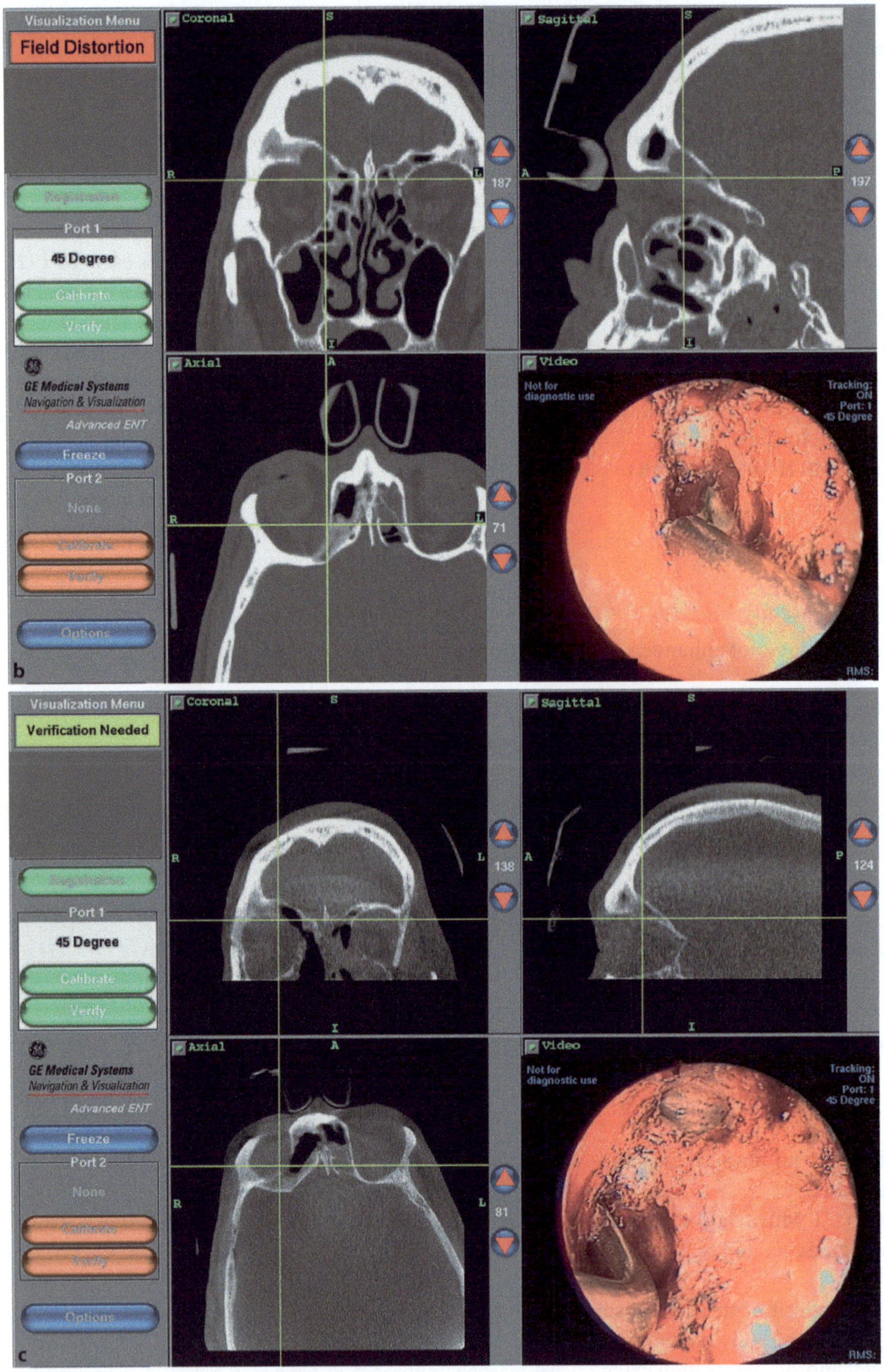

Fig. 22.1 (*continued*) **b** Intraoperative computed tomography (CT) scan and real-time updating of image-guidance was performed to confirm that the mucocele was completely marsupialized (**c**)

- The overall goal of revision mucocele surgery includes complete adjacent sinusotomy followed by wide-field marsupialization of the cyst wall to minimize the risk of scarring and entrapment of residual secretory mucosa.

If significant intraorbital or intracranial extension is present, utilization of MRI and image-guidance technologies is advocated. An open approach including craniotomy may be required in select cases [18]. If the technology is available, intraoperative CT scanning with real-time update of computer-aided systems is valuable for difficult cases, especially when the confines of the mucocele are more difficult to visualize (Fig. 22.1).

Frontal Sinus Mucoceles

Adequate drainage of frontal mucoceles to establish long-term patency requires a thorough knowledge of frontal recess anatomy and its variants. All air cells encroaching on the frontal sinus outflow tract, such as agger nasi cells anterolaterally or suprabullar cells posteriorly, are removed in their entirety to increase the chance of long-term frontal patency.

- A common set-up for recurrence is a reliance on image-guidance technology in the absence of technical skill and a comprehensive understanding of frontal recess anatomy.

Evacuating a frontal sinus mucocele using image-guidance-based suction without performing a complete frontal recess dissection invites a recurrence (Fig. 22.2). All endoscopic frontal recess dissections are more easily performed with 45 or 70 4-mm nasal endoscopes for visualization. If there is little osteoneogenesis present, the frontal recess should be dissected with frontal sinus hand instruments in an attempt to drain the mucocele into the nose. Careful attention is paid to preserving the mucosa surrounding the outflow tract to help increase long-term patency. In cases with abundant osteoneogenesis, a 70 diamond burr is helpful during the dissection. When the drill is needed or in the case of small frontal openings, an intraoperative decision must be made to extend the operation to a Draf IIB or Draf III (modified endoscopic Lothrop) procedure. If the patient has a recurrent mucocele in the presence of a prior osteoplastic flap with obliteration, a Draf III is an option to unobliterate the frontal sinuses. Stenting after endoscopic frontal sinusotomy is of controversial benefit and is often left to surgeon prefer-

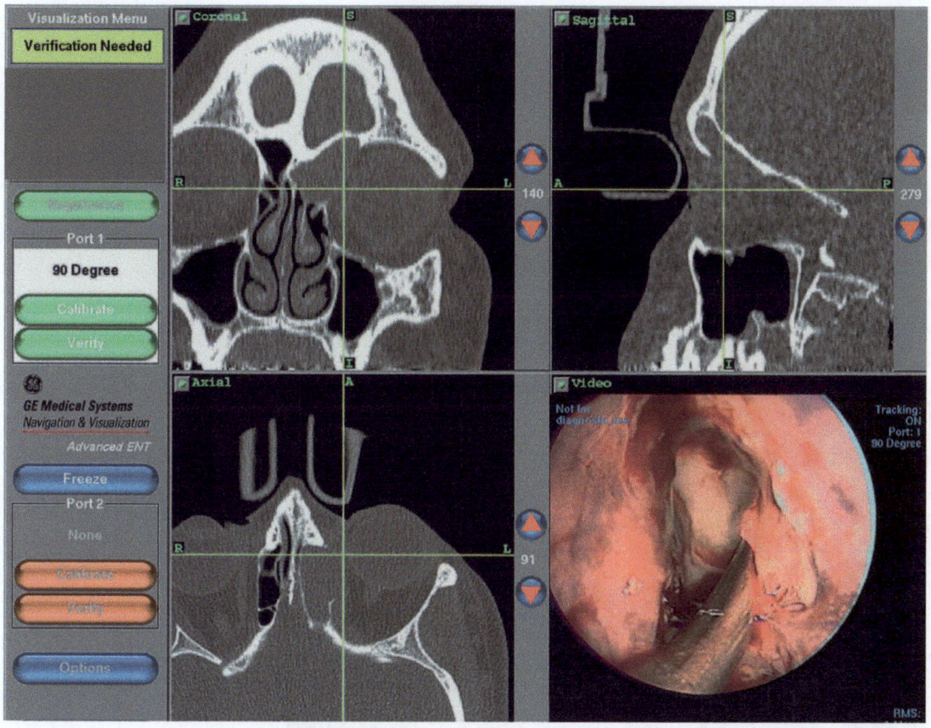

Fig. 22.2 Frontal sinus mucocele. Triplanar CT imaging and endoscopic view following complete frontal sinusotomy for a recurrent frontal sinus mucocele. The prior surgeons did not fully resect the uncinate process or adequately address the frontal recess

ence [9]. If stenting is used, it should be made from a soft, conformable material such as silastic and removed within 2–4 weeks to prevent bacterial biofilm formation on the stent itself, as this might create a nidus for inflammation.

Maxillary Sinus Mucoceles

- Mucoceles recurring in the maxillary sinus are treated with a partial (modified) endoscopic medial maxillectomy (Fig. 22.3) [19].

A middle meatal antrostomy is revised first, if necessary, with complete removal of the uncinate process. Using the turbinate scissors and through-biting forceps, an incision is carried through the anterior one-third of the inferior turbinate to the inferior portion of the maxillary antrostomy, directing the cut posterior to the distal end of the nasolacrimal duct (Hasner's valve). The anterior portion of the medial maxillary wall is then incised using the down-biting forceps to make the anterior cut. Using turbinate scissors, an inferior cut along the junction of the nasal floor and floor of the maxillary sinus is taken back flush with the posterior maxillary wall, followed by posterior cuts to remove the medial maxillary wall and inferior turbinate. The entire cavity is then inspected with 45, 70 and 120 rigid endoscopes. Meticulous preservation of mucosa is attempted in all cases. The modified endoscopic medial maxillectomy permits wide marsupialization of the maxillary sinus to decrease the probability of recurrence and optimizes distribution of postoperative topical medications and mechanical irrigations.

Patients with a prior history of Caldwell-Luc operations typically had their maxillary mucosa stripped, which may result in a contracted, hypoplastic maxillary sinus with multiple recurrent loculated mucoceles within the sinus. Facial trauma patients may also develop laterally located mucoceles within the maxillary sinus. In these instances, a modified endoscopic medial maxillectomy can be performed in conjunction with a Caldwell-Luc procedure to effectively drain and marsupialize these lateral mucoceles.

Ethmoid and Sphenoid Sinus Mucoceles

Recurrent ethmoid mucoceles are approached utilizing a complete ethmoidectomy with removal of the anteroinfe-

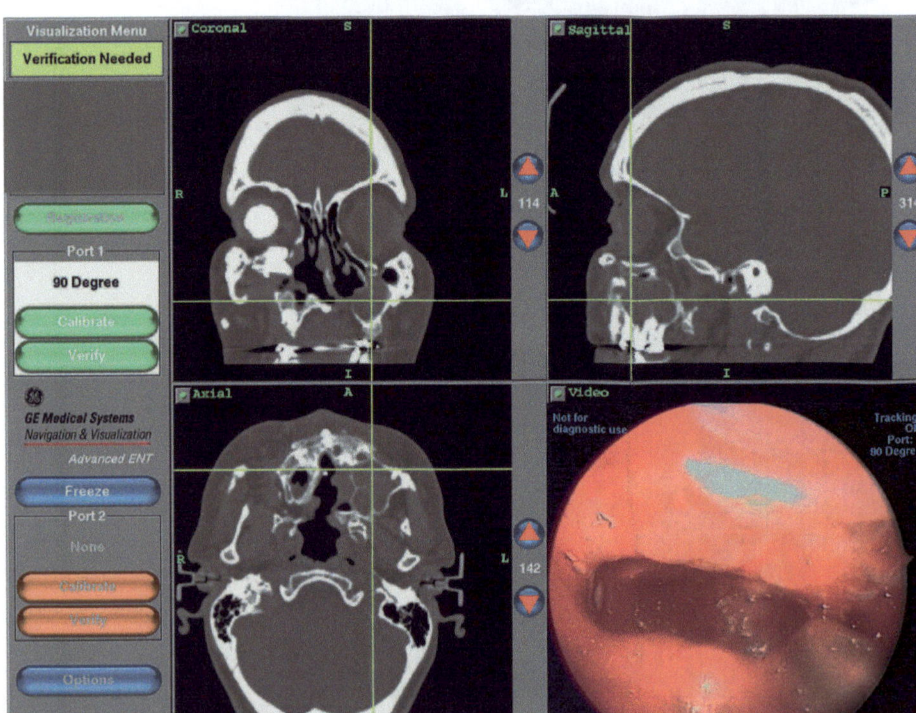

Fig. 22.3 Maxillary sinus mucocele. A patient with a history of massive facial trauma and multiple recurrent mucoceles. An inferiorly based left maxillary sinus mucocele is marsupialized with a modified medial maxillectomy

rior and medial aspects of the mucocele. Recurrent sphenoid mucoceles may be approached via either a transnasal/transseptal approach or a traditional transethmoid approach (Fig. 22.4). In both instances, locating the natural ostium of the sphenoid is the preferred entry point into the sphenoid. Recurrent lesions may be secondary to significant scarring and/or prior pituitary surgery, and thus are likely to have altered anatomy. The superior turbinate is the most reliable landmark if still present. The inferior aspect of the superior turbinate is removed to identify the natural ostium and a wide sphenoidotomy is performed.

Postoperative Care

Postoperatively nasal saline irrigation and topical nasal steroids are critical in helping to clear the operative site of debris and maintain patent ostia. Packing is generally not required. In the setting of mucopyocele or positive intranasal cultures, patients are placed on a culture-directed antibiotic regimen. Patients are monitored and debrided postoperatively until healing and reestablishment of normal mucociliary clearance pathways are complete.

Tips and Pearls to Avoid Complications

1. Carefully reexamine the CT scan just prior to surgery.
2. Potential landmarks should be identified on the CT in patients who have distorted anatomy due to prior surgery.
3. When chronic infection and inflammation is present, a preoperative course of oral antibiotic and steroid therapy helps reduce tissue inflammation and vascularity.
4. Provide careful topical and infiltrative vasoconstriction, minimize mucosal trauma (especially to the nasal mucosa anteriorly in the nose), and limit dissection in the region of the sphenopalatine artery branches. If during surgery, bleeding persists so that it interferes with visualization, it is safer to stop the procedure and if necessary, return at a later time.
5. Identify medial orbital wall and skull base early on in the dissection.
6. Avoid trauma to the anterior ethmoid artery. Identify by imaging preoperatively to avoid mistaking the artery for a bony septae of an ethmoid cell and attempting resection. Supraorbital ethmoid muco-

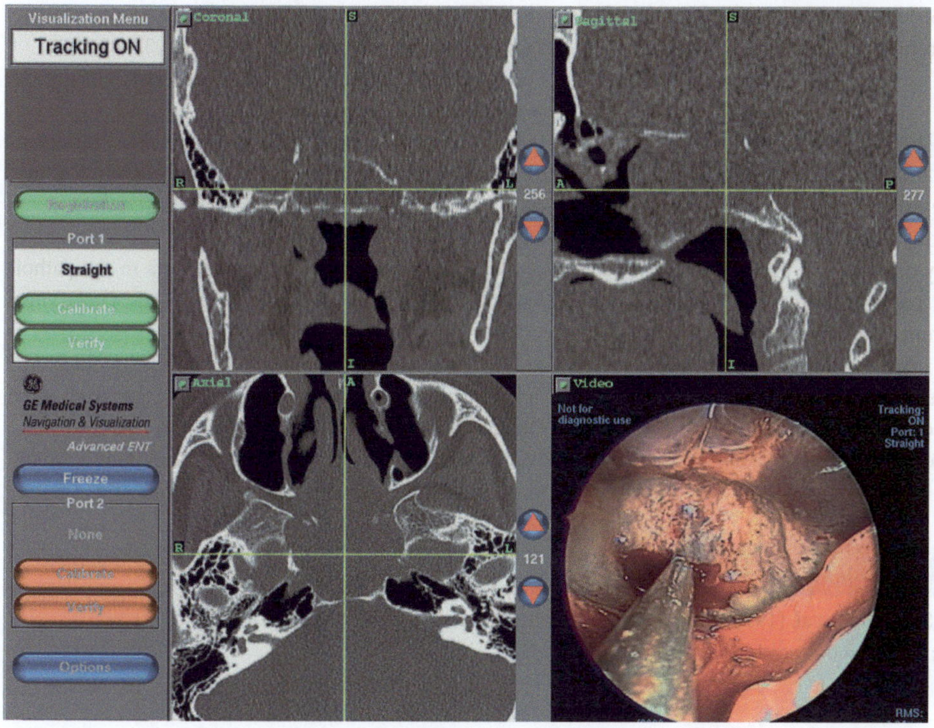

Fig. 22.4 Sphenoid sinus mucocele. This large mucocele with significant skull-base erosion recurred following sphenoidotomy at an outside institution. A transnasal/transseptal approach was performed to completely open the face of the sphenoid sinus

celes are particularly tricky as the artery often lies just posterior to this sinus.
7. Extruded orbital fat from a periorbital violation not only puts the orbit at risk, but can also obstruct the frontal outflow tract in the area of the frontal recess. Use extreme care near dehiscent lamina and avoid powered instrumentation as much as possible in these areas.
8. Preserve mucosa within the frontal recess.

Outcomes

In 1989, Kennedy et al. [12] successfully drained 16 of 18 complicated frontal mucoceles endoscopically, many of which had eroded the posterior table, extended into the orbit, or had associated Pott's puffy tumor. There were no mucocele recurrences after 42 months of follow-up. Har-El reported that 107 of 108 paranasal sinus mucoceles were successfully managed endoscopically with recurrence noted in only 1 patient (0.9%) [9]. This one recurrence was subsequently managed with an open procedure and obliteration. This case series had a median clinical follow-up of 4.6 years. Therefore, endoscopic drainage appears to be an effective technique with little morbidity in the proper hands. Mucocele recurrence rates with modern endoscopic techniques have been reported anywhere between 9 and 10%. However, given the scarcity, no larger series have been reported [9, 18].

Conclusion

Sinonasal mucoceles represent benign, expansile lesions that most often occur in the frontal and ethmoid sinus and can result in local bony destruction. In the era of endoscopic marsupialization complimented by high-resolution CT imaging, recurrences are rare. When they do occur, surgery should be directed toward creating a wide outflow tract with complete adjacent sinusotomy. In complex cases with significant orbital or intracranial involvement, open approaches may be required.

References

1. Arrue P, Thorn Kany M, Serrano E, et al. (1998) Mucoceles of the paranasal sinuses: Uncommon location. J Laryngol Otol 112:840–844
2. Batsakis JG (1980) Tumours of the Head and Neck. Williams and Wilkins, Baltimore
3. Brook I, Frazier EH (2001) The microbiology of mucopyocele. Laryngoscope 111:1771–1773
4. Delfini R, Missori P, Ianetti G, Ciappetta P, Cantore G (1993) Mucoceles of the paranasal sinuses with intracranial and intraorbital extension: report of 28 cases. Neurosurgery 32:901–906
5. al-Dousary S, al-Kaharashi S (1996) Maxillary sinus mucopyocele in children: a case report and review of literature. Int J Pediatr Otol 36:53–60
6. Garston JB (1968) Frontal sinus mucocele. Proc R Soc Med 61:549–551
7. Guttenplan MD, Wetmore RF (1989) Paranasal sinus mucoceles in cystic fibrosis. Clin Pediatr 28:429–430
8. Hardy JM, Montgomery WW (1976) Osteoplastic frontal sinusotomy: an analysis of 250 operations. Ann Otol Rhinol Laryngol 85:523–532
9. Har-El G (2000) Endoscopic management of 108 sinus mucoceles. Laryngoscope 111:2131–2143
10. Har-El G, Dimaio (2000) Histologic and physiologic studies of marsupialized sinus mucoceles. J Otolaryngol 29:195–198
11. Howarth WG (1921) Mucocele and pyocele of the nasal accessory sinuses. Lancet 2:744–746
12. Kennedy DW Josephson JS, Zinreich SJ, Mattox DE, Goldsmith MM (1989) Endoscopic sinus surgery for mucoceles: a viable alternative. Laryngoscope 99:885–895
13. Lloyd G, Lund VJ, Savy L, Howard D (2000) Optimum imaging for mucoceles. J Laryngol Otol 114:233–236
14. Lund VJ, (1991) Fronto-ethmoidal mucoceles: a histopathologic analysis. J Laryngol Otol 105:921–923
15. Lund VJ, Harvey W, Meghji S, Harris M (1988) Prostaglandin synthesis in the pathogenesis of fronto-ethmoidal mucoceles. Acta Otolaryngol 106:145–151
16. Lund VJ, Henderson B, Song Y (1993) Involvement of cytokines and vascular adhesion receptors in the pathology of fronto-ethmoidal mucoceles. Acta Otolaryngol 113:540–546
17. Rubin JS, Lund VJ, Salmon B (1986) Frontoethmoidectomy in the treatment of mucoceles. A neglected operation. Arch Otolaryngol Head Neck Surg 112:434–436
18. Weitzel EK, Hollier LH, Calzada G, Manolidis S (2002) Single stage management of complex fronto-orbital mucoceles. J Craniofac Surg 13:739–745
19. Woodworth BA, Parker RO, Schlosser RJ (2006) Modified endoscopic medial maxillectomy for chronic maxillary sinusitis. Am J Rhinol 20:317–319

Chapter 23

Allergy and the Patient Requiring Revision Sinus Surgery

23

Li-Xing Man and Berrylin J. Ferguson

Core Messages

- Allergic rhinitis is an IgE-mediated response to allergens including pollens, fungi, animal danders, insects, and dust mites.
- The role of allergic rhinitis in the pathogenesis of chronic rhinosinusitis is poorly understood, but the association is strong.
- Persistent sinonasal symptoms after endoscopic sinus surgery may indicate the need for management of an underlying allergy. Evaluation of allergy is therefore an important component in the evaluation of the patient considering revision sinus surgery.
- Typical symptoms of allergic rhinitis include nasal congestion, itching, sneezing, rhinorrhea, and postnasal discharge.
- Pharmacotherapy for allergic rhinitis should be targeted toward the specific symptom profile of the individual patient. Immunotherapy can benefit patients who fail to achieve symptom relief with environmental controls and pharmacotherapy, or who have perennial symptoms.

Contents

This chapter explores the role of allergy in chronic rhinosinusitis and reviews the diagnosis and treatment of allergic rhinitis in the patient undergoing revision sinus surgery.

Introduction

Evaluation of allergy is an integral part of the assessment of all patients with sinonasal complaints. Allergic rhinitis affects 10–40% of the population worldwide [30]. In the largest and most comprehensive national survey to date, approximately 14% of the adult population in the United States has been diagnosed with allergic rhinitis [28]. In terms of overall economic burden of illness in the United States, allergic rhinitis ranks fifth overall, with an estimated twofold increase in medication costs and physician visits, 3.5 million lost workdays, and 2 million lost schooldays [11, 12, 22].

Allergy and the Pathogenesis of Chronic Rhinosinusitis

Allergic rhinitis is a symptomatic nasal disorder characterized by IgE-mediated inflammation of nasal membranes triggered by exposure to an allergen [1]. Diagnosing allergic rhinitis in patients with chronic rhinosinusitis is difficult due to shared symptoms such as nasal congestion and rhinorrhea. Atopy, a state in which elevated levels of IgE antibodies to allergens can be detected by skin-prick, or specific IgE to antigens, can be determined objectively; however, atopic individuals may not have clinical manifestations of allergic rhinitis [18, 27]. In addition, only a subset of patients with rhinitis symptoms has disease attributable to atopy [18, 27, 35].

The role of allergic rhinitis in the pathogenesis of chronic rhinosinusitis is unclear. It has been hypothesized that allergen-mediated nasal mucosal inflammation may obstruct the sinus ostia, leading to poor sinus drainage and ventilation, mucus retention, and bacterial growth, but the evidence remains unconvincing [2]. The estimated prevalence of allergy in patients undergoing endoscopic sinus surgery ranges from 20 to 84% [6, 8, 13, 19, 23, 26, 27, 31, 32]. Few studies, however, tested all patients for atopy using in vivo assays (typically skin-prick tests) or in vitro assays for serum IgE antibody to allergens (Table 23.1). Some studies suggest that atopic patients have more severe disease when assessed by computed tomography scan appearance and have less improvement in symptoms and quality of life after endoscopic sinus surgery [3, 6, 14, 15, 23]. Other studies found no association between atopy and either preoperative severity of sinus disease or postoperative symptomatic improvement [19, 25–27, 31, 32].

Few studies have explored the role of allergy in the patient requiring revision sinus surgery. Several analyses have noted no difference in the rate of revision endoscopic sinus surgery between allergic and nonallergic patients [19, 25, 27]. One series demonstrated a reduction in prescription antihistamine use after revision endoscopic sinus surgery that was not statistically significant [4]. Another study of patients undergoing revision sinus surgery showed a nonsignificant trend toward allergic patients being more likely to require further surgical management [25].

The persistence of sinonasal symptoms in patients with allergy after endoscopic sinus surgery may reflect the need for more intensive or specific allergy management [19]. In a review of 190 consecutive patients with chronic rhinosinusitis refractory to medical management and who subsequently underwent endoscopic sinus surgery, none had received preoperative immunotherapy, but 84% tested positive for inhalant allergies [8]. Evaluation of allergy is an integral part in the assessment of all patients considering revision sinus surgery.

Allergic Rhinitis

Diagnosis

- The diagnosis of allergic rhinitis is suggested by a history of typical symptoms and confirmed by skin or blood testing for allergies. Symptoms of allergic rhinitis include:
  1. Nasal congestion.
  2. Fatigue.
  3. Postnasal discharge.
  4. Rhinorrhea.
  5. Sneezing.

Many of these symptoms are typical of chronic rhinosinusitis. The diagnosis of allergic rhinitis is more likely if the patient can relate a history in which symptoms resolve in different localities and recur with a return to the home or local environment. Patients with seasonal allergic rhinitis have often already made the diagnosis on their own, but those with perennial allergic rhinitis are often unaware that they have an allergy.

Table 23.1 Prevalence of allergy in patients undergoing endoscopic sinus surgery for chronic rhinosinusitis. *NA* Data not available

Study	Number of patients	Number tested for allergy (%)	Prevalence of allergy	Method of diagnosis for allergy
Newman et al. [23]	104	95 (91.3%)	20.0%	In vitro testing
Robinson et al. [27]	193	193 (100.%)	30.1%	Skin or in vitro testing[a]
Smith et al. [31]	119	NA	34.5%	Patient history
Sobol et al. [32]	393	NA	34.6%	Skin testing
Dursun et al. [6]	130	67 (51.5%)	36.2%	Skin testing and history
Marks et al. [19]	115	0	54.5%	Self-reported on survey
Ramadan et al. [26]	141	NA	54.6%	Patient history[b]
Kennedy [13]	120	NA	57.5%	Skin or in vitro testing
Emanuel and Shah [8]	190	190 (100.%)	83.7%	Skin or in vitro testing

[a] Skin testing of 10% and in vitro testing of 90% of patients (Wormald 2007, personal communication)

[b] Study population comprised children aged 3–13 years

23

- Allergy testing is valuable in the management of patients with chronic nasal symptoms for two reasons:
  1. Allergy testing can identify allergens that the patient did not previously suspect so that environmental controls can be directed.
  2. Allergy testing provides the basis for formulation of allergen vials for immunotherapy.

- Immunotherapy is the only treatment modality that has the potential to cure the patient with allergic rhinitis. Indications for immunotherapy include patients who:
  1. Fail to achieve relief from targeted pharmacotherapy.
  2. Have symptoms over half of the year so immunotherapy becomes a cost-effective alternative.

In-vitro (blood) testing and skin testing are the two major forms of allergy testing. There are multiple in-vitro tests available for allergy testing including, but not limited to, radioallergosorbent test (RAST), modified RAST, and the Pharmacia CAP System. There are two types of skin testing for allergy: intradermal dilutional testing (IDT) and prick testing. A serum total IgE level is not an adequate screen for allergy, as it can often be within normal limits and yet the patient will have significant specific IgE-mediated hypersensitivity to a few antigens.

In-Vitro Screens

A mini-allergy screen of six antigens using RAST batteries of one grass (Timothy), one weed (common ragweed), one tree (oak), two molds (*Alternaria* and *Helmithosporium*), and one dust mite (*Dermatophagoides pteronyssinus*) – with epidermals (i.e., cat, horse, etc., added if indicated by history – has a predictive value of 75%. If the testing battery is expanded to a total of nine antigens by including a second grass (Bermuda), an additional tree (mountain cedar), and an additional mold (*Cladosporium*), the predictive value increases to 95% compared to a 13-antigen screen [16]. The population for this study comprised patients living in southwest Texas. Practitioners in other locales should tailor the antigens to the most prevalent and likely allergens in their particular region. Pollen maps, available from many of the testing companies, can help guide the selection of these antigens.

Skin Testing

IDT, also known as skin endpoint titration, is the most sensitive allergy test and is able to establish a safe starting dose for immunotherapy. Usually a screen using dust mite, cat, dog, mold mix, tree mix, and grass mix is performed initially and additional IDTs within the subgroups are performed if the respective mix is positive. There is a wide selection of prick-testing devices. The Multitest II device is one of the most popular, most reproducible, and fastest to apply. A negative Multitest using 14 antigens plus histamine and glycerin controls indicates that significant inhalant allergy is unlikely. A positive Multitest may require additional in vitro or IDT testing [17].

- The simplest screen for allergies involves either an in-vitro allergen screen of 6–9 allergens or a Multitest II prick test. As they are most often associated with chronic rhinosinusitis, the allergen screen should be focused on perennial allergens:
  1. Dust mite.
  2. Cockroach.
  3. Molds.
  4. Cat (if applicable).

The patient probably does not have inhalant allergy if the screen is negative. If the screen is positive, the patient may be allergic to multiple other allergens and may require further, more detailed investigation.

Medical Therapy for Allergic Rhinitis

It is essential to control the symptoms of rhinitis in the allergic patient requiring revision sinus surgery. Management of allergic rhinitis in the patient considering revision sinus surgery has four components: allergen avoidance, pharmacotherapy, immunotherapy, and surgery.

The ideal treatment of allergic rhinitis is avoidance of allergens that provoke symptoms. Common environmental agents that trigger IgE-mediated allergic rhinitis symptoms include dust mites, pollens, molds, animal danders, and insect allergens [7]. In very specific circumstances, environmental control can be as effective as pharmacologic therapy [9]. For example, a pet linked to a patient's allergy can be removed from the home. There is evidence that a home-based, total environmental control program benefits patients with dust mite and cockroach sensitivity [21, 24, 29]. Other interventions, such as avoidance of the outdoors, keeping windows closed, and air conditioning during peak pollen seasons are often more difficult to achieve. Avoidance of all offending allergens is unrealistic for many patients [20].

When environmental controls are impractical or incompletely effective, pharmacotherapy is introduced. A wide variety of medications is available for the treatment of allergic rhinitis. The choice of pharmacologic agent is tailored to the individual patient's symptoms. Medications and their relative efficacy toward specific symptoms are outlined in Table 23.2.

- Medications effective for treating allergic rhinitis include:
  1. Topical and systemic steroids.
  2. Topical and oral antihistamines.
  3. Topical and oral decongestants.
  4. Leukotriene receptor modulators.
  5. Mast cell stabilizers.
  6. Anticholinergics.
  7. Saline nasal washes.
  8. Anti-IgE.

Nasal steroid sprays provide the most comprehensive relief of allergic rhinitis symptoms with the least amount of morbidity and are recommended as first-line therapy [5, 9]. Nasal steroid sprays are distinct from the other classes of pharmacotherapy since they control all of the major nasal symptoms of allergic rhinitis: sneezing, rhinorrhea, itching, and congestion. In a meta-analysis of 16 randomized trials, nasal steroid sprays were significantly better than oral antihistamines at relieving nasal symptoms [33]. Nasal steroid sprays may begin to take effect within 12 h after dosing, but efficacy may not be maximal until 1–2 weeks after initiation of therapy. Patients should always be educated in directing the steroid spray away from the septum and toward the lateral wall of the nose to minimize septal excoriation, bleeding, and the very rare complication of septal perforation.

Azelastine is a topical antihistamine nasal spray that has a symptom relief profile similar to that of nasal steroid sprays. Onset of action is within a day. Its use is limited by a bad taste appreciated by approximately 30% of users, and a slight sedation potential.

Oral antihistamines can be divided into sedating and nonsedating drugs. Fexofenadine, loratadine, and desloratadine at recommended doses do not cause sedation and are effective for nasal itching and sneezing symptoms, but have little impact on nasal congestion. For this reason, antihistamines are often paired with a decongestant. Sedating antihistamines are available over-the-counter and have anticholinergic properties, which thickens nasal secretions and may over-dry the nose in some patients. The utility of oral antihistamines in patients with chronic rhinosinusitis is limited due to the failure of antihistamines to significantly reduce congestion.

Topical decongestants may be used for short periods of time to decongest the nose and to optimize drainage. Prolonged use can lead to rebound swelling. This may be diminished with concurrent use of a topical nasal steroid spray [10]. Most practitioners do not recommend long-term use of oral decongestants because of the side effects of tachycardia, tremors, and insomnia.

The leukotriene receptor antagonist montelukast is moderately effective in relieving symptoms of rhinorrhea, congestion, sneezing, and nasal itching. Overall, it is less effective than nasal steroid sprays [34]. Certain patients, however, may respond markedly to montelukast.

The cromone cromolyn is available over-the-counter as a nasal spray. The efficacy data for this product are inconsistent and the effects on nasal symptoms are modest.

It is often difficult to predict which pharmacologic therapy will be the most effective, but initial treatment should be directed according to symptom profile. The senior author currently practices a cost-effective method whereby samples of several classes of pharmacologic agents are given to the patient to try serially. Prescriptions are filled only if the drug is found to provide relief. This reduces the number of prescriptions and frequency of clinic visits. Patients who have incomplete relief with monotherapy may require combination therapy with several classes of drugs.

Table 23.2 Medications and their relative efficacy in allergic rhinitis

Medication	Congestion	Sneezing	Rhinorrhea	Nasal itching	Eye symptoms
Nasal steroid	+++	+++	+++	+++	+
Antihistamine					
Sedating	+/–	++	++	++	++
Nonsedating	+/–	++	–	++	++
Decongestant	+++	–	–	–	–
Leukotriene receptor antagonist	++	+	+	+	+
Mast cell stabilizer	+	+	+	+	+/–
Ipratropium	–	–	+++	–	–

Allergen immunotherapy is the only treatment modality with the potential for disease modification. Immunotherapy should be considered in patients who continue to have significant symptoms despite pharmacotherapy, who require systemic corticosteroids, or who have comorbid conditions such as asthma [7]. Typical candidates for immunotherapy have severe seasonal symptoms that return or worsen each year, or perennial symptoms. Subcutaneous allergen immunotherapy typically consists of weekly doses of a solution containing the culpable allergens that are gradually increased to an optimal maintenance dose. Immunotherapy can be stopped after 1 year if there are no noticeable improvements.

Patients who continue to have residual nasal congestion after endoscopic sinus surgery should be evaluated for turbinate hypertrophy. In patients who have chronic hypertrophy of the inferior turbinate with nasal symptoms refractory to pharmacotherapy, surgery to reduce the inferior turbinate may be a useful treatment option. Several inferior turbinate reduction techniques have been described.

Conclusion

Allergic rhinitis is a common comorbidity in patients with chronic rhinosinusitis. Many patients who continue to have symptoms of rhinosinusitis despite endoscopic sinus surgery have not been adequately evaluated and treated for allergic rhinitis. The diagnosis of allergic rhinitis is based on history, and on in vitro or skin allergy testing. Optimal therapy of allergic rhinitis includes the identification and elimination of allergen exposure. Pharmacotherapy should be targeted toward allergic symptoms. Immunotherapy can be utilized in patients who failed to achieve adequate symptom relief with environmental controls and pharmacotherapy, or who have perennial symptoms. Inferior turbinate reduction can provide relief from nasal congestions in patients with chronic turbinate hypertrophy.

References

1. Bachert C, van Cauwenberge P, Khaltaev N (2002) Allergic rhinitis and its impact on asthma. In collaboration with the World Health Organization. Executive summary of the workshop report. 7–10 December 1999, Geneva, Switzerland. Allergy 57:841–855
2. Bachert C, Vignola AM, Gevaert P, et al. (2004) Allergic rhinitis, rhinosinusitis, and asthma: one airway disease. Immunol Allergy Clin North Am 24:19–43
3. Berrettini S, Carabelli A, Sellari-Franceschini S, et al. (1999) Perennial allergic rhinitis and chronic sinusitis: correlation with rhinologic risk factors. Allergy 54:242–248
4. Bhattacharyya N (2004) Clinical outcomes after revision endoscopic sinus surgery. Arch Otolaryngol Head Neck Surg 130:975–978
5. Bousquet J, Van Cauwenberge P, Khaltaev N (2001) Allergic rhinitis and its impact on asthma. J Allergy Clin Immunol 108:S147–S334
6. Dursun E, Korkmaz H, Eryilmaz A, et al. (2003) Clinical predictors of long-term success after endoscopic sinus surgery. Otolaryngol Head Neck Surg 129:526–531
7. Dykewicz MS, Fineman S, Skoner DP, et al. (1998) Diagnosis and management of rhinitis: complete guidelines of the Joint Task Force on Practice Parameters in Allergy, Asthma and Immunology. American Academy of Allergy, Asthma, and Immunology. Ann Allergy Asthma Immunol 81:478–518
8. Emanuel IA, Shah SB (2000) Chronic rhinosinusitis: allergy and sinus computed tomography relationships. Otolaryngol Head Neck Surg 123:687–691
9. Ferguson BJ (1997) Allergic rhinitis. Options for pharmacotherapy and immunotherapy. Postgrad Med 101:117–120, 123–116, 131
10. Ferguson BJ, Paramaesvaran S, Rubinstein E (2001) A study of the effect of nasal steroid sprays in perennial allergic rhinitis patients with rhinitis medicamentosa. Otolaryngol Head Neck Surg 125:253–260
11. Goetzel RZ, Long SR, Ozminkowski RJ, et al. (2004) Health, absence, disability, and presenteeism cost estimates of certain physical and mental health conditions affecting U.S. employers. J Occup Environ Med 46:398–412
12. Kay GG (2000) The effects of antihistamines on cognition and performance. J Allergy Clin Immunol 105:S622–S627
13. Kennedy DW (1992) Prognostic factors, outcomes and staging in ethmoid sinus surgery. Laryngoscope 102:1–18
14. Kountakis SE, Arango P, Bradley D, et al. (2004) Molecular and cellular staging for the severity of chronic rhinosinusitis. Laryngoscope 114:1895–1905
15. Krouse JH (2000) Computed tomography stage, allergy testing, and quality of life in patients with sinusitis. Otolaryngol Head Neck Surg 123:389–392
16. Lehr AJ, Mabry RL, Mabry CS (1997) The screening RAST: is it a valid concept? Otolaryngol Head Neck Surg 117:54–55
17. Levine JL, Mabry RL, Mabry CS (1998) Comparison of Multi-Test device skin testing and modified RAST results. Otolaryngol Head Neck Surg 118:797–799
18. Lilja G, Wickman M (1998) Allergy–atopy–hypersensitivity – a matter of definition. Allergy 53:1011–1012
19. Marks SC, Shamsa F (1997) Evaluation of prognostic factors in endoscopic sinus surgery. Am J Rhinol 11:187–191

20. Marple BF, Fornadley JA, Patel AA, et al. (2007) Keys to successful management of patients with allergic rhinitis: focus on patient confidence, compliance, and satisfaction. Otolaryngol Head Neck Surg 136:S107–S124
21. Morgan WJ, Crain EF, Gruchalla RS, et al. (2004) Results of a home-based environmental intervention among urban children with asthma. N Engl J Med 351:1068–1080
22. Nathan RA (2007) The burden of allergic rhinitis. Allergy Asthma Proc 28:3–9
23. Newman LJ, Platts-Mills TA, Phillips CD, et al. (1994) Chronic sinusitis. Relationship of computed tomographic findings to allergy, asthma, and eosinophilia. JAMA 271:363–367
24. Platts-Mills TA, Vaughan JW, Carter MC, et al. (2000) The role of intervention in established allergy: avoidance of indoor allergens in the treatment of chronic allergic disease. J Allergy Clin Immunol 106:787–804
25. Ramadan HH (1999) Surgical causes of failure in endoscopic sinus surgery. Laryngoscope 109:27–29
26. Ramadan HH, Hinerman RA (2006) Outcome of endoscopic sinus surgery in children with allergic rhinitis. Am J Rhinol 20:438–440
27. Robinson S, Douglas R, Wormald PJ (2006) The relationship between atopy and chronic rhinosinusitis. Am J Rhinol 20:625–628
28. Schulman, Ronca, and Bucuvalas, Inc (2006) Allergies in America: A Landmark Survey of Nasal Allergy Sufferers. Executive Summary. Available at: http://www.myallergiesinamerica.com/executive-summary.php. Accessed August 6, 2007. Altana Pharma US, Florham Park, NJ
29. Sheikh A, Hurwitz B, Shehata Y (2007) House dust mite avoidance measures for perennial allergic rhinitis. Cochrane Database Syst Rev:CD001563
30. Sly RM (1999) Changing prevalence of allergic rhinitis and asthma. Ann Allergy Asthma Immunol 82:233–248; quiz 248–252
31. Smith TL, Mendolia-Loffredo S, Loehrl TA, et al. (2005) Predictive factors and outcomes in endoscopic sinus surgery for chronic rhinosinusitis. Laryngoscope 115:2199–2205
32. Sobol SE, Wright ED, Frenkiel S (1998) One-year outcome analysis of functional endoscopic sinus surgery for chronic sinusitis. J Otolaryngology 27:252–257
33. Weiner JM, Abramson MJ, Puy RM (1998) Intranasal corticosteroids versus oral H1 receptor antagonists in allergic rhinitis: systematic review of randomised controlled trials. BMJ 317:1624–1629
34. Wilson AM, O'Byrne PM, Parameswaran K (2004) Leukotriene receptor antagonists for allergic rhinitis: a systematic review and meta-analysis. Am J Med 116:338–344
35. Zacharasiewicz A, Douwes J, Pearce N (2003) What proportion of rhinitis symptoms is attributable to atopy? J Clin Epidemiol 56:385–390

Chapter 24

Staging of Disease after Sinus Surgery Failure

24

Valerie J. Lund

Core Messages

- Despite many suggested methods of staging for chronic rhinosinusitis, there are intrinsic difficulties in finding the "perfect" solution.
- Most staging systems have relied on computed tomography (CT) scoring, endoscopic findings, symptom scores or combinations thereof and have concentrated on patients undergoing primary surgery rather than patients with recurrent symptoms awaiting revision surgery.
- Whilst a correlation can be shown between CT and endoscopic findings, the correlation between CT changes and symptoms is generally poor in either circumstance.
- The purpose of staging in inflammation/infection in contrast to malignancy may relate more to demonstration of the disease and as an inclusion criterion for clinical research than as a predictive tool.

Contents

Introduction

"Staging: the determination of the particular stage which a progressive disease or condition has reached.".
Oxford English Dictionary 2003

"A staging system is necessary to have meaningful results".
Caldwell 1893 [11]

"A judgement on prognosis requires an objective assessment of the anatomical extent of the disease".
TNM: Classification of Malignant Tumours [23]

Throughout medicine considerable effort has been made to quantify and qualify disease processes to facilitate clinical management and research. In rhinology, this has proved remarkably difficult despite several objective tests and investigations, and none more so than in the assessment of patients after surgical treatment. Part of the problem has lain with inter- and intra-individual variation, partly with the cost, availability and the technical requirements of some of these tests, but above all with the difficulty in correlating results with symptoms. There is clearly a need for a universally accepted method of assessing disease extent that might provide criteria for further therapeutic intervention and allow comparison of results of treatment between centres. However, this presupposes that the purpose of staging is to correlate extent of disease with outcome, using the same premise as that on which the TNM classification is based. Whilst the majority of work in this area has focused on inflammatory conditions such as chronic rhinosinusitis (CRS) and nasal polyposis (NP) where the outcomes are ultimately less finite than in cancer, some mention will also be made of staging in relation to other conditions such as benign and malignant neoplasia where recurrence and revision surgery are frequently required.

CRS and NP

- Rhinosinusitis (including NP) is defined [18] as inflammation of the nose and the paranasal sinuses characterised by two or more of these symptoms, one of which should be either nasal blockage/obstruction/congestion or nasal discharge (anterior/posterior nasal drip):

1. ± Facial pain/pressure.
2. ± Reduction or loss of smell.

and either

3. Endoscopic signs of:
   a. Polyps and/or;
   b. Mucopurulent discharge primarily from the middle meatus and/or;
   c. Oedema/mucosal obstruction primarily in the middle meatus.

and/or

4. Computed tomography (CT) changes: mucosal changes within the ostiomeatal complex and/or sinuses.

It would therefore seem sensible to use some, if not all of these criteria to stage disease, particularly as virtually all patients will be undergoing symptom assessment, endoscopy and imaging if they have recurrent problems and are being considered for revision surgery.

Subjective assessment of symptoms generally considers the degree and duration of those directly associated with the condition and it has been shown that in a general population of patients with CRS/NP, some of whom had undergone previous surgery, their symptoms could be divided into mild, moderate and severe based on a total severity visual analogue scale (VAS) score (0-10 cm; see below) [39].

Not troublesome |———————| Worst thinkable troublesome

10 cm

Subjective assessment of symptoms. A VAS >5 affects patient quality of life:

1. Mild = VAS 0–3
2. Moderate = VAS > 3–7
3. Severe = VAS > 7–10

- To evaluate the total severity, the patient can be asked to indicate on a VAS the answer to the question: "How troublesome are your symptoms of rhinosinusitis?" This can be factored into any staging of disease as a measure of symptom severity (Table 24.1a).

Other consensus documents have recommended a 0–7 scale [45] where:

1: None to an occasional limited episode.
2–3: Mild-steady symptoms but easily tolerable.
4–5: Moderately bothersome – symptoms are difficult to tolerate and may interfere with activities of daily living and/or sleep.
6–7: Very severe – symptoms are so bad that they cannot function all of the time.

However, it should be noted that the "normal" population do not score zero, with a mean of 8.8 being found in an ostensibly healthy sample versus a mean of 35.3 ($p = 0.0001$) in those with CRS [62].

When considering duration of disease, one is reliant on the definition endorsed by various drugs and therapeutic agencies around the world, which were created largely for the purpose of providing inclusion criteria for trials in acute bacterial rhinosinusitis, and which are at best generalisations and at worst, arbitrary.

- Rhinosinusitis classification:
  1. Acute
     a. < 12 weeks.
     b. Complete resolution of symptoms.
  2. Chronic
     a. > 12 weeks symptoms.
     b. Without complete resolution of symptoms.

CRS may also be subject to exacerbations (i.e. acute on chronic). It would be implicit in an individual requiring further surgery that their symptoms had lasted for at least 3 months, and therefore the duration has little utility in staging.

Considerable debate surrounds the relationship between CRS and NP, with many researchers believing that the two are distinct conditions with a different pathophysiology and inflammatory profile, which may have a bearing on staging. However, others prefer to consider NP as part of a spectrum of inflammation that can be generically referred to as CRS. From a practical point of view in the clinical setting, it is probably best to consider the condition as CRS without polyps and CRS with polyps, a distinction that can usually be made on endoscopy.

- Definition of CRS with/without polyps in individuals who have not had previous surgery:
  1. CRS without NP: no visible polyps in the middle meatus, if necessary following administration of decongestant.
  2. CRS with nasal polyposis: polyps bilateral, visualised endoscopically in the middle meatus.

This definition accepts that there is a spectrum of disease in CRS that includes polypoid change in the sinuses and/or middle meatus but excludes those with polypoid disease presenting in the nasal cavity to avoid overlap.

Table 24.1a The Lund-MacKay scoring system [42]: symptom scores using the visual analogue method. Each category is scored on a scale of 0–10 according to the degree of symptom severity, where 0 = symptoms not present and 10 = greatest possible severity

Symptom	Pre-surgery	After operation	After 3 months	After 6 months	After 1 year	After 2 years
Nasal blockage or congestion						
Headache						
Facial pain						
Problems of smell						
Nasal discharge						
Sneezing						
Overall						
Total points						

Table 24.1 b Lund-MacKay scoring system: endoscopic appearances scores

Characteristic	Baseline and follow-up
Polyp left (0,1,2,3)[a]	
Polyp, right (0,1,2,3)[a]	
Oedema, left (0,1,2,)[b]	
Oedema, right (0,1,2,)[b]	
Discharge, left (0,1,2)[c]	
Discharge, right (0,1,2)[c]	
Postoperative scores to be used for outcome assessment only Scarring, left (0.1,2)[d]	
Scarring, right (0.1,2)[d]	
Crusting, left (0,1,2)[e]	
Crusting, right (0,1,2)[e]	
Total points	

[a] 0 = Absence of polyps; 1 = polyps in middle meatus only; 2 = polyps beyond middle meatus but not blocking the nose completely; 3 = polyps completely obstructing the nose

[b] Oedema: 0 = absent; 1 = mild; 2 = severe

[c] Discharge: 0 = no discharge; 1 = clear, thin discharge; 2 = thick, purulent discharge

[d] Scarring: 0 = absent; 1 = mild; 2-severe

[e] Crusting: 0 = absent; 1 = mild; 2 = severe

Table 24.1 c Lund-MacKay scoring system: CT scoring system

Sinus system[a]	Left	Right
Maxillary (0,1,2)		
Anterior ethmoids (0,1,2)		
Posterior ethmoids (0,1,2)		
Sphenoid (0,1,2)		
Frontal (0,1,2)		
Ostiomeatal complex (0 or 2 only)*		
Total points		

[a]0 = no abnormalities; 1 = partial opacification; 2 = total opacification

Table 24.1 d Lund-MacKay scoring system: radiological grading of anatomic variants

Anatomic variant[a]	Left	Right
Absent frontal sinus		
Concha bullosa		
Paradoxical middle turbinate		
Everted uncinate process		
Haller cells		
Agger nasi cells		
Total points		

[a]Scoring: 0 = no variant, 1 = variant present

Table 24.1 e Lund-MacKay scoring system: surgery scores

Surgery[a]	Left	Right
Uncinectomy		
Middle meatal antrostomy		
Anterior ethmoidectomy		
Posterior ethmoidectomy		
Sphenoidectomy		
Frontal recess surgery		
Reduction of the middle turbinate		
Total points each side		

[a]Score: 0 = no procedure done; 1 = surgery done. The maximum score is 14 (7 each side)

Unfortunately the situation is more difficult once surgery has altered the anatomy of the lateral wall. Under these circumstances, it has been proposed that the presence of polyps is defined as bilateral pedunculated lesions as opposed to cobblestoned mucosa >6 months after surgery on endoscopic examination.

- Any mucosal disease without overt polyps should be regarded as CRS.

It should be remembered that other conditions may occur concomitantly with CRS/NP and may significantly alter the prognosis, and thus the validity of staging systems, for example cystic fibrosis, gross immunodeficiency (congenital or acquired), congenital mucociliary problems (e.g. primary ciliary dyskinesia), non-invasive and invasive fungal disease, systemic vasculitis and granulomatous diseases, cocaine abuse and neoplasia.

Endoscopy

This may be performed with or without decongestion and some form of local anaesthesia. Schemes have proposed semi-quantitative scores [41] for polyps, oedema, discharge, crusting and scarring, such as that shown in Table 24.1b, which are designed to provide a baseline score and can be repeated at regular intervals following therapeutic interventions (e.g. at 3, 6, 9 and 12 months). The most important factor is the ease with which a particular staging system can be taught, performed and reproduced, and this particular one has a high inter-rater concordance [1] and can be used in the presence of recurrent disease and both prior and following revision surgery. In the system shown, which has been widely adopted, polyps are scored on a scale of 0–3. However, there are at least three other systems ranging from 0–2, 0–4 and 0–7 (Tables 24.2 and 24.3) [30, 38, 42]. Johansson showed good correlation between a 0-3 scoring system and their own system in which they estimated the percentage projection of polyps from the lateral wall and the percentage of the nasal cavity volume occupied by polyps. However, they did not find a correlation between the size of polyps and symptoms.

Imaging

It is widely accepted that plain sinus x-rays play no part in the diagnosis and thus staging of sinus disease, and we have come to rely on CT scanning as the modality of choice in inflammation and infection (Figs. 24.1 and 24.2). It is therefore not surprising that this has proved the mainstay of staging despite the many protocols and interest in reducing radiation exposure. All were originally designed with the evaluation of primary chronic disease in mind but can be adapted to the presence of recurrence. However, there are no published scoring systems for acute bacterial rhinosinusitis. At least nine systems have been published (Tables 24.1 and 24.4–24.11), some of which formulate a number of stages, usually 0–4 (e.g. Kennedy [34]), whereas others produce a score (e.g. the Lund-MacKay system [42]). This latter system has probably gained the greatest currency, largely due to its simplicity and reproducibility. However, few have specifically addressed the issue of the patient undergoing revision surgery.

The Lund-MacKay system relies on a score of 0–2 dependent upon the absence, partial or complete opacification of each sinus system and of the ostiomeatal complex, deriving a maximum score of 12 per side (Table 24.1c). It can be used following surgery, but the extent of surgical disruption will affect its application. Nonetheless, the presence of mucosal thickening and opacification of extant sinuses may still be scored. Previous surgery, such as Caldwell-Luc, may lead to permanently thickened mucosa, although this may be fibrotic rather than evidence of ongoing inflammation. However, this does not preclude the application of a numerical score in a patient whose symptoms have warranted a scan.

It should be noted that incidental abnormalities are found on scanning in up to one-fifth of the "normal" population [40]. Mean Lund-MacKay scores of 4.26 in adults [2] and 2.81 in children aged 1–18 years [25] have been reported. In addition, for ethical reasons a CT scan is generally only performed post-operatively when there are persistent problems, and therefore CT staging or scoring is best regarded as an inclusion criterion for studies rather than as an outcome assessment.

This system also allows for a radiological grading of anatomic variants (Table 24.1d), some of which may still be present post-surgery and provides a method of scoring extent of the operation itself (Table 24.1e), which again may be of use in the revision case.

The Lund-MacKay system has been validated in several studies [50] and shown to have a high inter- and intra-rater reproducibility. As a consequence it was adopted by the Rhinosinusitis Task Force Committee of the American Academy of Otolaryngology Head and Neck Surgery in 1996 [53] as well as several subsequent consensus documents and guidelines [16, 18]. CT and endoscopic scores correlate well in CRS both with and without polyps [24, 56, 60], but as previously indicated, the correlation between CT findings and symptom scores has generally been shown to be poor and is not a good indicator of outcome [9, 10, 26, 59]. However, Wabnitz and colleagues did find a correlation between a total VAS based on the sum of five sinonasal symptoms and CT score, although

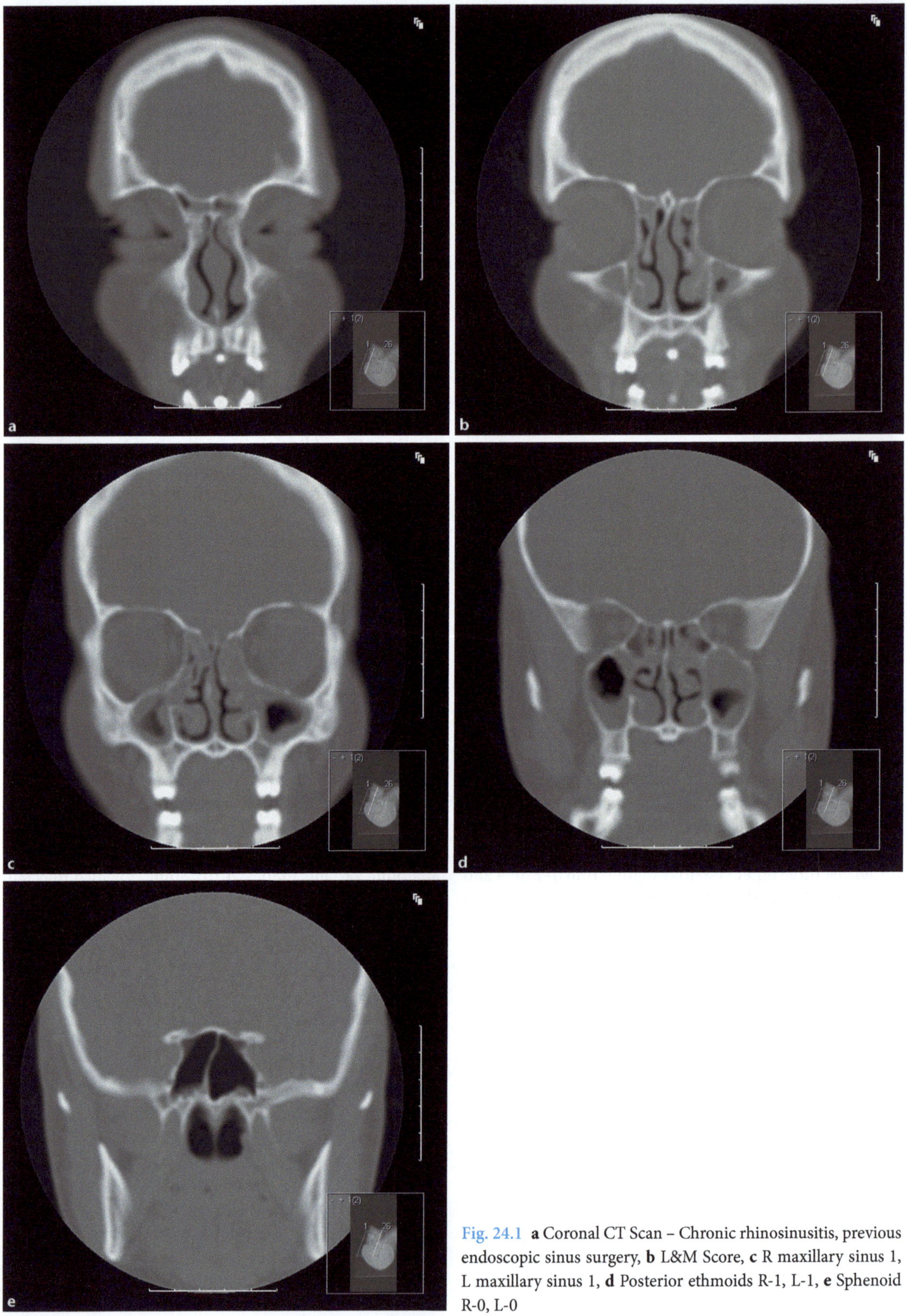

Fig. 24.1 **a** Coronal CT Scan – Chronic rhinosinusitis, previous endoscopic sinus surgery, **b** L&M Score, **c** R maxillary sinus 1, L maxillary sinus 1, **d** Posterior ethmoids R-1, L-1, **e** Sphenoid R-0, L-0

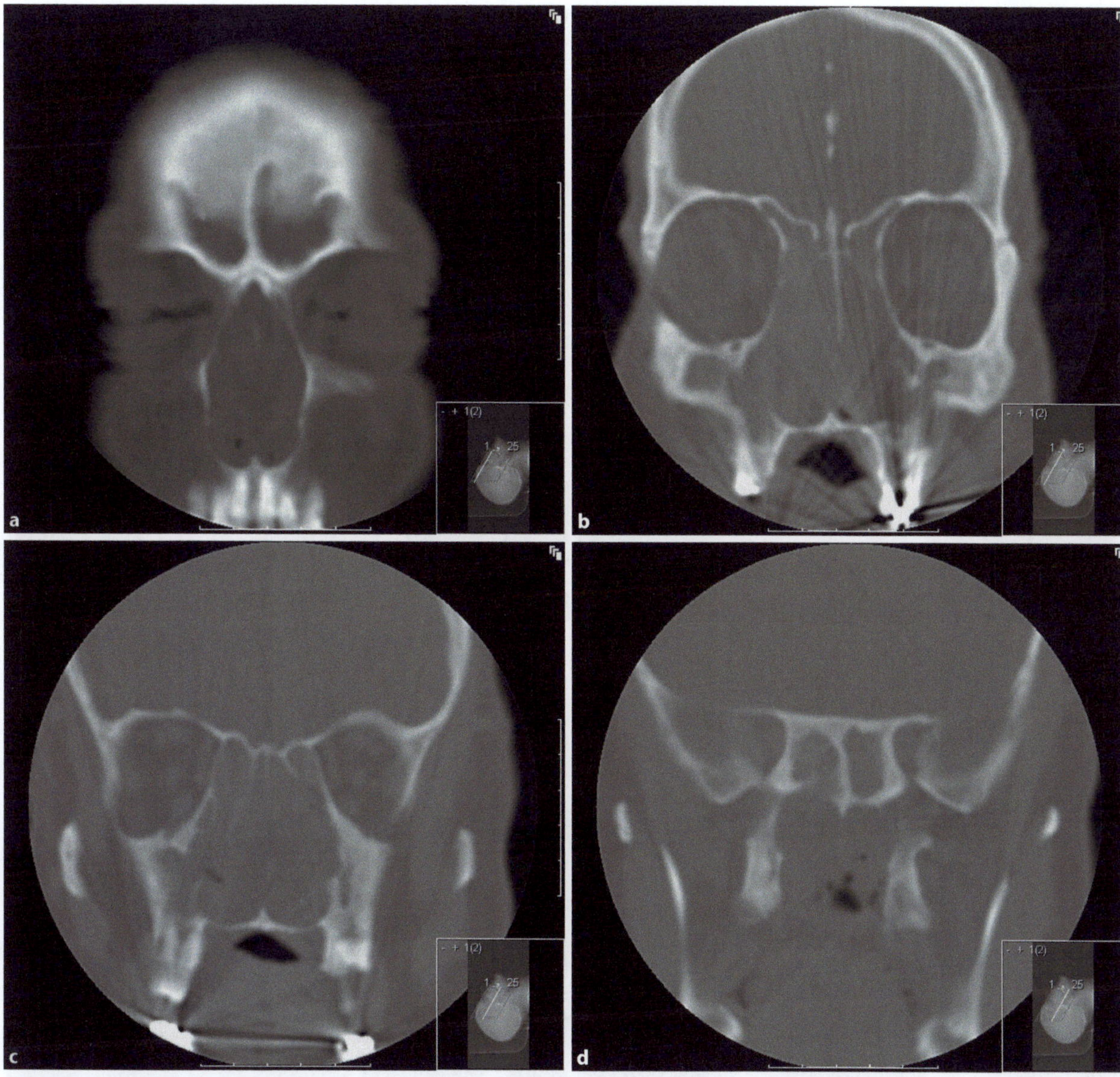

Fig. 24.2 **a** Coronal CTScan – Chronic rhinosinusitis with nasal polyps, **b** Anterior ethmoids R-2, L-2, **c** Posterior ethmoids R-2, L-2, **d** Sphenoid R-2, L-2

Table 24.2 Lildholt et al. [38]: semi-quantitative scoring of nasal polyps

0	None
1	Cobblestoned
2	Pedunculated polyps only visible endoscopically
3	Pedunculated polyps not protruding below the middle turbinate (equivalent to the back of the inferior turbinate when the middle turbinate has been resected)
4	Pedunculated polyps below the middle turbinate

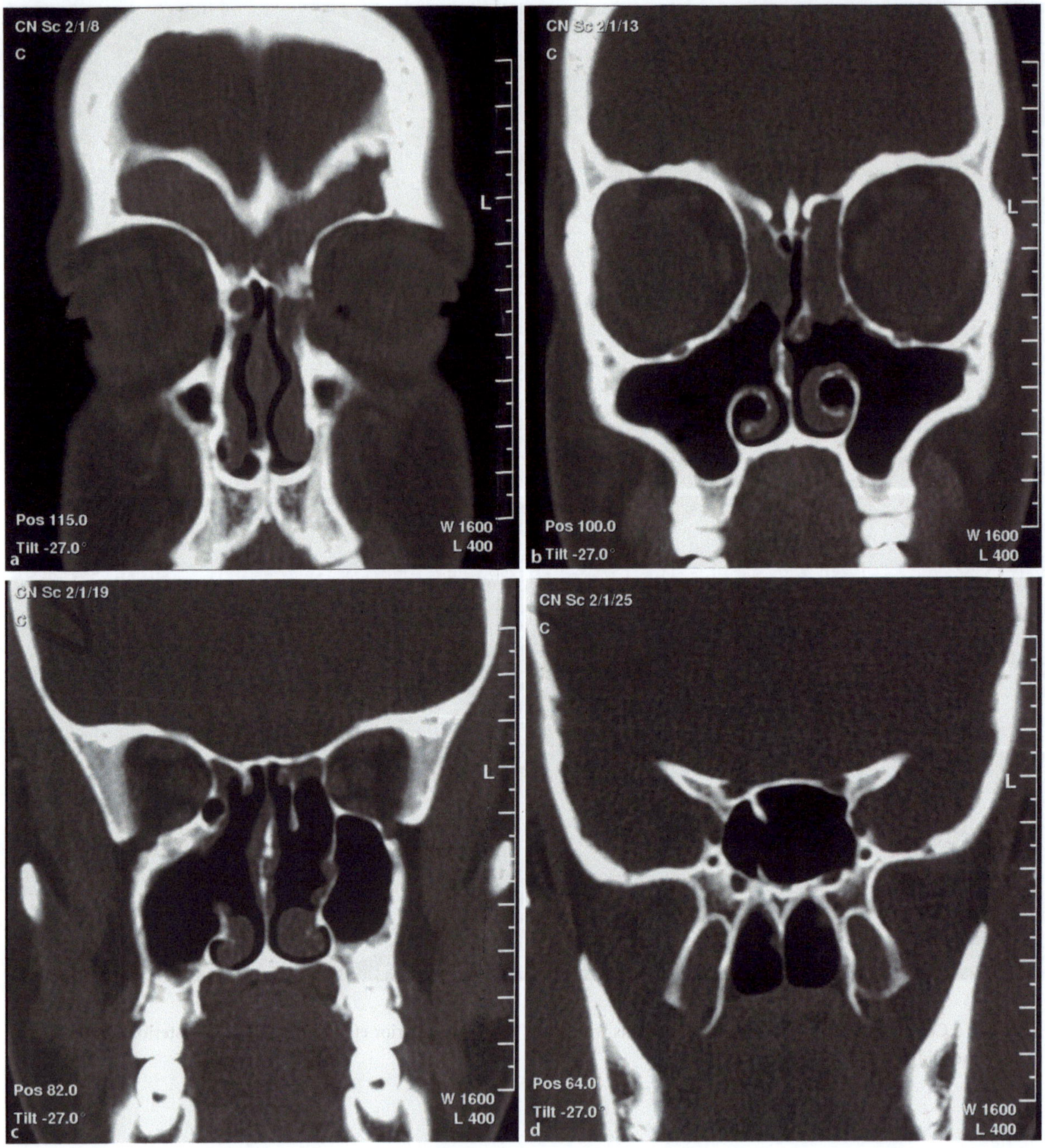

Fig 24.3 **a** Coronal CT scans: Chronic rhinosinusitis with previous nasal polyposis, one previous endoscopic operation, **b** Anterior ethmoid cavities R-2, L-2, **c** Posterior ethmoidal cavities R-1, L-1, **d** Sphenoid R-0, L-0

Table 24.3 Johansson et al. [30]: semi-quantitative scoring of nasal polyps

4	As before
5	Polyps medial to the middle turbinate
6	Polyps medial and lateral to the middle turbinate
7	Nasal cavity completely filled with polyps

Table 24.4 The staging system of Friedman et al. [19]

Stage 0	Normal
Stage I	Single-focus disease (involving a single focus or sinus unit)
Stage II	Multifocal disease (includes bilateral or multiple areas of disease that are not confluent or are diffuse throughout the ethmoid labyrinth, bilateral middle-meatal polyps)
Stage III	Diffuse disease (extensive bilateral involvement of multiple sinuses) without bony changes
Stage IV	Diffuse disease associated with bony changes

Table 24.5 The staging system of Kennedy [34]

Stage 0	Normal
Stage I	Anatomic abnormalities All unilateral sinus disease Bilateral disease limited to ethmoid sinuses
Stage II	Bilateral ethmoid disease with involvement of one dependent sinus
Stage III	Bilateral ethmoid disease with involvement of two or more dependent sinuses on each side
Stage IV	Diffuse sinonasal polyposis

Table 24.6 The staging system of Levine and May [37]

Stage 0	Normal
Stage I	Disease limited to the ostiomeatal complex
Stage II	Incomplete opacification of one or more major sinuses (frontal, maxillary, sphenoid)
Stage III	Complete opacification of one or more major sinuses, but not all
Stage IV	Total opacification of all sinuses

Table 24.7 The staging system of Gliklich and Metson [22]

Stage 0	Normal (< 2 mm of mucosal thickening on any sinus wall)
Stage I	All unilateral disease or anatomic abnormality
Stage II	Bilateral disease limited to ethmoid or maxillary sinuses
Stage III	Bilateral disease with involvement of at least one sphenoid or frontal sinus
Stage IV	Pansinusitis

Table 24.8 Radiological scoring system of Jorgensen [31]

Structure	Left	Right
Frontal-sinus opacification[a]		
Maxillary-antrum opacification[a]		
Anterior ethmoidal-labyrinth opacification[a]		
Posterior ethmoidal-labyrinth opacification[a]		
Sphenoid-sinus opacification[a]		
Maxillary-antrum polyp[b]		
Hiatus-semilunaris occlusion[c]		
Maxillary-sinus ostium occlusion[c]		
Frontal-recess occlusion[c]		
Ethmoidal-infundibulum occlusion[c]		

[a]Score for opacification: none = 0; mild = 1; moderate = 2; marked = 3; complete = 4

[b]Score for size of maxillary sinus polyp: none = 0; small = 1; medium = 2; large = 3

[c]Score for occlusion: none = 0; mild = 1; moderate = 2; complete = 3

Table 24.9 Worksheet for the radiological grading system of Newman et al. [48]

Structure	Left	Right
Maxillary sinus[a]		
Frontal sinus[a]		
Sphenoid sinus[a]		
Ethmoidal sinus[b]		
Ostiomeatal complex[c]		
Nasal passages[c]		
Hiatus-semilunaris occlusion[c]		
Maxillary-sinus ostium occlusion[c]		

Table 24.9 (*continued*)

Structure	Left	Right
Frontal-recess occlusion[c]		
Ethmoidal-infundibulum occlusion[c]		

[a] Mucosal thickening scores: 0 (0–1 mm); 1 (2–5 mm); 2 (6–9 mm); 3 (>9 mm)

[b] Mucosal thickening scores: 0 (0 mm) 1 (0–1 mm); 2 (2–3 mm); 3 (>3 mm)

[c] Degree of obstruction scores: 0 (none); 1 (mild); 2 (partial); 3 (complete)

Table 24.10 Gaskins [20]: stages of surgical sinus disease

Stage 0: Score = 0	No surgical sinus disease
Stage I: Score < 1.3	
Site	Inflammation limited to the ostiomeatal complex area
Surgery	No prior sinus/nasal surgery except septoplasty and/or inferior meatal antrostomies
Polyps	No polyps or localised to < 10% of the sinus space
Infection	Well-controlled infection with no active mucopurulent drainage
Immunology	No underlying immunologic disease except well-controlled allergy
Stage II: Score + 1.2–2.3	
Site	Inflammation confined to the maxillary/ethmoid/ostiomeatal areas
Surgery	Prior Caldwell-Luc or polypectomy
Polyps	Polyp disease, with involvement of 10–50% of the nasal/sinus cavities
Infection	Persistent, localised infection with some active purulent drainage
Immunology	Low-grade immune disorder or fair allergy control
S tage III: Score 2.3–4.0	
Site	Pansinus involvement (unilateral or bilateral); isolated sphenoid disease
Surgery	Prior anterior ethmoidectomy/middle-turbinate surgery
Polyps	Nasal/sinus polyposis filling more than 50% of the nasal and sinus cavities
Infection	Poorly controlled multisinus infection with active muco-purulent drainage; active fungal sinusitis
Immunology	Poorly controlled allergic rhinitis or significant immune disorder; history of long-term steroid treatment
Stage IV: Score > 4.0	
Site	Sinus disease with extranasal/sinus extension, orbital or intracranial; frontal disease above the nasofrontal duct

Table 24.10 (*continued*)

Surgery	Prior complete ethmoidectomy or sphenoidectomy
Polyps	Inverting papilloma or other potentially malignant nasal/sinus neoplasms
Infection	Osteomyelitis or infection eroding into the orbit or cranium; mucormycosis
Immunology	End-stage immunologic disease; profoundly immunocompromised patient

Table 24.11 Lehman et al. [36]: endoscopic staging worksheet for revision cases. *OMC* Ostiomeatal complex

Section A: *Select the endoscopic classification (for the right and left sides separately), that best describes your patient's endoscopic examination*			
Points	**Endoscopic Findings**	**Right Side**	**Left Side**
0	**Normal mucosal membranes** *in all the opened sinuses: otherwise normal remnants of the OMC or sphenoethmoidal recess structures*		
1	**Mild edema** *of the anterior or posterior sinus cavities (or remnants of the OMC and sphenoethmoidal recess structure) with the other being normal*		
2	**Mild edema** *of the anterior and posterior sinus cavities (or remnants of the OMC and sphenoethmoidal recess structure)*		
3	**Marked edema or polypoid changes** *limited to the anterior or posterior sinus cavities (or remnants of the OMC and sphenoethmoidal recess structure)with the other being normal*		
4	**Marked edema or polypoid changes** *of the anterior and posterior sinus cavities cavities (or remnants of the OMC and sphenoethmoidal recess structure); or marked edema in one and mild edema in the other*		
5	**Frank polyps limited** *to the anterior or posterior sinus cavities (or remnants of the OMC and sphenoethmoidal recess structure), but not extending outside the confines of the cavities or meatal area*		
6	**Frank polyps limited** *to the anterior and posterior sinus cavities (or remnants of the OMC and sphenoethmoidal recess structure), but not extending outside the confines of the cavities or meatal area*		
7	**Frank polyps extending outside the limits** *of the anterior and/or posterior sinus cavities or OMC remnants, but not completely obstructing the nasal cavity; a visible airway is seen along the inferior nasal cavity; through which the nasopharynx can be examined*		
8	**Frank polyps completely obstructing** *the nasal cavity; no visible airway*		

Table 24.11 (*continued*)

Points	Endoscopic Findings	Right Side	Left Side
Section A: *Select the endoscopic classification (for the right and left sides separately), that best describes your patient's endoscopic examination*			
Section B: *Check off the endoscopic findings below (for the right and left side separately), if the patient has discolored mucus or allergic mucin*			
2	**Discolored mucus or allergic mucin**		
Total Score for sections A & B (Maximum of 20 points):			
Check the stage that matches the total points score above:			
– Stage I (Mild disease: 1–6)			
– Stage II (Moderate disease: 7–13)			
– Stage III (Severe disease: 14–20)			

not between CT score and quality of life (QoL) as measured with the Chronic Sinusitis Score [61].

Bhattacharyya compared three staging systems with the Rhinosinusitis Symptom Inventory [7] and found the Lund-MacKay score to correlate best with nasal scores, but the degree of correlation remained low.

It has been suggested that an attempt to quantify the percentage of the sinus occupied by inflammatory disease might improve its sensitivity [46], although it would not necessarily be easy to reproduce or indeed apply to the post-operative situation. The extent of sinus opacification is calculated from the sum of the scores of the five major sinuses (frontal, maxillary, anterior and posterior ethmoid, and sphenoid), each scored on a five-point opacification scale, where 0 = 0%; 1 = 1–25%; 2 = 26–50%; 3 = 51–75%; 4 = 76–99%; 5 = 100%. Alternatively, both CT [52] and magnetic resonance imaging (MRI) might be used to assess the volume of inflamed mucosa, but interpretation could be difficult due to the reproducibility of the scans, and in the case of MRI, the effect of the nasal cycle and the high incidence of incidental changes renders it oversensitive. As with CT, there is a similar lack of correlation between rhinological symptoms and MRI changes [44].

The University of Miami staging system, which includes CT and endoscopic assessment, has also been assessed by its creators for inter-rater reliability [36]. Inter-rater reliability for the CT and endoscopic arms were good for patients undergoing either primary or revision surgery. The correlation between endoscopic findings and CT staging was also high, again in both primary and revision cases.

In a study from Switzerland [21], the Kennedy CT Staging system I–III was used in 77 patients with CRS without polyps, and showed that the likelihood of revision was greatest in those with higher-staged disease.

Bhattacharyya has considered the role of the predictive value of symptoms and extent of disease on CT in both primary and revision endoscopic sinus surgery (ESS) for CRS [7, 8], again confirming that extent of disease using the Lund-MacKay, Kennedy or Harvard systems correlates poorly with symptoms either pre- or post-operatively. However, he was able to show that a scoring system such the Lund-MacKay could be applied to the revision patient, with similar scores before the primary and secondary procedure (10.5 vs. 9.7, $p = 0.38$) [5].

In a study considering clinical outcomes after revision ESS, the Lund-MacKay CT score confirmed the presence of disease (mean score 12.6) and allowed a comparison of results with patients undergoing primary surgery to be matched according to the extent of their inflammatory change on imaging [6]. Results were similar in this group of refractory CRS patients to that found in the primary population.

Other Methods of Assessment

A range of investigative tools have been applied to the CRS/NP patient, including measures of mucociliary clearance, olfaction and airway, but these are not universally available and may be subject to intra-individual variation. Consequently, these have generally not featured in most staging systems. However, an increasing number of studies have used validated questionnaires, considering QoL and quantification of symptoms. Kountakis and colleagues attempted a correlation of the level of tissue and systemic eosinophilia and degree of polymorphisms of the leukotriene C4 synthase gene with endoscopy, CT and a validated sinonasal questionnaire [35]. As expected, tissue eosinophilia was associated with polyps, asthma, allergy, and higher CT and symptom scores. Stratification was proposed, with those with polyps, tissue and blood eosinophilia representing the most severe, and those without these features being the least severe. It is probable that this would apply to patients irrespective of their surgical status, but has not been used widely in clinical practice.

General (generic) measurements such as the Medical Outcomes Study Short Form 36 [63] enable the comparison of patients suffering from CRS with other patient groups, but have not been used to any degree in the stratification of CRS, especially not in recurrent problems. In addition, there are several disease-specific questionnaires for CRS that may be more sensitive than general health status instruments, but again have not generally been utilised in staging the extent of disease [3, 4, 33, 51, 54].

Use of Staging in Outcome Research

Any attempt at staging, particularly after the anatomy has been distorted by previous surgery, is open to criticism. Both the endoscopic appearances and particularly the scan represent a snapshot at a particular moment and may be influenced by the medical treatment that patients receive. It is difficult enough to devise schemes to stage primary disease [18, 46] that few have grappled with the complexities of staging recurrent disease, although they may have considered studies to prevent disease recurrence in chronic disease.

Requirements of a staging system [45]:

1. Provide an objective means of quantifying the volume of inflammatory mucosa and opacification.
2. Be easy to use and require no formal training.
3. Have high reproducibility, as demonstrated by interobserver and intra-observer studies.
4. Be able to quantify the patency of the ostiomeatal passageways.

This does not mention a relationship to outcome, but also does not address the issue of revision surgery in recurrent disease.

Validated questionnaires that cover some health-related QoL aspects, such as the 20-item Sino-Nasal Outcome Test (SNOT-20 and SNOT-22) have been used in several studies to assess outcome, but have not been used specifically as part of a stratification or staging process, nor in general focused on a revision population [9, 27]. Nonetheless, this approach might reward further investigation, particularly in those patients likely to relapse (e.g. CRS+polyps), and the SNOT-20 is regarded as one of the most useful [47].

One of the few studies to consider staging instruments in revision ESS by McMains and Kountakis [43] utilised the Lund-MacKay CT score, endoscopic score, VAS and SNOT-20. CT scores in this group were similar to those seen in patients undergoing primary surgery (13.4±0.7), and the score served principally to quantify disease, whereas the other measures could be used to quantify outcome and confirmed overall improvement. Those patients with polyps, not surprisingly, constituted the majority of failures.

In a study by Smith et al. [57] concerning predictive factors in ESS for CRS, 119 patients with CRS and a mean follow-up of 1.4 years were evaluated prospectively. This group included patients who had undergone surgery. Contributory medical conditions, CT and endoscopy scores as well as QoL were considered. As usual, CT scores were worse in the presence of polyps, but interestingly the CT score was not affected by prior sinus surgery, whereas endoscopic scores were significantly worse. Nonetheless, these patients had the greatest improvement in endoscopy score, and CT scores approached significance in predicting worse outcome. However, other factors such as aspirin sensitivity and depression were associated with worse outcome, suggesting that this information needs to be factored into any staging in both primary and revision surgery.

If staging based on CT does not correlate well with symptoms, does it assist in determining other outcomes, such as complication rates? The Sino-Nasal Audit undertaken by the Royal College of Surgeons of England on 3128 consecutive patients undergoing all forms of sinonasal surgery for CRS ± NP confirmed by multivariate analysis that the complication rate was linked to extent of disease measured in terms of CT score (Lund-MacKay) as well as symptom severity, health-related QoL, extent of polyposis and the presence of co-morbidity, but interestingly not on extent of surgery. However, this group was a heterogeneous mix of those having primary and revision surgery [28].

Virtually all of the systems have been developed for an adult population, possibly recognising the changing development of the sinus system in the paediatric population and the high frequency of opacification due to common upper-respiratory-tract infections [15].

Staging for Neoplasia

Even in the area of neoplasia, staging in the nose and sinuses has proved problematic. A variety of systems has been devised for malignant tumours, but these systems are generally of less prognostic use than elsewhere in the head and neck. The nose and sinuses represent an area of great histological diversity, each with a unique natural history, which undermines the value of 5-year survival rates as malignant tumours can recur many years, even decades later. This combined with late presentation, the complexity of the anatomy and proximity to skull base and orbit means that most patients present with advanced local disease, but rather less often with dissemination, so staging is of much less relevance in determining prognosis. The standard systems such as TNM [23] are relatively crude and do not take into account the many different histopathologies; nor are they based on the findings of modern imaging and histology. Cantu et al. compared the 1997 and 2002 American Joint Committee on Cancer–Union Internationale Contre le Cancer systems and their own classification system, perhaps not surprisingly, finding their own to be superior [13].

There have been several attempts to classify according to extent (e.g. Kadish et al. [32], staging for olfactory neuroblastoma), but again these have been relatively crude. Histological classification based on degree of differentiation may be of some help in predicting prognosis (e.g. in adenocarcinoma). With the increasing use of endoscopic resection of skull-base tumours, this situation will need to be addressed, as not only can the origin of the tumour be more accurately determined, but the subtleties of dural and orbital periosteal invasion assessed. Unfortunately, a significant proportion of these patients will relapse and require revision surgery. To date, none of the staging systems have addressed this aspect.

There have been several studies based on large personal series that have considered some of the more common benign tumours, such as inverted papilloma and juvenile angiofibroma. Inverted papilloma is associated with a recurrence rate that varies in the literature from 0 to 75%. However, virtually all "recurrence" actually represents residual disease and requires further surgical intervention. Attempts at staging have utilised CT, MRI and endoscopic findings [12, 49, 55, 58] to stratify according to site of involvement, but as usual they focus on initial presentation and treatment rather than considering those with recurrence/residual papilloma.

Juvenile angiofibroma has been previously crudely staged using systems such as those of Chandler et al. [14] or Fisch [17] into stage I–III, which overlooked one of the most essential determinants of "recurrence", invasion of the basisphenoid. Since this issue has been fully realised through careful analysis of imaging studies and addressed surgically, the "recurrence" rate and need for revision surgery has dropped dramatically from ~25% to <2% [29].

Conclusion

Staging in inflammatory disease is helpful in confirming its presence and extent, corroborating the endoscopic findings and clinical diagnosis and serving as inclusion criteria and for case matching in clinical research. Few systems have considered the situation when recurrent disease is present or revision surgery contemplated. In contrast to neoplastic disease, conventional staging does not serve as a strong indicator of prognosis, as symptoms correlate poorly with extent of disease in both primary and recurrent CRS/nasal polyposis. Perhaps it is simply useful to confirm one's own prejudice and bias!

References

1. Annamalai S, Kumar NA, Madkour MB, et al. (2003) An association between acquired epiphora and the signs and symptoms of chronic rhinosinusitis: A prospective case-control study. Am J Rhinol 17:111–114
2. Ashraf N, Bhattacharyya N (2001) Determination of the "incidental" Lund score for the staging of chronic rhinosinusitis. Otolaryngol Head Neck Surg 125:483–486
3. Atlas SJ, Gallagher PM, Wu YA et al. (2005) Development and validation of a new health-related quality of life instrument for patients with sinusitis. Qual Life Res 14:1375–1386
4. Benninger MS, Senior BA (1997) The development of the Rhinosinusitis Disability Index. Arch Otolaryngol Head Neck Surg 123:1175–1179
5. Bhattacharrya N (1999) Computed tomographic staging and the fate of the dependent sinuses in revision endoscopic sinus surgery. Arch Otolaryngol Head Neck Surg 125: 994–999
6. Bhattacharyya N (2004) Clinical outcomes after revision endoscopic sinus surgery. Arch Otolaryngol Head Neck Surg 130:975–978
7. Bhattacharyya N (2005) A comparison of symptom scores and radiographic staging systems in chronic rhinosinusitis. Am J Rhinol 19:175–179
8. Bhattacharyya N (2006) Radiographic stage fails to predict symptom outcomes after endoscopic sinus surgery for chronic rhinosinusitis. Laryngoscope 116:18–22
9. Bradley DT, Kountakis SE (2005) Correlation between computed tomograph scores and symptomatic improvement after endoscopic sinus surgery. Laryngoscope 115:466–469

10. Browne JP, Hopkins C, Slack R, et al. (2006) Health-related quality of life after polypectomy with and without additional surgery. Laryngoscope 116:297–302
11. Caldwell GW (1893) Diseases of the accessory sinuses of the nose and an improved method of treatment of suppuration of the maxillary sinus. N Y Med J 58:526–528
12. Cannady SB, Baztra PS, Sautter NB, et al. (2007) New staging system for sinonasal inverted papilloma in the endoscopic era. Laryngoscope 117:1283–1287
13. Cantu G, Solero CL, Miceli R, et al. (2005) Which classification for ethmoid malignant tumors involving the anterior skull base? Head Neck 27:224–231
14. Chandler JR, Goulding R, Moskowitz L (1984) Nasopharyngeal angiofibromas: staging and managements. Ann Otol Rhinol Laryngol 93:322–329
15. Clement PA, Bijloos J, Kaufman L, et al. (1989) Incidence and etiology of rhinosinusitis in children. Acta Otorhinolaryngol Belg 43:523–543
16. Fokkens W, Lund VJ, Bachert C et al. European Academy of Allergology and Clinical Immunology (2005) European position paper on rhinosinusitis and nasal polyps. Rhinol Suppl 18:1–87
17. Fisch U (1983) The infratemporal fossa approach for nasopharyngeal tumours. Laryngoscope 93:36–44
18. Fokkens W, Lund VJ, Mullol J, et al. (2007) European position paper on rhinosinusitis and nasal polyps 2007. Rhinology Suppl 20:1–136
19. Friedman WH, Katsantonis GP, Bumpous JM (1995) Staging of chronic hyperplastic rhinosinusitis: treatment strategies. Otolaryngol Head Neck Surg 112:210–214
20. Gaskins RE (1992) A surgical staging system for chronic rhinosinusitis. Am J Rhinol 6:5–12
21. Giger R, Dulguerov P, Quinodoz D, et al. (2004) Chronic panrhinosinusitis without nasal polyps: long-term outcome after functional endoscopic sinus surgery. Otolaryngol Head Neck Surg 131:534–541
22. Gliklich R, Metson R (1994) A comparison of sinus computed tomography (CT) staging systems for outcomes research. Am J Rhinol 8:291–297
23. Greene FL, Compton CC, Fritz AG, Shah JP, Winchester DP (eds) (2006) American Joint Committee on Cancer: Cancer Staging Atlas. Springer, Berlin, Heidelberg, New York
24. Guerrero J, Molina B, Echeverría L, et al. (2007) Endoscopic sinonasal surgery: study of 110 patients with nasal polyposis and chronic rhinosinusitis. Acta Otorhinolaringol Esp 58:252–256
25. Hill M, Bhattacharyya N, Hall TR, et al. (2004) Incidental paranasal sinus imaging abnormalities and the normal Lund score in children. Otolaryngol Head Neck Surg 130:171–175
26. Holbrook EH, Brown CL, Lyden ER, et al. (2005) Lack of significant correlation between rhinosinusitis symptoms and specific regions of sinus computer tomography scans. Am J Rhinol 19:382–387
27. Hopkins C, Browne JP, Slack R, et al. (2006) The national comparative audit of surgery for nasal polyposis and chronic rhinosinusitis. Clin Otolaryngol 31:390–398
28. Hopkins C, Browne JP, Slack R, et al. (2006) Complications of surgery for nasal polyposis and chronic rhinosinusitis: the results of a national audit in England and Wales. Laryngoscope 116:1494–1499
29. Howard DJ, Lloyd G, Lund VJ (2001) Recurrence and its avoidance in juvenile angiofibroma. Laryngoscope 111:1509–1511
30. Johansson L, Akerlund A, Holmberg K, et al. (2000) Evaluation of methods for endoscopic staging of nasal polyposis. Acta Otolaryngol 120:72–76
31. Jorgensen RA (1991) Endoscopic and computed tomographic findings in ostiomeatal sinus disease. Arch Otolaryngol Head Neck Surg 117:279–287
32. Kadish S, Goodman M, Wang C (1976) Olfactory neuroblastoma: a clinical analysis of 17 cases. Cancer 37:1571–1576
33. Kay DJ, Rosenfeld RM (2003) Quality of life for children with persistent sinonasal symptoms. Otolaryngol Head Neck Surg 128:17–26
34. Kennedy DW (1992) Prognostic factors, outcomes and staging in ethmoid sinus surgery. Laryngoscope 57: 1–18
35. Kountakis SE, Arango P, Bradley D, et al. (2004) Molecular and cellular staging for the severity of chronic rhinosinusitis. Laryngoscope 114:1895–1905
36. Lehman DA, Casiano RR, Polak M (2006) Reliability of the University of Miami chronic rhinosinusitis staging system. Am J Rhinol 20:11–19
37. Levine H, May E (eds) (1993) Rhinology and Sinusology. Thieme, New York, p 261
38. Lildholdt T, Rundcrantz H, Lindqvist N (1995) Efficacy of topical corticosteroid powder for nasal polyps: a double-blind, placebo-controlled study of budesonide. Clin Otolaryngol 20:26–30
39. Lim M, Lew-Gor, S. Darby Y, et al. (2007) The relationship between subjective assessment instruments in chronic rhinosinusitis. Rhinology 45:144–147
40. Lloyd GA (1990) CT of the paranasal sinuses: study of a control series in relation to endoscopic sinus surgery. J Laryngol Otol 104:477–481
41. Lund VJ, Kennedy DW (1997) Staging for rhinosinusitis. Otolaryngol Head Neck Surg 117:S35–S40
42. Lund VJ, MacKay IS (1993) Staging in rhinosinusitis. Rhinology 31:183–184
43. McMains KC, Kountakis SE (2005) Revision functional endoscopic sinus surgery: objective and subjective surgical outcomes. Am J Rhinol 19:344–347

44. McNeill E, O'Hara J, Carrie S (2006) The significance of MRI findings for non-rhinological disease. Clin Otolaryngol 31:292–296; discussion 296
45. Meltzer EO, Hamilos D, Hadley JA, et al. (2004) Rhinosinusitis: establishing definitions for clinical research and patient care. Otolaryngol Head Neck Surg 131:S1–S62
46. Meltzer EO, Hamilos DL, Hadley JA, et al. (2006) Rhinosinusitis: developing guidance for clinical trials. Otolaryngol Head Neck Surg 135:S31–S80
47. Morley AD, Sharp HR (2006) A review of sinonasal outcome scoring systems – Which is best? Clin Otolaryngol 31:103–109
48. Newman LJ, Platts-Mills TAE, Phillips DC, et al. (1994) Chronic sinusitis relationship of computed tomographic findings to allergy, asthma and eosinophilia. JAMA 271:363–367
49. Oikawa K, Furuta Y, Oridate N (2003) Pre-operative staging of sinonasal inverted papilloma by magnetic resonance imaging. Laryngoscope 113:1983–1987
50. Oluwole M, Russell N, Tan L, et al. (1996) A comparison of computerized tomographic staging systems in chronic sinusitis. Clin Otolaryngol Allied Sci 21:91–95
51. Piccirillo JF, Merritt MG Jr, Richards ML (2002) Psychometric and clinimetric validity of the 20-Item Sino-Nasal Outcome Test (SNOT-20). Otolaryngol Head Neck Surg 126:41–47
52. Ponikau JU, Sherris DA, Weaver A, et al. (2005) Treatment of chronic rhinosinusitis with intranasal amphotericin B: a randomised, placebo-controlled, double-blinded pilot trial. J Allergy Clin Immunol 115:125–131
53. Report of the Rhinosinusitis Task Force Committee Meeting (1997) Alexandria, Virginia, August 17, 1996. Otolaryngol Head Neck Surg 117:S1–S68
54. Revicki DA, Leidy NK, Brennan-Diemer F, et al. (1998) Development and preliminary validation of the multiattribute Rhinitis Symptom Utility Index. Qual Life Res 7:693–702
55. Savy L, Lloyd G, Lund VJ, Howard DH (2000) Optimum imaging and diagnosis for inverted papilloma. J Laryngol Otol 114:891–893
56. Smith TL, Batra PS, Seiden AM, Hanley M (2005) Evidence supporting endoscopic sinus surgery in the management of adult chronic rhinosinusitis: A systematic review. Am J Rhinol 19:537–543
57. Smith TL, Mendolia-Loffredo S, Loehrl TA, et al. (2005) Predictive factors and outcomes in endoscopic sinus surgery for chronic rhinosinusitis. Laryngoscope 115:2199–2205
58. Stamm AC (2000) Surgical grading system for inverted papillomas. In: Stamm AC, Draf W (eds) Micro-endoscopic Surgery of the Paranasal Sinuses and the Skull Base. Springer, Berlin, Heidelberg, New York, pp 147–152
59. Stewart MG, Sicard MW, Piccirillo J, et al. (1999) Severity staging in chronic sinusitis: are CT scans findings related to patient symptoms. Am J Rhinol 13:161–167
60. Toros SZ, Bölükbasi S, Naiboğlu B, et al. (2004) Comparative outcomes of endoscopic sinus surgery in patients with chronic rhinosinusitis and nasal polyps. Laryngoscope 114:1895–905
61. Wabnitz DAM, Nair S, Wormald PJ (2005) Correlation between preoperative symptom scores, quality-of-life questionnaires, and staging with computed tomography in patients with chronic rhinosinusitis. Am J Rhinol 19:91–96
62. Walker FD, White PS (2000) Sinus symptom scores: what is the range in healthy individuals. Clin Otolaryngol 25:482–484
63. Ware JE Jr, Sherbourne CD (1992) The MOS 36-item short-form health survey (SF-36) I. Conceptual framework and item selection. Med Care 30:473–483

Chapter 25

Headache and the Patient who Failed Primary Sinus Surgery

25

William H. Moretz III and Stilianos E. Kountakis

Core Messages

- Headache is a common symptom in patients diagnosed with chronic rhinosinusitis.
- The diagnosis of primary and secondary headache disorders is important to avoid unnecessary revision surgery.
- Headache symptoms attributable to persistent or recurrent rhinologic disease may be addressed surgically if medical therapy has failed.
- Headache symptoms secondary to rhinologic disease have shown significant improvement following endoscopic sinus surgery.

Contents

Introduction

Headache is a common symptom in patients diagnosed with chronic rhinosinusitis (CRS), being present in up to 83% of patients [1]. The severity of headaches has been reported to be one of the highest among the most common symptoms associated with CRS [2]. Persistent headache symptoms after primary functional endoscopic sinus surgery (FESS) for CRS may create an unhappy patient and a frustrated physician. An appropriate understanding of the differential diagnoses of headache is important for treating patients presenting to a rhinology practice.

In 1997, the American Academy of Otolaryngology – Head and Neck Surgery Rhinosinusitis Task Force published recommendations for symptom-based criteria for the accurate diagnosis of CRS [8, 20]. Headache is considered a minor diagnostic symptom using these criteria.

- The Rhinosinusitis Task Force suggests that headache alone should not constitute a suggestive history for rhinosinusitis without major nasal symptoms or signs.

The Rhinosinusitis Initiative, consisting of five national societies, created a guideline for evidence-based research of rhinosinusitis in 2004 [11]. This guideline included headache as a relevant symptom of CRS and recommended its severity documentation for treatment assessment. Accordingly, the Rhinosinusitis Initiative has recommended including headache as one of the 11 symptoms scored for efficacy assessment in clinical trials studying CRS [11,12].

The treatment of headache associated with CRS is challenging, as its underlying cause is unknown and its severity associated with multiple factors. Concomitant headache, inappropriately associated with CRS, will not improve following FESS. As such, a rhinologist should rely on a comprehensive history and physical examination, along with objective endoscopic and radiologic findings, to ensure appropriate headache management.

Differential Diagnosis

Understanding nonrhinologic headache is important, as patients may be referred to otolaryngologists for presumed rhinosinusitis without subjective or objective findings to support the diagnosis.

- Primary headache disorders include:
  1. Migraine.
  2. Tension-type headache.
  3. Cluster headaches.
  4. Other less common entities, including primary thunderclap headache and hemicrania continua.

Secondary headache disorders are associated with underlying central nervous system pathology [6,15].

Primary Headache Disorders

Migraine Headaches

Migraine headaches are common and underdiagnosed [9]. Approximately 28 million Americans are affected, with the 1-year prevalence of 18% in women and 6% in men [9, 24]. Migraine is an episodic neurovascular headache disorder involving moderate to severe attacks lasting 4–72 h, with a pulsating quality [6].

- Migraine headaches are:
  1. Usually associated with nausea.
  2. Associated with sensitivity to light, sound, or movement.
  3. Often unilateral.
  4. With pain described over the frontal and temporal regions.
  5. Pain can also be described in the parietal, occipital, and high cervical regions [5].

The pathogenesis of pain in migraine is not completely understood; however, it is thought to be a neurovascular disorder resulting in nerve activation from vascular dilation. The diagnostic criteria defined by the International Headache Society (IHS) in 2004 are presented in Table 25.1 [6].

Migraine headaches are divided into two major subtypes, migraine with and without aura. Aura is defined as a reversible focal neurological symptom that usually develops gradually over 5–20 min and lasts for less than 60 min [6]. The aura occurs at the onset or just prior to a migraine headache. Auras may include visual symptoms, including flickering lights, sensory symptoms, which may involve numbness or sensation of pins and needles, or dysphasic speech disturbance.

A recent analysis by Perry et al. [17] was performed on patients with headaches presenting to a tertiary rhinology practice without evidence of rhinosinusitis on CT or endoscopic evaluation.

- The majority of patients with headache as a chief complaint were diagnosed with migraine upon further evaluation by a neurologist [17].

Other studies have shown similar findings in patients seeking treatment for "sinus headaches." Schreiber et al. reported that 80% of 2991 patients with "sinus headaches" presenting to primary care physicians fulfilled IHS migraine criteria [21].

Tension-Type Headaches

- Tension-type headaches are the most common type of primary headache, affecting up to 78% of the general population [6].

The etiology of tension-type headaches is unknown. Subtypes of tension-type headache have been described, dividing the headaches into episodic or chronic, and with or without pericranial tenderness on manual palpation. Pericranial tenderness is a distinguishing characteristic of tension-type headaches, but does not necessarily need to be present for its diagnosis.

Diagnostic criteria for episodic tension-type headaches have been outlined by the IHS. Episodic tension-type headaches last from 30 min to 7 days, are usually bilateral, and have a pressing/tightening quality. These headaches occur for at least 3 months, averaging less than 15 days out of the month, and are not aggravated by routine physical activity. Chronic tension-type headaches typically last hours or may be continuous, occur for at least 3 months, averaging 15 or more days per month, and have the same characteristics of episodic tension-type headaches [6].

- Perry et al. [17] found that 6% of patients with nonrhinologic headache presenting to their rhinology practice with a chief complaint of headache were diagnosed with tension-type headache upon subsequent evaluation by a neurologist.

Cluster Headaches

The IHS describes the cluster headache as a severe, unilateral pain located at the orbital, supraorbital, or temporal areas, lasting 15–180 min and occurring from once every other day to eight times a day. Cluster headaches typically

Table 25.1 Revised International Headache Society criteria for chronic migraine

Grade	Criteria
A	Headache (tension-type and/or migraine) on ≥15 days/month for at least 3 months
B	Occurring in a patient who has had at least five attacks, fulfilling criteria for 1.1 migraine without aura
C	On ≥8 days/month for at least 3 months headache has fulfilled C1 and/or C2 below, that is, has fulfilled the criteria for pain and associated symptoms of migraine without aura: 1. Has at least two of a–d: a. Unilateral location; b. Pulsating quality; c. Moderate or severe pain intensity; d. Aggravation by or causing avoidance of routine physical activity (e.g. walking or climbing stairs) and at least one of i or ii: i. nausea and/or vomiting ii. photophobia and phonophobia 2. Treated and relieved by triptan(s) or ergot before the expected development of C1 above.
D	No medication overuse and not attributed to another causative disorder

occur together, lasting for weeks or months, and are separated by remission periods lasting months or years.

- Cluster headache attacks are associated with:
  1. Ipsilateral nasal congestion.
  2. Rhinorrhea.
  3. Facial sweating.
  4. Conjunctival injection.
  5. Lacrimation.
  6. Miosis.
  7. Eyelid ptosis.
  8. Eyelid edema.

A sense of restlessness and agitation has been reported by patients during cluster headaches, and episodes of cluster headaches may be provoked by alcohol, histamine, or nitroglycerine. Cluster headaches show autosomal dominant inheritance in 5% of cases and are most common in adults aged 20–40 years, with prevalence rates 3–4 times higher in men than women [6].

Other Primary Headaches

Hemicrania continua describes headaches that are strictly unilateral and last for over 3 months. These headaches occur daily and are unremitting without treatment. Ipsilateral conjunctival injection, lacrimation, nasal congestion, rhinorrhea, ptosis, or miosis are associated with hemicrania continua. Complete response is achieved with indomethacin.

Thunderclap headache is a high-intensity headache of acute onset, reaching maximum intensity in less than 1 min and lasting from 1 h to 10 days. Thunderclap headache is a diagnosis of exclusion after appropriate work-up is performed to rule out intracranial disorders, such as subarachnoid hemorrhage, arterial dissection, and pituitary apoplexy.

Primary stabbing headache, cough headache, exertional headache, headache associated with sexual activity, and hypnic headache have also been described in the IHS classification system of primary headache disorders.

Secondary Headache Disorders

Headaches caused by underlying central nervous system pathology are considered secondary.

- Eight categories of secondary headaches are classified in the IHS system and include those attributed to [6]:
  1. Head and neck trauma.
  2. Cranial or cervical vascular disorder.
  3. Nonvascular intracranial disorder.
  4. Substance abuse or its withdrawal.
  5. Infection.
  6. Disorder of homeostasis.
  7. Disorder of a facial or cranial structure.
  8. Psychiatric disorder.

Headaches attributed to rhinosinusitis are considered secondary headaches by IHS classification, defined as pain in one or more regions of the face, developing simultaneously with the onset or acute exacerbation of rhinosinusitis, and resolving within 7 days of successful treatment [6].

- Life-threatening pathology presenting with headache should always be considered and include intracranial hemorrhage, cerebral infarction, meningitis, and intracranial neoplasm.

Approximately 50% of patients with brain tumors report headache as their primary complaint. A tumor could be suspected if the headache is associated with confusion, seizures, or neurologic deficit. Other findings that raise the possibility of an intracranial mass lesion include a progressive nature of headache, new onset in adult life (>40 years), a change in headache pattern, or a worsening of headache with changes in posture or Valsalva maneuver [18]. Fortunately, headache alone is a rare presentation of an intracranial neoplasm.

Rhinologic Headache

Although headache does not generally suggest rhinosinusitis in the absence of other symptoms, it may present as the sole symptom with signs of rhinosinusitis.

- Anatomic abnormalities associated with rhinologic headache include:
  1. Nasal septal deviation.
  2. Concha bullosa.
  3. Paradoxical middle turbinate.
  4. Large ethmoid bulla.
  5. Prominent agger nasi cells.

Nasal endoscopy and computerized tomography (CT) evaluation accurately identify anatomic abnormalities in the nasal cavities (Figs. 25.1 and 25.2). Success rates for endoscopic sinus surgery have been reported as high as 83% for patients with anatomic abnormalities and a primary symptom of headache [3]. In a separate study of prospectively collected data on 201 patients with CRS, a 91.9% improvement in headache severity was shown after primary FESS [13]. This improvement in headache severity is consistent with other studies of CRS patients undergoing FESS [16, 22].

Theories suggest that mucosal contact between these areas result in the release of substance P. Substance P is a neuropeptide found in high concentrations within the sensory nerve endings of the nasal mucosa and has been proposed to play a prominent role in pain transmission [4, 23]. The orthodromic impulse from intranasal stimuli does not localize well to higher cortical centers, resulting in referred pain to sites in the distribution of the ophthalmic and maxillary divisions of the trigeminal nerve. An antidromic impulse results in the release of substance P at the nasal mucosa, causing mast cell degranulation, neurogenic edema, and hypersecretion, resulting in other common symptoms associated with CRS [4, 23].

Revision Endoscopic Sinus Surgery

Revision endoscopic sinus surgery (RESS) is thought to have a lower success rate than primary FESS because

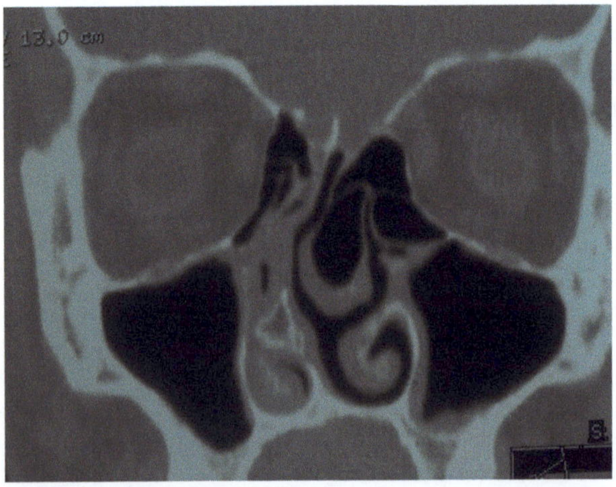

Fig. 25.1 Coronal sinus computed tomography scan showing significant septal deviation with a septal spur pushing against the right lateral nasal wall

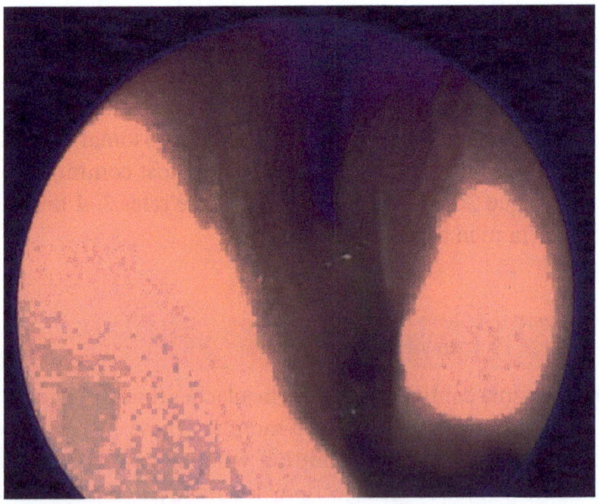

Fig. 25.2 Endoscopic picture of a septal spur "stabbing" the left inferior turbinate

of the associated recurrent rhinologic disease states including nasal polyposis and allergic fungal rhinossinusitis, as well as challenges inherent to distorted anatomic landmarks. Success rates for RESS have been reported at between 50 and 93.6% [7, 10, 14], with several studies showing significant improvement in symptom scores following RESS.

The initial evaluation of a patient with persistent symptoms following primary FESS should include a detailed history of symptoms, including those prior to the primary surgery. If possible, the initial CT should be evaluated as well as the documented endoscopy findings to identify evidence of disease. Persistent headache symptoms with relatively normal CT and endoscopy prior to initial FESS should raise suspicion that headache symptoms may not be associated with CRS. Proceeding with RESS to treat persistent headaches in this scenario is not recommended.

Patients referred to a rhinologist with "sinus headaches" following primary FESS should be carefully evaluated for concurrent headache disorders. Pynnonen and Terrell [19] evaluated 186 consecutive patients presenting to a tertiary care rhinology clinic for the evaluation of CRS-like symptoms; 40% of these patients had no evidence of CRS. In this group, 19% were subsequently diagnosed with head or facial pain, including tension headache, migraine headache, and temporomandibular dysfunction [19]. Careful evaluation of headache symptoms can prevent unnecessary revision surgery.

Summary

The evaluation of patients with headache symptoms following FESS should include a detailed history of headache-specific symptoms as well as an analysis of objective findings prior to surgery. The diagnosis of primary and secondary headache disorders in these patients is important to avoid unnecessary surgery. Several effective medical treatment regimens exist for headache disorders. Accordingly, evaluation and treatment by a headache specialist is appropriate for these complicated, and often unhappy, patients. Headache symptoms attributable to persistent or recurrent rhinologic disease may be addressed surgically if medical therapy has failed. Headache symptoms secondary to rhinologic disease have shown significant improvement following endoscopic sinus surgery.

References

1. Bhattacharyya N (2003) The economic burden and symptom manifestations of chronic rhinosinusitis: symptoms and surgical outcomes. Laryngoscope 144:1932–1935
2. Bhattacharyya N (2006) Clinical and symptom criteria for the accurate diagnosis of chronic rhinosinusitis. Laryngoscope 116:1–22
3. Chow JM (1994) Rhinologic headaches. Otolaryngol Head Neck Surg 111:211–218
4. Clerico DM (1995) Sinus headaches reconsidered: referred cephalgia of rhinologic origin masquerading as refractory primary headaches. Headache 35:185–192
5. Goadsby PJ, Lipton RB, Ferrari MD (2002) Migraine–current understanding and treatment. N Engl J Med 346:257–270
6. Headache Classification Committee, et al. (2006) New appendix criteria open for a broader concept of chronic migraine. Cephalalgia 26:742–746
7. Jiang RS, Hsu CY (2002) Revision functional endoscopic sinus surgery. Ann Otol Rhinol Laryngol 111:155–159
8. Lanza DC, Kennedy DW (1997) Adult rhinosinusitis defined. Otolaryngol Head Neck Surg 117:S1–S7
9. Lipton RB, Diamond S, Reed M, Diamond ML, Stewart WF (2001) Migraine diagnosis and treatment: results from the American Migraine Study II. Headache 41:638–645
10. McMains KC, Kountakis SE (2005) Revision endoscopic sinus surgery: objective and subjective surgical outcomes. Am J Rhinol 19:344–347
11. Meltzer EO, Hamilos DL, Hadley JA, et al. (2004) Rhinosinusitis: establishing definitions for clinical research and patient care. Otolaryngol Head Neck Surg 131:S1–S62
12. Meltzer EO, Hamilos DL, Hadley JA, et al. (2006) Rhinosinusitis: developing guidance for clinical trials. Otolaryngol Head Neck Surg 135:S31–S80
13. Moretz WM, Kountakis SE (2006) Subjective headaches before and after endoscopic sinus surgery. Am J Rhinol 20:305–307
14. Moses RL, Cornetta A, Atkins JP Jr, et al. (1998) Revision endoscopic sinus surgery: the Thomas Jefferson University experience. Ear Nose Throat J 77:190–202
15. Olesen J (2005) The International Classification of Headache Disorders, 2nd edition: application to practice. Funct Neurol 20:61–68
16. Parsons DS, Batra PS (1998) Functional endoscopic sinus surgical outcomes for contact point headaches. Laryngoscope 108:696–702
17. Perry BF, Login IS, Kountakis SE (2004) Nonrhinologic headache in a tertiary rhinology practice. Otolaryngol Head Neck Surg 130:449–452
18. Purdy RA (2001) Clinical evaluation of a patient presenting with headache. Med Clin North Am 85:847–863
19. Pynnonen MA, Terrell JE (2006) Conditions that masquerade as chronic rhinosinusitis. Arch Otolaryngol Head Neck Surg 132:748–751
20. Rhinosinusitis Task Force Committee (1997) Report of the Rhinosinusitis Task Force Committee Meeting. Alexandria, Virginia, August 17, 1996. Otolaryngol Head Neck Surg 117:S1–S68

21. Schreiber CP, Hutchinson S, Webster CJ, et al. (2004) Prevalence of migraine in patients with a history of self-reported or physician-diagnosed "sinus" headache. Arch Intern Med 164:1769–1772
22. Senior BA, Kennedy DW, Tanabodee J, et al. (1998) Long-term results of functional endoscopic sinus surgery. Laryngoscope 108:151–157
23. Stammberger H, Wolf G (1988) Headaches and sinus disease: the endoscopic approach. Ann Otol Rhinol Laryngol 97:3–23
24. Stewart WF, Lipton RB, Celentano DD, Reed ML (1992) Prevalence of migraine headache in the United States: relation to age, income, race, and other sociodemographic factors. JAMA 267:64–69

Chapter 26

Complications in Revision Sinus Surgery: Presentation and Management

26

John Scianna and James Stankiewicz

Core Messages

- Revision surgery holds the same potential hazards and complications as primary sinus surgery.
- Revision surgery offers additional difficulties in that landmarks may be obscured and natural barriers dehiscent.
- Orbital musculature injury, acute orbital hemorrhage, delayed orbital hemorrhage, blindness, carotid injury, and cerebrospinal fluid leak are potential complications.
- Prevention remains the best treatment; however, early recognition of a complication, appropriate intra- and postoperative management, and consultation with colleagues can minimize the adverse outcomes associated with a complication.

Contents

Introduction

"The time to worry is before you place your bet, not after they spin the wheel."

Lou Holtz [7]

- As Coach Holtz so correctly stated, concerns regarding complications should be considered and understood well before they ever happen.

Sinus surgery is fraught with potential significant complications including orbital injury, acute/delayed orbital hemorrhage, optic nerve injury, cerebral spinal fluid (CSF) leak, carotid injury, and skull-base penetration [16]. Many of these complications can have catastrophic adverse effects including blindness, double vision, stroke, coma, and even death [14].

Avoiding these potential adverse outcomes requires knowledge of the significant and intricate anatomy of the paranasal sinuses. This intricate anatomy generally provides the surgeon with essential landmarks; in revision sinus surgery, however, this is not the case [31]. The loss of the virginity of the nasal anatomy associated with primary sinus surgery can significantly complicate revision sinus surgery [9]. In understanding that the expected may be absent, and more importantly that the unexpected may be present, the revision sinus surgeon can navigate safely within the nose [17].

Despite the greatest of understanding, consideration, and expertise, complications will still occur [30].

- An outline to limiting the adversity of a complication:
  1. Prompt recognition.
  2. Acute management.
  3. Appropriate follow up and consultation.

With this outline to the management of complications, the sinus surgeon is better prepared to successfully perform revision sinus surgery.

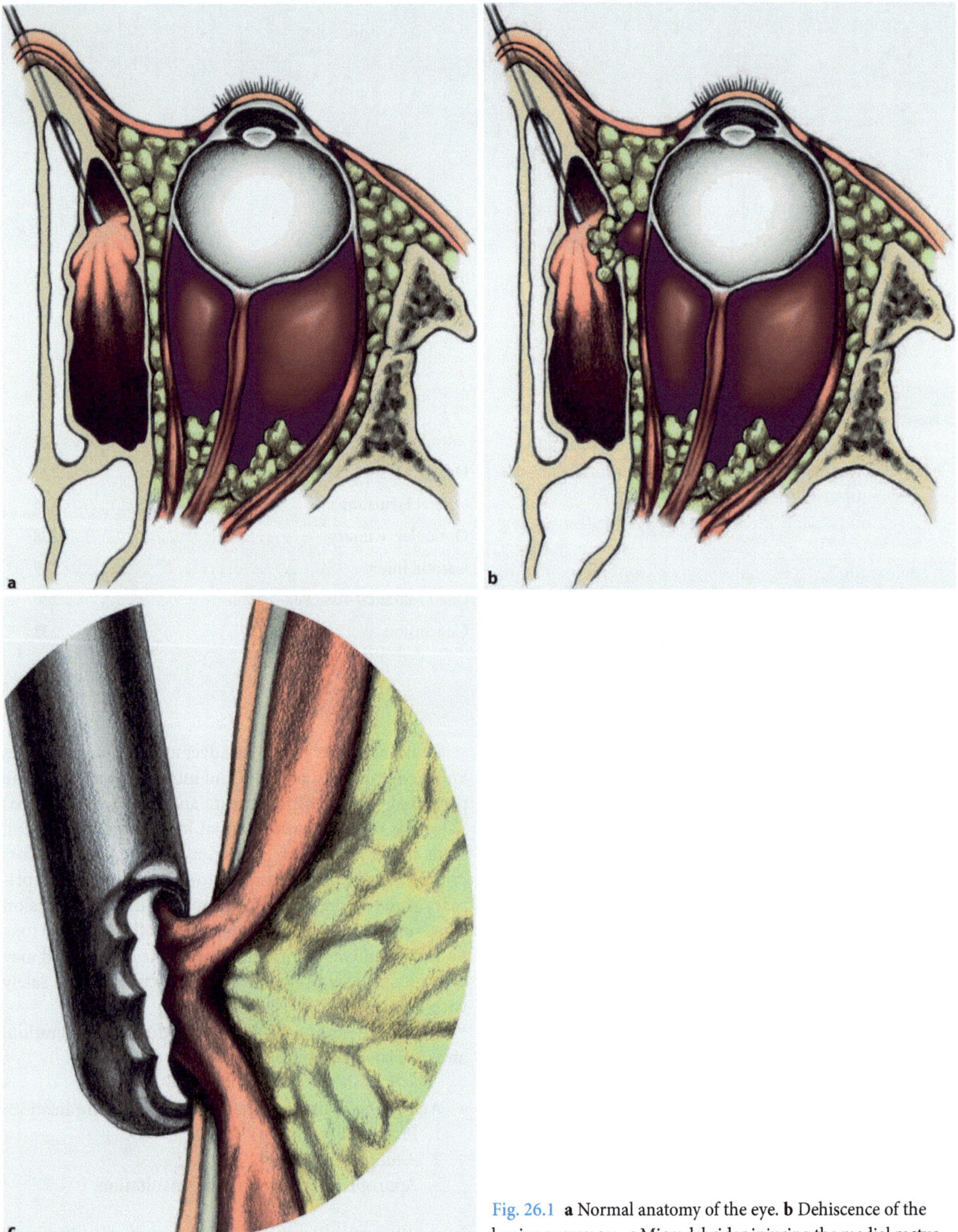

Fig. 26.1 **a** Normal anatomy of the eye. **b** Dehiscence of the lamina papyracea. **c** Microdebrider injuring the medial rectus

Orbital Musculature Injury

- To limit the risk of orbital complications:
  1. Evaluate the integrity of the lamina papyracea.
  2. Frequently palpate the orbit and keep it visible in the surgical field.
  3. Keep powered instrumentation pointed away from the lamina.

The anatomic division between the orbital contents and the paranasal sinuses inherently puts the orbit, and more specifically the orbital musculature, at risk of injury [11]. The lamina papyracea, so named for its "paper thin" character, is the only bony barrier between the medial orbital musculature and the nose. While the periorbita, a fibrous sheath, encases the orbital fat and musculature, it provides little protection in the face of powered instrumentation. In cases of revision sinus surgery, in particular, preexisting dehiscence of the lamina papyracea and/or preexisting damage to the periorbita places the patient at potentially increased risk to have inadvertent damage to the orbital contents, specifically the medial rectus (Fig. 26.1) [21].

Damage to the medial rectus and orbital contents when performing endoscopic sinus surgery can generally occur in one of two ways. First of all, when attempting to remove any residual uncinate process, the lamina papyracea and the periorbita can be violated. In revision cases, the unresected uncinate process can be adherent or scarred to the lateral nasal wall/lamina papyracea. When attempting to remove this process with a back-biting forceps, it is feasible to inadvertently puncture the lamina papyracea and tear the periorbita. If orbital dehiscence is unrecognized at the time of occurrence, the introduction of powered debriders can result in suction of orbital fat and muscle through this dehiscence/puncture and result in injury to the medial rectus. This exact scenario is what can also happen when unrecognized dehiscence in any area of the lamina papyracea is preexisting in revision cases [23].

Prevention of such an injury is accomplished primarily with careful preoperative review of the available imaging and intraoperative inspection and palpation [27]. Preoperative examination of the coronal and axial images of the sinuses, specifically with a bone window available, can alert the surgeon to a possible lateralized uncinate or a dehiscence. Intraoperative examination and palpation of the orbit while examining the lateral nasal wall (the so-called Stankiewicz maneuver or orbital press test) can further demonstrate a potential hazard (Fig. 26.2) [29]. In addition, the endoscopic sinus surgeon should be well versed in the yellow appearance of orbital fat and how this differs from typical sinonasal pathology and tissue. Prior to performing an uncinectomy, a Lusk probe or other blunt, beaded probe can be use to palpate the edge of the uncinate process and can peal the uncinate away from the medial orbital wall. Finally, when performing an uncinectomy with a back-biting forceps, maintaining the forceps at an acute angle (Fig. 26.3) will avoid spearing of the fully opened instrument through the lamina and into the periorbita. If using a sickle knife or elevator to incise the uncinate process, especially in a revision case, close observation for orbital fat prolapse is necessary.

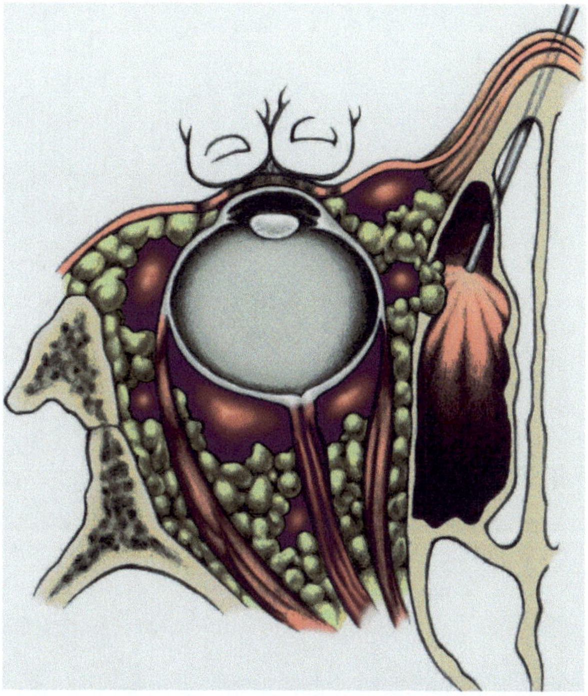

Fig. 26.2 Orbital press test (Stankiewicz maneuver)

If the lamina papyracea or the periorbita is injured, immediate recognition will aid in preventing a more significant injury to the medial rectus. Again, the orbital press test can aid in demonstrating a dehiscence [29]. Avoidance of the use of a microdebrider around this area may help in preventing the suction of orbital contents into the debrider blade and the resultant damage. Without question, in cases of dehiscence the debrider window should be turned upward or away from the orbit [5]. Proper prepping and draping of a patient, with exposure of the eyes, and with the eyelids taped along the lateral canthus allows for the scrub assistant to notice any unusual bruising or, of greater concern, movement of the eye during surgery. The use of a properly registered computer image guidance probe may also be useful in identifying an area of dehiscence or damage [24]. If, however, the medial rectus is inadvertently damaged or severed, consultation with an ophthalmologist, or more specifically, an oculoplastic surgeon, is appropriate. Immediate repair or delayed repair of the injury by suturing the cut ends of the muscle have been described with mixed results [8].

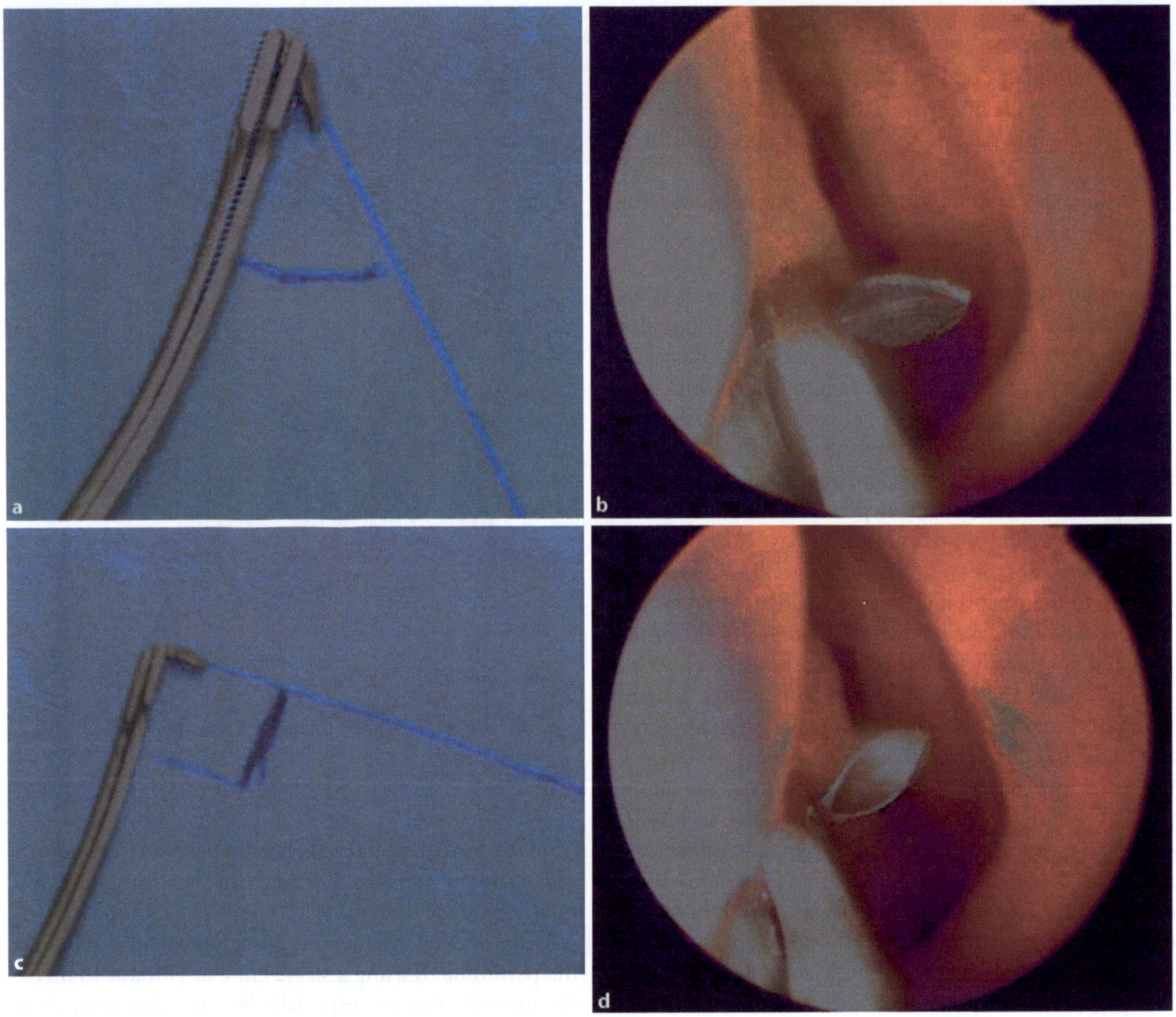

Fig. 26.3 **a** Microdebrider at the correct acute angle. **b** Endoscopic view of the correct angle. **c** Microdebrider at an incorrect 90 angle. **d** Endoscopic view of the incorrect angle

When such an injury occurs, it is important that the appropriate colleagues are consulted for postoperative observation and follow up. Proper and complete documentation is important. Involvement of tertiary care centers and "experts" in the field may prove beneficial to patient outcome. Observation of the patient overnight in a setting where vision and the eye can be routinely assessed should also be considered, as any damage to the orbital contents can result in an orbital hematoma.

Orbital Hematoma

- For the management of orbital hematoma:

1. Understand that arterial and venous orbital bleeding differ significantly in presentation and treatment.
2. Always be prepared to perform a lateral canthotomy.

Two separate categories of orbital hematoma exist: immediate and delayed. As described above, the proximity of the orbital anatomy and the sparse separation of the orbital contents from the paranasal sinuses puts the orbit at risk. Penetration and damage to the existing barrier to the orbit has been described. An acute or delayed hemorrhage and resultant orbital hematoma can ultimately result in blindness [29].

A delayed or slow-forming orbital hematoma can occur when there has been damage to the periorbita and orbital fat. The orbital fat has a significant venous blood supply, and a slow bleeder within the orbital cone may result in the slow formation of a hematoma. While generally less catastrophic than an unrecognized/untreated acute orbital hematoma, a significant rise in ocular pressure can occur with as little as 5 ml of blood in the orbit and may ultimately result in compromise of the retinal blood supply and blindness [35].

As will be repeated many times, early recognition of damage to the lamina papyracea and periorbita will alert the surgeon to a potential complication. Early periocular bruising can also alert the surgeon to a possibility of a slowly forming hematoma. In the face of either of these circumstances, nasal packing should be used sparingly, as heavy packing can block an intranasal evacuation path that the bleeding can follow. Palpation of the orbit may demonstrate increased ocular pressure. If high ocular pressure is a concern, then an ophthalmology consult is appropriate. Gentle external palpation of the orbit may also result in evacuation of the formed hematoma into the nasal cavity. If hematoma formation is noted intraoperatively, one can consider a medial orbital decompression via endoscopic or external approaches. In this procedure the remainder of the lamina papyracea is removed endoscopically and the periorbita is incised using a sickle knife. This procedure allows for an adequate drainage path of blood into the nasal cavity and can prevent increasing intraocular pressure. It is generally not advisable to cauterize within the orbital contents as this can result in heat damage to the musculature and unwanted scarring [20].

Acute orbital hematoma, as opposed to a delayed hematoma, has a separate mechanism of action. Acute orbital hematoma is the result of an arterial bleed within an intact orbital cone. The anterior ethmoid artery is most often to blame in the cases of such an occurrence. The anterior ethmoid artery is an end artery of the internal carotid system as opposed to the majority of the nasal blood supply, which is derived from the external carotid system. The anterior and posterior ethmoid arteries represent branches of the ophthalmic artery, a direct branch of the internal carotid artery (ICA). As the ophthalmic artery courses medial to the medial rectus muscle, branches extending through the periorbita enter into the superiormost aspect of the ethmoidal sinuses.

It is this lateral-to-medial course of the anterior ethmoid artery that potentiates its role as the cause of an acute orbital hematoma. Occasionally dehiscent as it passes through the ethmoids and to its ultimate branching to the dura, intranasal damage can result in retraction of the severed artery into the boney orbital cone and/or deep to the periorbita. Here, unopposed arterial bleeding will result in the rapid formation of an orbital hematoma, acutely and greatly increasing intraocular pressures. Left unattended, the retinal arterial supply and venous drainage will be compromised, ultimately resulting in blindness in a relatively short period of time (< 90 min) [4].

Preventing such a complication starts with reviewing the coronal sinus imaging preoperatively. Generally, the anterior ethmoid artery peak or "nipple" can be identified on coronal computed tomography imaging (Fig. 26.4) [18]. Recognizing this area and determining if a possible dehiscence of the anterior ethmoid artery exists, can signal the sinus surgeon to use considerable care when performing an anterior ethmoidectomy. In addition to recognizing this preexisting anatomic potential, proper prepping and draping of the patient should allow for visualization and palpation of the orbit during surgery. It is a good habit to routinely palpate the orbit of the patient at the start of the case, occasionally throughout the case, and at the termination of the procedure prior to extubation. This allows for routine assessment of a potential orbital hematoma.

In the face of a high-pressure orbital hematoma, immediate reaction is required [19]. As mentioned, high intraocular pressures can quickly be reached resulting in retinal ischemia. Two immediate options exist: lateral

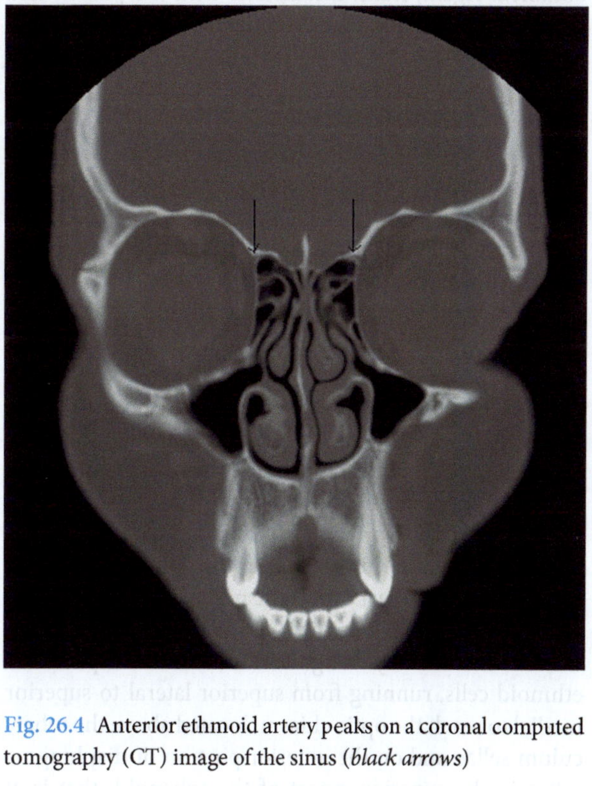

Fig. 26.4 Anterior ethmoid artery peaks on a coronal computed tomography (CT) image of the sinus (*black arrows*)

canthotomy and medial orbital decompression. The technique of medial orbital decompression has been described previously and can allow for adequate drainage and decompression of the orbit [20]. While a medial decompression can be challenging for some, it does offer an excellent, nonexternal alternative to a lateral canthotomy. All sinus surgeons should be capable of performing a lateral canthotomy. This simple, external procedure decreases intraocular pressures and can significantly decompress the orbit. A lateral canthotomy requires two instruments, a hemostat, and curved Metzenbaum or Mayo scissors. Initially the hemostat is place in the lateral canthus and extended until the boney orbital rim is felt. The hemostat is then used to crush the blood supply to the lateral canthus. After this is accomplished, the scissors are used to make a cut from the lateral canthus to the boney rim, directed laterally. The scissors are then angled inferiorly and used to cut the lateral attachment of the periorbita [19]. If this fails to relieve high pressures within the eye, then medial orbital decompression should be pursued.

Clearly, if either or both of the aforementioned procedures are necessary, consultation with the ophthalmologist is a necessity. Postoperative evaluation and monitoring in a unit where vision and the eye can be assessed should be routine. Repeat ocular and visual examinations by the ophthalmologist should be done. Cosmetic repair, if necessary, of the lateral canthotomy site can be sought well after the safety and security of the patient's vision is obtained. Again, frank discussions with the patient and proper documentation are essential in such cases.

Optic Nerve Injury

- To minimize optic nerve injury in revision sinus surgery:
  1. Be aware that optic nerve dehiscence can occur up to 4% of the time.
  2. Enter the sphenoid sinus medially and inferiorly.
  3. Recognize the presence of Onodi cells.

The second cranial nerve, the optic nerve, comprises a series of fibers extending from the orbit, through the optic foramen to the optic chiasm where the fibers continue to form the optic tracts leading to the primary visual centers of the brain. Approximately 20–30 mm of optic nerve length is present from the orbit to the optic foramen. An additional 10 mm carry the optic nerve from the foramen to the optic chiasm. It is this 10 mm of optic nerve, which extend intracranially along the skull base in the posterior ethmoid cells, running from superior lateral to superior medial to reach the optic chiasm, located above the tuberculum sellae and on the anterior portion of diaphragma sellae in the superior aspect of the sphenoid, that is at greatest risk for direct damage during endoscopic sinus surgery [1].

The optic nerve is at risk of being damaged at three points during complete functional endoscopic sinus surgery: the maxillary antrostomy, the sphenoidotomy, and the total ethmoidectomy. While a rarity, the orbit can be entered through the maxillary sinus, resulting in direct injury to the optic nerve. More commonly, the sphenoidotomy or ethmoidectomy places the optic nerve at greatest risk.

When identifying the natural os of the sphenoid sinus it should be found at 7 cm from the nasal sill, at the level of the maxillary sinus and immediately medial to the middle turbinate [12]. It is not uncommon to be deeper in the ethmoid or sphenoid sinus than anticipated. The use of a measuring device or computer image guidance is especially helpful in revision cases. In revision cases, scarring, absence of the middle turbinate, or an unnatural accessory os may be noted. When opening the sphenoid sinus, opening in a superior and lateral direction with any instrument may result in inadvertent damage to the optic nerve. In addition, with the optic nerve being dehiscent within the sphenoid sinus approximately 4–6% of the time, using power instrumentation (or any instrumentation) blindly within the sphenoid sinus may result in severing or directly damaging the optic nerve [34].

Direct damage to the optic nerve can also occur during a posterior ethmoidectomy. As mentioned earlier, the optic nerve courses intracranially directly superior to the lateral and superior extent of the ethmoid air cells. Overaggressive cleaning of the skull base in these areas can result in skull-base damage and compromise the integrity of the optic nerve. In addition, a variant of the posterior-most ethmoid cell, known as the Onodi cell, can extend superior to the actual sphenoid sinus. The Onodi cell, recognized by the horizontal bar seen within the sphenoid sinus on a coronal or sagittal image, may be mistaken as the sphenoid sinus and thus lead to unwarranted proximity to the posterior, superior, lateral skull base and the optic nerve (Fig. 26.5) [32]. Again, with the suction associated with powered instrumentation and damage that can be done with biting or grasping instruments, unplanned contact with the optic nerve can result in catastrophic damage.

Careful review of the axial and coronal computed tomography images prior to surgical intervention can alert the surgeon to the presence of the Onodi cell and/or the possibility of a dehiscent optic nerve within the sphenoid sinus. Identification of the os of the maxillary sinus will provide the level of the natural os of the sphenoid sinus and prevent the sinus surgeon from carrying a posterior ethmoid dissection high into the posterior skull base. The os of the maxillary sinus also allows for identification of the lamina papyracea, which represents the lateral extent of the dissection. Use of computer image guidance, prop-

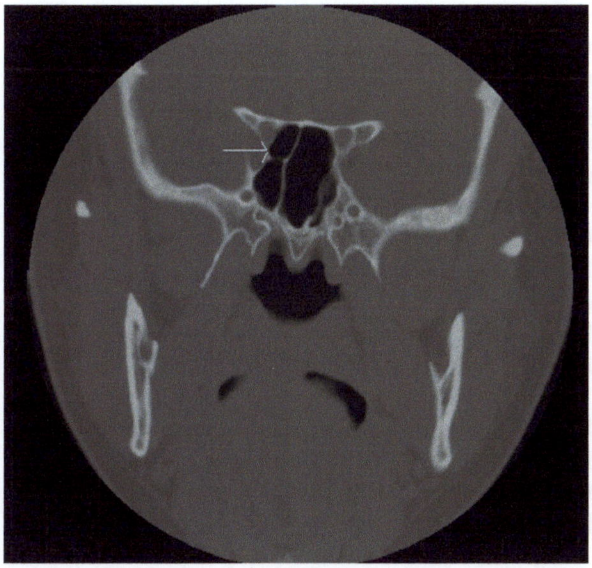

Fig. 26.5 Coronal CT with Onodi cell (*white arrow*); note the proximity of the optic nerve to roof of the Onodi cell

erly calibrated, can provide additional reinforcement of the location of the skull base and the depth of dissection. Routinely entering the sphenoid sinus in its inferior- and medial-most aspect continues to be the safest means by which to enter the sphenoid sinus, providing the greatest distant between any instrumentation and the superior, lateral course of the optic nerve.

Unfortunately, damage to the optic nerve is unlikely to be forgiving. Severing or disrupting the fibers of the optic nerve will more than likely result in permanent visual compromise. Heat damage or swelling related to manipulation of an area around the optic nerve sheath can be treated with high-dose oral steroids and/or an optic nerve decompression (however, this is usually unsuccessful). An optic nerve decompression relies upon endoscopic release of the optic sheath along its entire course to the annulus of Zinn [15]. In either case, consultation with ophthalmology and documentation of the patient's vision immediately post-injury and after any intervention is essential. Postoperative monitoring in a unit where routine monitoring of vision can be accomplished is essential.

Carotid Injury

- To avoid injury to the carotid artery in revision sinus surgery:
  1. Recognize that carotid dehiscence occurs up to 25% of the time.
  2. Avoid powered instrumentation or biting/grasping instrumentation within the sphenoid sinus (especially posterior and lateral) without proper visualization.

The potentially catastrophic complication of ICA injury can result in life-threatening hemorrhage, hemispheric stroke, coma, or death [33]. The anatomic relationship of the cavernous portion of the ICA in the sphenoid sinus results in a potential risk of injury during endoscopic sinus surgery. Ascending toward the posterior clinoid process and passing forward by the side of the body of the sphenoid bone, the ICA curves upward and perforates the dura mater, forming the roof of the sphenoid sinus. It is in this lateral and posterior aspect of the sphenoid sinus that iatrogenic injury can occur.

As one enters the sphenoid sinus, the ICA can be dehiscent approximately 20–25% of the time along some portion of its course [34]. Entering in the lateral, posterior aspect of the sphenoid sinus with a blunt instrument can pierce the uncovered ICA. In addition, blindly placing a powered debrider or other grasping/biting instrument into the posterior and lateral aspect of the sphenoid sinus may result in carotid artery damage.

Visualization, preparation, and finesse will aid the surgeon in preventing this potentially lethal complication. Identifying a preexisting dehiscence when examining the axial computed tomography images will alert the surgeon to a potential hazard. Proper visualization and location of the natural os of the sphenoid sinus as it has been described will also aid in prevention. As mentioned earlier, the safest method by which to widen the sphenoid sinus is identification of the natural os and opening the sinus in its medial- and inferior-most aspect. Avoiding placement of any powered instrumentation or grasping/biting instrument in the posterior and lateral aspect of the sphenoid sinus is highly recommended. Routine placement of an oropharyngeal throat pack in any patient having sphenoid or sinus surgery offers the benefit of potential complete oronasopharyngeal tamponade in the case of carotid injury and uncontrolled bleeding.

Identification of a compromise to the integrity of the ICA is generally not difficult. Occasionally, however, subendothelial damage to the ICA may result in a delayed aneurysm, pseudoaneurysm, or delayed rupture of the carotid artery [26]. For small, pinhole-type injuries where visualization can be accomplished, placement of small piece of Gelfoam or an epinephrine-soaked pledget over the area can allow for clot formation. Gentle packing around this area and use of fibrin sealants can also help control a small manageable defect. Notably, vasospasm of the ICA can still occur with this manipulation, resulting in hemispheric stroke [22].

More significant bleeding, however, will quickly obscure endoscopic visualization. In such a case, immediate packing of the nasal cavity will be required. Placement of a Foley catheter or other into the posterior nasal pharynx and inflating the balloon, in combination with providing counterpressure to the balloon anteriorly allows for tight packing within the nasopharynx, tamponading the hemorrhage. With an oropharyngeal throat pack in place, any significant nasopharyngeal packing can provide the required pressure to slow or halt a carotid bleed. Immediate transfer to an institution/location where endovascular procedures are performed is a necessity. A neurovascular interventional radiologist may be able to control such damage with endovascular coiling or other hemostatic measures. Such procedures can result in hemispheric stroke or blindness; however, this risk is overshadowed by the alternative – a fatal hemorrhage [22].

After control of the hemorrhage is achieved, neurological assessment must be accomplished and documented. Involvement of the neurologist is a necessity. Discussions with the patient's family as to the seriousness of this potentially lethal complication should be undertaken. Observation in an appropriate hospital unit is a necessity.

CSF Leak/Skull-Base Penetration

- To prevent and manage anterior skull-base injuries:
  1. Recognize high-risk areas of the fovea ethmoidalis, cribriform plate, and the anterior, medial, superior sphenoid sinus.
  2. Avoid operating medially, superior to the middle turbinate.
  3. Recognize the presence of CSF as a warning sign that the skull base has been penetrated.

Clearly, the anatomy of the paranasal sinuses places the endoscopic sinus surgeon millimeters from the intracranial contents of the anterior cranial fossa. The roof of the nasal cavity represents the floor of the anterior skull base. The thin lateral lamella connecting the cribriform plate with the fovea ethmoidalis provides a fragile barrier between the nasal cavity and the intracranial contents. Posteriorly, the sloping extension of the planum sphenoidale represents a potential entry point into the intracranial cavity.

Injury to the skull base in any of theses areas can occur in a variety of ways. Initially, failure to identify the level of the skull base at any point can enable puncture of the skull base with sharp, dull, or powered instrumentation [13]. An ethmoidectomy carried too far medial and superior can result in penetration of the lateral lamella of the cribriform plate or fovea ethmoidalis. It should be mentioned that the medial fovea ethmoidalis is up to ten times thinner than the lamina papyracea. Aggressive management of a middle turbinate that inserts into the lateral lamella can result in a fracture of the skull base in this area and resultant CSF leak. Entrance into the sphenoid sinus or Onodi-type cell medially in too high a manner can also result in skull-base penetration. With regard to revision surgery, the high-speed cutting drills used in revision frontal sinus surgery can easily be misplaced or skip into areas adjacent to the frontal sinus recess, resulting in skull-base injury [28].

Prevention begins with careful review and identification of the skull base on preoperative imaging. Evaluation for preexisting dehiscence and determination of the level of the skull base is mandatory. Three-dimensional imaging can aid in this endeavor. However, basic coronal imaging is generally used for determining the skull-base level. Multiple classifications have been used to describe the height of the skull base. While the measurements of the Keros classification can be extremely useful, a practical means of evaluating the skull base can be accomplished by comparing the level of the cribriform to the orbit [3]. A high skull base is at the superior aspect of the orbit, whereas a low skull base is located at one-third to one-half of the horizontal plane into the orbit. Any skull base at the level of the medial rectus or below is hazardous (Fig. 26.6). In addition to understanding the height associated with the skull base, understanding that in some individuals the fovea ethmoidalis slopes toward the cribriform plate, whereas in other individuals the fovea ethmoidalis is more vertical forming a "goblet" shape (Fig. 26.7) [10].

Beyond preoperative review of imaging, care must be taken during revision surgery not to accidentally puncture the skull base. Computer image guidance can be used to confirm the level of the skull base, understanding that visualization of the skull base as it slopes away from the surgeon supersedes computer imaging. In addition, the posterior level of the skull base is generally no more than 7 cm from the nasal sill and slopes in an arc anteriorly. Care must be taken in the areas of the superior aspect of the sphenoid sinus, the cribriform plate, and the fovea ethmoidalis. In revision cases, the middle turbinate may be absent. If present, one must avoid operating superiorly medial to the middle turbinate as this is a key "danger" zone and can easily lead to skull-base penetration. addition, scraping, using a bone rongeur, or aggressively cleaning the skull base in a variety of ways can result in a CSF leak. Understanding that sinus disease does not require resection to the skull-base mucosa, and allowing for a 2- to 3-mm cushion zone, even in revision cases, should adequately ensure avoidance of skull-base penetration, CSF leak, and complication.

CSF leak is the first sign that the skull base has been penetrated; it also represents a clear warning not to proceed any further with powered or other instrumentation. The endoscopic sinus surgeon should be well versed in the appearance of the skull base and recognize the white color of the dura. CSF rhinorrhea seen at the time of surgery is generally evident as gush of clear fluid that washes

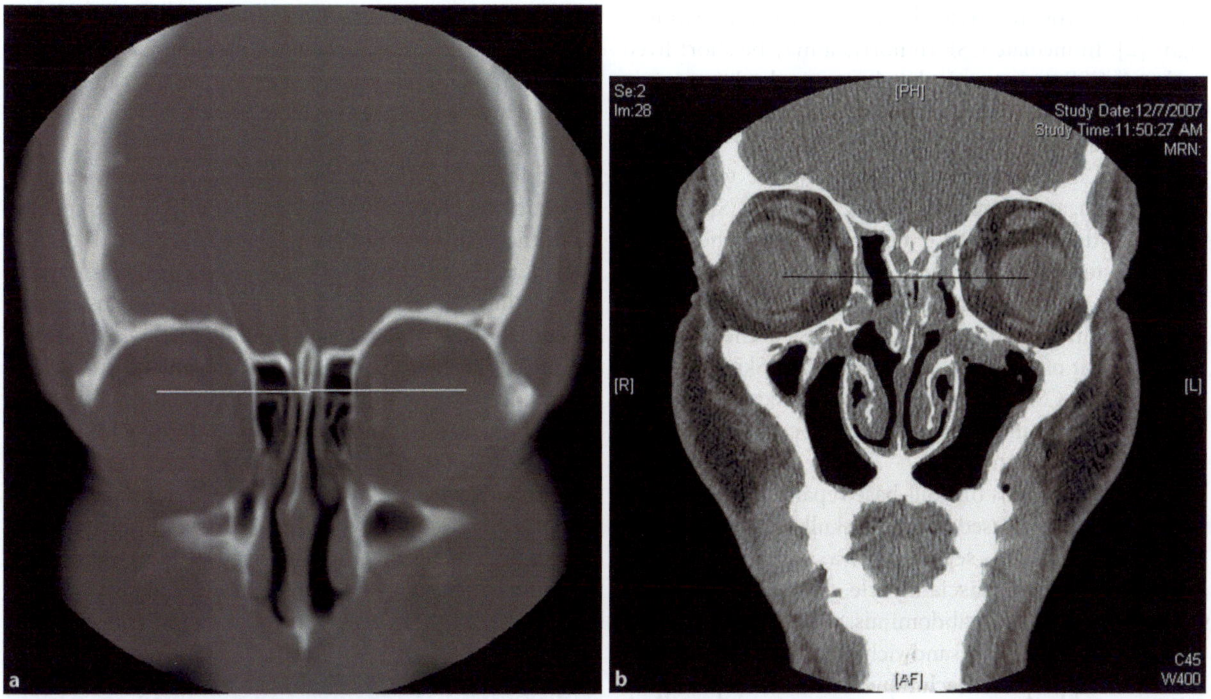

Fig. 26.6 **a** High skull base: the *white line* indicates the skull base above the upper third of the orbit. **b** Low-lying skull base: the *black line* indicates the skull base at the lower half of the orbit

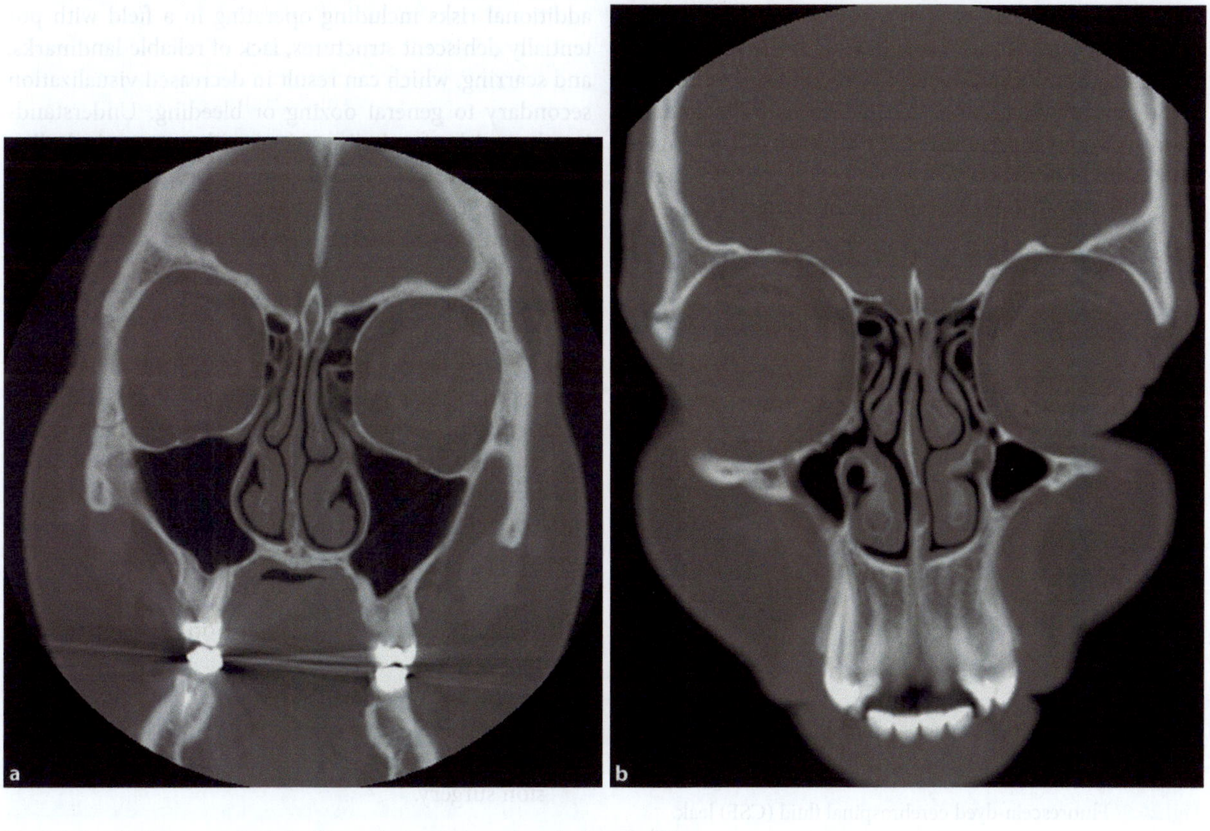

Fig. 26.7 **a** Goblet or vertical skull base. **b** Bowl-shaped or sloping skull base

away blood from the area. This is known as the "washout sign" [2]. Immediate CSF rhinorrhea may be short lived in that as CSF stores are depleted or as cerebral tissue prolapses into the defect, the rhinorrhea may resolve.

When it is evident that the skull base has been penetrated, intervention must occur. While with skull-base trauma, approximately 95% of the time CSF rhinorrhea is evident within the 3 months of injury, there is no literature to date that outlines the time line for identifying skull-base injury as a result of only endoscopic-sinus-surgery-induced trauma [25]. Regardless of the timing of injury, repair of the skull base is necessary. Skull-base dehiscence and CSF rhinorrhea unrecognized or untreated can result in chronic headache, pneumocephalus, meningitis, coma, and even death.

Multiple methods of skull-base repair exist. A variety of materials can be used to graft a skull-base injury: synthetic dura materials, septal mucosa, septal or turbinate cartilage, temporalis fascia/muscle, fat, and vascularized tissue such as rectus abdominus. Additionally, on-lay, over-lay, under-lay, and sandwich grafts have all been described as appropriate techniques for endoscopic repair of a skull-base defect. A traditional open, anterior cranial approach to the skull base can also be considered in cases where endoscopic repair fails. Endoscopic repair, however, is associated with a high success rate (approximately 90%) and considerably lower mortality [6]. Associated with repair of a skull-base defect, the use of CSF-reducing medications such as acetazolamide, and the use of lumbar drains have been advocated. In addition, with leaks found in a delayed fashion, the off-label use of intrathecal fluorescein at a concentration of one-tenth of 1 ml mixed with 10 ml of preservative free 0.9% saline or the patient's own CSF can aid in the localization of a defect. While not essential and requiring a separate consent indicating that a risk of seizure and/or chemical meningitis is associated with intrathecal fluorescein injection, its use can be quite helpful in isolating the area of a CSF leak (Fig. 26.8, Video 26.1) [25].

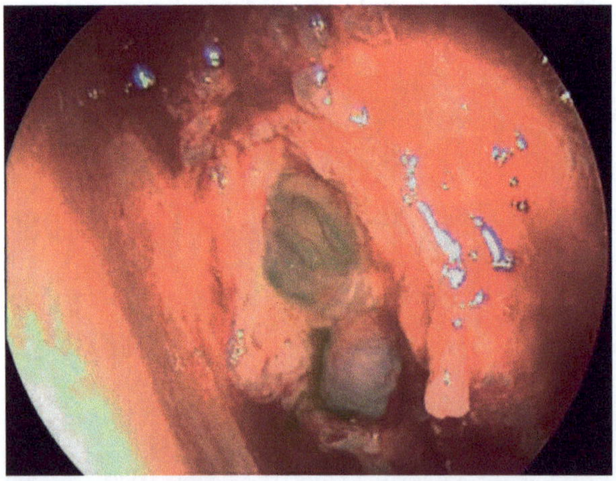

Fig. 26.8 Fluorescein-dyed cerebrospinal fluid (CSF) leak

In addition to repair, a consultation with neurosurgeon is indicated, especially if a lumbar drain is contemplated. If intraoperative skull-base penetration is noted, discussion with the anesthetist about avoiding positive-pressure ventilation, which may result in pneumocephalus, should occur. The following measures should also be considered: no heavy lifting/strenuous activity, avoidance of straws, avoidance of nose blowing, and an initial period (24 h) of strict bed rest at minimal (< 15°) incline with gradual increase to a 90° position. If cortical injury is suspected, discussions with a neurosurgeon and neurologist as appropriate are required together with obtaining appropriate radiographic imaging. A period of observation in a monitored setting of at least 24 h should be provided.

Conclusion

All surgery is fraught with potential complications. Endoscopic sinus surgery as described herein involves high-risk territory with multiple vital structures in the immediate vicinity. Revision sinus surgery poses significant additional risks including operating in a field with potentially dehiscent structures, lack of reliable landmarks, and scarring, which can result in decreased visualization secondary to general oozing or bleeding. Understanding these risks, frank discussions with patients including well-documented informed consent, proper preoperative evaluation, radiographic evaluation, and intraoperative evaluation are mandatory. Avoidance of complications remains the best treatment. However, early recognition of a complication can help prevent a minor complication from becoming a major complication. The ability to appropriately intervene when a complication becomes evident relies on surgical skill, anatomic knowledge, and experience. Involving appropriate colleagues and specialists can be an invaluable asset. Observation and diligence postcomplication is essential. Finally, open discussions with patients and their families can help prevent legal sequelae associated with surgical complications.

Tips/pearls to avoid complications in revision sinus surgery:

1. Always obtain a detailed informed consent.
2. Always obtain appropriate preoperative imaging.
3. Computer image guidance can be helpful in revision surgery.

4. Always review all available imaging and previous operative reports and have them available in the operating suite.
5. Recognize areas of potential complication prior to surgery.
6. Maintain visualization throughout all endoscopic procedures.
7. Identify key landmarks when available: middle turbinate, maxillary antrostomy, sphenoid os, nasopharynx.
8. Recognize complications as early as possible.
9. Intervene appropriately and definitively when complications occur.
10. Involve appropriate colleagues and experts, transferring patients when necessary.
11. Always discuss complications, treatments, and required interventions with patients and their family.

References

1. Buus DR. Farris BK (1990) Ophthalmic complications of sinus surgery. Ophthalmology 97:612–619
2. Cumberworth VL, Sudderick RM, MacKay IS (1994) Major complications of functional endoscopic sinus surgery. Clin Otolaryngol 19:248–253
3. Gauba V, Saleh G, Dua G, et al. (2006) Radiological classification of anterior skull base anatomy prior to performing medial orbital wall decompression. Orbit 25:93–96
4. Graham SM, Nerad JA (2003) Orbital complications in endoscopic sinus surgery using powered instrumentation. Laryngoscope 113:874–878
5. Hackman TG, Ferguson BJ (2005) Powered instrumentation and tissue effects in the nose and paranasal sinuses. Curr Opin Otolaryngol Head Neck Surg 13:22–26
6. Hegazy HM, Carrau RL, Snyderman CH, et al. (2000) Transnasal endoscopic repair of cerebrospinal fluid rhinorrhea: a meta-analysis. Laryngoscope 110:1166–1172
7. Holtz L (2006) Wins, Losses and Lessons: an Autobiography. Harper Collins, New York
8. Huang CM, Meyer DR, Patrinely JR, et al. (2003) Medial rectus muscle injuries associated with functional endoscopic sinus surgery: characterization and management. Ophthal Plast Reconstr Surg 19:25–37
9. Jiang RS, Hsu Cy (2002) Revision functional endoscopic sinus surgery. Ann Otol Rhinol Laryngol 111:155–159
10. Jones TM, Almahdi JM, Bhalla RK, et al. (2002) The radiological anatomy of the anterior skull base. Clin Otolaryngol 27:101–105
11. Kim HJ, Kim CH, Song MS, Yoon JH (2004) Diplopia secondary to endoscopic sinus surgery. Acta Otolaryngol 124:1237–1239
12. Kim HU, Kim SS, Kang SS, et al. (2001) Surgical anatomy of the natural ostium of the sphenoid sinus. Laryngoscope 111:1599–1602
13. Lee JC, Song YJ, Chung YS, et al. (2007) Height and shape of the skull base as risk factors for skull base penetration during endoscopic sinus surgery. Ann Otol Rhinol Laryngol 116:199–205
14. Lund VJ, Wright A, Yiotakis J (1997) Complications and medicolegal aspects of endoscopic sinus surgery. J Roy Soc Med 90:422–428
15. Luxenberger W, Stammberger H, Jebeles JA, Walch C (1998) Endoscopic optic nerve decompression: the Graz experience. Laryngoscope 108:873–882
16. Maniglia AJ (1991) Fatal and other major complication of endoscopic sinus surgery. Laryngoscope 101:349–354
17. May M, Schiatkin B, Kay SL (1994) Revision endoscopic sinus surgery: six friendly surgical landmarks. Laryngoscope 104:766–767
18. McDonald SE, Robinson PJ, Nunez DA (2007) Radiological anatomy of the anterior ethmoidal artery for functional endoscopic sinus surgery. J Laryngol Otol 122:264–267
19. McInnes G, Howes DW (2002) Lateral canthotomy and cantholysis: a simple, vision-saving procedure. Can J Emerg Med 4:49–52
20. Metson R, Pletcher SD (2006) Endoscopic and optic nerve decompression. Otolaryngol Clin North Am 39:551–561
21. Meyers RM, Valvassori G (1998) Interpretation of anatomic variation of computed scan of the sinuses: a surgeon's perspective. Laryngoscope 108:422–425
22. Park AH, Stankiewicz JA, Chow J, Azar-Kia B (1998) A protocol for management of a catastrophic complication of functional endoscopic sinus surgery: internal carotid artery injury. Am J Rhinol 12:153–158
23. Rene C, Rose G, Lenthall R, Moseley I (2001) Major orbital complications of endoscopic sinus surgery. Br J Ophthalmol 85:598–603
24. Sadoughi B, Brown SM, Nachlas NE, Fried MP (2006) Image guided surgery. E-medicine. Available at http://www.emedicine.com/ent/topic396.htm
25. Scianna JM, Stankiewicz JA (2006) CSF Rhinorrhea. E-medicine. Available at http://www.emedicine.com/ent/topic332.htm
26. Sood S, Timothy J, Anthony R, et al. (2000) Extracranial internal carotid artery pseudoaneurysm. Am J Otolaryngol 21:259–262
27. Stankiewicz JA (1989) Blindness and intranasal ethmoidectomy: prevention and management. Otolaryngol Head Neck Surg 101:322–329
28. Stankiewicz JA (1991) Cerebrospinal fluid fistula and endoscopic sinus surgery. Laryngoscope 101:250–256
29. Stankiewicz JA, Chow JM (1999) Two faces of orbital hematoma in intranasal (endoscopic) sinus surgery. Otolaryngol Head Neck Surg 120:841–846

30. Stankiewicz JA (1987) Complications of endoscopic nasal surgery: occurrence and treatment. Am J Rhinol 1:45–49
31. Streitmann MJ, Otto RA, Sakai CS (1994) Anatomic considerations in complications of endoscopic and intranasal surgery. Ann Otol Rhinol Laryngol 103:105–109
32. Thanaviratananich S, Chaisiwamongkol K, Kraitrakul S, et al. (2003) The prevalence of an Onodi cell in adult Thai cadavers. Ear Nose Throat J 82:200–204
33. Weidenbecher M, Huk WJ, Iro H (2005) Internal carotid artery injury during functional endoscopic sinus surgery and its management. Eur Arch Otorhinolaryngol 262:640–645
34. Yanagisawa E (2002) The optic nerve and internal carotid artery in the sphenoid sinus. Ear Nose Throat J 81:611–612
35. Yung CW, Moorthy RS, Lindley D, et al. (1994) Efficacy of lateral canthotomy and cantholysis in orbital hemorrhage. Ophthalmol Plast Reconstr Surg 10:137–141

Chapter 27

Revision Dacryocystorhinostomy

27

Metin Onerci

Core Messages

- A small and inappropriately placed bony opening, inadequate and improperly opened rhinostomy, excessive scar tissue production, anatomical abnormalities, and concomitant paranasal sinus infections are the most important causes for the failure of dacryocystorhinostomy (DCR) surgery.
- The endonasal approach is well suited for revision DCR surgery because the residual lacrimal sac can be directly accessed through the previous bony ostium created at the time of the primary DCR.
- During revision external surgery, the bony ostium is more easily enlarged through the endonasal approach.
- In revision cases a detailed examination should be performed to find the possible causes and the site of pathology.
- The rhinostomy from the sac into the lateral nasal wall should be created at the correct location and with the correct size, which should be over 5 mm wide.
- A low rhinostomy may not bypass a midsac or upper-sac obstruction. A high rhinostomy leaves the nasolacrimal duct as a blind pouch that is not adequately drained. Despite a patent anastomosis, retention produces sump syndrome.
- A larger rhinostomy removing enough bone (15 mm × 15 mm) may prevent sump syndrome.
- Any nasal or paranasal abnormalities should be corrected during DCR surgery.
- If the rhinostomy is placed in a wrong location in the previous surgery, the new rhinostomy should be opened in the correct location.
- The success rate is directly related to the appropriate technique — inadequate surgical training and the lack of proper instrumentation decrease the success rate.

Contents

Introduction

Epiphora is one of the most prevalent functional disabilities of the ocular system. Various techniques (Table 27.1) have been developed to treat lacrimal diseases, to eliminate the infection, and to reconstruct a functional drainage pathway using very sophisticated instruments.

The practice of lacrimal surgery has been done by an external approach for a long time. Despite much debate, many ophthalmologists still believe that external DCR provides higher success rates than endoscopic DCR. The surgical treatment of DCR is very closely related to the inside of the nose. The problem of an endonasal approach was the difficulty in visualizing the endonasal anatomy. The introduction of microscopes and endoscopes into medicine opened the door for visualization of the interior of the nose, and endoscopic or microscopic endonasal

Table 27.1 The surgical approaches to the nasolacrimal sac

1. Endocanalicular	(a) Lacrimal endoscopy (b) Balloon dacryocystoplasty (c) Endocanalicular laser-assisted dacryocystorhinostomy
2. Endonasal approach	(a) Transseptal approach (b) Transnasal (classical) approach (c) Transnasal (endoscopic or microscopic) approach (d) Endonasal laser-assisted dacryocystorhinostomy
3. Paranasal approach	(a) Transantral approach (b) Paranasal approach
4. External approach	(a) Dacryoethmoidostomy (b) Falk's operation (c) Toti operation (d) Modifications of Toti operations

lacrimal surgery has become more popular in recent times [21]. Long-term success rates with endonasal techniques have been equivalent to that achieved with external DCR [10]. However, it is difficult to make evidence-based determinations about the efficacy of endonasal or external approaches. Each approach has its own advantages and disadvantages (Tables 27.2–27.5).

The endonasal approach is well suited for revision DCR surgery because the residual lacrimal sac can be accessed directly through the previous bony ostium created at the time of primary DCR, and the bony ostium is more easily enlarged [28]. The endoscopic DCR in revision cases also offers several other advantages including a complete exposure of those anatomical anomalies or inflammatory changes of the normal structures that commonly hinder conventional external surgery. Before revision surgery, a detailed preoperative evaluation is necessary.

Preoperative Evaluation

Although the tear drainage system appears very simple, draining the tears through the nasolacrimal system with the help of gravity is indeed an intricate process. Drainage of tears depends on the volume of tear production, eyelid position, pump mechanisms, anatomy of the lacrimal system, gravity, and nasal air convection currents. Although clinical evaluation of gross lacrimal function is not difficult and can be made on the basis of history, determination of the cause may be extremely difficult and requires a variety of diagnostic procedures [7].

Lacrimal drainage dysfunction can be due to an anatomic obstruction, such as nasolacrimal duct fibrosis, or physiologic dysfunction from a failure of functional mechanisms (for example lacrimal pump inadequacy caused by poor orbicularis muscle tone); therefore, the diagnosis of the cause of epiphora is important. A list of tests required for the diagnosis of epiphora is given in Table 27.6.

The routine preoperative evaluation includes dacryoscintigraphy or dacryocystography. Dacryocystography is a safe, quick, and easy procedure using a radio-opaque material. It is widely established for the demonstration of stenosis. This procedure should not be performed in the presence of active dacryocystitis. Dacryocystography may be useful in demonstrating localized stricture, par-

Table 27.2 The advantages of the external approach

- Unsurpassed exposure of the lacrimal drainage system
- Intraoperative inspection of suspected or unsuspected anomalies
- Biopsies performed easily
- Easy to suture the adjacent flaps of lacrimal and nasal mucosa to provide a patent with an epithelium-lined tract for tear drainage

Table 27.3 The disadvantages of external dacryocystorhinostomy (DCR)

- Cutaneous scar
- Disturbance of the nasolacrimal pump system
- Bleeding
- Acute dacryocystitis with abscess formation

Table 27.4 The advantages of the endonasal DCR procedure

- Less disruption of medial canthal anatomy
- Preservation of lacrimal pumping function
- No external incision, with improved cosmesis
- Decreased postoperative morbidity and enhanced recovery
- No hospital stay required
- Operating under direct vision with minimal trauma
- Addressing the nasal and paranasal sinus abnormalities through the same surgical approach
- Can be performed in patients with acute dacryocystitis with abscess formation
- Endoscopic postoperative evaluation for persistent or recurrent disease
- Decreased operative time
- Excellent visualization
- Ability to evaluate the location and size of the rhinostomy site
- Decreased intraoperative hemorrhage
- Can be used for previously radiated patients
- Can be used for pediatric patients
- Revision procedures

Table 27.5 The disadvantages of the endonasal dacryocystorhinostomy procedure

- Suspicion of lacrimal system neoplasia
- Technical difficulty in patients who have sustained severe midfacial trauma with secondary hyperostosis, or altered anatomy involving the bones surrounding the lacrimal sac
- High equipment cost
- Steep learning curve

tial obstruction, lacrimal diverticuli, fistulae, dacryoliths, and extrinsic and intrinsic tumors of the lacrimal drainage system [7].

The disadvantage of dacryocystography is that it provides restricted functional information, as in dysfunction of the canalicular muscle pump, slight narrowing of the ductal lumen and mucous membranes, since intubation of the canaliculi and active injection of the contrast material may overcome stenosis. Dacryoscintigraphy is also a simple, noninvasive physiologic test. Dacryoscintigraphy may provide information about physiological function. Limiting factors are the methodologically inherent minimal morphologic information and relatively large variations of normal transit times. Dacryocystography gives finer anatomic detail; however, dacryoscintigraphy is a more physiologic assessment since no instrumentation is necessary [7, 14]. In revision cases, functional dysfunction and canalicular obstruction should be considered in the differential diagnosis of epiphora before surgery.

Table 27.6 Diagnostic tests for the lacrimal system

Dye (fluorescein) disappearance test
Primary Jones dye test (Jones I and Jones II)
Lacrimal irrigation
Ultrasonography
Dacryocystography
Radionuclide dacryoscintigraphy
Computed tomography
Computed tomography dacryocystography
Magnetic resonance imaging
Magnetic resonance dacryocystography
Lacrimal endoscopy

Revision Dacryocystorhinostomy

Reasons for Failure

Failure of dacryocystorhinostomy (DCR) is attributable to a variety of causes (Table 27.7). The majority of cases were found to be related to internal nasal problems. A small and inappropriately placed bony opening, inadequate and improperly opened rhinostomy, excessive scar tissue production, anatomical abnormalities, and concomitant paranasal sinus infections are the most important causes for the failure of DCR surgery.

Functional obstruction can be diagnosed with dacryoscintigraphy. If it is due to dysfunction of the lacrimal pump system , the patient should be informed about the prognosis. Narrowing of the nasolacrimal canaliculus apparatus sometimes mimics the functional dysfunction. However, these patients may benefit from the surgery; at the very least their symptoms improve after surgery [41].

Surgical Approach

Endonasal endoscopic or microscopic DCR is generally the preference of many authors in instances of failed DCRs [8, 22, 28]. The angled instruments developed for endoscopic sinus surgery allow the occluded ostium to be relatively safely evaluated under direct endoscopic visualization. Under direct endoscopic or microscopic visualization, the ostium can be enlarged and properly positioned to increase the likelihood of continued patency [19]. Granulations can be easily trimmed and cauterized, adhesions are cut together with resection of the anterior end of the middle turbinate. A small, high rhinostomy may cause sump syndrome. The sac should not be opened very high up without opening it inferiorly in order to prevent sump syndrome (Figure 27.1). Placement of the ostium too close to the middle turbinate results in subsequent adhesion and occlusion,. The endonasal approach is a one-stage procedure that permits correction of associated nasal disorders, such as septal deviation, middle-

Table 26.7 Reasons for failure

- Improper placement of the ostium
- Creating a small bony ostium
- Sump syndrome
- Insufficient membranous rhinostomy
- Scar formation in the area of rhinostomy
- Scarring at the canaliculi–sac junction
- Small cicatrized sacs
- Associated nasal or paranasal abnormalities
- Development of adhesions between the rhinostomy and the middle turbinate or rarely the nasal septum
- Granuloma formation
- Insufficient removal of periosteum
- Leaving bony spicules in the operating area
- Lacrimal pump insufficiency
- Persistence of a lacrimal sac diverticulum that was not drained
- Previous surgery, chemotherapy, or radiotherapy for paranasal sinus malignancy

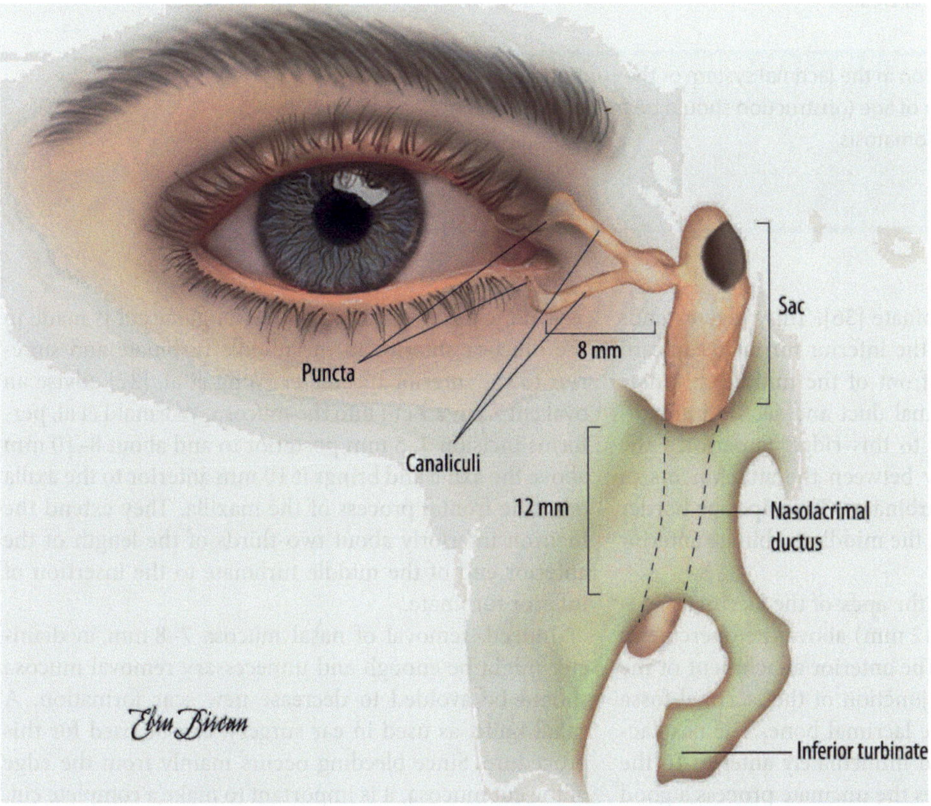

Fig 27.1 High and small rhinostomies may cause sump syndrome. The sac should not be opened very high up without opening it inferiorly in order to prevent sump syndrome. (Courtesy of TESAV)

turbinate hypertrophy, or polypoidal disease, which may be a causative factor in the failure of DCR [8].

Surgical Technique for Revision Cases

If it is done under general anesthesia, hypotensive anesthesia is preferred. The inside of the nose is decongested. The head is elevated by bringing the table 20° or 30° in a reverse Trendelenburg position. The lateral nasal wall and previous rhinostomy site are examined carefully endoscopically for potential structural issues that may have contributed to the failure of initial procedure [38]. The mucosa anterior to the middle turbinate may be infiltrated with 1 ml lidocaine with 1:100,000 epinephrine. The disadvantage of this infiltration is that it may obscure the bulging of the nasolacrimal sac. It is important not to traumatize the nasal mucosa, since bleeding prevents visualization. At this stage any septal deviation, concha bullosa, or paradoxical middle turbinate obstructing the view must be corrected. Occasionally, the head of the middle turbinate needs to be removed to expose the sac area. Chronic maxillary rhinossinusitis or pansinusitis should be addressed simultaneously by the same endonasal route. In revision cases, before starting the operation the lacrimal probe is introduced through the superior canaliculus and passed into the area of rhinostomy. In most cases a fibrous membrane is noted to occlude the previously created channel. The extent of the previous rhinostomy and the size of the bony opening are determined [39]. Active Wegener's granulomatosis or benign or malignant lesions of the lacrimal sac or the neighboring structures are absolute contraindications for DCR (Table 27.8).

Localization of the Lacrimal Sac and Duct

The key initial landmark is the posterior border of the frontal process of the maxilla, which is usually identifiable as a ridge or an indentation into the nasal airway just

Table 27.8 Contraindications to DCR

• Benign or malignant lesion in the lacrimal system or the surrounding tissues
• Children less than 1 year of age (obstruction should be treated by probing)
• Active Wegener's granulomatosis
• Canalicular obstruction
• A functional sac

anterior to the middle turbinate [36]. This ridge extends from the highest point of the inferior turbinate upward and ends immediately in front of the middle turbinate attachment. The nasolacrimal duct and sac lie immediately lateral and posterior to this ridge. Superiorly, the duct joins the sac halfway between the attachments of the middle and inferior turbinates. The superior border of the lacrimal sac is above the middle-turbinate anterior attachment.

The average position of the apex of the lacrimal sac is 6.10 ± 2.02 mm (range, 2–12 mm) above the opercule of the middle turbinate [9]. The anterior attachment of the uncinate process is at the junction of the lacrimal fossa and the orbital plate of the lacrimal bone. The nasolacrimal sac is always situated immediately anterior to the uncinate process and makes the uncinate process a good landmark in DCR operations. It is important not to enter beyond this point in a lateral direction since it may cause orbital penetration. A 20-gauge fiberoptic light pipe may also be used to identify the location of the sac and is inserted into the lacrimal sac through either of the lacrimal canaliculi. The light is visualized endonasally with a rigid endoscope.

Mucosal Incision

Soft tissue rather than bony occlusion of the surgical ostium is one of the most frequent causes of failure of external DCR. The most common identified obstruction results from lacrimal sac cicatrization, granulation tissue, fibrosis, and synechia between the opening and adjacent middle-turbinate mucosa [8]. The nasal mucosal incision is made slightly more anterior on the frontal process of maxilla. Approximately one-half of the lacrimal sac fossa lies anterior to the location of the maxillary line; this supports the recommendation that the nasal mucosal incision be placed anterior to this landmark [38, 39] The periosteum is identified and elevated. The anterior edge of the previous bony rhinostomy site is found. In some cases it is not possible to identify the rhinostomy opening either due to wrong placement of the ostium or reclosure of the ostium. In such situations DCR is performed as is done in the usual way. A rectangular cut is made in the mucosa anterior to the middle turbinate and superior to the inferior turbinate. Wong et al. [37] advise an oval cut 2 cm × 1 cm into the mucosa. Wormald et al. performs incision 3–5 mm posterior to and about 8–10 mm above the axilla and brings it 10 mm anterior to the axilla onto the frontal process of the maxilla. They extend the incision inferiorly about two-thirds of the length of the anterior end of the middle turbinate to the insertion of inferior turbinate.

Indeed, removal of nasal mucosa 7–8 mm in diameter might be enough and unnecessary removal mucosa should be avoided to decrease new scar formation. A canal knife, as used in ear surgery, can be used for this procedure. Since bleeding occurs mainly from the edge of the cut mucosa, it is important to make a complete cut, and not to pull and tear the mucosa [24]. After the cut is completed through the mucoperiosteum all the way down to the bone, the mucosa is elevated off the bone and removed or can be used as a posteriorly based flap. It does not appear to be necessary to apply special mucosal flaps [13]. If needed, through-cutting forceps may be used instead of Blakesley forceps to avoid tearing of the mucosa. To prevent recurrences it is important to remove the periosteum with the nasal mucosa and to remove all bony partitions and spicules. The periosteum induces new bone formation and in turn leads to narrowing or closure of the ostium. If the edge of the previous rhinostomy opening is found, the mucosa around it is elevated and the bone is drilled in such a way that the new rhinostomy be at the correct location. It is important to prepare the sac completely exposed.

Bone Removal

Inadequate bone removal is a common cause of failure in DCR. In all revision operations agger nasi cells should be checked. In approximately 8% of patients there is an agger nasi cell in this area. In some cases, agger nasi ethmoid cells may extend under the fossa causing confusion during surgery, and removal of bone results in opening into the ethmoid cell rather than the lacrimal fossa. If the agger nasi cell has not been opened yet, it will be necessary to open the agger nasi cell up and go through it before going through the lateral wall and the lacrimal bone into the sac.

If the anterior edge of the previous bony rhinostomy site is found, it is widened so as to create a proper rhinostomy. If there can be found no bony rhinostomy opening, the surgical procedure should be as in primary DCR operation. The sac and duct junction is above the insertion of inferior turbinate, 6 mm below the operculum. Woog et al. suggest removing the bone overlying the common canaliculus completely and achieving a rhinostomy with at least 6–8 mm vertical dimension in adults. The medial side of the bone of the maxillary portion of the lacrimal fossa can be removed either from posterior to anterior or from anterior to posterior. Since it is thinner in the posterior part, it makes sense to start from posterior. However, it is really challenging to remove the bone with conventional endoscopic sinus instruments alone. There are currently no bone-removing instruments specifically designed for this location. Kerrison forceps or backbiting forceps may be used for this purpose [40]. The surgeon may feel safer if he/she starts from the anteromedial part of the bony sac, identifies the sac, and continues posteriorly. The use of a laser takes more time and may cause thermal injury. The laser can only ablate the much thinner lacrimal bone. Removal of part of the frontal process of the maxilla gives better access and visualization of the lacrimal sac, but a laser cannot ablate this thick bone.

Weidenbecher et al. [33] suggest removing the entire medial bony covering of the sac. Whittet et al. [36] insert a Leibrich lacrimal probe into the inferior canaliculus, direct it against the medial wall of the lacrimal sac in order to tent, and decide how much bone to remove after this procedure. They advocate leaving approximately 5 mm free of bone around the canaliculus, especially at the junction of attachment of the middle turbinate and the lateral nasal wall, a point that demarcates the floor of the lacrimal fossa. Woog et al. [38, 39] suggest creating a generous rhinostomy that extends from above the middle-turbinate attachment to the level of the midpoint of the maxillary line inferiorly. Welham and Wulc [35] think that the ideal osteotomy should involve the removal of all of the bone between the medial wall of the sac and the nose. Drills specifically designed for intranasal use make it easier to remove the bone but may be associated with thermal injury and damage to the surrounding mucosa. The bony opening should start a few millimeters above the operculum, and the medial half of the bony nasolacrimal sac should be removed in such a way that after the surgical bony opening it should be 10–17 mm in diameter (average 11.75 mm). A functional result can be achieved with a fistula of 6 mm^2. No statistical correlation was found between the size of the ostium at the surgery and after healing [18]. Iliff [15] removed a 10-mm diameter piece of bone, with 1 failure out of 87 cases. The mean diameter of the healed ostium was 1.8 mm, representing an area only 18% of that of the initial anastomosis. So the aim is not to create a very large bony osteotomy, but a functioning osteotomy of efficient size.

The entire medial bony covering of the sac can be removed under endoscopic or microscopic control. If a chisel is used, attention should be given to removing all bony fragments, since if left they may cause obstruction later. Previously irradiated patients should be handled carefully owing to healing problems and anatomic derangements. However, in revision cases using drills is more advocated. Thus, following DCR, the sac and the duct should coexist as anatomic structures and be incorporated into the nose.

Removal of the Medial Mucosal Wall of the Sac

The vascularized white color of the sac is characteristic and can easily be identified. The medial part of the lacrimal sac should be fully exposed. A lacrimal probe may be used to identify the lacrimal sac. A lacrimal probe is passed through a canaliculus and directed medially into the obstructed sac. The fibrous tissue is tented into the nasal cavity with probes to provide a broad soft-tissue region under tension. The tenting of the medial sac wall by the probe is visualized endonasally. While it is tented by the lacrimal probe, the sac mucosa is incised with a sickle knife. Mucopus, residual contrast material, may drain from the sac, or dacryoliths may be seen in the interior of the sac. Once the sac has been entered, the lacrimal probe may be seen. Using Bellucci scissors, one can extend the incision and use through-cutting instruments to enlarge the intranasal opening. Blakesley forceps are not through-cutting and may tear the sac mucosa; for this reason, through-cutting forceps are preferred. A carbon dioxide laser can also be used. As much of the medial wall of the sac should be removed as possible. Metson [19] advises enlarging of intranasal opening to a diameter of approximately 10 mm, allowing free passage of the lacrimal probes into the nose from both superior and inferior canaliculi. In some failed DCRs there is a large sac remnant seen in DCG whereas in others a small cicatrized sac is present. In patients with small cicatrized sacs it may be difficult to achieve lacrimal and nasal mucosal anastomosis. If there exists any problem to appose the mucosal edges, the nasal mucosal flap is trimmed to fit the size of the lacrimal ostium [28]. According to Woog et al. [39] an adequate rhinostomy should permit easy passage of lacrimal probes and removal of the medial wall of the lacrimal sac in the area of common canaliculus should be confirmed by direct visualization of the internal common punctum with angled endoscopes.

In revision procedures orbital soft tissues and internal common punctum may be incorporated into the scar tissue. Vigorous avulsion of this cicatrix may cause injury to orbital soft tissues, medial canthal ligament, and internal common punctum. Woog et al. [38, 39] recommend to observe the medial commissure while gentle traction is placed on the tissue to be removed at the rhinostomy site. Excessive movement of the medial commissure by this maneuver may signify that deeper tissues than desired are being grasped by the forceps.

Silicone Tubing

A silicone tube is placed through the upper and lower canaliculi into the nasal cavity, the ends of the tubing are grasped with forceps, guided out of the nose, and are tied and trimmed so that the knot lies within the nasal cavity. The tubing thus forms a continuous loop, which passes through the intranasal ostium and is unlikely to become dislodged [19]. The knot may be fixed by a suture or a vessel clip. Wong et al. [37] use a black silk suture to tie round the silicone tubes. According to Allen and Berlin [1] and Bartley [2], silk sutures can produce pyogenic and giant cell granulomas. Packing of the nose is unnecessary unless bleeding is a problem.

Silicone intubation may be recommended in cases with canalicular stenosis, a small scarred lacrimal sac, a tight upper nasal cavity, in reoperations, and if the flaps of the lacrimal sac and nasal mucosa are not sutured. In other cases it is the surgeon's preference to use silicone tubes or not. Silicone tubing may serve to dilate constricted passages in patients with canalicular or common internal punctual stenosis and marks the site of the intranasal ostium [6]. Kohn [17] believes that silicone tubing keeps the anterior and posterior flaps separate, and also discourages cicatricial closure of the bony ostium. Some reports [1, 23] give less favorable results when tubes are inserted. Allen and Berlin [1] believe that intubation may be the reason for failure. Tubes may cause inflammation, granulation, and slit the canaliculus. Silicone tubing may incite granulomatous inflammation at the internal ostium, chronic infection, or canalicular laceration. Walland and Rose [30] did not find any difference in failure rates or inflammation with or without silicone intubation. Insertion of silicone tubes is generally encouraged [3]. Snead et al. [26] showed that silicone intubation did not increase canalicular inflammation in animals. Walland and Rose [31] found no significant difference in the rate of failure or soft-tissue infection between silicone-intubated and nonintubated patients. Wormald et al. placed tubes to dilate the common canaliculus opening into the lacrimal sac; this is especially important for patients who have functional epiphora rather than to keep the sac open. In revision cases intubation with silicone tubes is generally recommended.

How Long Should the Silicone Tubes Be Kept in Place?

It is advised to keep silicone stents in place for 2–6 months; however, tubes kept in place over 3 months are associated with inflammation and granulation. Wong et al. [37] and Weidenbecher et al. [33] advise removing the tubes after 6 weeks. El Guindy et al. [8] keep the tubes for only 2 months and recommend early removal (at 2 months) because silicone tubing may incite a granulomatous reaction. Hartikainen et al. [10] keep the tubes in place for 6 months. Hausler and Caversaccio [11] use the tubes in place for the long term and they have several cases where silicone tubes have been used for over 3 years without any complications. They even suggest leaving the tubes permanently in persistent cases and think that the silicone tubing produces a maximal dilatation of the canaliculi and a natural aspiration of tear liquid by capillary force. However, keeping silicone tubes for at least 2 months is generally advocated in revision cases.

Mitomycin C

Mitomycin C, an antiproliferative agent that is widely used in pterygium excision and trabulectomy with favorable results, was also used to inhibit fibrous tissue growth and scarring at the osteotomy site and to decrease the failure rate. Cottonoids soaked with 0.2 mg/ml mitomycin C are applied to the osteotomy site. Kao et al. [16] reported that mytomicin C improved success rates; Zilelioğlu et al. [42] found no benefit in using mitomycin C. Use of mitomycin C needs further investigation.

Complications

Soft-tissue infection after open lacrimal surgery occurs in 8% of patients. It is reduced fivefold with routine administration of antibiotics [31]. Vardy and Rose [29] demonstrated that intraoperative or postoperative broad-spectrum antibiotics reduced the incidence of cellulitis after open primary lacrimal surgery. Tsirbas and McNab [27] reported 3.8% of cases with secondary hemorrhage after DCR. The incidence of bleeding was higher in patients taking nonsteroidal anti-inflammatory drugs. Severe nasal hemorrhage requiring nasal packing was also reported

[22, 34]. Orbital complications were also mentioned [25, 32]. Orbital emphysema can be prevented by asking patients not to blow their nose for at least 2 weeks following surgery. Prolapsed tubes, punctal widening, corneal irritation, and intranasal discomfort are the complications related to silicone tubing [5]. There are rare reports of cerebrospinal fluid leaks and meningitis [4, 12, 20]. Meticulous surgery avoiding unnecessary mucosal trauma may prevent intranasal adhesions.

Tips and Pearls

1. The sac should not be opened very high up without opening it inferiorly in order to prevent sump syndrome. High and small rhinostomies may cause sump syndrome.
2. Preservation of as much mucosa as possible is of paramount importance to decrease scarring.
3. The bony osteotomy should be as big as the mucosal opening (7–10 mm) and the periosteum should be removed with mucosa (since new bone formation requires the presence of periosteum).
4. The bone in the region of the lacrimal fossa may be thicker following a midfacial fracture owing to callus formation.
5. The medial membranous sac wall should be removed. Only puncturing the medial membranous wall decreases the success rate.

Conclusion

A small bony ostium, inadequate rhinostomy, excessive scar tissue production, anatomical abnormalities, and concomitant paranasal sinus infections are the most important causes of the failure of DCR surgery. The endonasal approach is well suited for revision DCR surgery because the residual lacrimal sac can be accessed directly through the previous bony ostium created at the primary DCR. The bony ostium is more easily enlarged through the endonasal approach. It preserves the pump function of the sac and avoids an external scar. It allows sinus surgery to be performed in the same sitting if needed. The success of the surgery depends on accurate diagnosis ruling out canalicular and functional obstruction, and meticulous surgery, avoiding trauma to the mucosa and neighboring structures.

References

1. Allen K, Berlin AJ (1989) Dacryocystorhinostomy failure: association with nasolacrimal silicon intubation. Ophthalmol Surg 20:486–489
2. Bartley GB (1992) Acquired lacrimal drainage obstruction: an etiologic classification system, case reports, and a review of the literature. Part 1. Ophthal Plast Reconstr Surg 8:237–242
3. Beigi B, Westlake W, Chang B, Marsh C, Jacob J, Chatfield J (1998) Dacryocystorhinostomy in South West England. Eye 12:358–362
4. Beiran I, Pikkel J, Gilboa M, Miller B (1994) Meningitis as a complication of dacryocystorhinostomy. Br J Ophthalmol 78:417–418
5. Brookes JL, Oliver JM (1999) Endoscopic endonasal management of prolapsed silicone tubes after dacryocystorhinostomy. Ophthalmology 106:2101–2105
6. Burns JA, Cahill KV (1985) Modified Kinosian dacryocystorhinostomy. Ophthalmic Surg, 16:710–716
7. Dutton JJ (1988) Diagnostic tests and imaging techniques. In: Linberg JV (Ed) Lacrimal Surgery. Churchill Livingstone, New York, pp 19–48
8. El-Guindy A, Dorgham A, Ghoraba M (2000) Endoscopic revision surgery for recurrent epiphora occurring after external dacryocystorhinostomy. Ann Otol Rhinol Laryngol 109:425–430
9. Fayet B, Racy E, Assouline M, Zerbib M (2005) Surgical anatomy of the lacrimal fossa. A prospective computed tomodensitometry scan analysis. Ophthalmology 112:1119–1128
10. Hartikainen J, Antila J, Varpula M, Puukka P, Seppa H, Grenman R (1998) Prospective randomized comparison of endonasal endoscopic dacryocystorhinostomy and external dacryocystorhinostomy. Laryngoscope 108:1861–1866
11. Hauslaer R, Caversaccio M (1998) Microsurgical endonasal dacryocystorhinostomy with long term insertion of bicanalicular silicone tubes. Arch Otolaryngol Head Neck Surg 124:188–191
12. Heerman J Jr (1991) Rhinologische Aspekte bei Traenenwegstenosen. Otorhinolaryngol Nova 1:227–232
13. Hosemann WG, Weber RK, Keerl RE, Lund VJ (2002) Minimally Invasive Endonasal Sinus Surgery. Georg Thieme Verlag, Stuttgart, pp 66–70
14. Hurwitz JJ (1996) The Lacrimal System. Lippincott Raven, Philadelphia
15. Iliff CE(1971) A simplified dacryocystorhinostomy. Arch Ophthalmol 85:586–591
16. Kao SCS, Liao CL, Tseng JHS, Chen MS, Hou PK (1996) Dacryocystorhinostomy with intraoperative mitomycin C. Ophthalmology 104:86–91
17. Kohn R (1988) Ophthalmic Plastic and Reconstructive Surgery. Lea Febiger, Philadelphia
18. Lindberg JV, Anderson RL, Bumsted RM, Barreras R (1982) Study of intranasal ostium after external dacryocystorhinostomy. Arch Ophthalmol 100:1758–1762
19. Metson R (1990) The endoscopic approach for revision dacryocystorhinostomy. Laryngoscope 100:1344–1347

20. Neuhaus RW, Baylis HI (1983) Cerebrospinal fluid leakage after dacryocystorhinostomy. Ophthalmology 90:1091–1095
21. Onerci M (2002) Dacryocystorhinostomy. Rhinology 40:49–65
22. Orcutt JC, Hillel A, Weymuller EA Jr (1990) Endoscopic repair of failed dacryocystorhinostomy. Ophthal Plast Reconstr Surg 6:197–202
23. Psilas K, Eftaxias V, Kastaniondakis J, Kalogeropoulos C (1993) Silicon intubation as an alternative to dacryocystorhinostomy for nasolacrimal drainage obstruction in adults. Eur J Ophthalmol 3:71–76
24. Shun-Shin GA (1998) Endoscopic dacryocystorhinostomy. Eye 12:467–470
25. Slonim CB, Older JJ, Jones PL (1984) Orbital hemorrhage with proptosis following a dacryocystorhinostomy. Ophthalmic Surg 15:774–775
26. Snead JW, Rathbun JE, Crawford JB (1980) Effects of silicone tube on the canaliculus. An animal experiment. Ophthalmology 87:1031–1036
27. Tsirbas A, McNab AA (2000) Secondary hemorrhage after dacryocystorhinostomy. Clin Exp Ophthalmol 28:22–25
28. Tsirbas A, Davis G, Wormald PJ (2005) Revision dacryocystorhinostomy, Am J Rhinol 19:322–325
29. Vardy SJ, Rose GE (1999) Prevention of cellulitis after open lacrimal surgery. Ophthalmology 107:315–317
30. Walland MJ, Rose GE (1994) The effect of silicone intubation on failure and infection rates after dacryocystorhinostomy. Ophthal Surg 25:597-600
31. Walland MJ, Rose GE (1994) Soft tissue infections after open lacrimal surgery. Ophthalmology 101:608–611
32. Weber R, Draf W, Kolb P (1993) Die endonasale mikrochirurgische Behandlung von Traenenwegsstenosen. HNO 41:11–18
33. Weidenbecher M, Hosemann W, Buhr W (1994) Endoscopic endonasal dacryocystorhinostomy. Ann Otol Rhinol Laryngol 103:363–367
34. Welham RA, Hughes SM (1985) Lacrimal surgery in children. Am J Ophthalmol 99:27–34
35. Welham RAN, Wulc AE (1987) Management of unsuccessful lacrimal surgery. Br J Ophthalmol 71:152–157
36. Whittet HB, Shun-Shin GA, Awdry P (1993) Functional endoscopic transnasal dacryocystorhinostomy. Eye 7:545–549
37. Wong RJ, Glicklich RE, Rubin PAD, Goodman M (1998) Bilateral nasolacrimal duct obstruction managed with endoscopic techniques. Arch Otolaryngol Head Neck Surg 124:703–706
38. Woog JJ, Sindwani R(2006) Endoscopic dacryocystorhinostomy and conjuctivodacryocystorhinostomy. Otolaryngol Clin N Am 39:1001–1017
39. Woog JJ, Kennedy RH, Custer PL, Kaltreider SA, Meyer DR, Camara JG (2001) Endonasal dacryocystorhinostomy: a report by the American Academy of Ophthalmology. Ophthalmology 108:2369–2377
40. Yung MW, Logan BM (1999) The anatomy of the lacrimal bone at the lacrimal bone at the lateral wall of the nose. Clin Otolaryngol 24:262–265
41. Wormald PJ (2006) Powered endoscopic dacryocystorhinostomy. Otolaryngol Clin North Am 39:539–549
42. Zilelioğlu G, Uğurbaş SH, Anadolu Y, Akıner M, Aktürk T (1998) Adjunctive use of mytomicin C on endoscopic lacrimal surgery. Br J Ophthalmol 82:63–66

Chapter 28

Revision Endoscopic Transsphenoidal Hypophysectomy

28

Karen A. Kölln and Brent A. Senior

Core Messages

- A multidisciplinary team should be utilized including an endocrinologist and neuro-ophthalmologist, in addition to the neurosurgeon and otolaryngologist who will be performing the procedure, to maximize perioperative treatment.
- Computed tomography and magnetic resonance imaging should be used as complementary imaging studies.
- Intraoperative stereotactic image guidance is crucial for safe revision endoscopic approaches to the sella.
- Revision endoscopic transsphenoidal hypophysectomy is associated with an increased risk of cerebrospinal fluid leak irrespective of the prior method of resection.

Contents

Introduction

Approaches to the sella have varied greatly over the past 100 years, with Schloffer performing the first transsphenoidal approach to the pituitary in 1907. This was later modified by Cushing in 1914 when he described the sublabial transseptal approach to the sella, but he eventually abandoned this approach secondary to concern for high recurrence rates. With the advent of fluoroscopy and the operating microscope, the sublabial transseptal approach again came into favor in the 1970s, decreasing the overall morbidity associated with accessing the sella via a frontal craniotomy [3]. The next major advancement came in 1992 when Jankowski et al. first reported the successful use of 0 and 30 endoscopes to approach the sella via a transnasal approach, and since that time numerous reports have outlined the surgical technique and overall safety of the procedure [1, 5, 6, 12]. The aim of this chapter is to review revision endoscopic transsphenoidal hypophysectomy, focusing specifically on the indications and preoperative considerations, surgical technique, and complications.

Indications for Surgery

The indications for revision pituitary surgery are similar to those for primary surgery. Recurrence of pituitary lesions can occur months to years following primary resection. Surgical intervention is generally reserved for:

1. Pituitary adenomas that are nonresponsive to medical management.
2. Pituitary masses that cause visual impairment.
3. Lesions that are increasing in size, as evidenced with serial imaging.
4. Pituitary apoplexy.

Pituitary apoplexy is considered a surgical emergency and occurs when necrosis or hemorrhage into pituitary lesions causes abrupt vision loss, headache, cranial neuropathies, and sometimes acute adrenal insufficiency.

Contraindications for Revision Endoscopic Pituitary Surgery

Exclusively suprasellar tumor. Relative contraindications are:

1. Prior craniotomy.
2. Multiply recurrent tumor.

Preoperative Evaluation

Prior to transsphenoidal hypophysectomy a patient should be evaluated by a multidisciplinary team to ensure proper management in the perioperative period. In addition to the neurosurgeon and otolaryngologist who will be performing the procedure, this team should include an endocrinologist and neuro-ophthalmologist.

- Preoperative anesthesia consultation should be considered, especially in those patients with acromegaly and Cushing's disease.

Excessive growth hormone affects the heart, leading to cardiac myopathy, as well as pharyngeal tissue, leading to hypertrophy of the base of tongue and redundant mucosa, creating a potentially difficult intubation, and may require tracheotomy. Patients with Cushing's disease have increased intraoperative anesthetic risk due to their multiple comorbidities including obesity, diabetes, obstructive sleep apnea, and hypertension.

As mentioned, patients with acromegaly may require a temporary tracheotomy to establish a safe airway, and this should also be considered in patients with severe obstructive sleep apnea, as these patients will not be able to use continuous positive airway pressure (CPAP) postoperatively. In addition, the negative pressure from deep breaths associated with an apneic event can lead to pneumocephalus postoperatively. Similarly, wide swings in intracranial pressure occurring during apneic events may increase the risk of postoperative cerebrospinal fluid (CSF) leak.

A detailed history and physical examination should be performed. Special care should be taken to note any history of sinonasal complaints including nasal congestion or obstruction, hyposmia/anosmia, rhinorrhea, postnasal drip, past nasal trauma, and headache. In addition, history of other medical problems that could impact the surgical outcome should be specifically queried including diabetes, hypertension, and obstructive sleep apnea. Review of old operative reports should be performed, noting the type of approach (sublabial transseptal, frontal craniotomy, or endoscopic endonasal), side of approach when applicable, and any perioperative complications. A detailed physical examination should be completed specifically to evaluate for visual field deficits, visual acuity, stigmata of endocrine dysfunction, and cranial neuropathies. Sinonasal endoscopy should be performed in all patients preoperatively to evaluate for septal deviation, nasal polyposis, and purulence.

- Imaging is of utmost importance in preoperative, as well as intraoperative, surgical planning in revision surgery, as scarring can lead to distortion of the anatomy including medialization of the carotid arteries.

Imaging should include the complementary studies of a noncontrasted computed tomography (CT) of the paranasal sinuses with fine (< 3-mm) cuts and a magnetic resonance imaging (MRI) scan of the brain with gadolinium enhancement, including special focus on the pituitary gland. CT of the paranasal sinuses is used to better define the bony anatomy, pneumatization of the sphenoid, presence of a concha bullosa, position and possible dehiscence of the carotid artery, location of the intersinus septum, presence of an Onodi sinus, and extent of postsurgical scarring (Fig. 28.1). MRI of the brain should be used to define the extent and location of the tumor, including cavernous sinus involvement and impingement of the optic nerve/chiasm, and very importantly, to assess for any vascular abnormalities and the location of the carotid arteries (Fig. 28.2). These images should then be fused for intraoperative stereotactic guidance.

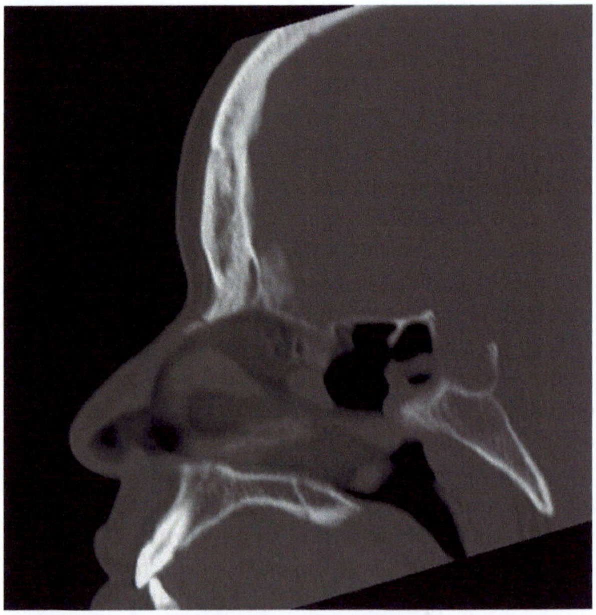

Fig. 28.1 Computed tomography, sagittal view, demonstrating previous resection and scar within the sphenoid

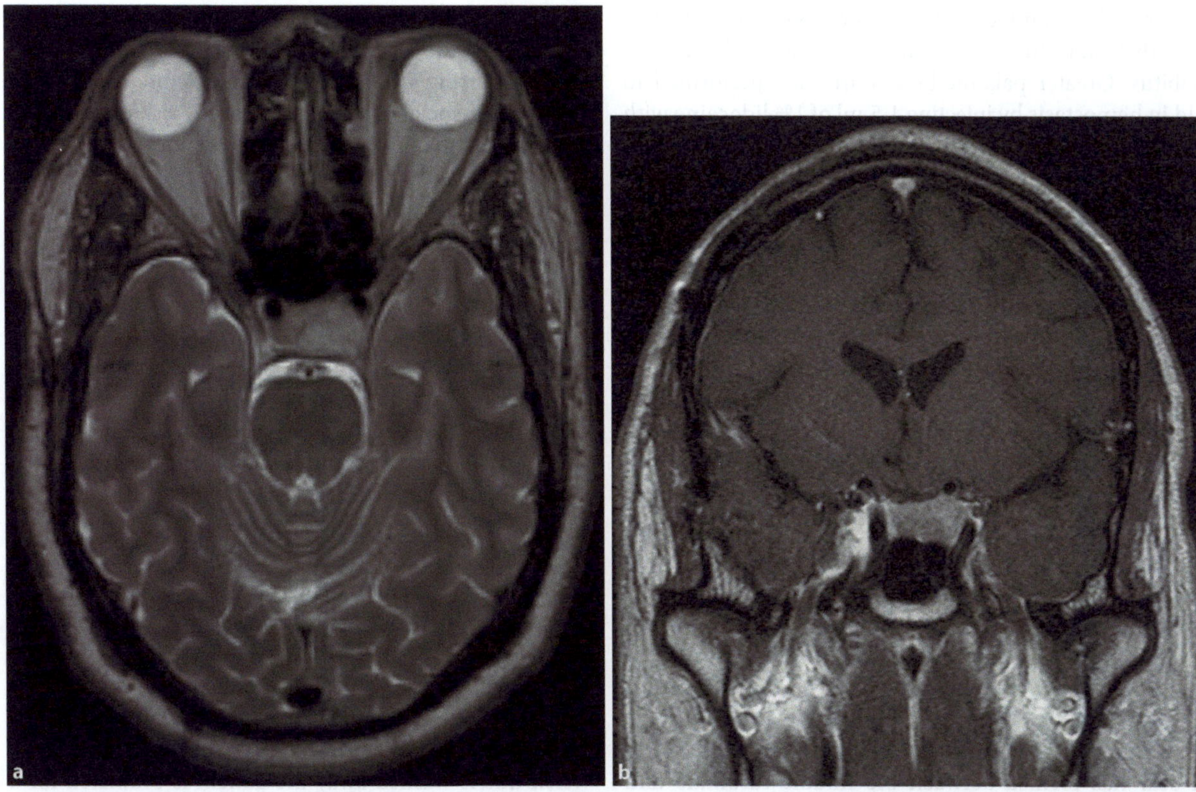

Fig. 28.2 Magnetic resonance image (**a**) axial and (**b**) coronal views of recurrent pituitary adenoma, note the displacement of the carotid arteries

Laboratory data including complete blood count, and a comprehensive metabolic panel to evaluate for hyponatremia, hypokalemia, hypercalcemia and hyperglycemia as well as other metabolic abnormalities should be obtained. Coagulation studies including partial thromboplastin time, prothrombin time, and international normalized ratio should be obtained if there is a family history of bleeding disorders. Endocrine evaluation of prolactin, insulin-like growth factor-1, adrenocorticotropic hormone, thyroid-stimulating hormone, thyroxine, follicle-stimulating hormone, luteinizing hormone, testosterone, morning cortisol, 24-h urine free cortisol, and 24-h urine free cortisol with low-dose dexamethasone suppression should occur as indicated by the clinical scenario [8]. In addition, all of our patients are placed on perioperative steroids due to decreased endogenous steroid production.

Surgical Technique

Standard-length 4-mm endoscopes fitted with scope irrigation are used to approach the sella, as they afford the best visualization and illumination. Angled (45 and occasionally 70) and longer telescopes can be useful in tumor resection and exploration of the sella. When approaching the sella, the surgeon can use a unilateral or bilateral approach. Early in our experience we preferred the unilateral approach, with the side of the approach determined primarily by nasal factors: the presence of septal deviation and concha bullosa, the degree of nasal congestion, and the location of the sphenoid intersinus septum. If all nasal factors are considered equal, the contralateral side usually confers the better angle of approach in lesions that are off the midline or that extend into the cavernous sinus.

- We have found with time that the bilateral approach is usually preferred as this allows wide access to the sella and the ability to use one side for the endoscope while the other is used for instrumentation. In addition, this can be requisite in patients with thin nasal cavities.

The patient is positioned in the "beach-chair" position with the head and torso elevated and the knees bent, and the patient's right arm is tucked by their side. The patient's head rests in a donut (gel or foam) and the head is rotated

15 toward the surgeon. It may be necessary to tilt the bed slightly toward the surgeon in a patient with a large body habitus. Greater palatine blocks are then performed to aid in hemostasis by injecting 1.5 ml of 1% lidocaine with 1:100,000 epinephrine transorally into each greater-palatine canal. The patient is then registered with the stereotactic computer guidance software to ensure safe tumor removal. The abdomen is prepped and draped in a sterile manner in case a fat graft is needed; however, the face is not prepped as the instruments are passed through a contaminated nasal cavity. Under endoscopic guidance, pledgets soaked with 0.05% oxymetazoline hydrochloride are placed into each nasal cavity for decongestion and then additional lidocaine is injected at the junction of the horizontal portion of the basal lamella and the lateral nasal wall to achieve a sphenopalatine artery block. The sphenoid ostium is then identified; a variable amount of scar tissue may be present both intranasally and at the face of the sphenoid.

- We rely heavily on image guidance to aid in the identification of the sphenoid, which can be entirely scarred over.

If scar has formed between the middle turbinate and septum, it is lysed with a cutting instrument. Stapes and J-curettes are utilized initially, and then the opening is serially enlarged using a mushroom punch or Kerrison rongeur. In some cases the sphenoid had been previously packed with fat and this must be carefully cauterized and resected using cutting instruments until the face of the sella is reached (Video 28.1).

- Great care must be taken when resecting tissue within the sphenoid, as the carotid and optic nerves can be dehiscent in 10 and 4% of individuals, respectively [11].

Once the sella has been adequately exposed, the mucosa on the posterior wall of the sphenoid sinus is coagulated with a bipolar cautery. Knowledge of the previous resection and presence of a CSF leak can aid the surgeon at this point for safe entry into the sella. There can be significant bone regrowth and it may be necessary to use a high-speed drill, or else a Kerrison may simply be needed to enlarge the previous opening into the sella. The edges of the window into the sella should be adequately exposed in any case, as demonstrated in Video 28.2. The endoscope is then attached to a fixed pneumatic holder, or an assistant can hold the scope, allowing the operating surgeon both hands for instrumentation. The dura is subsequently cauterized with bipolar cautery and a sickle knife is used to make a cruciate incision. This step again can be encountered with varying difficulty, as the dura may be scarred and it can be difficult to incise into the dura without causing a CSF leak. We have found that revision surgery is associated with an increased risk of CSF leak, regardless of the prior method of resection.

- In revision hypophysectomy the carotid arteries can be tethered medially; at this point the fused MRI and CT images are crucial for safe entrance into the sella and subsequent tumor removal.

The tumor generally bulges through the opening and samples are sent for frozen section. The remaining tumor is removed using neurosurgical ring curettes and suction (Video 28.3). In order to ensure complete tumor removal, the endoscope can be inserted inside the sella and angled telescopes can be used to examine the lateral crevices of the sella. The technique of "hydroscopy," the system of normal saline irrigation under pressure flooding the sella, can be utilized to push the diaphragma up, as well as to wash away debris and clot [13].

Following complete tumor removal, hemostasis is obtained by placing a hemostatic substance, such as microfibrillar collagen in thrombin, over the operative field. When this is washed away the patient is evaluated for a CSF leak.

- If no CSF leak is encountered we have found that reconstruction of the sella is not necessary.

In our report in 2003 we determined that there was no increase in the rate of postoperative leak (0.4% compared to reported rates of 0.8–6.4%) and there were no cases of meningitis or empty-sella syndrome [15]. If a CSF leak is encountered, we reconstruct the sella by using microfibrillar collagen and a fat graft bolstered by an absorbable miniplate cut to fit under the edges of the sella.

Tips to Avoid Complications

1. Meticulous dissection should be performed, as incomplete resection is associated with an increased risk of hemorrhage into the tumor.
2. Consider temporary tracheotomy in patients with obstructive sleep apnea to minimize the risk of postoperative pneumocephalus and reduce the risk of postoperative CSF leak. In addition, consideration for tracheotomy should be made since CPAP will not be able to be utilized during the postoperative period.
3. Perioperative steroids are critical in all patients, given the disruption in endogenous steroid production.

Complications

There are numerous complications associated with pituitary surgery, regardless of whether or not the patient has had previous surgery. The mortality rate associated with pituitary surgery is less than 1%, with the most common causes of death being (1) hemorrhage into an incompletely resected pituitary tumor and (2) medical complications (deep vein thrombosis, pulmonary embolus and myocardial infarction) [2]. Medical complications are found in patients with Cushing's disease, and these patients should be regarded with an increased risk of perioperative mortality.

Major complications of pituitary surgery include:

1. Carotid injury.
2. Intracranial hemorrhage.
3. Meningitis.

The carotid artery is at risk during pituitary surgery due to its tortuosity, and can be especially at risk during revision surgery where scarring can further distort its normal course along the skull base. Intraoperative damage to the carotid artery occurs with an incidence of 0.78–1.16% [7], and should it occur, the area should be packed and an angiogram should be emergently performed and intervention performed as deemed necessary. Even if the angiogram is initially normal, it should be repeated on postoperative day 6–10 to ensure there is no false aneurysm or carotid-cavernous fistula [10]. Intracranial hemorrhage occurs with an incidence of 0.4–3% and most commonly in the setting of incomplete removal of a macroadenoma, underscoring the need for meticulous and complete tumor removal [17].

Meningitis occurs with an incidence of 0.15–1.2% and has been associated with preoperative sinusitis and postoperative CSF leak. All patients should be evaluated for signs of acute sinusitis preoperatively, and if purulence is visualized the patient should be treated aggressively with antibiotics. If the procedure is considered elective, it should be postponed until the infection has resolved [16]. Chronic sinusitis does not increase the risk of meningitis per se; however, if there is any suspicious mucous within the nasal cavity a culture should be obtained and the patient should be treated.

The most common major complication that occurs following transsphenoidal pituitary surgery is CSF leak. This is especially common, as seen in our experience, in revision surgery. This is thought to be because the diaphragma has become scarred and tenuous and/or because more extensive resection is required due to the recurrent tumor itself. CSF leak has also been associated with large suprasellar tumors where the diaphragma becomes thin and incompetent. If the fistula is noted during the procedure, repair should be performed to decrease the risk of postoperative meningitis. When this occurs postoperatively, the patient may be treated conservatively with bedrest and head elevation, or more aggressively with lumbar puncture and/or surgical exploration. Some authors advocate early surgical intervention, proposing the following benefits: (1) decreased risk of developing meningitis for those who fail conservative management, (2) avoiding the risk associated with a lumbar drain, and (3) potentially a decreased hospital stay [14].

Endocrine complications are common in the postoperative period, with diabetes insipidus (DI) occurring with the highest frequency. Revision surgery is not a risk factor for developing DI; however, the presence of a Rathke's cleft cyst is, and these are apt to recur. In most instances DI is transient in nature and patients are able to sustain enough oral intake, negating the need for medical intervention. However, if it is sustained or symptomatic, DDAVP (desamino-8-arginine vasopressin) is used, and these patients should be followed closely by their endocrinologist after discharge from the hospital [9].

Finally, endonasal complications such as septal perforation, nasal obstruction, and sinusitis occur with a low frequency. We believe this is due to the fact the nose is left largely undisturbed, especially laterally, allowing for continued normal function of the paranasal sinuses. In addition, it has been found that patients undergoing revision endoscopic surgery who had undergone a prior sublabial approach found their recovery to be overall better with the endoscopic approach, with less pain and better nasal airflow. Also, those patients who had nasal packing in place postoperatively had a significantly worse postoperative experience than those who did not [4].

Conclusion

Endoscopic transsphenoidal hypophysectomy is overall a safe procedure. Revision surgery, although it may be technically challenging and is associated with an increased risk of CSF fistula, can also be performed in a safe and effective manner. Care should be taken, however, to avoid complications by meticulous preoperative preparation, intraoperative stereotactic image guidance, careful and thorough tumor resection, and heightened awareness of possible CSF fistula.

References

1. Cappabianca P, Cavall LM, de Divitiis E (2004) Endoscopic endonasal transsphenoidal surgery. Neurosurgery 55:933–941

2. Ciric I, Ragin A, Baumgartner C, et al. (1997) Complications of transsphenoidal surgery: results of a national survey, review of the literature and personal experience. Neurosurgery 40:223–237
3. Couldwell WT (2004) Transsphenoidal and transcranial surgery for pituitary adenomas. J Neurooncol 69:237–256
4. Dusick JR, Esposito F, Mattozo CA, et al. (2006) Endonasal transsphenoidal surgery: the patient's perspective – survey results from 259 patients. Surg Neurol 65:332–342
5. Jankowski R, Auque J, Simon C, et al. (1992) Endoscopic pituitary surgery. Laryngoscope 102:198–202
6. Jho HD, Carrau RL, Ko Y, et al. (1997) Endoscopic pituitary surgery: an early experience. Surg Neurol 47:213–223
7. Laws ER (1999) Vascular complications of transsphenoidal surgery. Pituitary 2:163–170
8. Nemergut EC, Dumont AS, Barry UT, et al. (2005) Perioperative management of patients undergoing transsphenoidal pituitary surgery. Anesth Analg 101:1170–1181
9. Nemergut ED, Zuo Z, Jane JA, et al. (2005) Predictors of diabetes insipidus after transsphenoidal surgery: a review of 881 patients. J Neurosurg 103:448–454
10. Raymond J, Hardy J, Czepko R, et al. (1997) Arterial injuries in transsphenoidal surgery for pituitary adenoma: the role of angiography and endovascular treatment. Am J Neuroradiol 18:655–665
11. Renn WH, Rhoton AL Jr (1975) Microsurgical anatomy of sellar region. J Neurosurg 43:288–298
12. Rosen MR, Saigal K, Evans J, Keane WM (2006) A review of the endoscopic approach to the pituitary through the sphenoid sinus. Curr Opin Otolaryngol Head Neck Surg 14:6–13
13. Senior BA, Dubin MG, Sonnenburg RE, et al. (2005) Increased role of the otolaryngologist in endoscopic pituitary surgery: endoscopic hydroscopy of the sella. Am J Rhinol 19:181–184
14. Shiley SG, Lionadi F, Delashaw JB, et al. (2003) Incidence, etiology and management of cerebrospinal fluid leaks following trans-sphenoidal surgery. Laryngoscope 113:1283–1288
15. Sonnenburg RE, White D, Ewend MG, et al. (2003) Sellar reconstruction: is it necessary? Am J Rhinol 17:343–346
16. van Aken MO, Feelders RA, de Marie S, et al. (2004) Cerebrospinal fluid leakage during transsphenoidal surgery: postoperative external lumbar drainage reduces the risk for meningitis. Pituitary 7:89–93
17. Woollons AC, Balakrishnan V, Hunn MK, et al. (2000) Complications of transsphenoidal surgery: the Wellington experience. Aust N Z J Surg 70:405–410

Chapter 29

Revision Image-Guided Functional Endoscopic Sinus Surgery

29

Martin J. Citardi and Pete S. Batra

Disclosure: Dr. Citardi was a member a consult for CBYON (Mountain View, CA) in 1999–2003. He has been a consultant for GE Healthcare Technologies (Waukesha, WI, USA) since 2003.

Core Messages

- Image-guided surgery (IGS) incorporates both computer-enabled review of preoperative imaging and intraoperative surgical navigation. Rhinologists have embraced IGS as a technological means to reduce surgical morbidity and improve surgical outcomes.
- All IGS systems share similar hardware (computer workstation, display monitor, tracking system, and surgical navigation) and software (data management, image review, surgical navigation) components.
- Registration is the process through which a surgical navigation system establishes a one-to-one mapping relationship between corresponding points in the operating field volume and the imaging data set volume.
- Registration protocols may be classified as paired-point, automatic, and contour-based.
- Surgical navigation is best assessed through determinations of target registration error (TRE). In the clinical realm, the surgeon estimates TRE by localizing against known anatomic landmarks.
- The American Academy of Otolaryngology – Head and Neck Surgery has issued a position statement that endorses the use of IGS at the discretion of the operating surgeon in sinus and skull-base surgery.
- Currently, IGS is commonly employed for revision endoscopic sinus surgery involving the ethmoid, frontal, and sphenoid sinuses. IGS is also useful in cases of sinonasal polyposis. In the setting of previous orbital and skull-base injury, IGS can provide critical information.
- Although prospective, randomized clinical trials for IGS have not been performed, published reports describe the consensus that IGS reduces morbidity and improves outcomes.

Contents

Introduction

Since its introduction more than two decades ago, functional endoscopic sinus surgery (FESS) [17,18] has emerged as the preferred surgical modality for the management of chronic rhinosinusitis (CRS) refractory to medical treatment. Even under ideal circumstances, approximately 10–15% of patients who undergo FESS will develop recalcitrant CRS [9], and an even smaller proportion of these patients will require one or more revision FESS procedures. Rhinologists universally acknowledge that these revision FESS procedures are technically more challenging and carry a greater risk of major and minor complications. Both significant inflammatory burden and previous procedures serve to obscure surgical landmarks. Thus, rhinologists have embraced computer-aided surgery (CAS) technology as a means to improve outcomes and reduce morbidity.

The term "image-guided surgery" (IGS) has come to refer to CAS in FESS. It should be remembered IGS incorporates computer-enabled review of preoperative imaging and intraoperative surgical navigation. Early IGS systems were cumbersome and their surgical navigation accuracy was suboptimal; however, more recent IGS platforms support a user-friendly interface and more robust navigation. In addition, the image quality has improved considerably compared with first-generation systems from more than 10 years ago. The availability of the technology is now quite good. Consequently, rhinologists now routinely incorporate IGS into most revision sinus surgery cases.

System Components

Image-guidance vendors often try to highlight the unique aspects of their respective systems. Although this may serve as a useful sales tactic, all IGS systems share certain similar components (Table 29.1).

Hardware

The computer workstation is the central component of all IGS systems as it supports the software that drives the entire process. The original operating system for many IGS systems was UNIX; newer systems utilize other operating systems, including Windows 2000, Windows XP, and LINUX. The keyboard and the standard computer mouse serve as input devices. A standard computer monitor allows for output of visual information from the system. Newer systems with high-resolution, flat-panel, liquid crystal display screens afford enhanced capabilities for review of image data sets.

The tracking system allows for monitoring of the relative position of the surgical instruments. Current commercially available systems rely on electromagnetic or optical tracking technology. For electromagnetic tracking, an electromagnetic receiver provides positional information in an electromagnetic field generated by a specific emitter attached to the patient. For an optical tracking system, an overhead camera array, termed the digitizer, tracks the position of light-emitting diodes (LEDs; or reflective spheres in a passive system).

Specific surgical instrumentation can be tracked in the operative field by its attachment to an intraoperative localization device (ILD). In an optical system, the ILD is an array of LEDs (or reflective spheres), and in an electromagnetic system, the ILD is an electromagnetic sensor. Almost any instrument can be adapted for intraoperative surgical navigation, including straight and curved suction, through-cutting forceps, soft-tissue shavers, and drills.

Data transfer hardware facilitates transfer of the preoperative dataset to the computer station. This can be achieved through network linking between the computer and the radiology department. Alternatively, the data can be transferred via commonly available digital media, including CD-ROM and DVD.

Table 29.1 Image-guided surgery (IGS) system hardware components

Item	Details
Computer workstation	Unix, Windows 2000, Windows XP, LINUX
Display system	Video monitor (cathode-ray tube monitor, high-resolution, flat-panel display)
Tracking system	Electromagnetic system, optical system
Surgical instrumentation	Straight and curved suction, cutting forceps, soft-tissue shavers, drills
Data transfer hardware	Computer network, CD-ROM, DVD

Software

User-friendly software is an integral component of a robust IGS system; it integrates the various hardware components for optimal surgical navigation and other related applications. In general, discussions surrounding IGS focus on intraoperative navigation. IGS offers numerous software tools that facilitate complex 3D manipulation of the preoperative data set. These software tools allow precise preoperative review of images to understand the vital 3D anatomic relationships that simply cannot be obtained by standard light-box review of radiographic images. This facilitates careful and detailed surgical planning, which can be instrumental for revision image-guided FESS (IG-FESS).

Registration

Registration is the process through which a surgical navigation system establishes a one-to-one mapping relationship between corresponding points in the operating field volume and imaging data set volume. Three basic paradigms for registration are commercially available: paired-point registration (PPR), automatic registration (AR), and contour-based registration (CBR; Table 29.2). Although specific approaches to registration are commonly associated with specific hardware, such an association is not intrinsic to the registration paradigm; rather, these associations reflect decisions made during the design of surgical navigation systems. Regardless of the registration paradigm, the principles that govern surgical navigation are similar.

Table 29.2 Registration paradigms

Registration paradigm	Concept	Steps
Paired-point registration	Manual mapping of corresponding points forms the basis for an alignment of the preoperative imaging volume and intraoperative surgical field volume	1. The surgeon selects fiducial points in the preoperative imaging volume (alternatively, software automatically locates external fiducial markers). 2. The surgeon places a tracking device on the patient. 3. The surgeon calibrates the surgical probe. 4. The surgeon localizes each corresponding fiducial point. 5. The computer calculates the registration. 6. The surgeon confirms surgical navigation accuracy.
Automatic registration	Patient wears a headset with built-in fiducial markers at the time of the preoperative imaging and surgery. The headset is designed so that it positioning is reproducible each time that it is placed upon the patient. Thus, the relationships between the fiducial points and the patient are the same during image acquisition and surgery. At surgery, the computer locates the fiducial points in the imaging data and calculates the registration.	1. The patient wears a special headset with fiducial markers during image acquisition and surgery. 2. The computer automatically locates the fiducial points in the imaging data set and then calculates the registration. 3. The surgeon places a tracking device on the patient. 4. The surgeon calibrates the surgical probe. 5. The surgeon confirms surgical navigation accuracy.
Contour-based registration	The computer builds a 3D model based upon the preoperative imaging. During registration, the surgeon localizes contours on the patient, and the computer fits the points on these contours to the contours defined by the 3D model.	1. The computer builds a 3D model of the patient. 2. The surgeon places a tracking system on the patient. 3. The surgeon calibrates the surgical probe. 4. The surgeon performs a rough paired-point registration. 5. The surgeon localizes points on contours on the patient. 6. The computer calculates the registration. 7. The surgeon confirms surgical navigation accuracy.

The term "calibration" should not be used interchangeably with the term "registration." Calibration is the process for confirming or defining the relationship of an instrument tip and a tracking device. Calibration must be performed independently of the registration process for intraoperative surgical navigation.

Paired-Point Registration

PPR requires three steps. First, the fiducial points must be identified in the preoperative imaging data set. Various types of fiducial markers may be used for PPR. External fiducial markers may be anchored to bone with screws or to skin with adhesive. Automated software routines may identify those external fiducial markers in the preoperative imaging data set, or the surgeon may manually identify the points at the computer workstation. Alternatively, the surgeon may select anatomic landmarks to serve as fiducial points. Next, the surgeon manually localizes each fiducial point in the patient volume with the navigation probe. Finally, the computer software performs the registration by aligning corresponding points in the preoperative imaging data set and the operative field volume.

Automatic Registration

AR depends upon the fiducial headset, which is designed so that its positioning on the patient is reproducible. Because of this unique feature, the relationship between the fiducial array built into the fiducial headset and the patient is the same each time the headset is placed upon the patient. For registration, the software automatically identifies the fiducial markers in the headset worn by the patient at the time of preoperative imaging, and then calculates registration. At the time of surgery, it is assumed that the positioning of the headset is functionally identical at the time of preoperative imaging and surgery.

Contour-Based Registration

CBR is similar to PPR in that the surgeon must manually map points in the surgical volume. For CBR, the computer builds a 3D model from the preoperative imaging data. Then, the surgeon must identify corresponding contours on the surface of the surgical volume. In most systems, this step requires an initial approximate PPR with three anatomic fiducial points; subsequently, the surgeon runs the surgical probe across contours on the surface of the surgical volume to identify 40–500 discrete points. Rather than a fixed probe, a laser-based device may also serve to identify this contour, or a flexible grid of LEDs may be placed on the surface. These devices serve simply to define a surface contour, much as the task of running a rigid tracked probe across a surface defines a contour. Finally, the software aligns corresponding contours in the preoperative imaging volume and the surgical field volume to create the registration.

Assessment of Surgical Navigation Accuracy

Registration error theory [24] provides a framework for the discussion of the assessment of surgical navigation accuracy. Target registration error (TRE) provides the most clinically useful information, since it describes the difference between the measured position of an instrument tip (i.e., the indicated position in the preoperative imaging volume) and its position in the real world. Unfortunately reports of surgical navigation error in the otolaryngology literature are quite inconsistent; thus, it can be difficult to summarize surgical navigation accuracy, because different reports often use different nomenclature and methods to measure and report accuracy [20]

In the operating room, the surgeon must visually estimate TRE at different anatomic regions throughout the case. TRE can differ in different parts of the operating field volume, and mechanical slippage of the headset and similar hardware issues may increase TRE. Thus, it is important to continuously assess surgical navigation, since an unrecognized increase in TRE can lead to catastrophic complications. Visual estimates of TRE can be problematic when one considers that they are obtained under endoscopic visualization, which only provides a 2D, wide-angled (i.e., with some spherical distortion) view of a complex 3D space. As a result, TRE should be estimated by assessing its individual vector components (x-axis, y-axis, z-axis) independently. For example, the medial orbit, superior maxillary wall (the orbital floor), and the posterior maxillary wall can provide TRE information for the x-axis (medial–lateral), y-axis (superior–inferior), and z-axis (depth) directions, respectively.

Most published reports present only TRE for specific systems. Representative studies are summarized in Table 29.3. Several recent reports have highlighted comparisons of registration protocols. Hardy et al. examined TRE for PPR with bone-anchored fiducial markers, CBR with skin contours, and PPR with anatomic fiducial landmarks in a cadaveric model for endoscopic sinus surgery using a VectorVision surgical navigation system (BrainLab, Munich, Germany) [14]. Both PPR with bone-anchored fiducial markers and CBR yielded mean TRE values that were lower than corresponding TRE values from PPR with anatomic fiducial points, but TRE values for PPR with bone-anchored fiducial markers and CBR were statistically similar. Metzger et al. compared PPR with bone-anchored fiducial markers, CBR with skin contours, PPR with bone anatomic landmarks, and PPR for a simulated intraoral appliance in a cadaveric model for three surgical navigation platforms: VectorVision (BrainLab, Munich, Germany), Voxim (IVS Solutions, Chemintz, Germany), and StealthStation (Medtronic, Jacksonville, FL, USA) [28]. They reported TRE values of 1.13 ± 0.05 mm, 2.03 ± 0.07 mm, 3.17 ± 0.10 mm, and 3.79 ± 0.13 mm respectively. Differences between registration protocols were deemed statistically significant; however, each surgical navigation platform yielded similar TRE values for each registration protocol. Admittedly, this project was optimized for assessing navigational errors for craniomaxillofacial surgery. However, it does provide TRE information that is also relevant for rhinologic surgery.

Empiric data, theoretical considerations and anecdotal evidence all corroborate common principles for reducing TRE [36]: (1) observed TRE will be lowest at the centroid (point whose *x,y,z* coordinates are the mean values of the *x,y,z* coordinates of the fiducial points); that is, the observed TRE will be lowest at the center of the space defined by the fiducial points, (2) fiducial points should be spread in 3D space to provide maximum information for registration, (3) similarly, distances between fiducial points should be maximized, and (4) greater numbers of fiducial points yield lower TREs, although the incremental benefit of additional points decreases as the number of points increases.

Preoperative Considerations and Surgical Indications

The American Academy of Otolaryngology – Head and Neck Surgery (AAO-HNS) has published an official position statement on the utility of IGS:

"The American Academy of Otolaryngology – Head and Neck Surgery (AAO-HNS) endorses the intraoperative use of computer-aided surgery in appropriately select cases to assist the surgeon in clarifying complex anatomy during sinus and skull-base surgery. There is sufficient expert consensus opinion and literature evidence base to support this position. This technology is used at the discretion of the operating surgeon and is not experimental or investigational. Furthermore, the AAO-HNS is of the opinion that it is impossible to corroborate this with Level 1 evidence. These appropriate, specialty-specific, and surgically indicated procedural services should be reimbursed whether used by neurosurgeons or other qualified physicians regardless of the specialty." [1]

The currently accepted indications for the use of IGS as advocated by AAO-HNS are listed in Table 29.4.

Specific Applications

Surgical navigation has emerged as an important part of revision FESS at most centers. Although it has been dif-

Table 29.3 Reported target registration error for commercially available IGS platforms for sinus surgery. *CBR* Contour-based registration, *N/A* registration protocol not available for the specific system, *PPR* paired-point registration

System (vendor)	Tracking hardware	Registration type	Reported accuracy
InstaTrak GE Navigation and Visualization Lawrence, MA, USA	Electromagnetic	Automatic	2.28 mm (95% CI 2.02–2.53) [12]
		PPR	1.97 mm (95% CI 1.75–2.23) [12]
		CBR with touch	1.5 ±0.3 mm [19]
Landmarx Medtronic Xomed Jacksonville, FL, USA	Optical	Automatic	N/A
		PPR	1.69 ± 0.38 mm [26]
		CBR	No report
Stryker Navigation System Stryker-Leibinger Kalamazoo, MI, USA	Optical	Automatic	N/A
		PPR	1.6 mm (range 0.6–3.7) [34]
		CBR ("Mask")	2.22 ± 0.91 mm [3]
VectorVision BrainLAB Hemstetten, Germany	Optical	Automatic	No report
		PPR	1.57 ± 1.1 mm [5]
		CBR with laser	2.4 ± 1.7 mm [4]

ficult to objectively document the positive impact of IGS on FESS (see "Outcomes" below), most rhinologic surgeons have concluded that it is helpful in most instances and thus routinely include it for the more complex cases. The utility of IGS for sinus surgery is best illustrated by considering specific cases that demonstrate the technology in action (Figs. 29.1–29.5).

It must be emphasized that the true value of IGS begins before surgery commences. IGS provides a platform for computer-enabled review of preoperative imaging and thus serves as a platform for preoperative surgical planning.

Ethmoid Surgery

During revision endoscopic ethmoidectomy, the surgeon completes a surgical dissection in a field that has been distorted by long-standing inflammatory processes as well as one or more surgical procedures. Achievement of the surgical objectives requires comprehension of the number, shape, and configuration of residual ethmoid cells (Fig. 29.1a). In addition, recognition of the limits of surgical dissection (i.e., the skull base and orbit) is critical (Fig. 29.1b).

Frontal Sinus Surgery

Numerous rhinologic surgeons have commented upon the complexity of endoscopic frontal sinusotomy, and daily anecdotal experiences easily corroborate these teachings. The key to successful endoscopic frontal sinusotomy is the appreciation of frontal recess pneumatization patterns. Today, those pneumatization patterns have been characterized in a clinically useful way through systematic study of frontal recess anatomy at a computer workstation with software for review of archived high-resolution computed tomography (CT) data [21]. Thus, it is logical to use the computer workstation for preoperative review of frontal recess anatomy.

During surgery, surgical navigation can greatly facilitate complete endoscopic dissection of an even heavily scarred frontal recess [8]. In many revision endoscopic frontal sinusotomy cases, the middle turbinate remnant fuses to a partially collapsed frontal recess. In this situation (as in others) the endoscopic view alone does not portray the anatomy "in depth;" that is, the endoscope alone cannot indicate the structures beneath a healed mucosal surface. The addition of surgical navigation gives the surgeon information about the structures beyond the healed mucosal surface. This can be especially important in the frontal recess, where residual frontal recess cells may be "stacked" (Fig. 29.2a). In some cases, the frontal recess may be obstructed by amorphous scarring that smoothly blends into the adjacent skull base and orbit; in this situation, intraoperative surgical navigation is invaluable (Fig. 29.2b).

IGS also has been incorporated into traditional techniques for frontal sinus surgery, including frontal sinus trephination and osteoplastic frontal sinusotomy. Melroy et al. analyzed the role of IGS for osteoplastic frontal sinusotomy in a cadaveric model that compared IGS, traditional Caldwell radiographs, and transillumination [25]. In this report, IGS was deemed more accurate than the two other alternatives in determining the extent of frontal-sinus pneumatization, and importantly, IGS did not seem to overestimate frontal size. In a clinical report, Zacharek et al. presented a series of 13 patients in whom placement of the frontal sinus trephine was planned through intraoperative surgical navigation [37].

Sphenoid Sinus Surgery

Surgical navigation also plays an important role in almost all endoscopic procedures performed on the sphenoid sinus [7]. Because of the asymmetry and variability of sphenoid anatomy as well as the proximity of critical adjacent structures, sphenoid surgery carries the risk of major complications. In the situation where there has been previous surgery, the potential for major complications is even greater. Surgical navigation gives localization above the relatively simple cues afforded by endoscopic visual-

Table 29.4 Clinical indications for the use of IGS

- Revision sinus surgery
- Distorted sinus anatomy of developmental, postoperative, or traumatic origin
- Extensive sinonasal polyposis
- Pathology involving the frontal, posterior ethmoid, and sphenoid sinuses
- Disease abutting the skull base, orbit, optic nerve, or carotid artery
- Cerebrospinal fluid rhinorrhea or conditions where there is a skull-base defect
- Benign and malignant sinonasal neoplasms

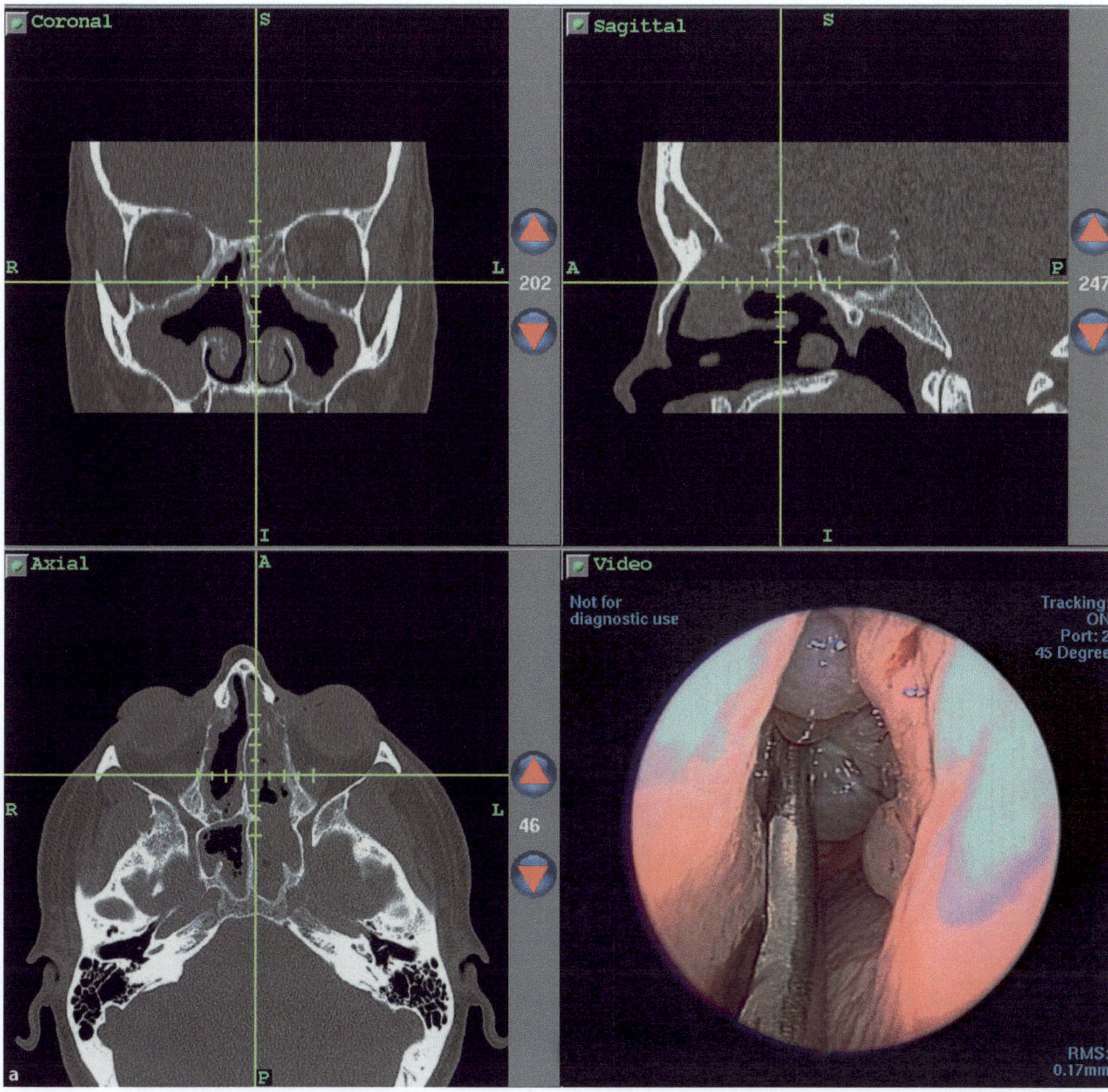

Fig. 29.1 **a** In this screen capture obtained with the InstaTrak 3500 Plus (GE Healthcare Navigation and Visualization, Lawrence, MA, USA) during revision endoscopic ethmoidectomy, the surgical aspirator is positioned in the posterior ethmoid. Simultaneous review of the coronal, sagittal, and axial computed tomography (CT) images provides information about the number, shape, and configuration of residual ethmoid partitions, as well as their relationship to the orbit and skull base. (*b continued next page*)

ization, and thus, it is an important tool for safe revision endoscopic sphenoidotomy (Fig. 29.3).

Previous Complications

Obviously any procedure performed on the paranasal sinuses may lead to disruption of the skull base and orbit with potentially catastrophic consequences. In most instances, appropriate recognition and treatment will minimize the immediate morbidity (and mortality) of these complications, but some of these patients will require revision procedures for persistent and recurrent inflammatory disease. In these instances, it is critical to recognize occult orbital and skull-base dehiscences, which can be found under intact mucosal boundaries. With surgi-

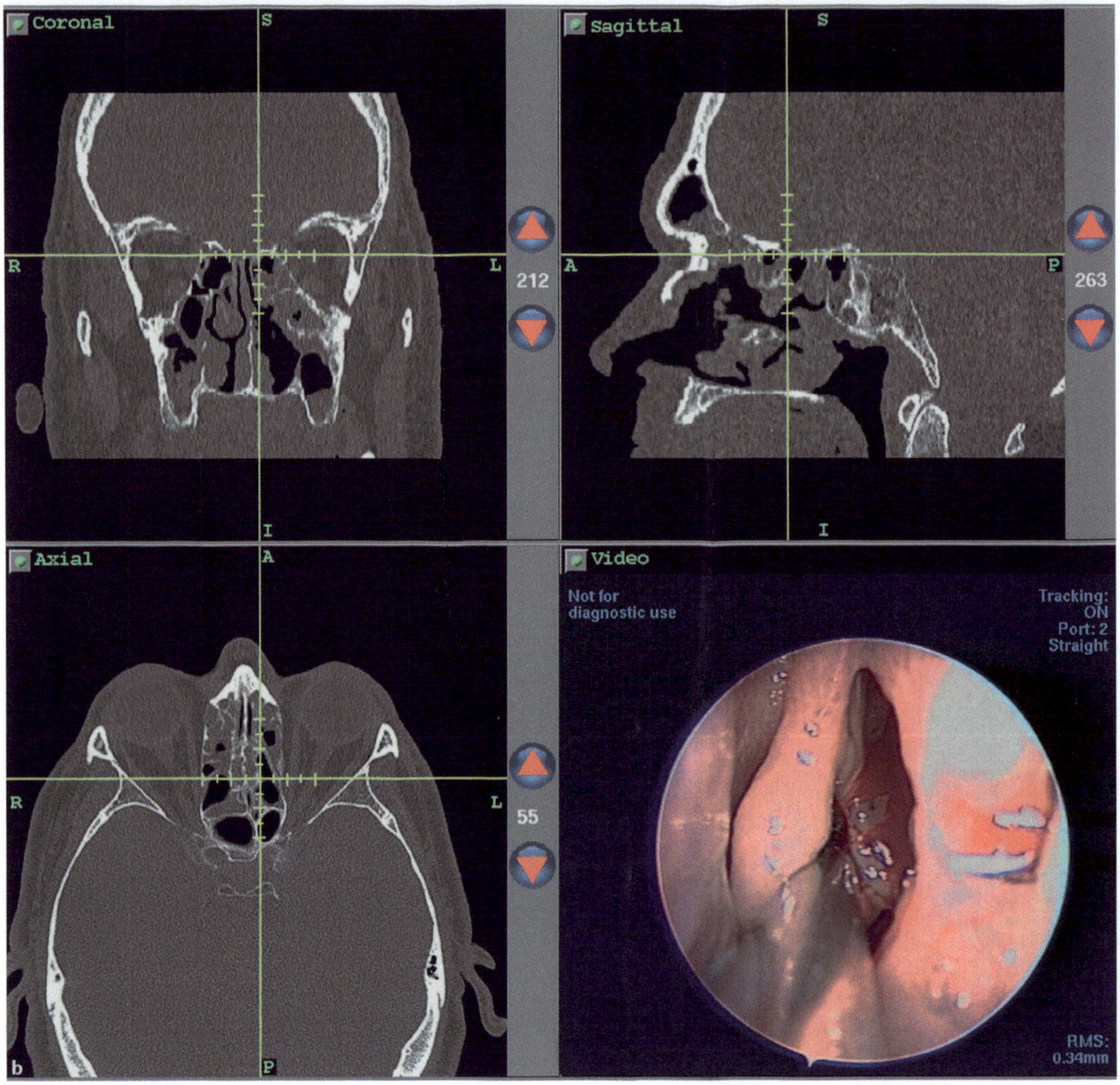

Fig. 29.1 (*continued*) **b** Skull-base identification is a critical step during revision endoscopic ethmoidectomy. In many cases it is possible to pass a tracked instrument through the previously dissected ethmoid to the skull base, as shown in this screen capture obtained with the InstaTrak 3500 Plus. This maneuver provides immediate information about depth, a cue whose importance is only recognized when one remembers that the view provided by the nasal endoscopes is only 2D

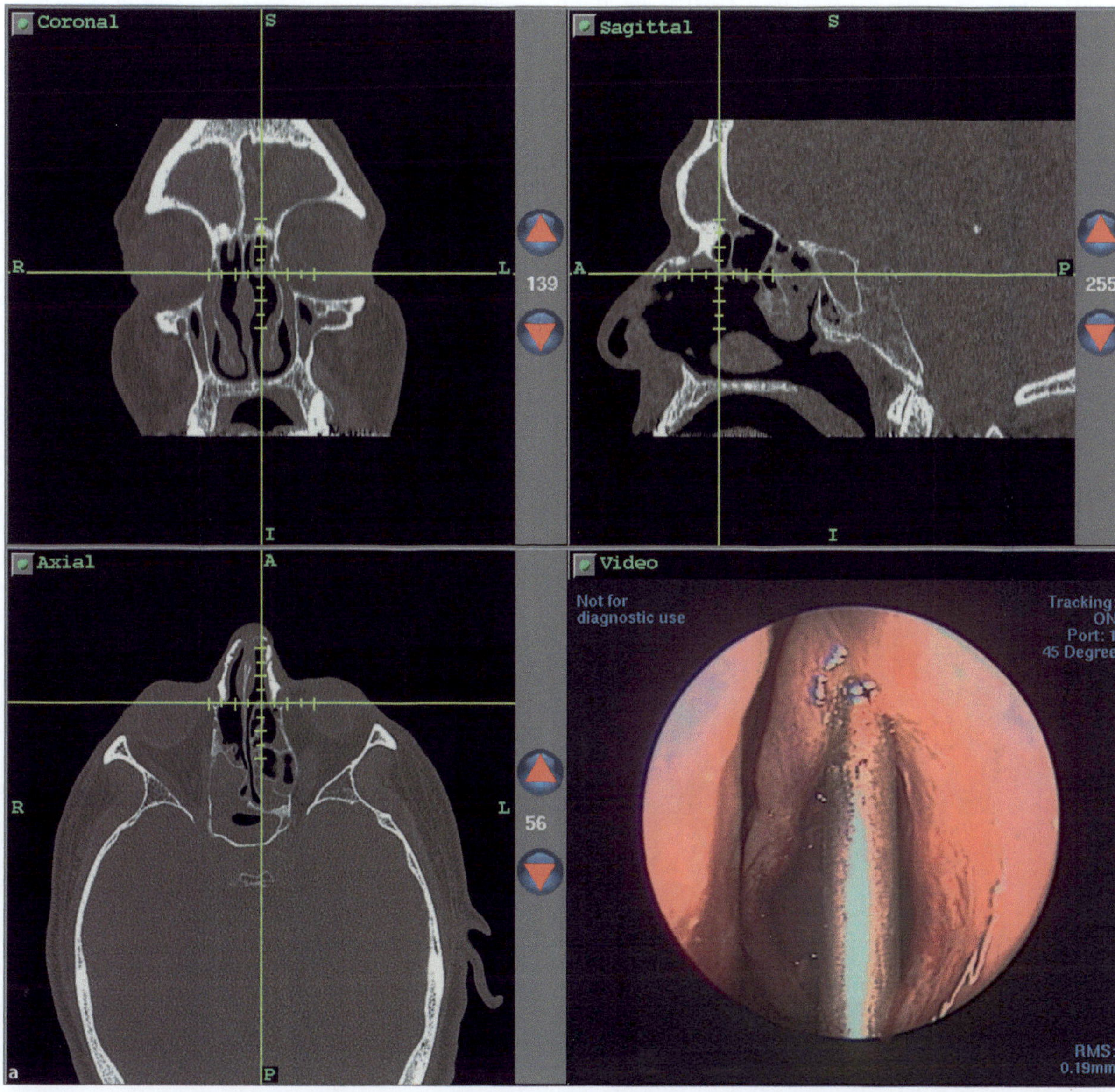

Fig. 29.2 **a** In this screen capture obtained with the InstaTrak 3500 Plus during revision endoscopic frontal sinusotomy, the instrument tip has been placed at the floor of the residual agger nasi cell. In the endoscopic view, it appears as if the instrument is resting upon the fusion point for a partial resected middle turbinate that has partially lateralized; however, the navigation views more accurately depict the true anatomy. *b continued next page)*

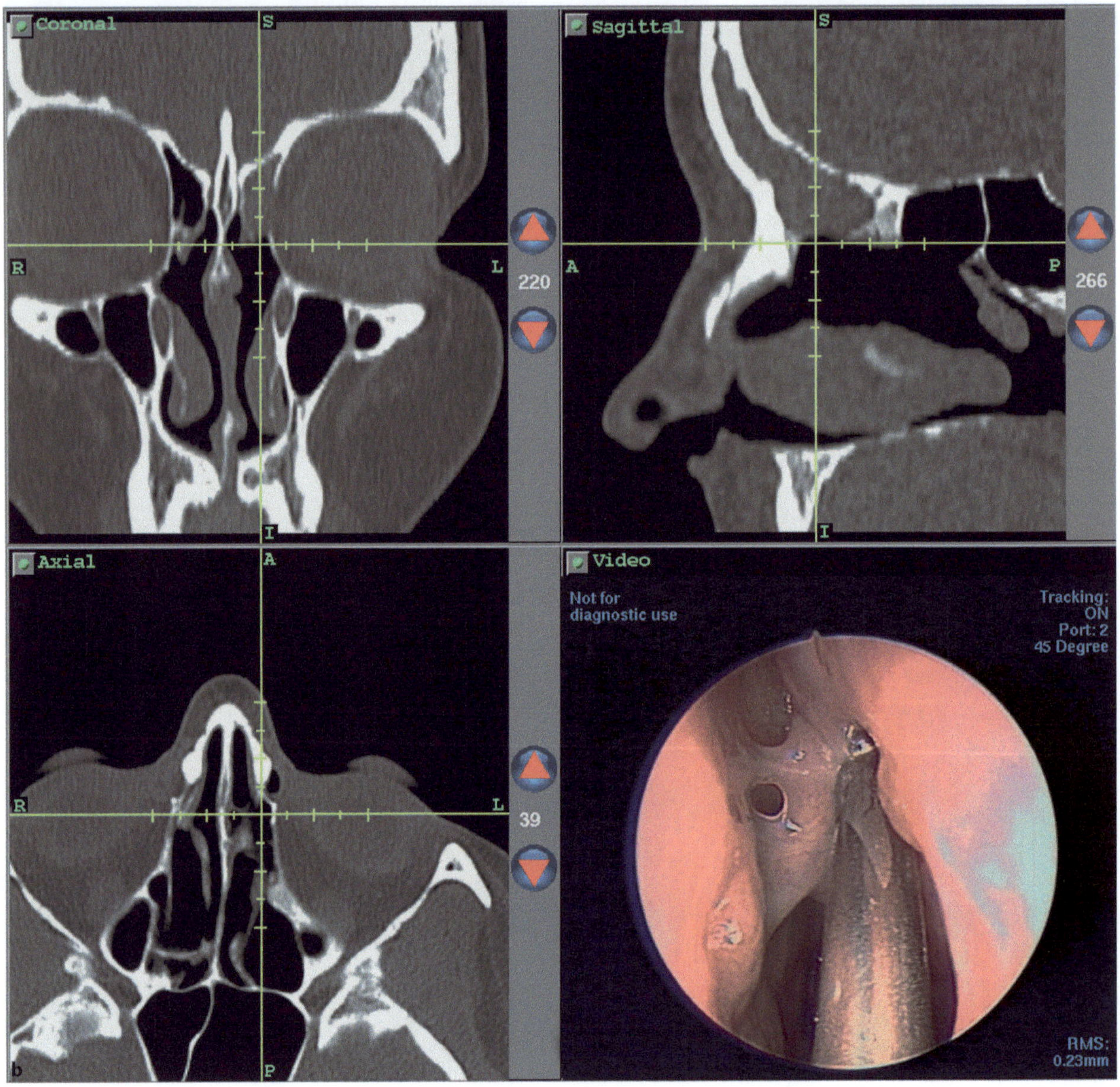

Fig. 29.2 (*continued*) **b** In this case, the left frontal sinus has been completely obstructed by scarring. The endoscopic view alone indicates a rather amorphous lump in the frontal recess; the key step is to distinguish the obstructed frontal recess tract (which is covered in scar) from the adjacent skull base and orbit. It is difficult to assess the entry point for revision endoscopic frontal sinusotomy from endoscopic visual cues alone. Surgical navigation can simplify this situation, since it can quickly demonstrate the position of the instrument tip relative to the obstructed frontal recess, the orbit, and the skull base, as demonstrated in this screen capture obtained with InstaTrak 3500 Plus

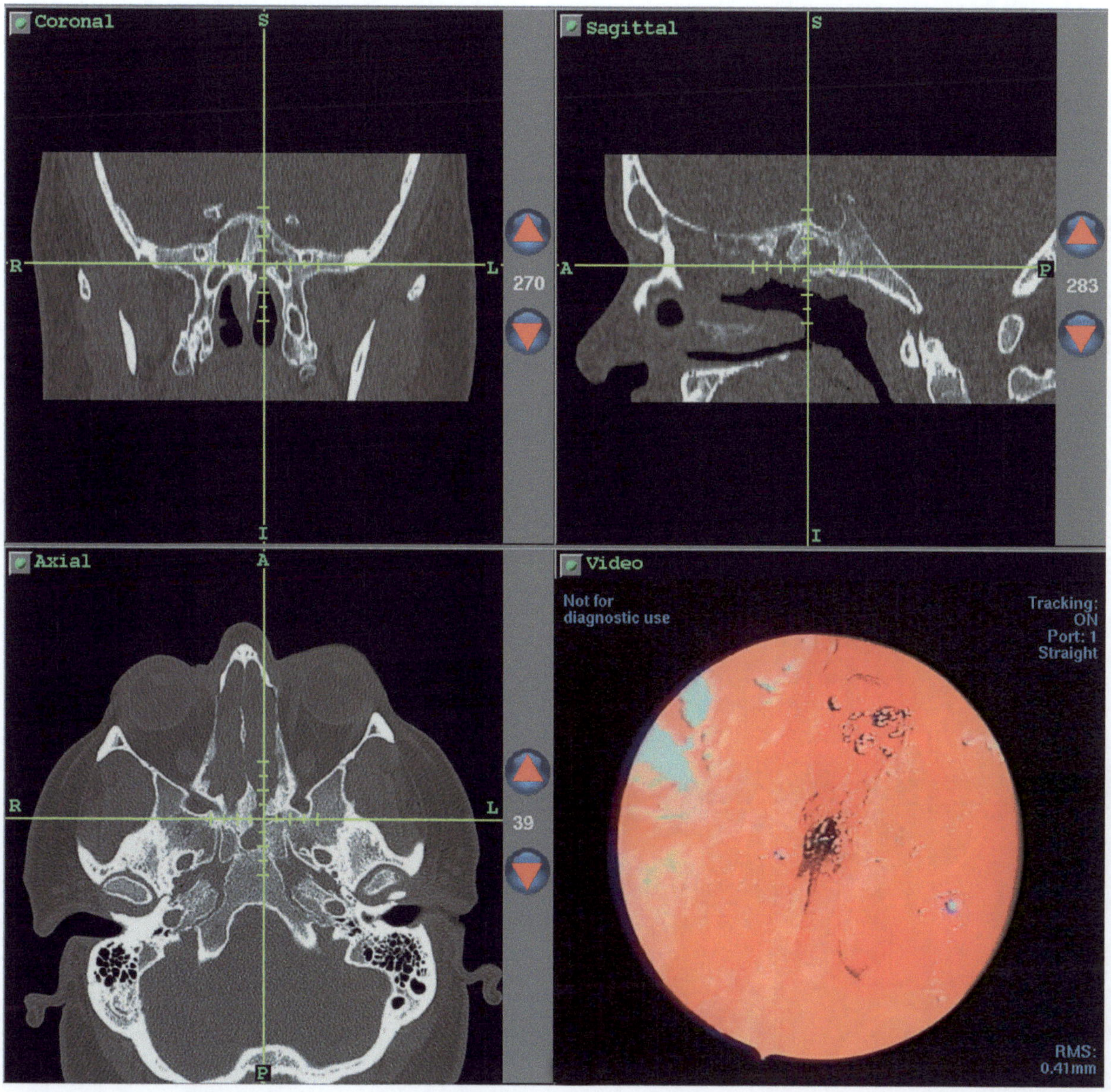

Fig. 29.3 In this patient, the sphenoid sinus has been become obstructed by reactive new bone formation. This screen capture, obtained with the InstaTrak 3500 Plus during revision endoscopic sinus surgery, shows the entry point into a small sphenoid sinus whose intraluminal volume has been contracted by so-called osteitic bone formation

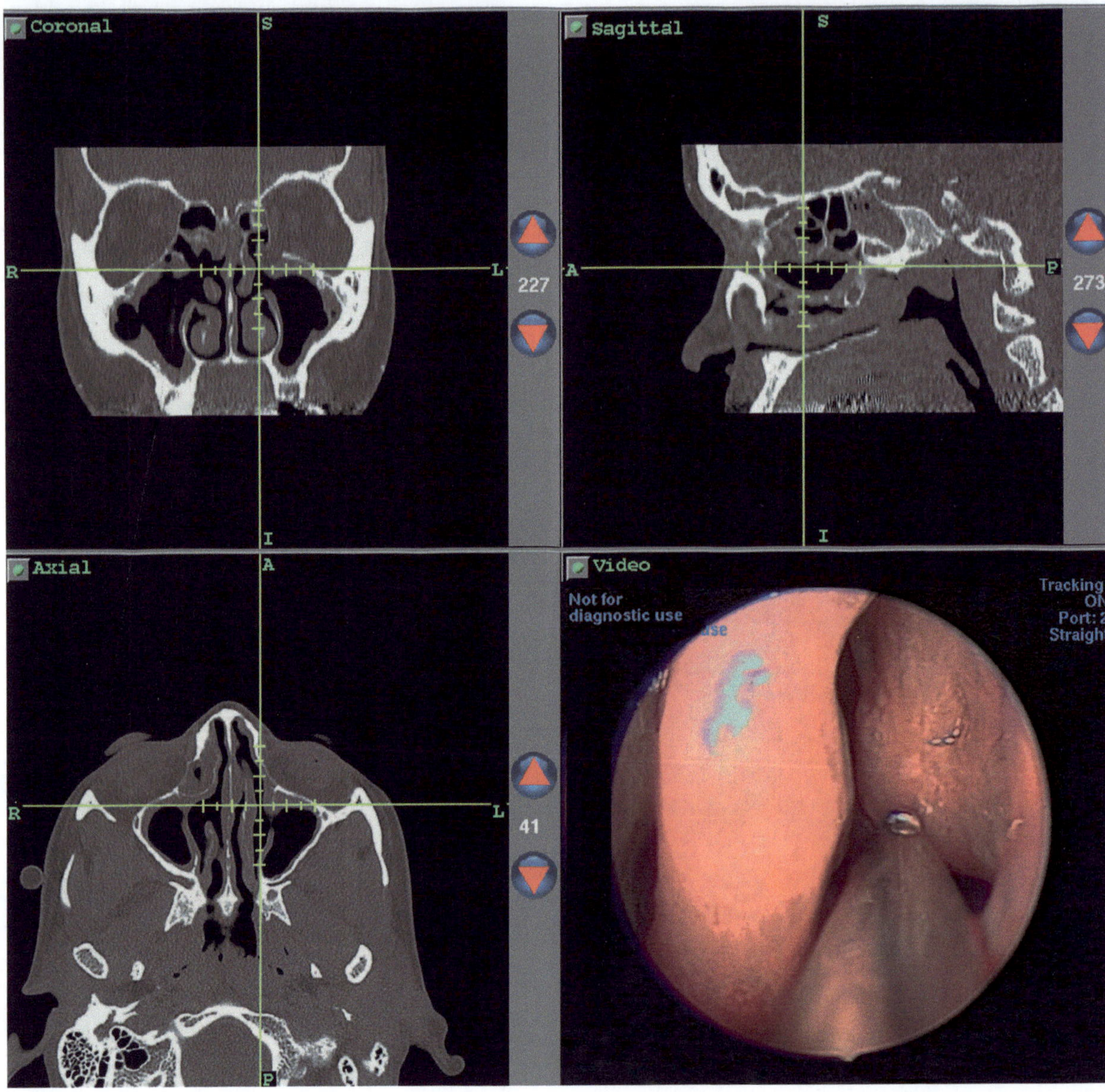

Fig. 29.4 In this screen capture, obtained with the InstaTrak 3500 Plus during revision endoscopic sinus surgery, the instrument tip rests upon an area of orbital dehiscence, through which a small amount of orbital fat has prolapsed. The endoscopic view alone suggests that this region is simply a residual anterior ethmoid cell; failure to recognize that this area is actually an orbital dehiscence from surgery performed in the distant past would have led to a potentially catastrophic orbital complication early in the revision procedure

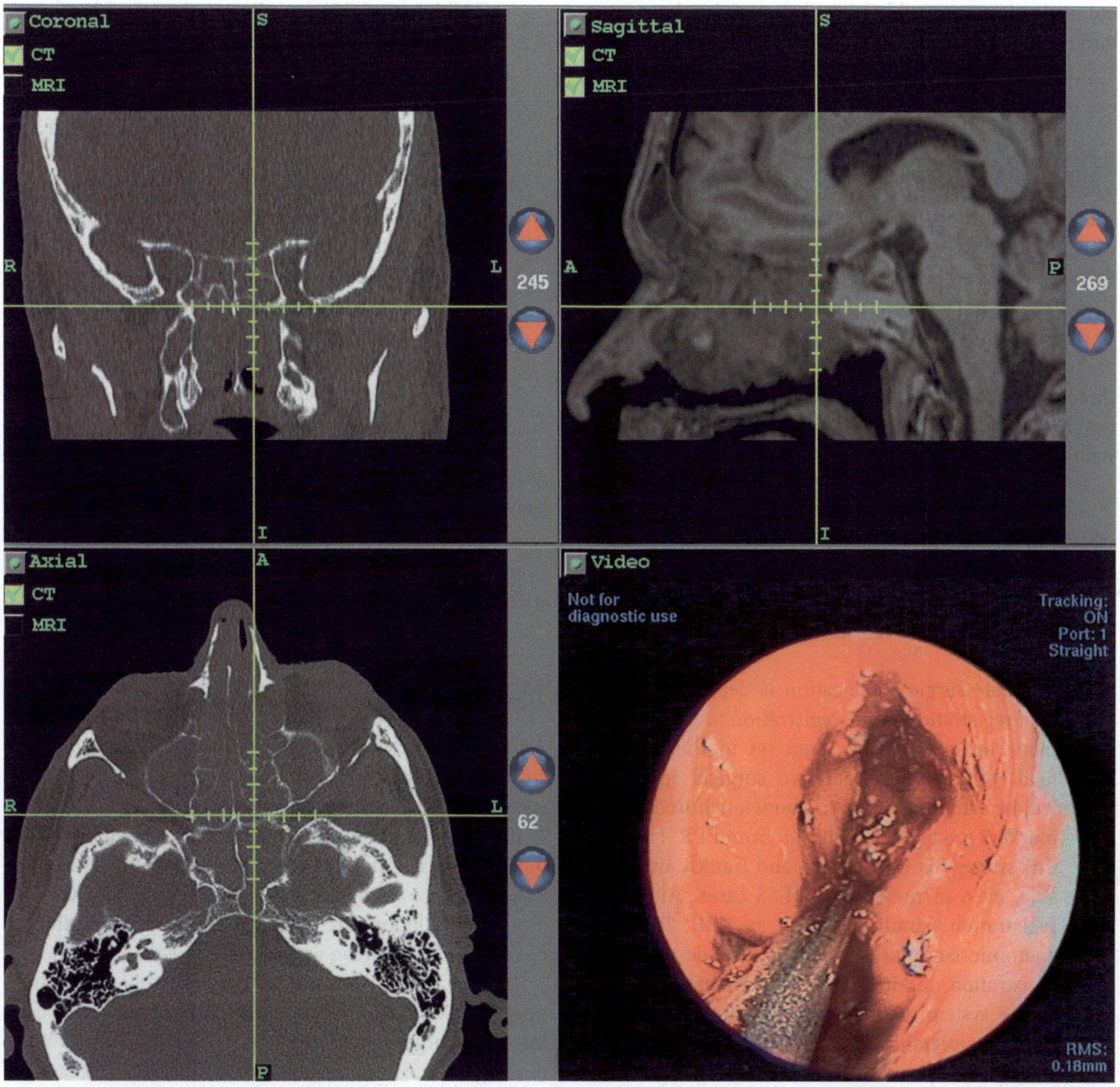

Fig. 29.5 Image fusion combines images obtained from the distinct imaging modalities of CT and magnetic resonance (MR). In this screen capture, obtained with the InstaTrak 3500 Plus during revision endoscopic sphenoidotomy, the upper right panel shows a fused CT-MR hybrid image that clearly demonstrates different signal characteristics within the opacified sphenoid sinus. In this instance, these findings were consistent with a mucocele. In other cases, the additional soft-tissue information can suggest the presence of an occult encephalocele or orbital dehiscence

cal navigation, it possible to easily recognize these issues and then simply work around them to achieve the desired surgical objectives (Fig. 29.4).

Sinonasal Polyposis

Endoscopic surgery for sinonasal polyposis is technically difficult. The inflamed polyp tissue tends to bleed so easily and profusely limiting the visualization that is among the prime advantages of surgical endoscopy. In the setting of revision surgery, previous surgery will also distort the anatomy. Surgical navigation, while not a substitute for direct visualization of a bloodless field, plays an important role in revision endoscopic sinus surgery in patients with sinonasal polyposis.

Limitations of Revision IG-FESS

- It is critical for otolaryngologists to recognize several inherent limitations of CAS when used in revision IG-FESS:
  1. Accurate surgical navigation is dependent on robust registration. If the registration protocol tightly maps the preoperative data set to the operative field, optimal intraoperative surgical navigation will be achieved. In theory, bone-anchored fiducial markers provide the best TRE from PPR. However, this strategy is impractical, and frankly unacceptable, even in revision IG-FESS cases. Alternative registration paradigms, such as CBR, PPR with anatomic landmarks, and AR provide acceptable registration, and importantly, increase the usability of the system. Given the importance of registration for successful surgical navigation, all surgeons should be capable of troubleshooting registration issues.
  2. Although IGS is a powerful surgical tool, it is not a substitute for surgical expertise and thorough understanding of the paranasal sinus anatomy. Thus, if a surgeon lacks the proper requisite training to perform revision IG-FESS cases, CAS systems will not improve the capabilities of the surgeon to complete this complex task. On the other hand, in the hands of a skilled surgeon, IGS may allow for better preoperative image assessment and surgical planning, resulting in a more complete surgical procedure with a decreased risk of complications.
  3. IGS platforms rely on preoperative imaging data sets. Thus, intraoperative surgical navigation cannot reliably account for changes in the anatomy incurred by surgical manipulation. The success of CAS in sinus surgery relies on the "rigid box" concept, which is ideal for surgical navigation based on the preoperative data set. The advent of intraoperative volume CT scanning may allow for real-time update of the image data set for revision IG-FESS cases.
  4. IGS is an enabling technology. It can facilitate revision IG-FESS procedures by providing detailed information about the 3D relationships. However, it does not change the nature of the procedure. The surgeon must still adhere to currently accepted surgical principles; in revision cases, functional, mucosal-sparing techniques are still paramount in successful execution of surgery.

Special IGS Techniques

Over the past several years, additional capabilities have been added to IGS systems. These new applications offer specific advantages in certain clinical situations.

Intraoperative CT and Fluoroscopy

An important criticism of surgical navigation is that the commonly available systems rely upon preoperative imaging and, as a result, the navigation is always relative to imaging that does not reflect anatomic changes made during surgery. This lack of real-time updating is a larger issue for more complex procedures in which greater surgical manipulations are performed. The incorporation of intraoperative imaging would overcome this limitation.

In the late 1990s, intraoperative magnetic resonance imaging (MRI) suites were introduced, and their uses for sinus surgery were explored [10, 154]. This strategy never gathered much traction for a variety of practical considerations. MRI surgical suites are expensive; in addition to the costs associated with the imaging technology, all instrumentation must be made MRI-compatible. Thus, the availability of this technology is limited due to the cost issues, which are considerable even under ideal circumstances. Furthermore, MRI does not provide good bony detail, which is desirable for most endoscopic sinus surgery procedures.

In contrast, intraoperative fluoroscopy is common and relatively inexpensive. Recent technical advances now permit the creation of CT-like images from fluoroscopy images, and in concept, these reconstructed fluoroscopic CT image sets can be used for surgical navigation. In a preliminary report Brown et al. report an initial series of cases in which fluoroscopic CT images were used during image-guided endoscopic sinus surgery; the authors describe the limitations of this technology in detail [4]. In addition to the costs and complexity associated with the extra equipment, the quality of the fluoroscopic CT is clearly below what most surgeons would deem acceptable, although technical modifications may partially ameliorate this problem. Fluoroscopic CT acquisition also entails additional radiation exposure to the patient and operating room (OR) staff. Nonetheless, as this technology matures, it may find a role in the most complex endoscopic procedures of the paranasal sinuses.

Most recently, intraoperative CT scanners have been introduced. With this technology, updated CT imaging can be used for intraoperative surgical navigation. Cumulative experiences with this approach are still sparse. Anecdotal reports suggest that intraoperative CT imaging is technically easy and may be useful in select cases. Of course, intraoperative CT imaging carries additional radiation exposure for both the patient and OR personnel. In addition, it must be remembered that sinuses filled with blood and irrigation fluid will appear as opacified on an intraoperative CT scan image, which will only highlight changes in bony anatomy.

CT-Magnetic Resonance Fusion

Through the process of image-to-image registration (IIR), computer software can fuse high-resolution CT and magnetic resonance (MR) images to create hybrid images that combine features of both CT and MRI. Then the fused data set can be during surgical navigation, allowing the surgeon to navigate with both preoperative CT and MRI information simultaneously [6, 23]. Navigation with CT-MR fusion is most advantageous during endoscopic skull-base surgery; it is especially helpful for tumor resection. This technology can also be useful for achieving adequate marsupialization of loculated mucoceles. Because the MR scan provides information about the position of the internal carotid artery (ICA), navigation with CT-MR fusion images has a role in endoscopic sphenoidal surgery. CT-MR fusion images provide information about the characteristics of the material within opacified sinuses; these images will help define mucoceles (as well as loculations within mucoceles) and encephaloceles (Fig. 29.5).

CT Angiography

Three-dimensional CT angiography (3D-CTA) provides information about the position of the ICA in the sphenoid sinus, since the image acquisition is performed as a contrast bolus fills the ICA at the skull base. High-resolution 3D-CTA images may be used for surgical navigation [22]. On some navigational platforms, it possible to segment a 3D model of the ICA and adjacent skull base and then incorporate this information into surgical planning and intraoperative surgical navigation. Obviously, surgical navigation with 3D-CTA plays a special role during complex endoscopic surgery of the sphenoid surgery and adjacent skull base.

Outcomes

Intuitively, IGS should improve surgical outcomes with a decrease in morbidity. Selected series in the literature have supported this concept. Almost all reports have been case series that highlighted the incorporation of IGS into endoscopic sinus surgery [2, 11, 27,29, 31]. Reardon compared a group of 400 patients whose sinus surgery was performed with IGS, to a second historical control group of 400 patients; no differences in major and minor complication rates were noted, although the IGS group cases included entry into more sinuses without an increase in operative time [30]. Fried performed a similar comparison of a group 97 patients whose endoscopic sinus surgery included IGS, to a historical control group of 61 patients whose surgery was performed before the availability of IGS; the rate for major complications was greater in the pre-IGS group compared to the IGS group (11.1% vs. 1%, $p<0.01$) [13].

Strauss et al. proposed a complex methodology for evaluating IGS utilizing surgical efficiency criteria [35]. A level of quality index was devised to evaluate the available information before and after FESS in 89 cases; the resultant change in the surgical strategy was measured. For a total of 792 applications with a surgical pointer, 47.9% of the applications yielded a change in the surgical strategy. Less-experienced surgeons used the navigation system more frequently in all cases and found the information to be more valuable than did more experienced surgeons. The information gained was felt to be greatest at the following locations: sphenoid sinus, orbital lamina, frontal base, and frontal recess. The authors also noted a higher adjustment rate in surgical strategy for more advanced cases, such as tumor resection and biopsies.

Kacker et al. reviewed a cohort of 110 patients undergoing endoscopic procedures utilizing IGS [16]. The indications included 85 cases of revision FESS; the remainder involved sphenoid and frontal disease and cerebrospinal fluid leak. No major complications were encountered in these series, helping support the concept that IGS may help minimize complications in revision cases. In addition, only 12 (11%) patients required revision surgery for persistent infection, which was reportedly a lower revision rate than without the use of IGS. Thus, the authors proposed that the use of IGS "may allow for more a complete sinus procedure and improve the efficacy of revision surgery."

More recently, Smith et al. have applied the evidence-based medicine paradigm to the application of IGS in sinus surgery [33]. After review of 105 articles, a total of 5 were identified that addressed the following two questions: (1) "Does image-guided sinus surgery reduce complication rates?", and (2) "Does image-guided sinus surgery improve clinical outcomes?" Four series were retrospective and were deemed level 4 evidence. One study was level 5 and reflected expert opinion. In general, these studies focused on complication and revision surgery rates, but none of the studies focused on patient-based outcomes such as quality of life.

To date, no prospective trials have been conducted to evaluate the efficacy of IGS for FESS or other advanced endoscopic applications. Many authors have acknowledged that this would likely be an insurmountable task given multiple ethical and logistical considerations. Smith et al. have reported that approximately 35,000 patients may need to be enrolled to show a statistical reduction in the rate of major complications, if one establishes a major complication rate of 0.25% for a clinical trial [33]. Moreover, it would be unethical to randomize patients away from IGS when clinical experience and data suggest that the technology would benefit the potential patient.

In a recent review titled "Parachute use to prevent death and major trauma related to gravitational challenge: systematic review of randomized controlled trials," Smith and Pell tackle the question of whether every intervention intended to prevent ill health must be subjected to the rigor of a randomized trial. They concluded that "advocates of evidence-based medicine have criticized the adoption of interventions evaluated by using only observational data. We think that everyone might benefit if the most radical protagonists of evidence-based medicine organized (sic) and participated in a double-blind, randomized, placebo-controlled, crossover trial of the parachute." [32].

Conclusion

With continued refinement and widespread acceptance, IGS has become a transformative technology in the realm of rhinology and other surgical disciplines. The application of IGS to revision sinus surgery, or revision IG-FESS, may allow for more complete surgery, with reductions in complication rates and less need for additional revision procedures. To optimize performance of IGS in revision FESS, surgeons must be intimately familiar with the hardware and software applications of the image-guidance technology. Careful preoperative review of CT images allows for a better understanding of the complex anatomic relationships and development of a surgical plan. Rigorous adherence to registration principles minimizes the risks of inaccurate navigation and allows for safe execution of the surgical strategy.

References

1. American Academy of Otolaryngology – Head and Neck Surgery (2007) AAO-HNS Policy on Intra-Operative Use of Computer-Aided Surgery. Retrieved August 12, 2007, 2007, from www.entlink.net/practice/rules/image-guiding.cfm
2. Anon JB (1998) Computer-aided endoscopic sinus surgery. Laryngoscope 108:949–961
3. Arapakis I, Hubbe U, et al. (2005) LED autoregistration in navigated endonasal sinus surgery. Laryngorhinootologie 84:418–425
4. Brown SM, Sadoughi B, et al. (2007) Feasibility of near real-time image-guided sinus surgery using intraoperative fluoroscopic computed axial tomography. Otolaryngol Head Neck Surg 136:268–273
5. Cartellieri M, Kremser J, et al. (2001) Comparison of different 3D navigation systems by a clinical user. Eur Arch Otorhinolaryngol 258:38–41
6. Chiu AG, Palmer JN, et al. (2005) Use of image-guided computed tomography-magnetic resonance fusion for complex endoscopic sinus and skull base surgery. Laryngoscope 115:753–755
7. Citardi M (2003) Computer-aided sphenoid sinus surgery. Oper Techn Otolaryngol Head Neck Surg 14:188–194
8. Citardi MJ (2001) Computer-aided frontal sinus surgery. Otolaryngol Clin North Am 34:111–122
9. Desrosiers M (2004) Refractory chronic rhinosinusitis: pathophysiology and management of chronic rhinosinusitis persisting after endoscopic sinus surgery. Curr Allergy Asthma Rep 4:200–207
10. Fried MP, Hsu L, et al. (1996) Image-guided surgery in a new magnetic resonance suite: preclinical considerations. Laryngoscope 106:411–417
11. Fried MP, Kleefield J, et al. (1997) Image-guided endoscopic sinus surgery: results of accuracy and performance in a multi-center clinical study suing an electromagnetic tracking system. Laryngoscope 107:594–601
12. Fried MP, Kleefield J, et al. (1997) Image-guided endoscopic surgery: results of accuracy and performance in a multicenter clinical study using an electromagnetic tracking system. Laryngoscope 107:594–601
13. Fried MP, Moharir VM, et al. (2002) Comparison of endoscopic sinus surgery with and without image guidance. Am J Rhinol 16:193–197
14. Hardy SM, Melroy C, et al. (2006) A comparison of computer-aided surgery registration methods for endoscopic sinus surgery. Am J Rhinol 20:48–52

15. Hsu L, Fried MP, et al. (1998) MR-guided endoscopic sinus surgery. AJNR Am J Neuroradiol 19:1235–1240
16. Kacker A, Tabaee A, et al. (2005) Computer-assisted surgical navigation in revision endoscopic sinus surgery. Otolaryngol Clin North Am 38:473–482
17. Kennedy DW (1985) Functional endoscopic sinus surgery (technique). Arch Otolaryngol Head Neck Surg 111:643–649
18. Kennedy DW, Zinreich SJ, et al. (1985) Functional endoscopic sinus surgery (theory and diagnostic evaluation). Arch Otolaryngol 111:576–582
19. Knott PD, Batra PS, et al. (2006) Contour and paired-point registration in a model for image-guided surgery. Laryngoscope 116:1877–1881
20. Labadie RF, Davis BM, et al. (2005) Image-guided surgery: what is the accuracy? Curr Opin Otolaryngol Head Neck Surg 13:27–31
21. Lee WT, Kuhn FA, et al. (2004) 3D computed tomographic analysis of frontal recess anatomy in patients without frontal sinusitis. Otolaryngol Head Neck Surg 131:164–173
22. Leong JL, Batra PS, et al. (2005) Three-dimensional computed tomography angiography of the internal carotid artery for preoperative evaluation of sinonasal lesions and intraoperative surgical navigation. Laryngoscope 115:1618–1623
23. Leong JL, Batra PS, et al. (2006) CT-MR image fusion for the management of skull base lesions. Otolaryngol Head Neck Surg 134:868–876
24. Maurer CR Jr, Rohlfing T, et al. (2002) Sources of error in image registration for cranial image-guided neurosurgery. In: Germano IM (ed) Advanced Techniques in Image-Guided Brain and Spine Surgery. Thieme, New York, pp 10–36
25. Melroy CT, Dubin MG, et al. (2006) Analysis of methods to assess frontal sinus extent in osteoplastic flap surgery: transillumination versus 6-ft Caldwell versus image guidance. Am J Rhinol 20:77–83
26. Metson R, Cosenza M, et al. (1999) The role of image-guidance systems for head and neck surgery. Arch Otolaryngol Head Neck Surg 125:1100–1104
27. Metson RB, Cosenza MJ, et al. (2000) Physician experience with an optical image guidance system for sinus surgery. Laryngoscope 110:972–976
28. Metzger MC, Rafii A, et al. (2007) Comparison of 4 registration strategies for computer-aided maxillofacial surgery. Otolaryngol Head Neck Surg 137:93–99
29. Olson G, Citardi MJ (2000) Image-guided functional endoscopic sinus surgery. Otolaryngol Head Neck Surg 123:188–194
30. Reardon EJ (2002) Navigational risks associated with sinus surgery and the clinical effects of implementing a navigational system for sinus surgery. Laryngoscope 112:1–19
31. Roth M, Lanza DC, et al. (1995) Advantages and disadvantages of three-dimensional computed tomography intraoperative localization for functional endoscopic sinus surgery. Laryngoscope 105:1279–1286
32. Smith GCS, Pell JP (2003) Parachute use to prevent death and major trauma related to gravitational challenge: systematic review of randomized clinical trials. Br Med J 327:20–27
33. Smith TL, Stewart MG, et al. (2007) Indications for image-guided sinus surgery: the current evidence. Am J Rhinol 21:80–83
34. Snyderman C, Zimmer LA, et al. (2004) Sources of registration error with image guidance systems during endoscopic anterior cranial base surgery. Otolaryngol Head Neck Surg 131:145–149
35. Strauss G, Koulechov K, et al. (2006) Evaluation of a navigation system for ENT with surgical efficiency criteria. Laryngoscope 116:564–572
36. West JB, Fitzpatrick JM, et al. (2001) Fiducial point placement and the accuracy of point-based, rigid body registration. Neurosurgery 48:810–816; discussion 816–817
37. Zacharek MA, Fong KJ, et al. (2006) Image-guided frontal trephination: a minimally invasive approach for hard-to-reach frontal sinus disease. Otolaryngol Head Neck Surg 135:518–522

Chapter 30

Revision Endoscopic Sinus Surgery in Children

30

Hassan H. Ramadan

Core Messages

- Chronic rhinosinusitis is a very common condition in children.
- Endoscopic sinus surgery (ESS) is gaining popularity in children.
- The failure rate of ESS ranges between 13–20%.
- Image-guided CT scan should be considered in children with failure of ESS.
- Revision surgery is recommended for children who fail medical treatment.

Contents

Introduction

Endoscopic sinus surgery (ESS) is the surgical procedure of choice for chronic rhinosinusitis (CRS) in adults [1–3]. Recently it has gained wide popularity as a surgical procedure in children. Despite the fact that it is not the first procedure of choice in CRS refractory to medical treatment in children, it is being performed more and more in these patients. The success of ESS in children is reported to be approximately 88% [4–6]. Unlike ESS in adults, the procedure in children is more conservative and is limited in most children to anterior ethmoidectomy and maxillary sinus antrostomy because those are the sinuses that are most commonly involved. Some authors even perform a maxillary sinus wash at the time of adenoidectomy, before ESS is performed [7]. Surgery on the septum and turbinates is not very common in these children. The main purpose in children is to restore ventilation and mucociliary clearance of the sinuses.

Children with severe nasal polyposis, allergic fungal sinusitis, or pansinusitis are rare and mainly have cystic fibrosis, ciliary dyskinesia, or immune deficiency. They usually require continued medical management and a more aggressive surgical intervention [8].

Although causes of revision surgery in adults include extent of disease, severe polyposis, and previous nonendoscopic sinus procedures, these causes are uncommon in children [9]. Extent of disease is limited mainly to the ethmoid and maxillary sinuses. Rarely are the frontal and sphenoid sinuses involved.

- ESS in children is not the primary surgical procedure for CRS. Adenoidectomy, and/or maxillary sinus washing with culture-directed antibiotics are usually performed prior to ESS [6, 7, 10].

Children who do not respond to these conservative measurements are then evaluated with a computed tomography (CT) scan and considered for ESS. The surgical procedure in these children consists of anterior ethmoidectomy in 88%, maxillary antrostomy in 100%, posterior ethmoidectomy in 28%, frontal sinusotomy in 6%, and sphenoidotomy in 4% [6].

30

Failure of ESS

Failure of ESS in children is reported to be in the range of 12–13%. Failure should be defined as those children who require another surgical procedure or those who continue to have signs and symptoms of CRS despite continued medical therapy. Causes of failure in children can be divided into two groups if we exclude those with cystic fibrosis, immune deficiency, or ciliary abnormalities [4–6]: (1) children who have a surgical cause of failure, and (2) children who failed because of their age, presence of asthma/allergy, or severity of their disease. These two groups differ in the cause of the failure; however, in some children it may be a combination of those factors. Knowledge of the surgical causes of failure, however, may help us reduce the failure rate for some of these children.

Surgical Causes of Failure of ESS

Reports on the surgical causes of failure of ESS in children are very rare. In 1992, Lazar et al. reported that the most common causes of failure in children were recurrence of disease, adhesions, and narrowing of the maxillary sinus ostium [11]. In adults, numerous articles are available concerning causes of failure after ESS, which include extent of disease, nasal polyposis, previous traditional sinus surgery, presence of allergy, and anatomical abnormalities such as a deviated septum [9].

Analysis of the author's experience between 1993 and 2005 showed that 243 children had ESS. Children with cystic fibrosis, immune deficiency/suppression, and ciliary abnormalities were excluded because the reasons of failure in those children are very well known. Data were available on 176 children with at least 1 year of follow up; 23 (13%) children required revision ESS.

Analysis of the data showed that in the 23 patients, 47 findings were present causing the failure. Patients may have had more than one finding. The most common finding in our revision cases was adhesions in 57% of the cases, followed by maxillary sinus ostium stenosis or missed maxillary sinus ostium in 52% of the cases (Figs. 30.1 and 30.2). In 39% of the cases there was recurrent disease requiring revision surgery in the sinuses that were operated on initially. Interestingly however, we found that in 26% of the revision cases surgery was needed because of disease that was present in nonoperated sinuses during the primary ESS (Fig. 30). Four (17%) of the patients required a limited septoplasty at the time of revision that was thought to be the cause of failure on the side of deviation. In 13% of the children revision was needed because of a mucocele, which was causing symptoms of sinusitis due to obstruction of the sinuses (Fig. 30.4).

Follow up was available on 19 patients with a range of 1–5 years and a mean of 3 years. Fifteen (79%) patients at last follow up were doing well and only 4 (21%) continue to have sinusitis requiring medical management. Three patients required 3 revisions, 14 required 2 revisions, and 6 required 1 revision.

Medical Causes of Failure in ESS

The success of primary ESS ranges between 88 and 92% [12]. Conversely, those who continue to exhibit problems can either be manifesting a surgical failure as discussed

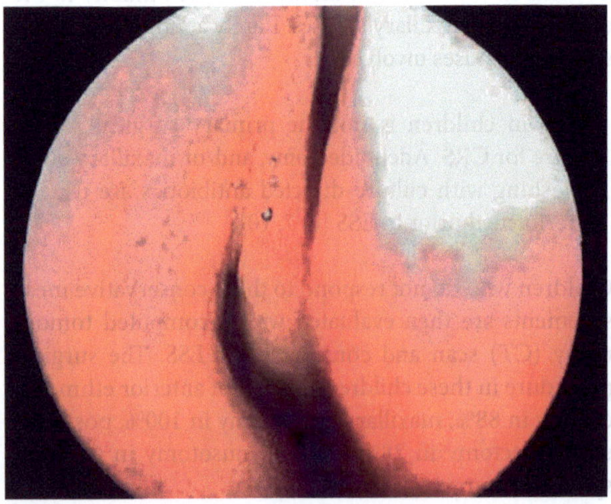

Fig. 30.1 Endoscopic view after endoscopic sinus surgery (ESS) showing deviated septum and adhesions between the middle turbinate and lateral nasal wall

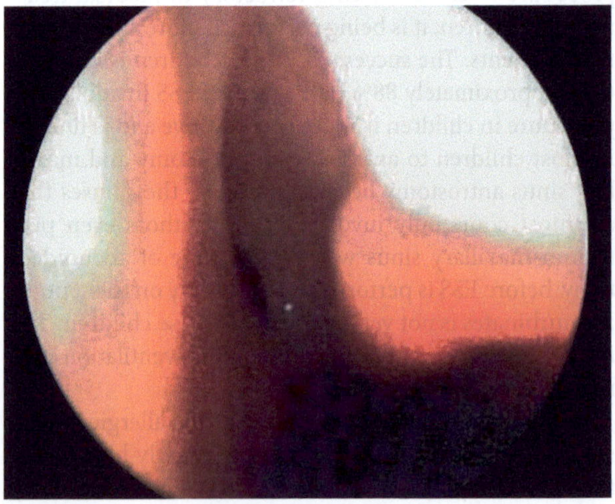

Fig. 30.2 Endoscopic view of a missed natural maxillary sinus ostium

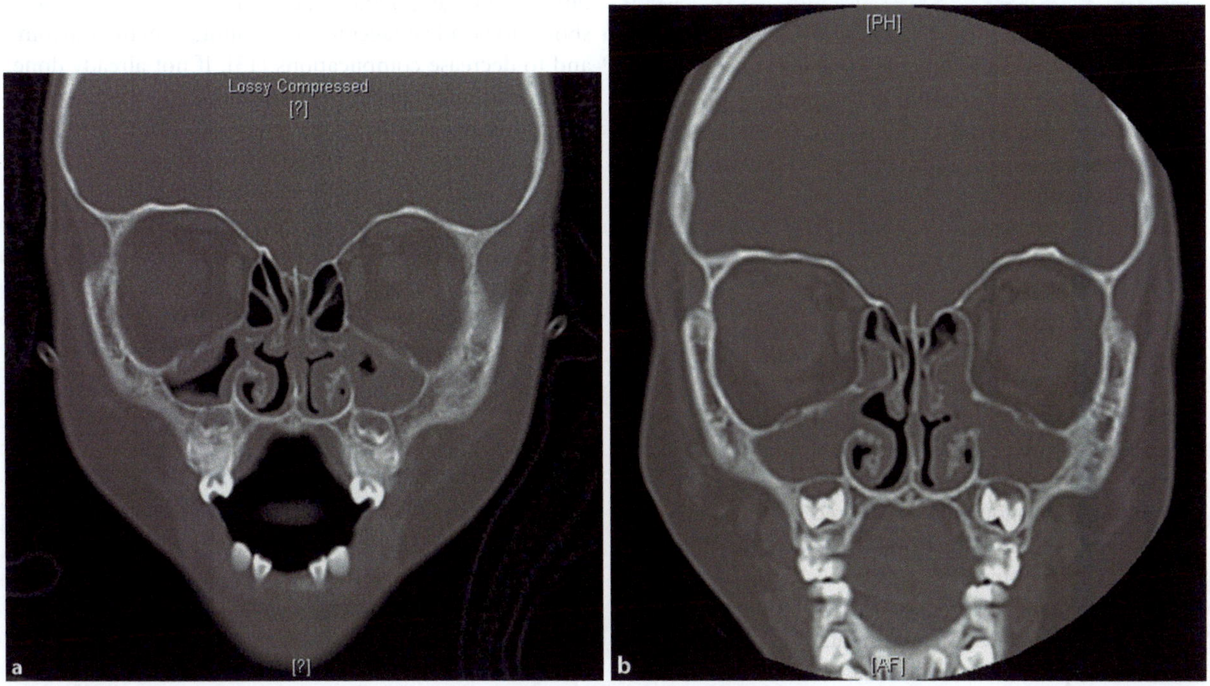

Fig. 30.3 **a** Coronal computed tomography (CT) scan of sinuses prior to primary sinus surgery showing maxillary sinus disease but clear sinuses. **b** Coronal CT sinuses before revision shows surgical changes at the maxillary sinus ostium, but now disease involving the ethmoid sinuses

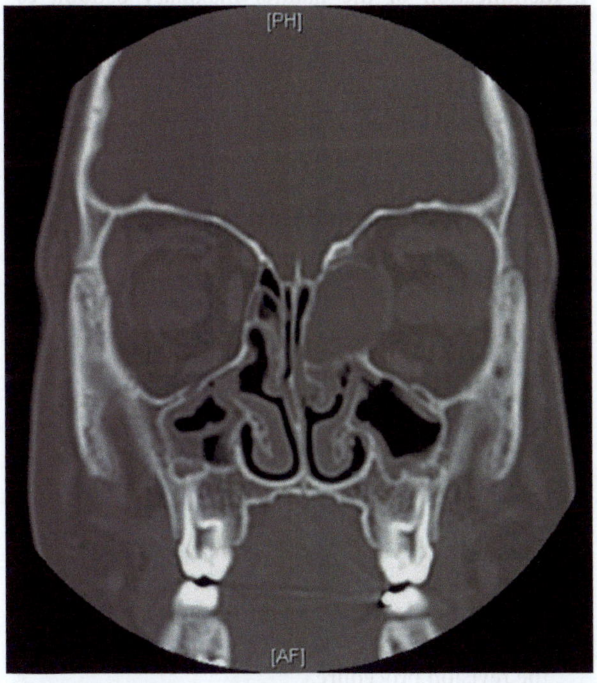

Fig. 30.4 Coronal CT scan sinuses shows a mucocele in the left ethmoid sinus eroding into the orbit post-ESS causing chronic rhinosinusitis symptoms

above, or they can be exhibiting certain medical morbidities. The most common cause of failure of ESS is asthma, followed by severity of sinus disease as evidenced by CT score. Age at time of surgery also plays a significant role in the outcome of surgery [6].

Asthma seems to impact outcome of ESS significantly. Children with asthma had a 62% success rate compared to 80% for those without asthma. Severity of disease as measured by CT score (Lund-McKay system) also seems to impact the outcome of ESS. Children with a higher CT score had a higher failure rate than those with a lower CT score. It was also noted that younger children (less than 6 years of age) had a higher failure rate with ESS than older children. Children who were older had an 84% success rate compared to 60% for the younger children. Allergy, smoke exposure, and day-care attendance have also been shown to influence the outcome of ESS, although to a lesser extent than asthma, age, and severity of disease. Children with cystic fibrosis, immune deficiency/suppression, and those with ciliary abnormalities can be included in this section.

Indications

Indications for revision ESS are similar to those of primary ESS. However, in children the primary procedure is usually very conservative. In revision cases the surgeon can be more aggressive in addressing the diseased sinuses, as done in adults.

Indications of revision sinus surgery in children include:

1. Complicated rhinosinusitis.
2. CRS symptoms not responsive to continued medical management for at least 3 months with antibiotics and ancillary medications.
3. Recurrent acute rhinosinusitis with periods of remission of at least 3 weeks between episodes. Children with four or more episodes of rhinosinusitis in a 6-month period should be considered for revision.
4. Presence of sinus disease on CT scans of the sinuses.
5. Allergic fungal sinusitis.
6. Antrochoanal polyp or presence of polyps not responding to medical management.
7. Mucocele present in the sinuses.

Contraindications

Contraindications can be relative and each surgeon should individualize depending on the status of his patient. Absolute contraindications can be children who are medically unfit for general anesthesia or those who have a terminal illness where the sinus disease is the least of their worries.

Relative contraindications for revision sinus surgery in children include:

1. Children with cystic fibrosis who did not respond to prior sinus surgery.
2. Children with developmental/mental delay whose symptoms do not cause any change in their quality of life.
3. Children with ciliary abnormalities who did not respond to prior sinus surgery.
4. Significant anatomical abnormalities with a high risk of complications; in these cases an open approach may be more desirable.
5. Disease that is present in the lateral aspect of the frontal sinus.

Preoperative Workup

The most important preoperative test in preparation for revision ESS in children is obtaining CT scan to identify disease and so that it can be used during the surgical procedure [6]. Image-guided surgery for revision ESS has been shown to be advantageous for obtaining a better outcome and to decrease complications [13]. If not already done, these children should have an immunology evaluation and allergy testing as part of their workup prior to revision ESS, and ciliary biopsy at the time of surgery. For those children with nasal polyposis, a course of oral steroids 1 week prior to surgery will help intraoperatively. Using preoperative antibiotics is controversial and is left to the discretion of the surgeon. If the child develops an infection a few days before surgery, it is advisable to treat the infection and defer the surgical procedure until the child is better.

Surgical Technique

The surgical technique is similar to that done during the primary procedure, as described elsewhere, especially for those sinuses that have not been operated on before [14].

Useful recommendations for revision sinus surgery in children:

1. Use of image-guided technology for a more complete procedure and decreased likelihood of complications.
2. Use of power tools, especially for cases of nasal polyposis and severe adhesions.
3. Care should be taken to identify the middle turbinate and to separate it from the lateral nasal wall intact if possible.
4. Identification of the natural maxillary ostium, especially in cases where a missed ostium is the cause of failure. Once identified it should be widened and joined to the accessory ostium.
5. If a deviated septum is thought to be the cause of failure then a limited endoscopic septoplasty should be performed.
6. Mucoceles and antrochoanal polyps can be easily identified and their excision is facilitated with power instruments.

Tips and Pearls to Avoid Complications

1. Obtain adequate accuracy with the image-guided system used.
2. Use a 4-mm scope for better visualization whenever possible. In most children a 4-mm scope can be used instead of a 2.7-mm scope.
3. Use the 0 and 30 scopes interchangeably during the procedure.
4. Identify and spare the middle turbinate; it is an important anatomical landmark for completing the revision procedure.
5. Extreme caution is needed while revising the maxillary antrostomy to avoid orbital fat herniation.

Complications

Complications are uncommon in children even in revision cases. They can be intraoperative or postoperative.

Intraoperative complications of revision sinus surgery in children include:

1. Cerebrospinal fluid (CSF) leak. This needs to be recognized during the procedure and repaired immediately.
2. Orbital entry with fat herniation. In most instances the procedure can be completed and no intervention is needed.
3. Orbital hemorrhage with increased pressure. An immediate lateral canthotomy should be performed with removal of all the packing on that side. An ophthalmology consult should be obtained.
4. Stripping of the maxillary sinus mucosa. This needs to be recognized otherwise, even though the bony ostium is open, the mucosa inside the sinus will be collapsed with no ventilation of the inside of the sinus.
5. Inadvertent injury to the middle turbinate. All attempts should be made to preserve it in place.
6. Bleeding. If bleeding is considerably impairing the surgeon's vision the procedure should be aborted. There is no need to put the patient at risk for blood transfusion. If the bleeding is excessive with respect to the blood volume of the child, the procedure should also be aborted.

Postoperative complications of revision sinus surgery in children:

1. Bleeding. In most instances it is self-contained. Rarely packing or exam in the operating room is needed.
2. Adhesions. Those can be very common depending on the age of the child. If they are not causing any symptoms, then they can be left alone. If symptomatic and severe, a reexamination to deal with them would be appropriate.
3. Orbital swelling and ecchymosis. If eye pressure is high, then proceed as in intraoperative increased pressure. If pressure is normal and the child is cooperative enough, remove the packing and observe.
4. CSF leak. Put the patient on complete bed rest, head elevation, and give stool softeners for 1 week. There is no support in the literature for a lumbar drain. If the CSF persists, then consider endoscopic repair.

Postoperative Care

1. All patients are given oral antibiotics for 10–14 days.
2. We recommend sleeping with the head elevated for 7 days.
3. We discourage blowing of the nose or use of nasal sprays for 1 week.
4. Absorbable packing is used. It will be absorbed by around 2–3 weeks, thus debridement in children is not necessary.

Outcomes

1. Success rate of revision ESS in children ranges between 77 and 82%.
2. Children may require more than one revision before achieving success.
3. Major complications in children are extremely rare.

References

1. Bhattacharyya N (2006) Surgical treatment of chronic recurrent rhinosinusitis: a preliminary report. Laryngoscope 116:1805–1808
2. Smith TL, Batra PS, Seiden AM, Hannley M (2005) Evidence supporting endoscopic sinus surgery in the management of adult chronic rhinosinusitis: a systematic review. Am J Rhinol 19:537–543
3. Dursun E, Korkmaz H, Eryilmaz A, Bayiz U, Sertkaya D, Samim E (2003) Clinical predictors of long-term success after endoscopic sinus surgery. Otolaryngol Head Neck Surg 129:526–531
4. Lusk RP, Muntz HR (1990) Endoscopic sinus surgery in children with chronic sinusitis. Laryngoscope 100:654–658
5. Parsons DS, Phillips SE (1993) Functional endoscopic surgery in children: a retrospective analysis of results. Laryngoscope 103: 899–903
6. Ramadan HH (2004) Surgical management of chronic sinusitis in children. Laryngoscope 114:2103–2109
7. Buchman CA, Yellon RF, Bluestone CD (1999) Alternative to endoscopic sinus surgery in the management of pediatric chronic rhinosinusitis refractory to oral antimicrobial therapy. Otolaryngol Head Neck Surg 120:219–224
8. Friedman EM, Stewart M (2006) An assessment of sinus quality of life and pulmonary function in children with cystic fibrosis. Am J Rhinol 20:568–572
9. McMains KC, Kountakis SE (2005) Revision functional endoscopic sinus surgery: objective and subjective surgical outcomes. Am J Rhinol 19:344–347
10. Ramadan HH (1999) Adenoidectomy vs endoscopic sinus surgery for the treatment of pediatric sinusitis. Arch Otolaryngol Head Neck Surg 125:1208–1211
11. Lazar RH, Younis RT, Long TE, Gross CW (1992) Revision functional endonasal sinus surgery. Ear Nose Throat J 71:131–133

12. Hebert RL 2nd, Bent JP 3rd (1998) Meta-analysis of outcomes of pediatric functional endoscopic sinus surgery. Laryngoscope 108:796–799
13. Dubin MG, Kuhn FA (2005) Stereotactic computer assisted navigation: state of the art for sinus surgery, not standard of care. Otolaryngol Clin North Am 38:535–549
14. Ramadan HH (2007) Pediatric sinus surgery. In: Kountakis SE, Önerci M (eds) Rhinologic and Sleep Apnea; Surgical Techniques. Springer, Heidelberg, pp 211–218

Chapter 31

Open Approaches after Failure of Primary Sinus Surgery

31

Mark C. Weissler

Core Messages

- Consider carefully the cause of failure before embarking on further open surgery.
- Osteoplastic frontal sinus surgery is the most common open sinus procedure to be required after failed primary surgery.
- External ethmoidectomy for failed primary endoscopic sinus surgery is rarely, if ever, indicated.

Contents

Introduction

The concept of "failed primary sinus surgery" itself requires some discussion. Obviously, surgery may fail because the infection one sought to cure was not cured. In the most obvious example, a patient with an intracranial abscess related to sinus infection may not be adequately drained and may go on to death; the patient with invasive mucormycosis of the sinonasal tract may not be adequately debrided and may die. In both examples, intensive medical therapy is equally as important as surgical drainage/debridement. Fortunately, however, such obvious examples of failure rarely occur. More commonly, when we speak of failed primary sinus surgery we are speaking about a patient who remains symptomatic after primary sinus surgery, or in whom continued objective evidence of ongoing inflammation persists after primary sinus surgery.

Several groups of failed patients can be identified:

1. The persistently symptomatic patient without objective evidence of sinonasal inflammation with or without anatomical derangement.
2. The persistently symptomatic patient with objective evidence of sinonasal inflammation with or without anatomical derangement.
3. The patient with a wholly new set of symptoms after primary sinus surgery that are felt to be iatrogenic in nature.
4. The patient for whom endoscopic surgery proved inadequate to achieve the necessary exposure and anatomical results.

The first question to be asked is whether or not the disease process in question is truly a surgical problem. Were the symptoms for which the patient initially underwent sinus surgery really related to sinonasal disease? Headache, for example, may have been the initial complaint and may have been due to some other factor such as migraine rather than sinonasal disease, or perhaps the migraine was exacerbated by sinonasal disease, but other factors are now causing persistent symptoms. Persistent mucosal inflammatory disease may or may not be amenable to surgical correction. It may instead be secondary to allergic rhinitis or other immune or inflammatory conditions related to environmental factors. Allergic fungal sinusitis is the most obvious of these conditions. Surgery may be necessary, but is not generally sufficient for control of the disease process. My subjective impression over the years is that often misguided initial surgery that is not successful in relieving a patient's symptoms may be followed by ever more aggressive surgical therapy that is equally misguided and ultimately results in iatrogenically created dysfunctional sinonasal cavities.

Ultimately, surgical intervention in diseases of the paranasal sinuses can change anatomy and drain infection.

It cannot intrinsically affect allergy, primary disease of the respiratory mucosa, the causes of nasal polyps, or alter mucosal sensitivity to the environment. If one must operate on the paranasal sinuses, one should set specific anatomic objectives and then aim to accomplish those objectives in as safe a manner as possible. The underlying mucosal disease must then be addressed medically. In the best of circumstances, recurrent or persistent localized sinus disease can be clearly related to an identifiable anatomic problem.

Particularly after failed primary sinus surgery, it behooves the surgeon to consider carefully and optimally treat underlying allergic and inflammatory conditions before embarking on further surgical treatment.

Indications

- Open approaches for failed endoscopic primary surgery are indicated primarily to correct specific anatomic abnormalities that are not accessible endoscopically.

The number of such abnormalities is increasingly limited. If primary surgery failed because of underlying mucosal disease rather than because of some anatomical aberration that prevented adequate aeration and drainage endoscopically, then there is no particular reason to believe that open surgery, aimed simply at creating drainage, would be any more likely to succeed.

Although it is anathema to some, another indication for open surgery might be to completely remove irreversibly condemned mucosa, with the intention of replacing it with nonrespiratory cuboidal epithelium and scar. The concept of "functional" endoscopic surgery was first predicated on the theory that no such irreversibly condemned mucosa existed, but rather that through aeration and drainage this mucosa could return to normal. Nonetheless, for practical purposes, it is debatable whether or not some patients might be better served in specific pathologic situations by removal of mucosa and obliteration of a sinus. True obliteration can only be adequately accomplished in the frontal and sphenoid sinuses. Attempts at obliteration of the maxillary sinuses with fat failed, but the end result after a Caldwell-Luc operation is essentially an obliteration of the maxillary sinuses that fill in with scar and cuboidal, nonrespiratory epithelium. In a recent review, Barzalai and Greenberg felt that the only remaining indications for the Caldwell-Luc operation were for fungal disease and in conjunction with endoscopic surgery for the treatment of inverting papilloma [1].

The most frequent indication for open surgery after failed primary endoscopic sinus surgery is for persistent or iatrogenically induced frontal sinus obstruction. This is probably because the frontal sinus is the most likely to present anatomical features that preclude adequate long-term drainage via an endoscopic approach. Overly aggressive removal of mucosa in the frontal recess may result in scarring and stenosis of the frontal sinus outflow tract, which is difficult to repair. Although an endoscopic Lothrop procedure may be possible in some cases, a narrow anteroposterior diameter of the frontal sinus outflow tract may preclude this approach. Failure to adequately remove an osteoma, inverted papilloma, or other neoplasm from this area endoscopically may also lead to the necessity of open surgery.

External ethmoid surgery is unlikely to have any real advantage in this day and age over revision endoscopic surgery for ethmoidal sinus disease. In addition, the Lynch procedure with attempted reconstruction of a functional nasofrontal outflow tract seems increasingly to be of historical interest only.

Procedures

Osteoplastic Frontal Sinus Obliteration

- Indications for osteoplastic frontal sinus obliteration:
  1. Failed primary endoscopic frontal sinus drainage procedures or failed Lynch or Lothrop procedures.
  2. Inability to adequately remove neoplasm such as inverted papilloma from the frontal sinus endoscopically.

- Contraindications: acute frontal sinusitis, as this may lead to infection of the bone flap.

The osteoplastic frontal sinus obliteration procedure remains an important part of the sinus surgeon's armamentarium. Although it can be carried out unilaterally, it is generally performed bilaterally (Fig. 31.1).

- The keys to success of frontal sinus obliteration are:
  1. *Complete* removal of *all* frontal sinus mucosa.
  2. Burring of the inner table of bone of the sinus cavity.

The sinus is generally obliterated with abdominal fat harvested from the left lower quadrant of the abdomen so as not to be confused in the future with an appendectomy incision. Montgomery has shown in cats, and personal experience corroborates, that fat can survive long term within the sinus cavity [2].

Preoperatively, the patient has a Caldwell view X-ray taken from 6 feet (approximately 2 m) away and the frontal sinus is cut out of the film to be used as a template during surgery. Alternatively, one can use intraoperative

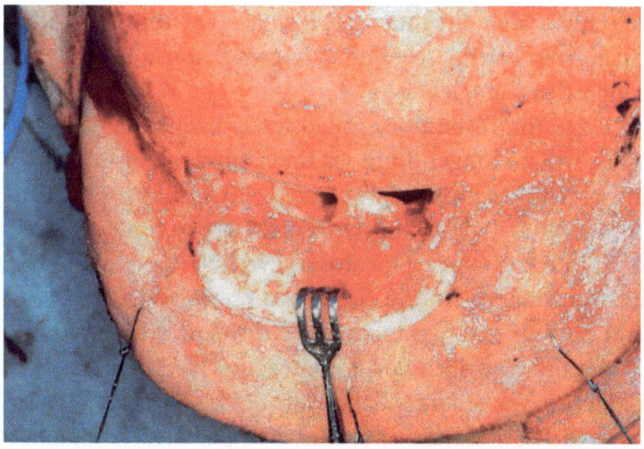

Fig. 31.1 Osteoplastic frontal sinus operation

computed tomography guidance or transillumination to delineate the borders of the frontal sinus. A coronal flap is elevated in a plane *superficial* to the periosteum, down to the supraorbital rim. The supratrochlear and supraorbital nerves are spared and may be released from the foramina as needed. Utilizing the template, or other method, the sinus is outlined and an oscillating or sagittal saw used to cut the frontal bone slightly inside the limits shown by the template. There is no need to follow the exact lateral contours of the sinus. The saw blade should be greatly beveled in toward the central sinus. At the supraorbital rims, the very thick bone must be completely transected; a horizontal bony incision is made at the nasal root. A fine osteotome is inserted through the superior bony kerf and used to divide the interfrontal sinus septum. The osteoplastic flap with vascularized periosteum adherent to its anterior wall is then fractured inferiorly through the roofs of the orbits. Next, all mucosa is painstakingly removed from the frontal sinus, and the lining cortical bone drilled with a cutting burr. Small, 1–2-mm burrs can be helpful in removing mucosa from small extensions of the sinus. The intersinus septum is completely drilled away. This dissection extends down into the nasofrontal drainage system. The sinus is copiously irrigated with saline or bacitracin solution. Small pieces of fat or separately harvested temporalis muscle are used to obliterate the nasofrontal drainage system and the frontal sinus filled with *atraumatically* harvested abdominal fat. The flap is then returned to anatomic position and fixed in position with small wires or miniplates. The periosteum is closed with absorbable suture and the coronal skin flap closed in layers over closed suction drains that exit separate stab-wound incisions laterally. In recent years, the necessity of keeping the bone flap vascularized by leaving the periosteum intact and pedicled inferiorly has been called into question. When performing craniofacial resection, the bone flap is routinely harvested without the periosteum, which is then used to reline the floor of the anterior cranial fossa as a periosteal flap. Bone necrosis is rarely a problem in these situations.

The Caldwell-Luc Procedure

- Indications of the Caldwell-Luc procedure:
  1. Chronic polypoid maxillary sinusitis unresponsive to conservative intranasal endoscopic procedures.
  2. Acute complicated maxillary sinusitis unresponsive to intranasal endoscopic procedures.
  3. As a route to biopsy of lesions not accessible transnasally:
     a. maxillary sinus mass
     b. infraorbital nerve.
  4. As an approach to the orbital floor when additional exposure is needed:
     a. to treat fracture
     b. for orbital decompression of Grave's ophthalmopathy.

The Caldwell-Luc procedure is a sublabial approach to the maxillary sinus through the anterior wall under the upper lip. Traditionally it was used to treat chronic maxillary sinusitis with irreversible changes of the maxillary sinus respiratory epithelium. During the procedure all the lining mucosa of the maxillary sinus is removed and will be replaced by a rind of scar tissue covered by cuboidal nonciliated epithelium as the sinus heals. Because there is no longer any active transport of mucous within the sinus, drainage must be created inferiorly through the inferior meatus. Since the floor of the maxillary sinus is lower than the floor of the nose, gravity does not serve entirely to drain the sinus. After a Caldwell-Luc procedure, plain films (Caldwell views) of the maxillary sinus will forever be abnormal with some degree of opacification. In recent times, it has been felt that creating aeration of the maxillary sinus via the natural ostium will allow for healing of the damaged mucosa of chronic sinusitis and reestablishment of the natural mucociliary transport system. Theoretically, respiratory epithelium within the sinus will regenerate. There may still, however, be a role for this operation in cases in which maximal medical and "functional" surgery of the sinus has failed to restore healthy mucosa to a sinus. Attempts have been made to obliterate the maxillary sinus with fat and other substances, but these have never been successful. After a well-performed Caldwell-Luc operation, the sinus is to some extent "obliterated" by the natural course of healing.

Other indications for a Caldwell-Luc approach include:

1. The treatment of oroantral fistulae.
2. The treatment of malignant exophthalmos.

3. As an approach to biopsy the infraorbital nerve in cases of suspected perineural invasion by cancer.
4. As an approach to the orbital floor in the treatment of trauma.
5. As an approach to the pterygomaxillary space for ligation of the internal maxillary artery in the treatment of resistant epistaxis.
6. As part of a larger operation to treat benign and malignant neoplasms of the lateral nasal wall, pterygomaxillary space, infratemporal fossa, and nasopharynx.

The operation is performed by retracting the upper lip superiorly, most effectively with a Johnson-type retractor. The soft tissues overlying the canine fossa are infiltrated with local anesthetic and epinephrine. An incision is made centered on the canine fossa, slightly convex inferiorly and extending from just short of the midline back to the second or third maxillary molar. The incision is kept at least 5 mm above the gingival edge to allow enough tissue for closure. The incision in carried down to bone and then elevated in a subperiosteal plane superiorly to expose the infraorbital foramen and nerve. This elevation is done most expeditiously by beginning with a McKenty or other small periosteal elevator and then pushing on a gauze sponge for further elevation. A 2-mm osteotome is used to create a small opening into the maxillary sinus above the level of the maxillary tooth roots; this is then enlarged with a Kerrison-type rongeur. Most of the enlargement occurs superiorly up to and even around the infraorbital nerve (Fig. 31.2). The offending maxillary sinus mucosa is then completely stripped from the sinus. The roof is saved for last, realizing that the infraorbital nerve is frequently dehiscent within the sinus. Great care is used to avoid damage to the infraorbital nerve. A variety of small curettes and pituitary-type forceps are used

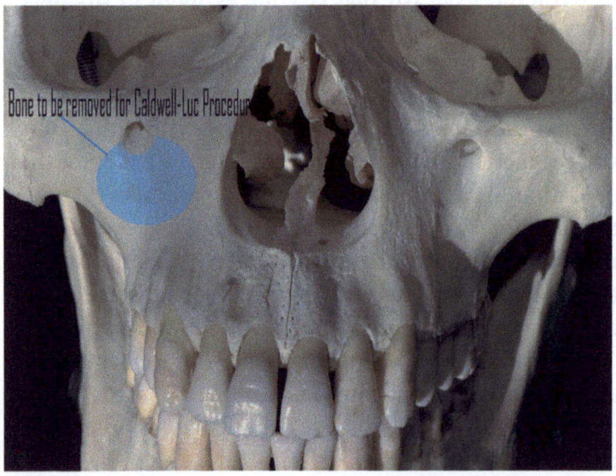

Fig. 31.2 Bony incision used for the Caldwell-Luc procedure

to remove all of the mucosa. Slow, steady traction is better than rapid tearing to remove large portions of the lining mucosa in a single piece.

Since the respiratory mucosa has been removed, the sinus will no longer drain via the natural ostium. A nasoantral window is therefore created via the inferior meatus. A mosquito-type clamp is inserted approximately 1 cm back into the inferior meatus to avoid the opening of the nasolacrimal duct. The clamp is directed toward the lateral canthus and bluntly inserted through the lateral wall of the inferior meatus, and spread. A rat-tail rasp, Kerrison forceps, or large Blakesly forceps is then used to enlarge the new ostium anteriorly and posteriorly to about 1.5–2.0 cm in diameter. If there is no significant bleeding, no packing is necessary. If bleeding persists, the sinus is packed with 0.5-inch (approximately 13 mm) gauze impregnated with antibiotic ointment, brought out via the nasoantral window. The gauze can be used as a file, much like dental floss, to smooth the opening of the new antrostomy by sliding it back and forth through the antrostomy. Finally, the sublabial incision is closed with interrupted simple absorbable sutures. If packing is used it is left for 1 or 2 days and then removed through the nose.

Although the open Lynch and Lothrop procedures are discussed here, they are increasingly of historic interest because they are not universally successful at creating long-term patency of a frontal sinus drainage system and are more cosmetically deforming than an osteoplastic frontal sinus procedure. Similarly, in the modern era it would be very unusual to resort to an external ethmoidectomy after failed endoscopic ethmoidectomy in the treatment of chronic rhinosinusitis.

The Lynch Procedure

- Indications for the Lynch procedure: failed primary surgery where hope still exists of reconstructing the frontal sinus outflow tract.

The Lynch procedure is used in the treatment of persistent frontal sinusitis in an attempt to reconstruct a large nasofrontal drainage pathway via an external approach. The operation begins with an external ethmoidectomy, but with the upper limb of the incision extending further laterally beneath the brow (Fig. 31.3). There are so many permutations of the "Lynch Procedure" that no single method is universally accepted. The original operation involved removal of the entire bony floor of the frontal sinus and stripping of all mucosa along with a complete ethmoidectomy and removal of the middle turbinate. Removal of the frontal sinus mucosa is difficult because of the limited exposure high and lateral. Eventually, many surgeons stopped trying to remove the mucosa and sim-

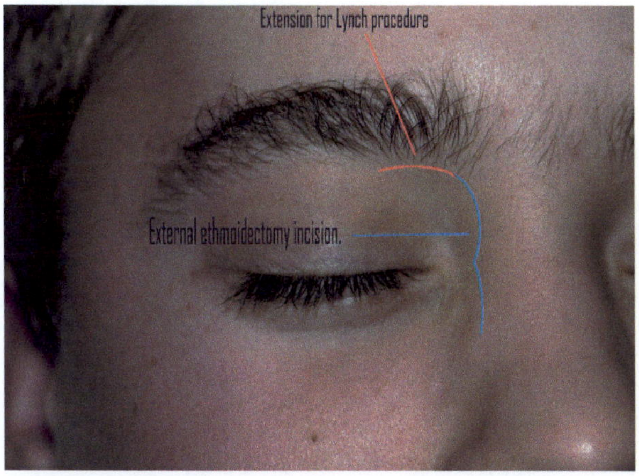

Fig. 31.3 Incisions for external ethmoidectomy (blue) and extension for Lynch procedure (red)

ply attempted to reconstruct the drainage system. A lateral nasal wall mucosal flap is fashioned with a superior base, and turned up at the conclusion of the operation to reline the nasofrontal drainage system medially. The reconstructed duct is stented for about 3 months with an endless variety of materials. The most popular is rolled silastic sheeting and cut portions of endotracheal tubes that are sewn to the nasal septum. The major complication of this procedure is restenosis of the nasofrontal drainage system and subsequent mucocele formation or recurrent frontal sinus obstruction and infection.

The Lynch procedure, like other "functional" operations is predicated on the belief that creating an adequate drainage system for the frontal sinus, in conjunction with medical therapy, can result in the return to normal of chronically diseased mucosa within the frontal sinus.

The Lothrop Procedure

- Indications for the Lothrop procedure: failed primary surgery where hope still exists of reconstructing the frontal sinus outflow tract.

The Lothrop procedure is performed via a unilateral or bilateral external anterior ethmoidectomy and middle turbinectomy. The frontal intersinus septum is resected along with the most anterosuperior portion of the nasal septum, creating a large drainage pathway. In cases of unilateral disease, the opposite nasofrontal drainage system could theoretically serve as a pathway for egress of frontal sinus secretions. Like its endoscopic counterpart, it works best in frontal sinuses with wide anteroposterior dimensions. Like the Lynch procedure, it assumes that "irreversibly damaged" mucosa does not exist within the frontal sinus.

Other Procedures

- Sometimes after failed attempts at endoscopic resection of cranial-base tumors or repair of extensive cerebrospinal fluid (CSF) leaks, it may be necessary to resort to an external approach.

Although unusual, it might at times prove necessary to resort to an external craniofacial approach to close a CSF leak or to resect tumors of the anterior skull base after failed attempts at endoscopic resection. This would most likely occur as a result of an error in judgment regarding the true extent of a tumor or the extent of a defect of the skull base. More commonly, these extensive lesions would be approached via an open approach initially, although this is beginning to change. It is important to remember that at times, endoscopic and open approaches are complementary and can be used in consort to achieve complete extirpation of particularly extensive lesions.

References

1. Barzilai G, Greenberg E, Uri N (2005) Indications for the Caldwell-Luc approach in the endoscopic era. Otolaryngol Head Neck Surg 132:219–220
2. Montgomery WW (1964) The fate of adipose implants in a bony cavity. Laryngoscope 74:816–827

Chapter 32

"Above and Below" Techniques in Revision Sinus Surgery

32

Timothy Haegen, Ryan M. Rehl, and Winston C. Vaughan

Core Messages

- Technological advances in endoscopic sinus surgery have limited the indications for external approaches to the frontal sinus. Despite this fact, certain conditions of the frontal sinus remain beyond the reach of the purely endoscopic approach.
- In selected cases, an "above and below" approach may allow access to pathologic diseases of the frontal sinus while minimizing morbidity.
- The addition of trephination to endoscopy may provide improved access to pathology of the lateral frontal sinus, assist in localizing the frontal recess, and allow postoperative irrigation in selected patients.

Contents

Background

Surgical management of the frontal sinus has been debated for over 250 years since Runge first described frontal sinus surgery [15]. In 1903, Killian changed the understanding of frontal sinus surgery by advocating the need to reconstitute the frontal recess, and he suggested the formation of a mucosal flap to help maintain patency [11]. Today, frontal sinus procedures reflect a rapid evolution of technology and a better understanding of sinonasal physiology. Functional endoscopic sinus surgery (FESS) has become the first-line approach for the majority of frontal sinus pathology. This trend has been facilitated by the introduction of image-guidance and endoscopic "extended" approaches to open the frontal sinus from below. Despite the dwindling number of indications for external frontal sinus techniques, procedures such as trephination, osteoplastic flap, or cranialization are considered when endoscopic techniques are unable to safely accomplish the goals of frontal sinus surgery. These more invasive procedures may have the disadvantage of increased morbidity [16].

Prior to electing a purely external approach, there remains the option of an "above and below" technique. The idea of a combined intranasal and external approach is not new. In 1914, Lothrop described the first combined intranasal and external approach to the frontal sinus [13]. After the introduction of advanced endoscopic instrumentation, Gross et al. popularized a completely endoscopic modification of the original Lothrop procedure. [10]. The current "above and below" technique includes an endoscopic sinus approach (below) and an external procedure (above). The early edition of the modern day "above and below" procedure was described by Wigand et al. to manage a fracture of the frontal sinus. This report by Wigand et al. included an osteoplastic flap [17]. The less invasive trephine was combined with an endoscopic procedure and later described by Bent et al. [3]. These combined approaches may provide improved visualization and access while theoretically minimizing overall risk and postoperative morbidity when compared with those of an osteoplastic flap. These procedures are also congruent with the basic tenets of treating frontal sinus pathology, which include: eradicate disease, restore function, minimize surgical risk, preserve cosmesis, and allow adequate surveillance.

Preoperative Workup

Patient history, office endoscopy, preoperative computed tomography (CT) scan with triplanar (axial, coronal, and sagittal) analysis, and surgeon experience are critical to surgical planning in frontal sinus surgery. It is also important to recognize that the decision to use the "above and below" approach may be made intraoperatively. Preoperative counseling regarding the possibility of an adjunctive trephine in the medial- or mid-brow area should be undertaken in patients with complex frontal recess anatomy or superior or lateral frontal sinus pathology. Procedures such as FESS, modified endoscopic Lothrop procedure (MELP), trephination, and an osteoplastic flap all have unique risks and benefits that require proper informed consent. Frank discussions regarding postoperative anosmia, bleeding, infection, frontal recess stenosis, cerebrospinal fluid (CSF) leak, orbital injury, meningitis, seizure, further surgery, pain, forehead hypoesthesia, cellulitis, brow hair loss, and scarring should occur.

Indications/Contraindications

Indications for the "above and below" approach include disease within laterally based frontal cells (some type III and most type IV), and laterally or superiorly based lesions in the frontal sinus. Frontal recess anatomy that has been altered by prior surgery, trauma, extensive inflammatory disease, or neoplasm might prevent adequate, safe frontal recess dissection.

- The trephination procedure provides the following benefits:
  1. Access to material for aspiration and culture.
  2. Access for irrigation from above to identify the frontal recess from below.
  3. Access for postoperative irrigation.
  4. Additional visualization of the frontal recess.
  5. Direct access for tissue manipulation or removal.

This approach has proven useful in the setting of mucocele, recalcitrant chronic sinusitis, inverted papilloma, osteoma, fibrous dysplasia, and pneumocephalus [1, 6, 7, 9, 12]. While absolute indications for the "above and below" approach have not been established, relative indications for the combined are listed here.

Indications for the "above and below" approach:

1. Chronic sinusitis of the frontal sinus associated with:
   a. Potts puffy tumor.
   b. Allergic fungal sinusitis with laterally impacted mucin.
   c. Lateral mucocele.
2. Distorted frontal recess anatomy secondary to:
   a. Iatrogenic or external trauma.
   b. Neo-osteogenesis.
   c. Obstructing or large-type III or IV frontal cells not amenable to endoscopic dissection.
3. Laterally based neoplasms/lesions:
   a. Osteomas
   b. Inverting papilloma
   c. Fibrous dysplasia
4. Contraindications to MELP:
   a. Narrow anteroposterior (AP) diameter of frontal sinus floor (<1.5 cm).
   b. Deep radix.
5. Evaluation of the posterior table of the frontal sinus in the setting of:
   a. Trauma
   b. CSF Leak
   c. Pneumocephalus

Chiu et al. discussed the role of the "above and below" approach in a report on their experience with frontal osteomas. They describe a grading system for frontal osteoma and three different surgical approaches (purely endoscopic, "above and below," and external). Chiu et al. present helpful guidelines for selecting the appropriate surgical procedure. They suggest that osteomas attached anterosuperiorly in the frontal sinus or those extending lateral to the lamina papyracea are best addressed with an "above and below" approach [6]. Dubin et al. reported indications for staged "above and below" treatment of frontal sinus inverted papilloma [7]. Four of six patients with frontal sinus inverting papilloma required a staged "below then above" approach consisting of an endoscopic frontal recess dissection followed by an osteoplastic flap at a separate operation. In addition to the size of the papilloma and location of the pedicle, a narrow frontal recess precluded successful purely endoscopic resection. One should note, however, there were no attempts at MELP or endoscopic Draf III in this series. The rest of this chapter addresses the combined "above and below" approach rather than the staged procedure described by Dubin et al.

In addition to the aforementioned indications, the "above and below" approach is useful when a Draf III is needed but the surgeon is not experienced with the endoscopic Draf III procedure or MELP, or when the surgeon feels these procedures would be contraindicated (deep radix, narrow AP diameter of frontal sinus floor). Benoit and Duncavage report similar safety and frontal recess patency rates with the "above and below" approach compared to the MELP [2]. Casiano and Livingston, reporting the University of Miami's experience with the MELP, highlighted the importance of obtaining an AP diameter of 8 mm or greater for the frontal sinus outflow tract. If the AP diameter of the frontal outflow tract is less than 8 mm at the conclusion of the surgery, postoperative stenosis is likely [4]. Unless the surgeon is confident that an 8-mm AP diameter can be obtained by the MELP, an "above and below" approach should be planned. The "above and below" approach need not exclude the MELP; however. Wormald et al. described a series of patients with mucoceles in previously obliterated frontal sinuses, who underwent a combination "above and below" unobliteration procedure. The below procedure in this series was a MELP [18]. As stated above, these are relative indications based on the preoperative evaluation of the patient and the surgeon's experience. This senior author has previously reported a series of ten patients with lateral frontal sinus lesions or supraorbital mucoceles. One patient failed and required the "above and below" approach later. Nine patients were successfully addressed by a purely endoscopic, image-guided procedure [5].

Contraindications to the "above and below" approach are similar to those of external frontal sinus surgery and include contraindications to general anesthesia. Trephination is contraindicated in an aplastic or markedly hypoplastic frontal sinus.

Contraindications to the "above and below" approach:
1. Medical disorders precluding general anesthesia.
2. Aplastic/hypoplastic frontal sinus.

Surgical Technique

The surgical technique may vary slightly depending on the triplanar CT scan findings (see Video 32.1).

- In preparation for the above and below" procedure, when reviewing CT images attention should be paid to:
  1. AP diameter of the frontal sinus floor.
  2. Pneumatization of the frontal sinuses.
  3. Integrity of the bony walls.
  4. Location of the pathology in the frontal sinus with respect to the lamina papyracea.
  5. Location of the superior attachment of the uncinate process.

The combined approach begins intranasally with adequate nasal decongestion. The patient is prepped after an image-guided system is calibrated and verified (if navigation is being used). Lidocaine with epinephrine is injected into the uncinate process, superior root of the middle turbinate and basal lamella of the middle turbinate when these structures are present and accessible. The endoscopic dissection begins with a complete uncinectomy. This improves frontal outflow tract endoscopic access. A maxillary antrostomy is done with identification of the superior roof of the maxillary sinus. The ethmoid bulla is removed and, if present, the suprabullar cell is also removed to identify the skull base and enlarge the frontal recess. A complete sphenoethmoidectomy is performed at this time if indicated. The skull base should be identified posteriorly at the sphenoid face and then followed anteriorly if a posterior ethmoidectomy is performed. Otherwise the skull base should be localized during the anterior ethmoidectomy. Important landmarks include the medial orbital wall and the anterior ethmoid artery. Coronal CT scans often reveal a medial dimpling of the lamina papyracea at the location of the anterior ethmoid artery. Careful preoperative review and intraoperative inspection with 30 , 45, or 70 endoscopy will demonstrate remaining anterior ethmoid, agger nasi, and frontal cells. These are identified and removed in a fashion described by Stammberger [14]. These cells are removed with mucosal-sparing techniques consisting of limited use of frontal sinus seekers, 90 curettes, curved mushroom punches, and giraffe forceps. Once the boundaries of the frontal recess (lateral, lamina papyracea; anterior, agger nasi; medial, superolateral surface of the middle turbinate; posterior, anterior skull base, anterior ethmoid artery, or the bulla lamella) have been identified, attention is turned to the frontal sinus pathology.

The 70 telescope is used to visualize the superior frontal recess and the frontal sinus. The author's group prefers a 70 telescope with a reverse light cable orientation, which allows easier instrument maneuvering below the eye piece and camera attachment. The 90 and 120 giraffe forceps, 90 curette, semimalleable suctions, and frontal seekers are used to marsupialize or remove the superior or lateral frontal sinus pathology. If the limits of endoscopic sinus surgery instruments are reached, a trephination is performed.

The trephine is placed to maximize surgical access of endoscopic instruments from above. Batra et al. stress the importance of a flexible location of the percutaneous incision and trephine, allowing entrance through the medial frontal sinus floor, medial anterior table, or lateral frontal sinus floor [1]. The incision and trephine may be medial or lateral to the supraorbital neurovascular bundle, as dictated by the sinus pathology. A 4-mm trephine is appropriate for frontal sinus pathology that requires only direct vision or in cases requiring aspiration or irrigation. In this instance, a percutaneous stab incision is more appropriate than a larger incision. For cases that require manipulation of frontal sinus pathology, a larger trephine may be needed. Typically a 6–8-mm trephine is used to place and manipulate both angled endoscopes and instruments.

This author's group prefers to place the trephine incision in the medial brow. This allows for excellent scar camouflage, even in the immediate postoperative period.

A transblepharoplasty incision is utilized by some authors. Knipe et al. described a series of five patients with frontal sinus disease and ophthalmologic manifestations [12]. These patients received a combined approach in which the percutaneous incision was through a transblepharoplasty approach. All five patients had the incision concealed in the upper eyelid skin crease with excellent postoperative cosmesis. Two of the five patients, however, eventually required revision endoscopic surgery.

Figures 32.1–32.4 show an "above and below" approach in a 26-year-old female flight attendant with recurrent severe, left-frontal headache during flying. Despite treatment with oral antibiotics, oral steroids, and topical therapy, her symptoms persisted. A CT scan following medical therapy revealed a lateral frontal spherical opacification that had decreased in size from her original CT scan at the time of initial presentation to the clinic. For the medial brow incision in the "above and below" approach, the appropriate eyebrow is prepped in a sterile fashion. The image-guidance system is used to assist in precise placement of the incision and point of entry into the sinus (Fig. 32.1). For the electromagnetic navigation system: after the incision has been planned and marked with the assistance of the image-guidance suction tip, the headset is temporarily removed or displaced to allow access to the medial brow. For cases in which image guidance is not used, the position and size of the frontal sinus may be aided with transillumination of the frontal sinus by flexible light, a 6-foot (approximately 2-m) PA Caldwell radiograph, or a prefabricated CT template [8]. The planned incision is infiltrated with lidocaine and epinephrine and a 1–2-cm incision is performed, beveled in a direction parallel to the hair shafts of the eyebrow. With the aid of a self-retaining retractor, the incision is carried down to bone (Fig. 32.2). A 4-mm drill bit is used to perform the boney trephination. The author's group uses the drill attachment for the powered sinus dissector (Fig. 32.3). Alternately, an otologic drill may be used. Care must be taken to keep the trajectory of the drill perpendicular to the frontal bone. The drill is applied until the mucosa is visible. If there is pulsation of the "mucosa," or it appears pale in color, it is important to reconfirm landmarks as this may be the dura. A fine-needle aspiration that produces air or mucous can be reassuring. The mucosa is carefully penetrated with sharp instrumentation. At this point, intranasal confirmation of successful

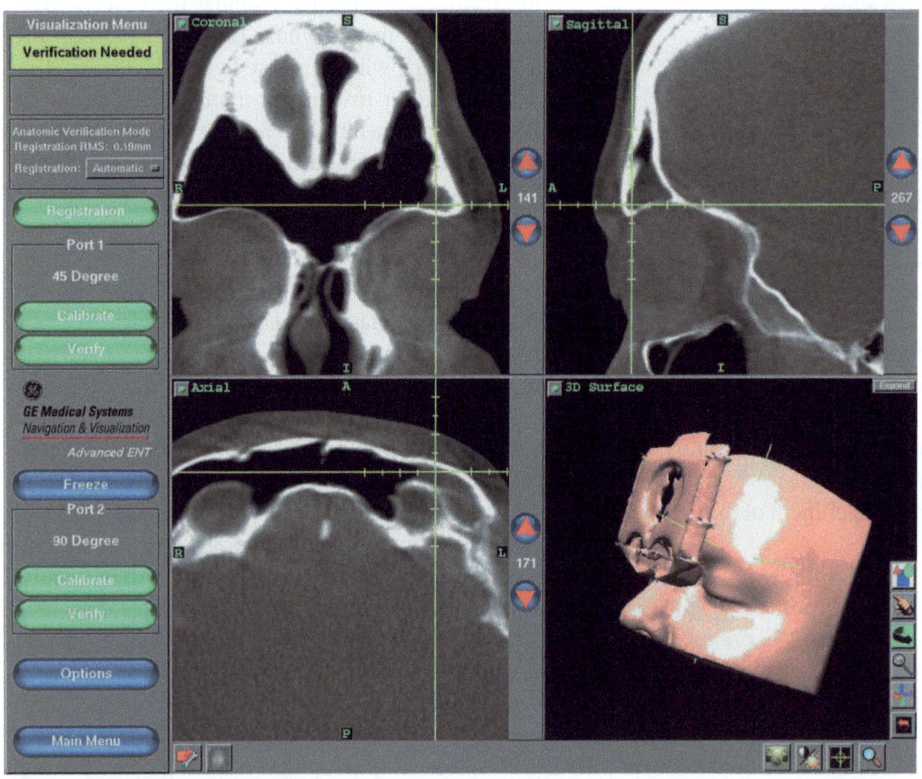

Fig. 32.1 After endoscopic frontal recess dissection, the image-guidance system is used to plan the location of trephination

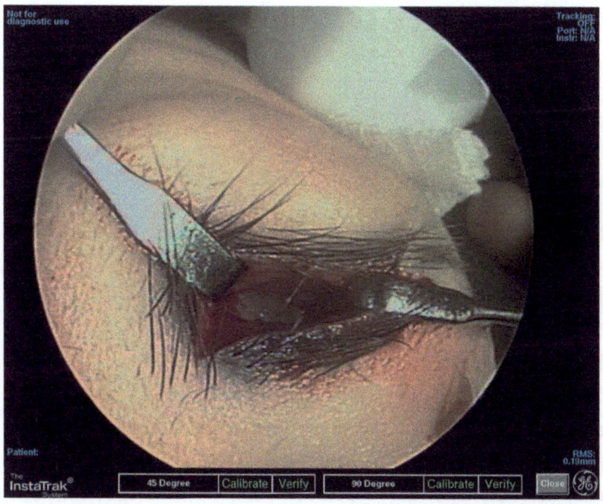

Fig. 32.2 An incision is made in the medial brow and blunt dissection is carried out down to the frontal bone. The periosteum is incised and a periosteal elevator is used to expose the area for drilling

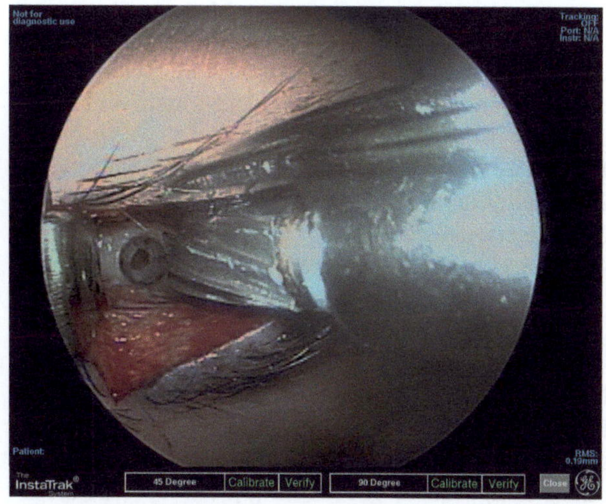

Fig. 32.3 The drill attachment on the powered sinus dissector is used for trephination

trephination is confirmed with irrigation from above. If the previous endoscopic dissection did not leave the frontal recess widely patent, intranasal identification of the frontal recess with irrigation may be facilitated by the addition of methylene blue to the saline irrigation. The trephine may then be enlarged with Kerrison rongeurs or the drill, as necessary. Once the frontal recess has been adequately opened, frontal sinus pathology including extensive type III cells, lateral type IV cells or tumors that can be manipulated under angled endoscopic visualization are addressed (Fig. 32.4). When possible, the posterior frontal sinus mucosa is everted down into the frontal recess along the anterior skull base or anterior ethmoid artery. If indicated, stents are placed from below and visualized from above. The external incision is then closed in a layered fashion. The skin is reapproximated with nylon or Prolene sutures. On occasion, a catheter may be left in the trephine and frontal sinus for approximately 2–5 days to allow postoperative irrigations.

Postoperative Care

As with all endoscopic frontal sinus surgery, meticulous postoperative debridement and medical management are mandatory for optimal surgical results. Skin sutures are removed at 1 week. Patients are followed every 1–2 weeks until the frontal recess demonstrates patency without crusting or inflammatory reaction. Patency is assessed with angled endoscopes, and gentle, atraumatic suction is used in a manner that limits granulation tissue formation. Proper office debridement is aided by 30 , 45 , and 70 telescopes, 90 semimalleable suctions, 90 curettes, and 45 and 90 giraffe forceps. Steroid sprays, drops, or irrigations are used routinely and culture-directed antibiotics are used for postoperative infection.

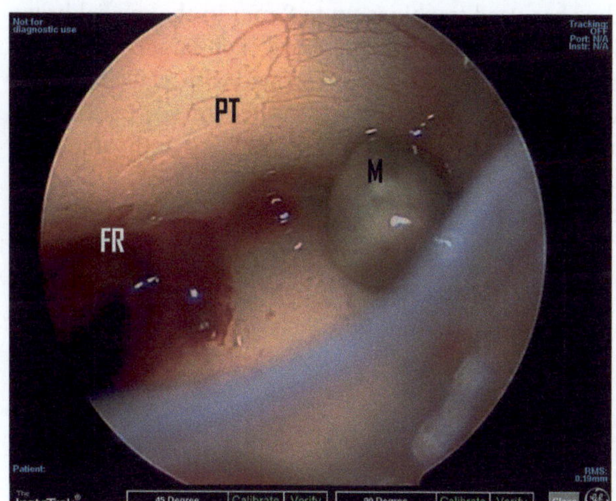

Fig. 32.4 A small mucopyocele is identified in the lateral and posterior portion of the frontal sinus. It was completely removed through the trephine with angled giraffe forceps. The patient's headache associated with flying resolved upon returning to work. *FR* Frontal recess, *M* mucocele, *PT* posterior table

32

Complications

Complications of the combined procedure include all the complications of routine endoscopic frontal sinus surgery:

1. Increases the risks of facial or periorbital cellulitis.
2. Posterior table CSF leak.
3. Cosmetic deformities.
4. Damage to the supraorbital and supratrochlear neurovascular bundle with subsequent anesthesia of the ipsilateral forehead.

In 62 consecutive "above and below" frontal procedures Benoit and Duncavage had no complications [2]. In the series reviewed by Batra et al., 3 of 22 patients developed minor complications of cellulitis [1]. There were no CSF leaks or cosmetic deformities. In a series of 22 minitrephinations by Gallagher and Gross, there were 2 patients with skin burns and 1 CSF leak from intracranial penetration [9]. Image guidance was not used in this series. Bent et al. had two localized cases of cellulitis in 11 patients treated with the "above and below" approach. Both complications were treated successfully with antibiotics [3]. Prevention is the best approach to complications. Minitrephination sets may be used in combination with image guidance to possibly decrease the risk of intracranial penetration. Prophylactic systemic and topical antibiotics may be used to decrease the likelihood of postoperative cellulitis.

Five millimeters has been recommended as the maximum diameter of an anterior table trephine to prevent soft-tissue prolapse and cosmetic deformity [3]. This author has used trephines up to 8 mm in the medial brow without any visible depressions. For larger trephines, bone replacement can be performed with available products. Although not reported in their series, Batra et al. also warn against anterior table trephine in the management of acute frontal sinusitis due to the risk of seeding the frontal bone and resulting osteomyelitis [1].

Tips and Pearls to Minimize Complications

1. Thorough analysis of frontal sinus anatomy on triplanar CT prior to performing the procedure.
2. Perform the endoscopic portion first and identify important landmarks.
3. Use image guidance to identify the trephine location.
4. Reduce damage to the supraorbital neurovascular bundle by blunt dissection and avoid monopolar cautery.
5. Limit trephines to 6–8 mm.
6. Use angled scopes and instruments from both directions.
7. As with FESS, mucosal preservation and eversion into the frontal recess/anterior ethmoid remain essential.
8. Consider a course of systemic antibiotics when the operative field is grossly involved by purulent material or in immunocompromised and diabetic patients.

Outcomes

In their report on 11 patients who underwent "above and below" procedures for frontal sinus mucoceles, Bent et al. found that all patients were free of disease or improved with a mean follow-up of 19 months. In this retrospective study, three patients did require reoperation. [3]. Benoit and Duncavage reported on 40 patients who underwent 62 "above and below" procedures with stent placement (a bilateral procedure was performed in 22 patients). Overall patency rates and subjective improvement were 79% and 78%, respectively after a mean follow up of 1 year. Five of their patients required reoperation after the "above and below" procedure. Four of those patients undergoing reoperation had the frontal sinus obliterated with fat [2]. Batra et al. reviewed the outcomes of 22 patients with complex frontal sinus pathology treated with the "above and below" approach in 2005. Resolution or improvement of headaches and orbital symptoms occurred in 82% and 88% of patients, respectively. In addition, confirmation of postoperative frontal recess patency was confirmed in 19 of 22 patients (86%). In one patient, frontal sinus patency could not be confirmed because of partial middle-turbinate lateralization. A CT scan on this patient revealed a well-aerated frontal sinus. Two patients had near-complete postoperative stenosis of the frontal outflow tract. Follow-up CT scans on these two patients revealed partial aeration of the frontal sinus without mucocele formation [1].

Conclusion

The "above and below" approach is a versatile technique that is intermediate in invasiveness between pure endoscopic frontal sinus surgery and external osteoplastic flap. In fact, it has been reported by some to be a reasonable option after obliteration has failed. The "above and below" procedure adheres to the basic tenets of frontal-sinus surgery, which include: remove disease, maintain the patency of the frontal recess, preserve the sinus mucosa, reduce the surgical risk, and facilitate endoscopic and radiographic surveillance. Although high-resolution CT, image guidance, and improved instrumentation have expanded the indications for pure endoscopic techniques, the "above and below" combined approach remains a valuable tool in the rhinologist's armamentarium.

References

1. Batra PS, Citardi MJ, Lanza DC (2005) Combined endoscopic trephination and endoscopic frontal sinusotomy for management of complex frontal sinus pathology. Am J Rhinol 5:435–441
2. Benoit CM, Duncavage JA (2001) Combined external and endoscopic frontal sinusotomy with stent placement: a retrospective review. Laryngoscope 111:1246–1249
3. Bent JP 3rd, Spears RA, Kuhn FA, et al. (1997) Combined endoscopic intranasal and external frontal sinusotomy. Am J Rhinol 11:349–354
4. Casiano RR, Livingston JA (1998) Endoscopic Lothrop procedure: the University of Miami experience. Am J Rhinol 12:335–339
5. Chiu AG, Vaughan WC (2004) Management of the lateral frontal sinus lesion and the supraorbital cell mucocele. Am J Rhinol 18:83–86
6. Chiu AG, Schipor I, Cohen NA, et al. (2005) Surgical decisions in the management of frontal sinus osteomas. Am J Rhinol 19:191–197
7. Dubin MG, Sonnenburg RE, Melroy CT, et al. (2005) Staged endoscopic and combined open/endoscopic approach in the management of inverted papilloma of the frontal sinus. Am J Rhinol 19:442–445
8. Fewins JL, Otto PM, Otto RA (2004) Computed tomography-generated templates: a new approach to frontal sinus osteoplastic flap surgery. Am J Rhinol 18:285–289; Discussion 289–290
9. Gallagher RM, Gross CW (1999) The role of mini-trephination in the management of frontal sinusitis. Am J Rhinol 13:289–293
10. Gross WE, Gross CW, Becker et al. (1995) Modified transnasal endoscopic Lothrop procedure as an alternative to frontal sinus obliteration. Otolaryngol Head Neck Surg 113:427–434
11. Killian G (1903) Die killianische radicaloperation chronischer strinhohleneiterungen: II. Weiteres kasuistisches material und zusammenfassung. Arch Laryngol Rhinol 12:59
12. Knipe TA, Gandhi PD, Fleming JC, et al. (2007) Transblepharoplasty approach to sequestered disease of the lateral frontal sinus with ophthalmologic manifestations. Am J Rhinol 21:100–104
13. Lothrop HA (1912) Frontal sinus suppuration. Ann Surg 59:937
14. Stammberger, H (2000) FESS "Uncapping the Egg" The Endoscopic Approach to Frontal Recess and Sinuses. A Surgical Technique of the Graz University Medical School. Endo-Press. Tuttlingen, Germany
15. Stevenson RS, Guthrie D (1949) History of Otolaryngology. Williams and Wilkins, Baltimore
16. Weber R, Draf W, Keerl R, et al. (2000) Osteoplastic frontal sinus surgery with fat obliteration: technique and long-term results using magnetic resonance imaging in 82 operations. Laryngoscope 110:1037–1044
17. Wigand ME, Steiner W, Jaumann MP (1978) Endonasal sinus surgery with endoscopical control: from radical operation to rehabilitation of the mucosa. Endoscopy 10:255–260
18. Wormald PJ, Ananda A, Nair S (2003) Modified endoscopic Lothrop as a salvage for the failed osteoplastic flap with obliteration. Laryngoscope 113:1988–1992

Chapter 33

Revision Endoscopic Skull-Base Surgery

Aldo C. Stamm, João Flávio, and Richard J. Harvey

33

Core Messages

- Revision skull-base surgery (SBS) should be practiced within a multidisciplinary team.
- Standard endoscopic sinus instrumentation is often inadequate for SBS and specialized equipment is required.
- Closure of large skull-base defects requires careful preoperative evaluation and planning of reconstructive options.
- The use of pedicled mucosal flaps and a multilayered reconstruction is the key to closing large skull-base defects.
- The potential for complications differs little from open SBS, but the ability for faster recovery and less morbidity is great.

Contents

Introduction

Skull-base surgery (SBS) evolved from a combination of craniofacial surgery and neurosurgery in the 19th century. Its earliest applications were for the removal of skull-base tumors and intracranial neurosurgery [39, 57]. Modern SBS now encompasses a diverse group of pathologies (Table 33.1) [54]. The use of endoscopes in surgery for skull-base lesions has been particularly successful. The management of sphenoid papilloma highlights the advantages of an endoscopic approach – minimal operative morbidity, direct access to pathology, and detailed visual assessment of anatomy and resection limits [14]. However, effective and safe treatment of lesions involving the skull base remains a challenging problem. Difficulties in endoscopic SBS and its revision include difficulty of access, the relationship between critical anatomy and pathology, and reconstructive techniques for large defects.

Revision SBS, either open or endoscopic, is a complex process with a significant risk of postoperative complications [12, 44]. In revision SBS, essential nasal landmarks are often missing. Reconstructive options may be limited and prior radiotherapy can further impede healing. Surgical success depends not only on technological advances, but also on a variety of factors, including intimate

33

Table 33.1 Endoscopic skull-base pathologies

- Cerebrospinal fluid leak
- Trauma
  - Optic nerve decompression
- Infection
  - Epidural abscess
  - Osteomyelitis
  - Inflammatory sinus disease
- Mucocele
- Allergic fungal sinusitis
- Benign neoplasms
  - Pituitary adenoma
  - Fibro-osseous lesions
  - Meningioma
  - Craniopharyngioma
  - Angiofibroma
- Malignant neoplasms
  - Sinonasal malignancies
  - Esthesioneuroblastoma
  - Chordoma
  - Chondrosarcoma
  - Metastases
- Miscellaneous
  - Rathke's cyst
  - Dermoid cyst
  - Arteriovenous malformation
  - Epidermoid

knowledge of the involved anatomy, adequate instrumentation, surgical experience, and a structured and appropriate surgical approach.

Why an Endoscopic Approach for Revision SBS?

The direct transnasal route is ideal for lesions of the anterior and central skull base. There is also increasing experience in endoscopic management of lateral pathology within the infra-temporal fossa [31, 49]. The entire ventral skull base can be accessed by a transnasal endoscopic route. Previous radiotherapy, surgery, and reconstructive efforts often complicate revision cases. An endoscopic route often allows minimal dissection of surgical planes. When the initial procedure was performed via an open approach, revision endoscopic SBS may provide fresh tissue planes with access to regions left untreated during previous surgeries [43]. In addition, postoperative recovery is generally shorter with endoscopic surgery [8] and morbidity is lower [3].

The Goals of Endoscopic SBS

There are a variety of indications for which revision endoscopic SBS may be performed. Removing recurrent disease is only one indication for those who need revision endoscopic SBS.

- Broadly, the goals of revision endoscopic SBS should include:
  1. Removal of disease.
  2. Treatment of the complications arising from previous SBS.
  3. Minimize functional loss:
     a. Vision
     b. Other cranial nerve integrity
     c. Pituitary/hypothalamic function
     d. Orbital function

An understanding of the significant complications associated with surgery, whether neurological, orbital, endocrine, or infectious, is paramount to an informed discussion with a patient considering revision endoscopic SBS.

The Multidisciplinary Approach

The team approach in the management of challenging pathology is still a relatively novel concept in medicine. Although the multidisciplinary team (MDT) has evolved only in the last few decades, complication rates from SBS, since the introduction of such an approach, have decreased [4]. The MDT approach should include neurosurgery, otolaryngology, intensive care, anesthesiology, pathology, endocrinology, and paramedical staff, such as skilled nursing to care for patients at risk of significant neurological sequelae [4, 32, 43, 46]. The MDT is even more applicable to the management of the revision SBS patient. With complication rates from open revision SBS approaching 30–50% in some series [12], the need for multiteam discussion and care is essential (Fig. 33.1).

- Indications:
  1. Disease:
     a. Removal of persistent disease.
     b. Decompression of cranial nerves with subtotal resection.
     c. Planned second stage.
  2. Common complications from prior SBS:
     a. Cerebrospinal fluid (CSF) leaks
     b. Frontal recess occlusion
     c. Sphenoid sinus obstruction
     d. Mucoceles
     e. Encephalocele formation

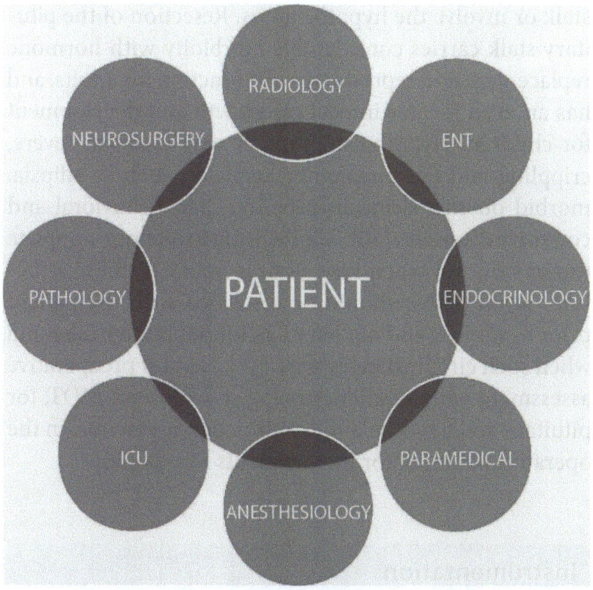

Fig. 33.1 The specialist groups involved in the care of the revision skull-base surgery patient (Reproduced with permission from Centro de ORL, Sao Paulo, Brazil)

f. Subdural hematoma
g. Osteoradionecrosis

- Contraindications:
  1. Acute/subacute rhinossinusitis.
  2. No MDT service.
  3. Lack of specialized equipment.

Preoperative Workup

Anatomy

Revision endoscopic SBS is often substantially more complex than primary surgery because essential nasal landmarks have frequently been removed or drastically altered. The skull base, lamina papyracea, and other natural barriers to complications may be eroded or removed from previous surgery. Posterior septectomy and partial or total amputation of the turbinates are common anatomical alterations from prior surgery. It is essential in the preoperative endoscopic evaluation to identify these changes in the skull base and nasal cavity. Pathology may, additionally, be hidden behind previous reconstructive efforts. A careful surgical plan for the reconstruction of any skull-base defect is very important. The use of pedicled or free mucosal grafts might be hindered by previous septum and turbinate removal. The loss of reconstructive options may be considerable.

Imaging

Imaging is crucial in the evaluation for revision SBS. This will almost always include both computed tomography (CT) and magnetic resonance imaging (MRI) modalities. A minimum slice thickness of 3 mm (preferably less) of coronal, axial, and sagittal CT images of the sinuses and skull base are essential in the assessment for surgery. In addition to diagnostic information, CT offers critical anatomical information such as [59]:

1. The presence and extent of erosions of the skull base.
2. The integrity of the medial orbital wall.
3. The position of anterior skull-base vessels.
4. The integrity and degree of aeration of paranasal sinuses (particularly the sphenoid sinus).
5. The location and presence of intersinus septae.
6. The position and erosion near internal carotid arteries (ICAs), optic nerves, and cavernous sinuses.
7. The relationship between the roof of the ethmoid sinuses and the cribriform plate.
8. The presence of Onodi cells.

MRI is the imaging study of choice to assess patients for recurrent skull-base tumor [66]. MRI is also particularly important when CT reveals soft-tissue densities adjacent to dehiscent bone in the skull base. The evaluation of dehiscent areas becomes even more crucial when located in the lateral sphenoid. Iatrogenic injury to this region can result in significant bleeding, the formation of a carotid pseudoaneurysm, or optic nerve injury.

- Anatomical areas that pose greater challenges to resection should be carefully evaluated. These include the:
  1. Cavernous sinus
  2. Meckel's cave
  3. Jugular foramen
  4. ICA.

The involvement of the carotid artery, the vertebrobasilar system, or dural sinuses should also alert the surgeon to additional risk to the intracranial vasculature [43].

Appropriate imaging sequences are essential in the correct interpretation of MRI changes. Previous SBS will often leave enhancing tissue that may be a combination of recurrent tumor, scar tissue, and reconstructive grafts.

- The use of T1-weighted images and fat saturation techniques before and after gadolinium enhancement will reduce misdiagnosis, such as changes related to free fat grafts used in prior reconstruction.

Scar and other high signal tissues may not be easily discernable from recurrent disease. Changes on serial examinations, after an early postoperative baseline study, may be the only characteristic features of residual pathology [43]. MRI also enables differentiation of tumor from retained secretions.

Magnetic resonance angiography or CT angiography (Fig. 33.2) [36] can be used to assess the structure of medium-to-large arteries in patients when erosion of the sphenoid and clivus has occurred. The relationship between the basilar arteries and ICAs to pathology is crucial in this area. Although conventional angiography is not routinely performed, it may verify the functional integrity of the circle of Willis, the extent of any carotid artery compromise, and differentiate aneurysm from tumor.

Endocrine and Hypothalamic Considerations

Even with the best preoperative imaging, the relationship between tumor and intracranial structures can be difficult to demonstrate. It is extremely difficult to evaluate before surgery whether some tumors are extra-arachnoidal, extrapial-subarachnoidal, or partially intraparenchymal-subpial [16]. This weighs heavily on considerations to obtain complete resection. Parasellar pathologies such as craniopharyngiomas may often encase the pituitary stalk or involve the hypothalamus. Resection of the pituitary stalk carries considerable morbidity with hormone replacement and reproductive dysfunction for adults, and has an even greater impact on growth and development for children. Hypothalamic injury may result in severe, crippling and life-threatening sequelae, such as adipsia, morbid obesity, sleep disturbances, and behavioral and cognitive disorders [56]. The decision to attempt complete tumor removal when resection or injury to these structures is inevitable should be discussed with the patient prior to surgery and not left to an intraoperative dilemma when such circumstances arise [17]. Careful preoperative assessment with an endocrinologist, within an MDT, for pituitary and hypothalamic dysfunction is essential in the operative planning for these patients [40, 48, 56].

Instrumentation

Endoscopic SBS is highly dependant on specialized instrumentation and its absence is an absolute contraindication to surgery. Dissection instruments and drills that are appropriately long enough to perform dissection beyond the sphenoid are essential. Similarly, high-quality endoscopes and video equipment are required. It is not appropriate to perform endoscopic SBS without camera equipment. An entire operative team needs to be visually informed of the state of surgery. A second surgeon, for bimanual dissection, and theater staff should be actively involved. The ability to maintain hemostasis and

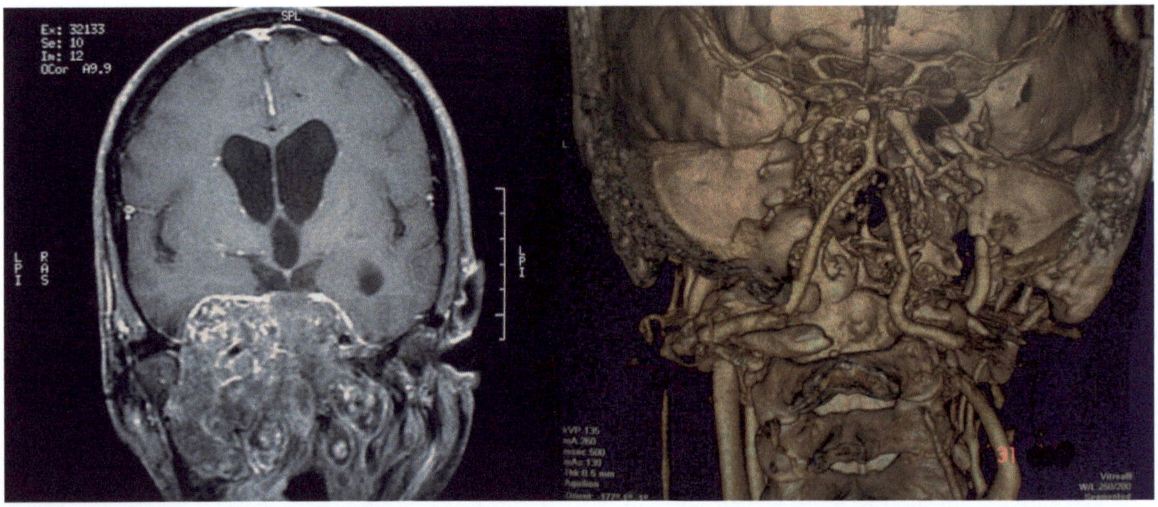

Fig. 33.2 Computed tomography angiogram of a recurrent clival chordoma. Note the laterally displaced position of the internal carotid arteries (ICAs). (Reproduced with permission from Centro de ORL, Sao Paulo, Brazil)

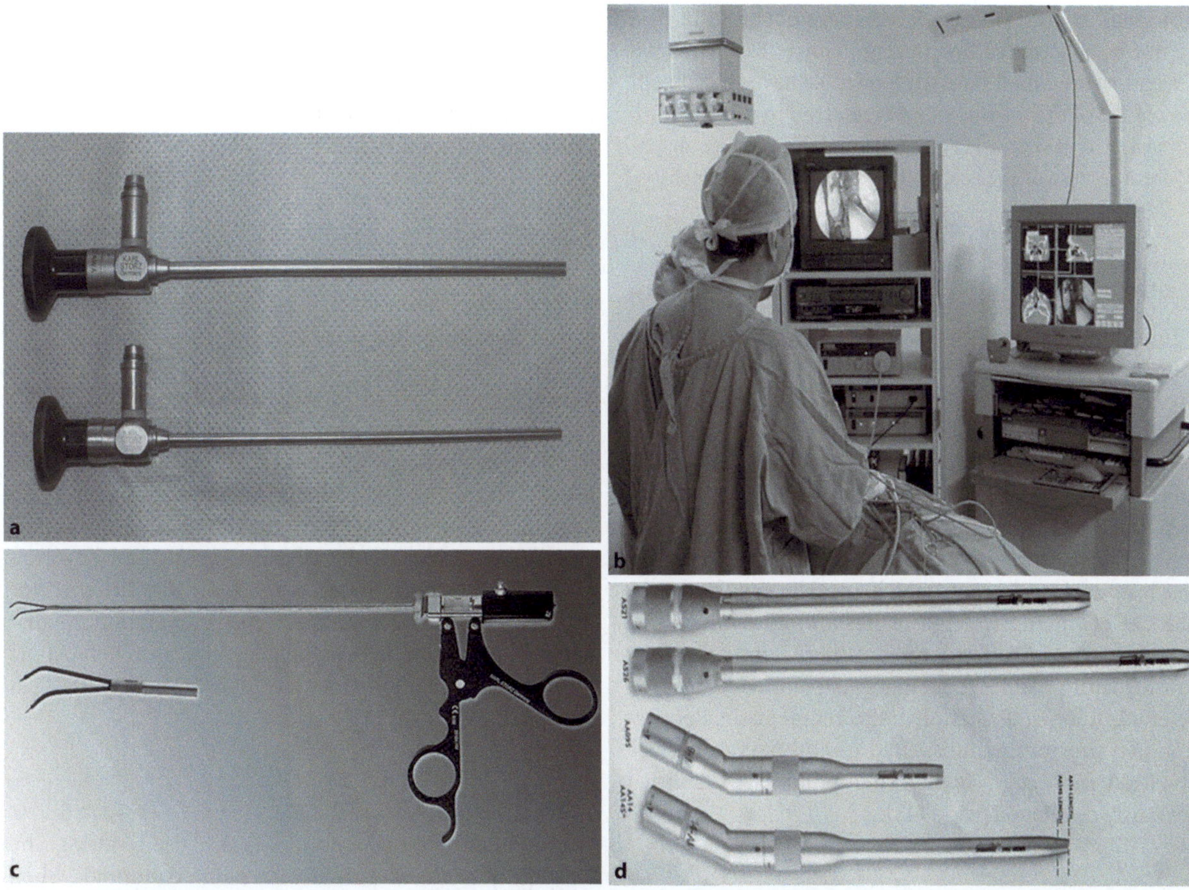

Fig. 33.3 Endoscopic skull-base surgery equipment. **a** 5.2-mm and 4-mm endoscopes. **b** Image-guidance systems. **c** Long bipolar forceps. **d** Long protected drill shafts. (Reproduced with permission from Centro de ORL, Sao Paulo, Brazil)

a workable operative field during prolonged surgery is a demanding aspect of extended endoscopic surgery. Long endoscopic bipolar forceps and hemostatic materials such as Surgicel or Avatine are essential to this process (Fig. 33.3) [28].

Previous Radiotherapy

Precise knowledge of previous radiotherapy fields will have significant impact on reconstructive options. In irradiated tissue, multilayered free graft repair of skull-base defects has a high dehiscence rate in our experience and elsewhere [45]. Reconstruction of the irradiated skull base almost always demands vascularized tissue. Pedicled mucoperiosteal and mucoperichondrial flaps are used for reconstruction. Radiotherapy may also thicken the pia-arachnoid tumor interface, obscuring dissection planes, and contribute to a greater risk of neural injury [43].

Surgical Techniques

General Principles

- The medial orbital wall, orbital apex, and prechiasmal optic nerve axis is a key landmark in revision SBS.
- Dissection should always proceed from known to unknown.

Endoscopic dissection in a previously operated skull base can be challenging due to the loss of traditional surgical landmarks. The use of image guidance has gained increasingly popularity since early reports of its use [6]. Improving the accuracy of image guidance has an associated learning curve [55] and occasional use may prove frustrating to the unfamiliar. Fusion MRI and CT guidance may provide more significant information for the surgeon operating on the skull base with extensive bone loss and altered soft-tissue structures [34]. However, detailed knowledge of the endoscopic anatomy of the skull base can not be substituted by image guidance [51]. The revision endoscopic skull-base surgeon must have an exquisite knowledge of the anatomy and is referred to two anatomical series by Jho and Ha [22–24] and Kassam et al. [29, 30] for a review of the relevant endoscopic relationships.

Dissection from the Cerebrovascular Structures

- Intradural dissection should be extra-arachnoid and preserve the arachnoid tissue and vessels – even for vessels much smaller than 1 mm in diameter.

The technical difficulties posed by reoperation in the anterior fossa, parasellar region, and posterior fossa are often the result of meningeal inflammation associated with previous dissection. The arachnoid can be diffusely tenacious and opalescent, which complicates the establishment of microdissection planes and may hinder the identification of vital structures. Where subtotal tumor removal with possible reoperation is planned, it may be preferable to resist dissection in the neural plane. Reoperation of a previously undissected tumor–nerve interface is typically more effective than attempting to reestablish a previously developed plane [43].

Staging the Resection

- Staged resection of benign lesions may allow safer dissection of the tumor capsule from critical cerebrovascular structures.

A planned staging of resection in cases of extensive benign skull-base tumors may be appropriate when pathologies involve critical structures or neurovascular planes [14]. This approach may assist with venous hemostasis, especially within the clivus.

Hemostasis

- The most important hemostatic technique, especially in venous bleeding, may be patience.

The principles of hemostasis in endoscopic SBS differ little from those of the microsurgical era. Prevention of bleeding is obviously the best solution. Tumor debulking, extracapsular sharp dissection, and countertraction using gentle suction still form the foundation of cerebrovascular control [28]. Standard neurosurgical bayonets are often not appropriate via the long surgical corridor of endoscopic SBS. Specialized instrumentation, as discussed previously, is essential. Examples of hemostatic techniques are demonstrated in Table 33.2.

Operative Basics

- Adrenaline-soaked cottonoids are used during the surgery but are replaced with saline cottonoids when intradural dissection proceeds.

Revision endoscopic SBS is performed under general controlled hypotensive anesthesia. Cottonoids containing epinephrine 1:1000 are placed in the nasal cavity over

Table 33.2 Endoscopic hemostatic techniques

- Electrocautery
  - Monopolar cautery (due to possible current dispersion, it should not be used within the sphenoidal sinus, on the skull base, or intracranially).
  - Bipolar cautery with endoscopic forceps
- Endoscopic clip applicators
  - Structured approach to ligating the anterior ethmoidal, sphenopalatine, or posterior ethmoidal artery with a Ligge Clip applicator prior to dissection [20].
- Hemostatic materials
  - Surgicell (Johnson and Johnson).
  - Avitene (Johnson and Johnson).
  - Floseal (Baxter International).
  - Syvek (Marine Polymer).
- Saline irrigation
  - Hot-water irrigation has been advocated for hemostasis in the nasal mucosa [60, 61] and warm saline is used in some skull-base centers [28].

the areas of surgical access for 10 min before the surgical procedure. If septectomy or mucosal flaps are planned, the septum is infiltrated with lidocaine with epinephrine 1:100.000. When the surgery includes the pterygopalatine and infratemporal fossa, the region of the sphenopalatine foramen is infiltrated with approximately 2.0 ml of the same concentration solution using an angulated 25-gauge spinal needle after first aspirating.

Avoiding Complications in Revision Endoscopic SBS

CSF Leak Closure

There are well established techniques for closing CSF leaks [68, 69]. The endoscopic management with free grafts is the first option for small defects (<1 cm) in primary and revision cases [18, 37, 41]. However, possible failure can be avoided by identification of benign intracranial hypertension, which is often characterized by empty sellae, multiple skull-base defects, or a broadly attenuated skull base. These patients and may require additional interventions, such as lumbar drains or CSF diversion, for success [52].

Transplanum/Transsphenoidal Surgery

Endoscopic revision surgery for pituitary adenoma is almost the standard care in many centers [5]. There are three important implications of previous surgery in this area. Firstly, the optic chiasm may lie superior or inferior to its original position and will often have fat from a previous repair adherent in the prechiasmatic position. Secondly, the anterior cerebral vessels may be adherent to the previous repair of a transplanum approach. If the arteries are adherent to fat or fascia then it may be prudent to leave an island of scar tissue on the vessel rather than attempt dissection (Fig. 33.4). Finally, the vasculature of the pituitary may be easily damaged if there is scar tissue involving the stalk. Most importantly, a recurrent superior hypophyseal artery may lie within the vasculature of the pituitary stalk and injury can result in optic nerve or pituitary injury (Fig. 33.5) [33, 65].

Transclival Surgery

The position of the ICA can be difficult to locate in revision SBS. Previous extensive bone removal can leave a long segment of the ICA in soft tissue. The ICAs usually remain in a lateral position after previous displacement by pathology (Fig. 33.6). Intraoperative micro-Doppler ultrasound can be used to help locate the vessels in such cases [10]. Prior radiotherapy, especially in chordoma, may make surgical planes difficult to identify. The role of CT angiography may be important in defining pathology from prior reconstruction (mainly fat) and the basilar arterial system (Fig. 33.2).

Reconstructive Options

- The ability to close large skull-base defects is perhaps the second greatest challenge to endoscopic SBS, after the management of cerebrovascular structures.

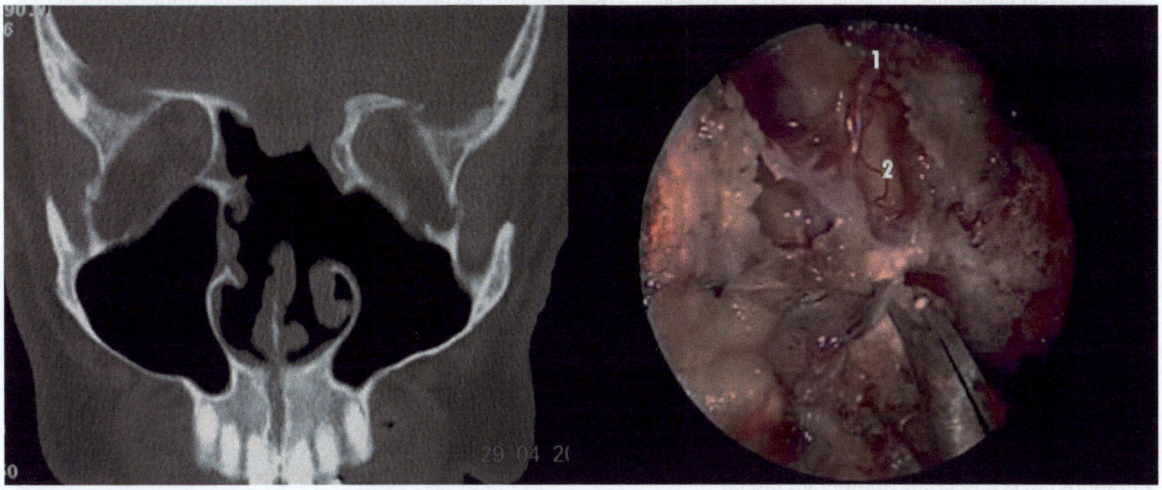

Fig. 33.4 Recurrent hemangiopericytoma. *1* Anterior cerebral vessels, *2* frontal gyrus. (Reproduced with permission from Centro de ORL, Sao Paulo, Brazil)

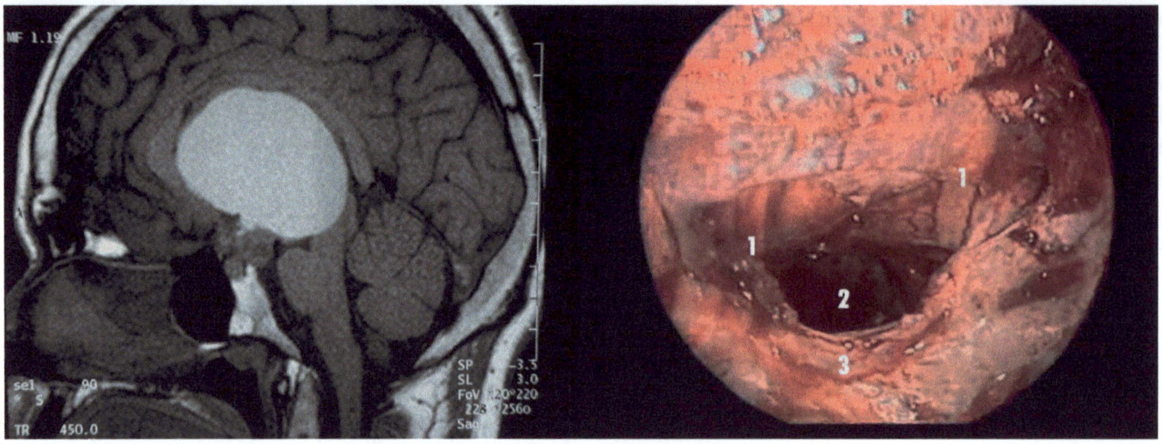

Fig. 33.5 Recurrent cystic craniopharyngioma. *1* Olfactory tract, *2* transplanum opening to cyst, *3* Sella. (Reproduced with permission from Centro de ORL, Sao Paulo, Brazil)

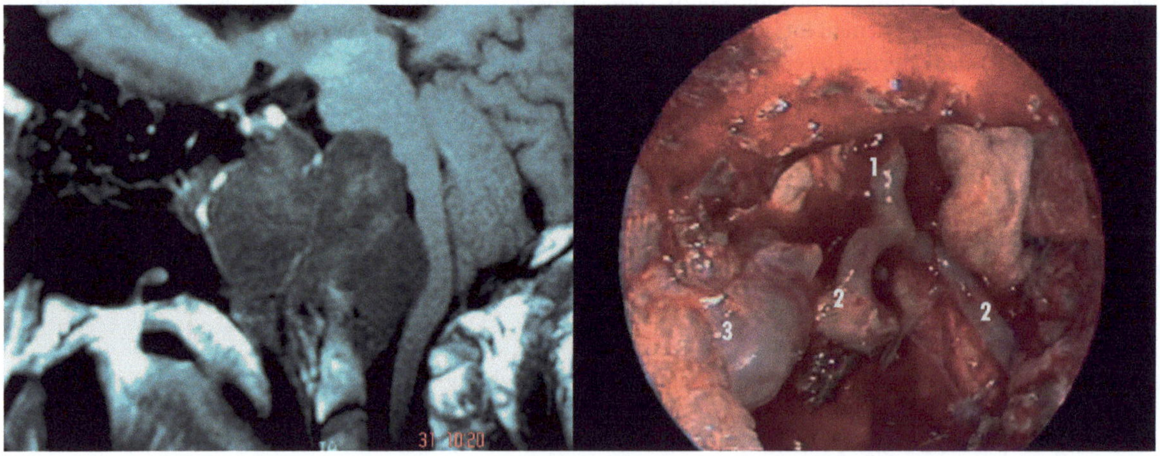

Fig. 33.6 Recurrent chordoma. *1* Basilar artery, *2* vertebral arteries, *3* tumor. (Reproduced with permission from Centro de ORL, Sao Paulo, Brazil)

Table 33.3 Graft materials used in reconstruction of skull-base defects

- Mucosal flaps
  - Posterior rotation septal flap (based on the septal branch of the sphenopalatine artery (SPA); Fig. 33.7a)
  - Contralateral transposition septal flap (based on ethmoidal arteries; Fig. 33.7b)
  - Inferior turbinate flap (based on turbinate branch of the SPA; Fig. 33.7c)
  - Nasal floor flap (based on branches of the SPA and Woodruff's plexus; Fig. 33.7d)
- Free mucosal or mucoperioteal grafts
  - Well-described series with closure of anterior skull-base defects with cerebrospinal fluid leaks but not with extensive dural resection [35]
- Tissue glues and substrates – BioGlue [13] Tisseel [27] DuraGen [9] and Duraseal
- Autologus fascia (fascia lata, temporalis fascia)
- Homologus fascia (Alloderm)
- Free fat grafts
- Free flaps [67] (usually requiring conversion to open skull-base surgery)
- Free bone or synthetic materials

- Multilayered reconstruction with pedicled mucosal flaps is the key to closing large skull-base defects.

A variety of reconstructive materials have been used (Table 33.3). The use of vascularized pedicled flaps has been the most significant advancement in our institution to reconstruct major skull-base defects (Fig. 33.7, Video 33.1). Pedicled mucosal flaps have been well described for a variety of reconstructive procedures such as septal perforation repair [47, 53], reconstructive rhinoplasty [2, 42], and choanal atresia repair [11, 58]. However, the use of vascularized mucosal flaps to repair large skull-base defects [19] or congenital defects [64] has been described only recently. Along with other centers, with endoscopic skull-base experience, we discourage the use of free bone grafts and synthetic materials (i.e., titanium mesh) as these may lead to poor healing and formation of sequestra [26].

Free fat grafts are used to fill dead space and form a buttress for a subdural fascial graft. This is covered with a combination of pedicled mucoperiosteal/chondrial flaps. Fibrin tissue glue is used to secure the repair. Gelfoam is layered to the area, followed by gauze packing. The packing is supported by a Foleys balloon catheter (Fig. 33.8).

Postoperative Care

If the procedure is intradural, recovery is performed with neurological observations in high dependency. CT is performed out our institution on the first postoperative day for evidence of hemorrhage. Antibiotics are used perioperatively and continued postoperatively while nasal packing remains in situ. Packing is left in place for 7–14 days as most grafts are adherent in bone in 1 week [50]. The onset of diabetes insipidus is monitored with serum and urine sodium/osmolality measurements. Patients are confined to bed/chair rest with toilet privileges for 48 hrs, have 30 ° head elevation, and avoid straining, Valsalva maneuvers, and nose blowing. Lumbar drains are not used unless there is an additional comorbidity such as raised intracranial hypertension or prior radiotherapy.

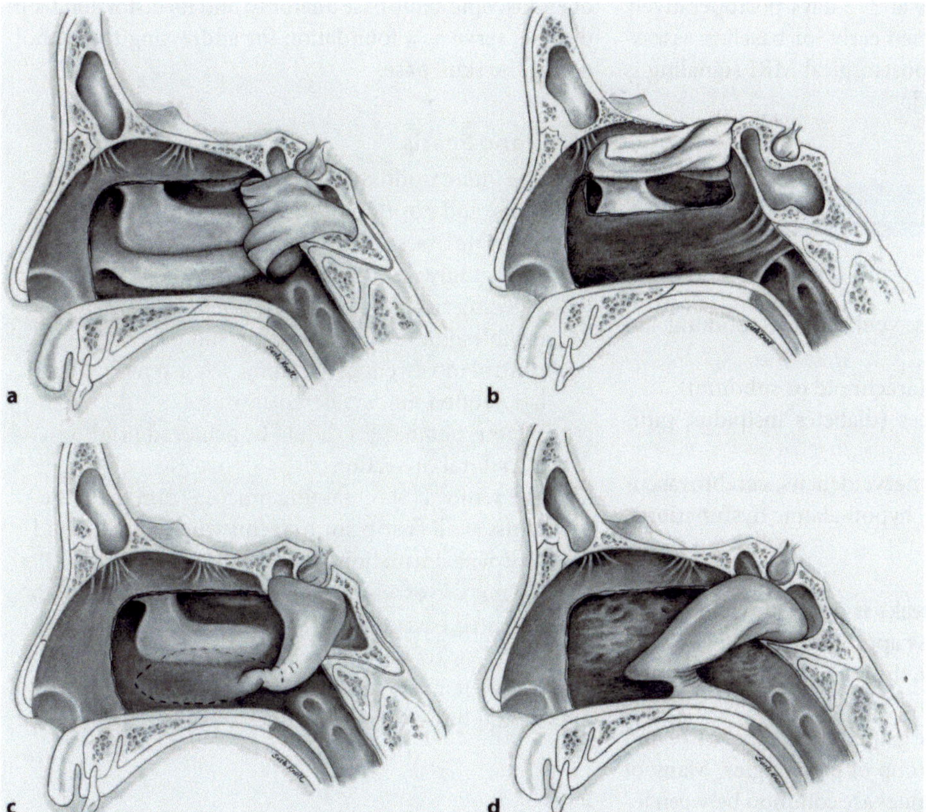

Fig. 33.7 Types of pedicled mucosal flaps for repair of large defects. **a** Posterior pedicled flap based on the septal artery. **b** Contralateral septal flap based on the ethmoid arteries, **c** Inferior turbinate flap based on the turbinate artery. **d** Nasal floor flap based on palatal and pharyngeal vessels. (Reproduced with permission from Centro de ORL, Sao Paulo, Brazil)

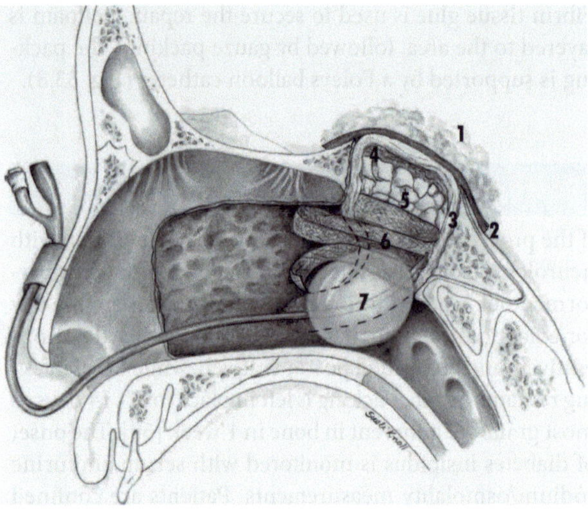

Fig. 33.8 A cross-section of the completed repair. *1* Fat, *2* subdural fascia, *3* mucosal flaps, *4* fibrin glue, *5* Gelfoam, *6* antibiotic-soaked gauze, *7* balloon catheter. (Reproduced with permission from Centro de ORL, Sao Paulo, Brazil)

Discharge usually occurs at 3–5 days postoperatively and an MRI scan is performed early for baseline assessment. This is important as postsurgical MRI signaling is often difficult to interpret [1].

Complications and Outcomes

- Major complications:
  1. Death.
  2. Infectious (meningitis, ventriculitis, subdural abscess).
  3. Intracranial bleeding (arachnoid or subdural).
  4. Endocrine disturbances (diabetes insipidus, pituitary).
  5. Neurological (cranial nerve deficits, cerebrovascular accidents, epilepsy, hypothalamic dysfunction).
  6. Pneumocephalus.

Endoscopic repair of CSF leaks is generally accepted as the standard of care. Success approaches 95% even with revision cases [21]. However, the incidence of many other skull-base pathologies is low. Most centers with endoscopic skull-base teams have gained their experience and skill by treating a diverse group of pathologies. Many of the surgical steps and techniques are common between lesions, but generating large populations for similar lesions is difficult. International collaborations, such as those for neoplastic disease, demonstrating an 88% 5-year survival for selected malignant skull-base pathologies, will be necessary to accrue sufficient patient numbers [38]. Outcomes for olfactory neuroblastoma have been the most widely reported, with survival rates in excess of 80% at about 3-year follow-up [7, 63]. Outcomes of recurrent chordoma, with or without proton beam radiotherapy, vary between 26% and 75% [15, 17, 62]. The results for recurrent craniopharyngioma vary even more, depending on the philosophy of the treating surgical team [25].

Conclusion

Endoscopic SBS has both neurosurgical and otorhinolaryngological origins. The ability of the surgical team to access the entire ventral skull base endoscopically greatly benefits patients with a variety of benign and malignant pathologies. Endoscopic revision SBS presents an even more challenging set of problems for treatment. The management of these complex problems should be firmly established within an MDT. Absolute familiarity with endoscopic techniques, the ability to control nasal vasculature, reconstruct skull-base defects, and manage cerebrovascular structures should be available to the operative team. These skills combined with a detailed knowledge of endoscopic skull-base anatomy, and its distortion from disease, serve as a foundation for addressing the pathology of the skull base.

Tips and Pearls

- The intercarotid distance, height of the sphenoid sinus, and position of sellar should be evaluated on CT to assess the dimensions for a transnasal craniotomy.
- Bleeding from the intercarvenous sinuses can be troublesome. Surgicel packing and patience will control most venous bleeding. Persistent manipulation often hinders hemostasis.
- Venous hemostasis should be achieved prior to intradural dissection.
- The removal of remaining mucosa from the bone of the skull base prior to reconstruction will avoid mucocele formation.
- Do not use excessive tissue glue as this will lead to potential barriers between reconstructive layers.
- Tight packing of the reconstructed area can occlude the vascular flow of pedicled grafts and should be avoided.

References

1. Anand VK, Arrowood JP Jr, Patel RB, et al. (1993) Significance of MRI changes after surgery of the skull base. Otolaryngol Head Neck Surg 109:35–45

2. Baker SR, Baker SR (1998) Nasal lining flaps in contemporary reconstructive rhinoplasty. Facial Plast Surg 14:133–144
3. Batra PS, Citardi MJ, Worley S, et al. (2005) Resection of anterior skull base tumors: comparison of combined traditional and endoscopic techniques. Am J Rhinol 19:521–528
4. Beals SP, Joganic EF, Holcombe TC, et al. (1997) Secondary craniofacial problems following skull base surgery. Clin Plast Surg 24:565–581
5. Carrau RL, Kassam AB, Snyderman CH (2001) Pituitary surgery. Otolaryngol Clin North Am 34:1143–1155
6. Carrau RL, Snyderman CH, Curtin HD, et al. (1996) Computer-assisted intraoperative navigation during skull base surgery. Am J Otolaryngol 17:95–101
7. Casiano RR, Numa WA, Falquez AM (2001) Endoscopic resection of esthesioneuroblastoma. Am J Rhinol 15:271–279
8. Casler JD, Doolittle AM, Mair EA (2005) Endoscopic surgery of the anterior skull base. Laryngoscope 115:16–24
9. Danish SF, Samdani A, Hanna A, et al. (2006) Experience with acellular human dura and bovine collagen matrix for duraplasty after posterior fossa decompression for Chiari malformations. J Neurosurg 104:16–20
10. de Divitiis E, Cappabianca P, Cavallo LM, et al. (2002) Endoscopic transsphenoidal approach: adaptability of the procedure to different sellar lesions. Neurosurgery 51:699–705
11. Dedo HH (2001) Transnasal mucosal flap rotation technique for repair of posterior choanal atresia. Otolaryngol Head Neck Surg 124:674–682
12. Donald PJ (1999) Complications in skull base surgery for malignancy. Laryngoscope 109:1959–1966
13. Dusick JR, Mattozo CA, Esposito F, et al. (2006) BioGlue for prevention of postoperative cerebrospinal fluid leaks in transsphenoidal surgery: a case series. Surg Neurol 66:371–376
14. Fakhri S, Citardi MJ, Wolfe S, et al. (2005) Challenges in the management of sphenoid inverted papilloma. Am J Rhinol 19:207–213
15. Foweraker KL, Burton KE, Maynard SE, et al. (2007) High-dose radiotherapy in the management of chordoma and chondrosarcoma of the skull base and cervical spine: Part 1 – Clinical outcomes. Clin Oncol (R Coll Radiol) 19:509–516
16. Frank G, Pasquini E, Doglietto F, et al. (2006) The endoscopic extended transsphenoidal approach for craniopharyngiomas. Neurosurgery 59:75–83
17. Frank G, Sciarretta V, Calbucci F, et al. (2006) The endoscopic transnasal transsphenoidal approach for the treatment of cranial base chordomas and chondrosarcomas. Neurosurgery 59: 50–57
18. Gassner HG, Ponikau JU, Sherris DA, et al. (1999) CSF rhinorrhea: 95 consecutive surgical cases with long term follow-up at the Mayo Clinic. Am J Rhinol 13:439–447
19. Hadad G, Bassagasteguy L, Carrau RL, et al. (2006) A novel reconstructive technique after endoscopic expanded endonasal approaches: vascular pedicle nasoseptal flap. Laryngoscope 116:1882–1886
20. Harvey RJ, Gallagher RM (2006) Endoscopic vascular control of the anterior skull base. Annual Scientific Conference 2006 March 25th; Melbourne, Australia: Australian Society of Otolaryngology, Head Neck Surgery
21. Hegazy HM, Carrau RL, Snyderman CH, et al. (2000) Transnasal endoscopic repair of cerebrospinal fluid rhinorrhea: a meta-analysis. Laryngoscope 110:1166–1172
22. Jho HD, Ha HG (2004) Endoscopic endonasal skull base surgery: Part 1 – The midline anterior fossa skull base. Minim Invasive Neurosurg 47:1–8
23. Jho HD, Ha HG (2004) Endoscopic endonasal skull base surgery: Part 2 – The cavernous sinus. Minim Invasive Neurosurg 47:9–15
24. Jho HD, Ha HG (2004) Endoscopic endonasal skull base surgery: Part 3 – The clivus and posterior fossa. Minim Invasive Neurosurg 47:16–23
25. Karavitaki N, Brufani C, Warner JT, et al. (2005) Craniopharyngiomas in children and adults: systematic analysis of 121 cases with long-term follow-up. Clin Endocrinol (Oxf) 62:397–409
26. Kassam A, Carrau RL, Snyderman CH, et al. (2005) Evolution of reconstructive techniques following endoscopic expanded endonasal approaches. Neurosurgery Focus 19:E8
27. Kassam A, Horowitz M, Carrau R, et al. (2003) Use of Tisseel fibrin sealant in neurosurgical procedures: incidence of cerebrospinal fluid leaks and cost–benefit analysis in a retrospective study. Neurosurgery 52:1102–1105
28. Kassam A, Snyderman CH, Carrau RL, et al. (2005) Endoneurosurgical hemostasis techniques: lessons learned from 400 cases. Neurosurgery Focus 19:E7
29. Kassam A, Snyderman CH, Mintz A, et al. (2005) Expanded endonasal approach: the rostrocaudal axis. Part I. Crista galli to the sella turcica. Neurosurgery Focus19:E3
30. Kassam A, Snyderman CH, Mintz A, et al. (2005) Expanded endonasal approach: the rostrocaudal axis. Part II. Posterior clinoids to the foramen magnum. Neurosurgery Focus19:E4
31. Kassam AB, Gardner P, Snyderman C, et al. (2005) Expanded endonasal approach: fully endoscopic, completely transnasal approach to the middle third of the clivus, petrous bone, middle cranial fossa, and infratemporal fossa. Neurosurgery Focus 19:E6
32. Kaylie DM, Wittkopf JE, Coppit G, et al. (2006) Revision lateral skull base surgery. Otol Neurotol 27:225–233
33. Krisht AF, Barrow DL, Barnett DW, et al. (1994) The microsurgical anatomy of the superior hypophyseal artery. Neurosurgery 35:899–903
34. Leong J-L, Batra PS, Citardi MJ (2006) CT-MR image fusion for the management of skull base lesions. Otolaryngol Head Neck Surg 134:868–876

33

35. Leong J-L, Citardi MJ, Batra PS (2006) Reconstruction of skull base defects after minimally invasive endoscopic resection of anterior skull base neoplasms. Am J Rhinol 20:476–482
36. Leong JL, Batra PS, Citardi MJ, et al. (2005) Three-dimensional computed tomography angiography of the internal carotid artery for preoperative evaluation of sinonasal lesions and intraoperative surgical navigation. Laryngoscope 115:1618–1623
37. Lindstrom DR, Toohill RJ, Loehrl TA, et al. (2004) Management of cerebrospinal fluid rhinorrhea: the Medical College of Wisconsin experience. Laryngoscope 114:969–974
38. Lund V, Howard DJ, Wei WI (2007) Endoscopic resection of malignant tumors of the nose and sinuses. Am J Rhinol 21:89–94
39. Maroon JC (2005) Skull base surgery: past, present, and future trends. Neurosurg Focus 19:E1
40. May JA, Krieger MD, Bowen I, et al. (2006) Craniopharyngioma in childhood. Adv Pediatr 53:183–209
41. McMains KC, Gross CW, Kountakis SE, et al. (2004) Endoscopic management of cerebrospinal fluid rhinorrhea. Laryngoscope 114:1833–1837
42. Murakami CS, Kriet JD, Ierokomos AP, et al. (1999) Nasal reconstruction using the inferior turbinate mucosal flap. Arch Facial Plast Surg 1:97–100
43. Nguyen-Huynh A, Blevins NH, Jackler RK (2006) The challenges of revision skull base surgery. Otolaryngol Clin North Am 39:783–799
44. Nibu K, Sasaki T, Kawahara N, et al. (1998) Complications of craniofacial surgery for tumors involving the anterior cranial base. Neurosurgery 42:455–461
45. Nishioka H, Haraoka J, Ikeda Y (2005) Risk factors of cerebrospinal fluid rhinorrhea following transsphenoidal surgery. Acta Neurochir (Wien) 147:1163–1166
46. Pieper DR, LaRouere M, Jackson IT (2002) Operative management of skull base malignancies: choosing the appropriate approach. Neurosurg Focus 12:e6
47. Presutti L, Ciufelli MA, Marchioni D, et al. (2007) Nasal septal perforations: our surgical technique. Otolaryngol Head Neck Surg 136:369–372
48. Puget S, Garnett M, Wray A, et al. (2007) Pediatric craniopharyngiomas: classification and treatment according to the degree of hypothalamic involvement. See comment. J Neurosurg 106:3–12
49. Robinson S, Patel N, Wormald PJ (2005) Endoscopic management of benign tumors extending into the infratemporal fossa: a two-surgeon transnasal approach. Laryngoscope 115:1818–1822
50. Schlosser RJ, Bolger WE (2006) Endoscopic management of cerebrospinal fluid rhinorrhea. Otolaryngol Clin North Am 39:523–538
51. Schlosser RJ, Bolger WE (2005) Image-guided procedures of the skull base. Otolaryngol Clin North Am 38:483–490
52. Schlosser RJ, Bolger WE (2003) Significance of empty sella in cerebrospinal fluid leaks. Otolaryngol Head Neck Surg 128:32–38
53. Schultz-Coulon H-J (2005) Three-layer repair of nasoseptal defects. Otolaryngol Head Neck Surg 132:213–218
54. Snyderman C, Kassam A, Carrau R, et al. (2007) Acquisition of surgical skills for endonasal skull base surgery: a training program. Laryngoscope 117:699–705
55. Snyderman C, Zimmer LA, Kassam A (2004) Sources of registration error with image guidance systems during endoscopic anterior cranial base surgery. Otolaryngol Head Neck Surg 131:145–149
56. Spoudeas HA, Saran F, Pizer B, et al. (2006) A multimodality approach to the treatment of craniopharyngiomas avoiding hypothalamic morbidity: a UK perspective. J Pediatr Endocrinol 19:447–451
57. Stamm AC (2006) Transnasal endoscopy-assisted skull base surgery. Ann Otol Rhinol Laryngol Suppl 196:45–53
58. Stamm AC, Pignatari SS (2001) Nasal septal cross-over flap technique: a choanal atresia micro-endoscopic surgical repair. Am J Rhinol 15:143–148
59. Stamm AC, Pignatari SSN, Vellutini E (2006) Transnasal endoscopic surgical approaches to the clivus. Otolaryngol Clin North Am 39:639–656
60. Stangerup SE, Dommerby H, Lau T, et al. (1996) Hot-water irrigation as a treatment of posterior epistaxis. Rhinology 34:18–20
61. Stangerup SE, Thomsen HK (1996) Histological changes in the nasal mucosa after hot-water irrigation. An animal experimental study. Rhinology 34:14–17
62. Tzortzidis F, Elahi F, Wright D, et al. (2006) Patient outcome at long-term follow-up after aggressive microsurgical resection of cranial base chordomas. Neurosurgery 59:230–237
63. Unger F, Haselsberger K, Walch C, et al. (2005) Combined endoscopic surgery and radiosurgery as treatment modality for olfactory neuroblastoma (esthesioneuroblastoma) Acta Neurochir (Wien) 147:595–601
64. Van Den Abbeele T, Elmaleh M, Herman P, et al. (1999) Transnasal endoscopic repair of congenital defects of the skull base in children. Arch Otolaryngol Head Neck Surg 125:580–584
65. van Overbeeke J, Sekhar L (2003) Microanatomy of the blood supply to the optic nerve. Orbit 22:81–88
66. Wallace RC, Dean BL, Beals SP, et al. (2003) Posttreatment imaging of the skull base. Semin Ultrasound CT MR 24:164–181
67. Weber SM, Kim J, Delashaw JB, et al. (2005) Radial forearm free tissue transfer in the management of persistent cerebrospinal fluid leaks. Laryngoscope 115:968–972
68. White DR, Dubin MG, Senior BA (2003) Endoscopic repair of cerebrospinal fluid leaks after neurosurgical procedures. Am J Otolaryngol 24:213–216
69. Wormald PJ, McDonogh M (2003) The bath-plug closure of anterior skull base cerebrospinal fluid leaks. Am J Rhinol 17:299–305

Chapter 34

Stenting in Revision Sinus Surgery

34

Seth J. Kanowitz, Joseph B. Jacobs, and Richard A. Lebowitz

Core Messages

- Long-term patency rates may be improved by postoperative stenting of the frontal sinus outflow tract.
- In cases of previous partial middle-turbinate resection, stenting of the frontal sinus outflow tract allows for stabilization of the remnant fragment during revision frontal sinusotomy.
- In cases of extended frontal sinus drillout procedures, stenting allows for improved mucosalization and aids in temporary inhibition of circumferential stenosis.
- Soft (Silicone) sheets or stents, either prefabricated or designed in the operating room, are superior to rigid stents.
- No absolute length of stenting exists and a determination should be made on a case-by-case basis.
- Postoperative stent management includes routine endoscopy with gentle debridement, culture-directed antibiotic therapy, and nasal irrigations. Nasal steroid spray is reserved for select cases.

Contents

Introduction

Revision frontal sinus surgery is a demanding challenge that incorporates a keen understanding of three-dimensional anatomy, surgical precision, and vigorous postoperative medical management aimed at maximizing long-term surgical success. Restenosis of the frontal sinus outflow tract (FSOT) is frustrating and can occur even under the best of circumstances. The concept of frontal sinus stenting to minimize postoperative stenosis, improve mucosalization, and allow for functional patency of the of the FSOT following frontal sinus surgery has been reported in the literature for over a century. In the initial description of the external frontoethmoidectomy that now bears his name, Lynch described postoperative stenting of the nasofrontal communication. Although many technological advances in sinus surgery including endoscopic visualization, high-resolution triplanar computed tomographic (CT) imaging, through-cutting frontal sinus instrumentation, and image-guided surgery have occurred since the original external approaches were described, prevention of FSOT restenosis after revision sinus surgery remains a difficult challenge.

Intrinsic host factors such as sinonasal polyposis, osteoneogenesis, ciliary dyskinesis, immunodeficiency, vasculitis, and other autoimmune phenomena may predispose the patient to a poor outcome regardless of the surgical technique. Extrinsic factors such as lateralization of the middle turbinate/middle turbinate remnant, postoperative sinus cavity infections, scarring, synechiae, and incomplete primary sinus surgery may also compromise postoperative healing and ultimately lead to FSOT stenosis. Historically, failure rates of nearly 30% have been reported in the literature – and because of this propensity for postoperative stenosis of the FSOT, stenting remains an important component in the surgical and postoperative management of chronic frontal sinusitis during revision endoscopic surgery.

Stenting Materials and Design

From a historical perspective, the initial descriptions of frontal sinus stenting usually involved external frontoethmoidectomy procedures followed by stenting of the FSOT with a wide variety of rigid or soft materials. Initially a gold tube, placed endonasally, was utilized by Ingals to stent the region of the FSOT until it was mucosalized [13]. In 1921, Lynch placed a firm rubber tube in the FSOT in 15 patients until postoperative day five. After 2.5 years of follow-up he reported a 100% success rate [15]. However, subsequent studies demonstrated a long-term failure rate of approximately 30% [17, 18].

The relative success of these early novel techniques led others to experiment with different stent materials in the 1940s and 1950s. Goodale, Harris, and Scharfe described their experiences with the use of tantalum, an inert basic element originally discovered by Eckenberg in 1802, for frontal sinus stenting [7, 8, 10, 22]. Goodale employed the material as a thin sheet sutured to the orbital periosteum during revision external frontoethmoidectomies as a way of minimizing circumferential granulation tissue and scarring [8, 9]. Extending on Goodale's work, Harris and Scharfe described their limited series of patients where tantalum tubes were placed from the frontal sinus into the nasal cavity [10, 22]. In all cases, patients demonstrated resolution of their symptoms and patency of their frontal sinus. Each author noted decreased scarring of the FSOT, improved epithelialization, and decreased granulation tissue formation. However, it should be noted that during the time of these procedures antibiotics were employed for the first time, and thus are probably partially responsible for the improved outcomes. Other materials, such as Dacron woven arterial graft have also been employed for similar indications and with similar results. However, Barton employed this material during a Lynch external frontal sinusotomy, for *permanent* stenting of the FSOT over a 17-year period in 34 patients [2]. No stents were removed and all patients were relieved of their frontal headache symptoms.

In contrast to today's modern soft materials, the original designs involved rigid materials likely employed out of convenience and limited by current technological standards. However, in 1976 Neel demonstrated the superiority of thin, pliable Silastic sheeting for the first time in a canine model [17]. In those treated with firm rubber stents, significant fibrosis and osteoblastic activity with little or no epithelialization resulted. In contrast, normal mucosal lining was observed on histological specimens in those ducts stented with thin Silastic sheeting. He attributed the difference to local ischemia, impaired drainage, and localized infection around the rigid tubes. He subsequently reviewed a series of patients after an average of 13.5 years of follow-up and reported a 29% failure rate with rubber tubing and a 17% failure rate with thin Silastic sheeting [18].

With the dawn of the endoscopic era, Schaefer and Close extended upon the ideas initially proposed by Neel and employed Silastic tubing for small endoscopic frontal sinusotomies (4–6 mm) in four patients [21]. However, a 50% stenosis rate resulted, which was attributed to a failure to maintain a postoperative communication between an air passage and the mucosa, thus resulting in massively hypertrophied mucosa and obstruction of the frontal sinus ostium. Since then, numerous authors have reported their experience with the external or endoscopic placement of Silicone tubes or rolled sheeting to help maintain patency of the FSOT (Fig. 34.1) [1, 3, 5, 6, 9, 11, 12, 14, 16, 20, 23–25].

In cases where an external approach is still necessary, there is some data supporting the role of frontal sinus stenting, although none of the reports are compared against nonstented controls. In a comprehensive review of 164 cases, Amble placed thin Silicone rubber sheeting to reconstruct the FSOT after a modified external Lynch procedure in which the frontal process of the superior maxilla was preserved [1]. Of the 164 patients studied, 79 of the patients had previous failed sinus surgical procedures addressing the frontal sinus and thus were undergoing a revision. After FSOT reconstruction with Silicone sheeting for 6–8 weeks, 96% achieved resolution of their symptoms at a mean follow-up of four years. Only 18% of the patients required a revision procedure to achieve 4 years during the study period.

Yamabosa also reported on his experience in placing a silicone T-tube in the FSOT via a Lynch incision in 18 patients presenting with frontoethmoid mucoceles [25]. Three of these patients had failed previous external frontal procedures, and all patients failed a transnasal approach at widening the FSOT due to thick bone formation. Removal of the tube was determined by aeration of the frontal sinus on CT imaging and lack of polypoid mucosa or mucous discharge on flexible endoscopic exam. Although the exact length of follow-up is unclear, 16 patients achieved patency of the FSOT and resolution of their symptoms. The two failures developed scar tissue and polyps of the FSOT at 3 and 5 months after stent removal.

As the endoscopic era began, more authors started to report their experience with endoscopic frontal sinus stenting. In a limited trial, Schaefer and Close endoscopically placed thin Silastic tubing as a frontal sinus stent in patients with small frontal sinusotomies (4–6 mm), resulting in a 50% failure rate in the four patients studied [21]. Weber retrospectively reviewed 12 patients who underwent various endoscopic Draf-type procedures for frontal sinusotomy followed by a 6-month course of FSOT stenting with either a Rains self-retaining Silicone tube, U-shaped Silicone tube, or an H-shaped Silicone tube [23]. While all patients had improvement or resolution of their headache symptom, only six FSOTs were endoscopically visible at a mean of 19.4 months of follow-up. Five other FSOTs were deemed functionally patent due to evidence of aeration on imaging studies. Hoyt reported similar results in 21 patients (32 stents) who had vented tubular plastic stents placed endoscopically over a guidewire for an average of 8 weeks [12].

Using the stent that now bears his name, Freeman placed a biflanged Silicone tube in an external or endoscopic fashion in 64 sinuses [19]. The Freeman frontal sinus stent is unique in that it requires an introducer and the distal flange is contained within a dissolving gel cap to allow for easier insertion. After a mean follow-up of 29 months, six sinuses eventually required fat obliteration due to return of polyposis or restenosis of the FSOT. Similarly, Rains endoscopically placed 102 stents (soft Silicone tube with a tapered collapsible bulb) in 67 patients for an average duration of 35 days [20]. After a follow-up of 8–48 months, a 94% endoscopic patency rate was reported, with allergic fungal sinusitis present in all failures.

Preoperative Assessment

- Carefully review the sinus anatomy on CT to determine the potential surgical diameter of the frontal sinus neo-ostium, as limited by the frontal beak, anterior skull base, medial orbit, and cribriform plate.
- Evaluate the preoperative CT for radiographic evidence of extensive sinonasal polyposis, allergic fungal sinusitis, and/or osteitis of the bone of the FSOT.
- Evaluate the preoperative CT for evidence of lateralization or scarring of the middle turbinate or middle turbinate remnant.
- Examine the FSOT with angled nasal endoscopes to determine the presence of polyposis or hyperplastic mucosa in the frontal recess, scarring or synechiae from prior surgery, and previous partial middle turbinectomy with lateralization of the remnant fragments.

Indications for Stenting

While many non-case-controlled reports of FSOT stenting demonstrating successful patency rates exist in the literature, no standardized indications exist to guide surgeons in the implementation of these devices.

- Routine stenting in uncomplicated cases is not recommended, and thus FSOT stents should be employed on a case-by-case basis based upon the surgeon's assessment of the patient's relative risk of postoperative FSOT stenosis.

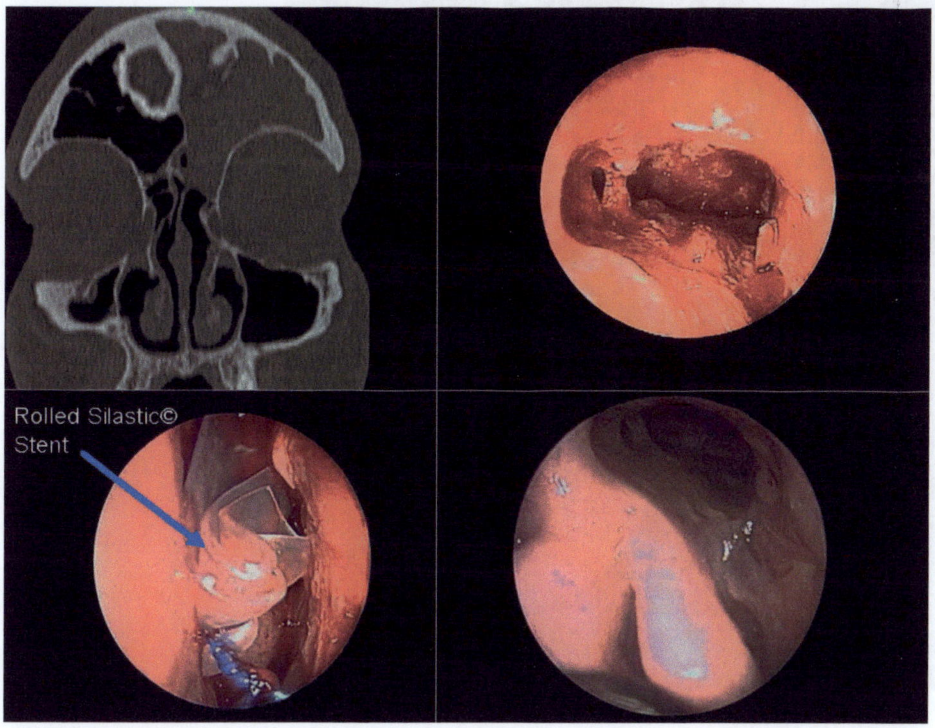

Fig. 34.1 Chronic left frontal sinusitis (left upper picture) requiring revision endoscopic frontal sinusotomy (right upper picture). A rolled Silastic stent (left lower picture) was placed in the frontal recess until mucosalization was complete (right lower picture)

Several intrinsic and extrinsic conditions need to be considered as risk factors for FSOT stenosis, and thus, as potential relative indications for stenting.

In one review, Hosemann demonstrated a doubling (16% vs. 33%) of the rate of FSOT stenosis when the intraoperative diameter of the neo-ostium was less than 5 mm. [11]. This is similar to the indications (4–6 mm) employed by Schafer and Close [21]. Therefore, a FSOT diameter of less than 5 mm at the completion of the frontal sinusotomy is often considered a relative indication for stenting. Other relative indications for FSOT stenting during revision frontal sinus surgery are listed below.

- Relative indications for FSOT stenting:
  1. Frontal sinus neo-ostium diameter less than 5 mm.
  2. Extensive or circumferential exposure of bone in the FSOT, which may lead to long-term postoperative crusting.
  3. Sinonasal polyposis or hyperplastic mucosa, which may lead to difficulty with postoperative endoscopic visualization and debridement
  4. Evidence of osteitic bone or osteo-neogenesis visualized on CT imaging or encountered intraoperatively (Fig. 34.2).
  5. Destabilized or lateralized middle turbinate or middle turbinate remnant.
  6. Draf III or tumor resection procedures with mucosal trauma and extensive bone exposure.
  7. Frontoethmoid mucoceles, which usually indicate long-standing chronic sinus disease or previous surgical failures.

Duration of Stenting

Similar to the indications for stenting, no prospective case-controlled studies have been performed to investigate the optimal duration of FSOT stenting. While most authors recommend a temporary period of stenting, Barton employed his Dacron woven arterial graft permanently over 17 years [2]. Whenever stent removal is deemed appropriate, all current authors report successful removal of the stenting material in the office using endoscopes and endoscopic sinus instrumentation.

The 6-week time frame that is often discussed comes from the canine model by Neel where he demonstrated histologically that re-epithelialization of the FSOT stented with thin Silicone rubber is complete within

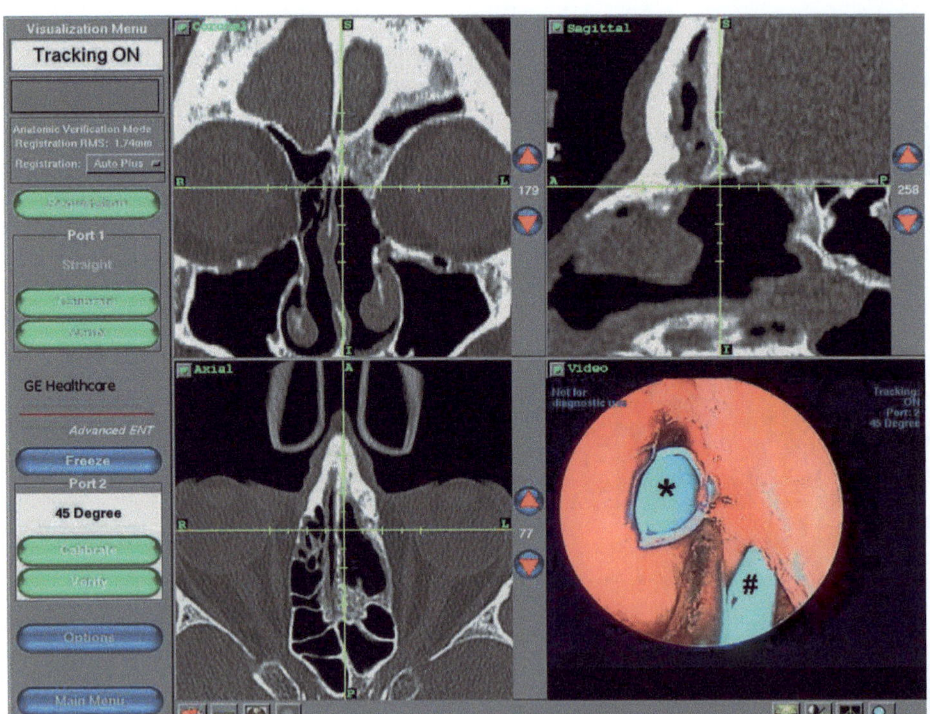

Fig. 34.2 Intraoperative surgical navigation with probe in stenotic left frontal sinus outflow tract during revision endoscopic frontal sinusotomy. The area of neo-osteogenesis has been removed by high-speed angled diamond burr and a Parrell frontal sinus stent (Medtronic) placed in the FSOT (*) as well as a large supraorbital ethmoid cell (#)

approximately 8 weeks [17]. He subsequently employed these findings to his patient population and removed Silastic sheeting stents beginning at a minimum of 6 weeks postoperatively (mean 6 months). After a 7-year follow-up period he reported an 80% success rate [18].

In many of the trials already outlined above, average stenting time with soft Silicone stents ranges from 4 to 8 weeks with a success rate of 80–90% [1, 3, 6, 13, 20, 21]. While the length of follow-up and definition of success or patency varies among authors, all arrive at similar conclusions. However, Weber recommended removal of the various stents he employed in revision endonasal frontal sinusotomy at 6 months and cited improved patency with a longer duration of stenting [23]. The 6-month duration was adapted from Montgomery tubes inserted during tracheal surgery, as it was felt many months were necessary to allow for stabilization of the subepithelial scar. Freeman also described a period of stenting after revision frontal sinus surgery lasting between 6 and 12 months for patients stented to correct FSOT stenosis [6]. However, the duration of stenting was once again determined arbitrarily.

More recently, Dubin and Kuhn reported their experience with the management of the FSOT after open and endoscopic procedures for the removal of frontal sinus osteomas [5]. Five of 12 patients (3 open, 2 endoscopic) were stented with rolled Silastic sheeting (0.01 inches, or 0.25 mm thick) for an average of 9.2 months (range 6–17 months). One patient developed a scarred frontal recess despite 12 months of stenting after an osteoplastic flap approach. Casiano employed similar methods (1-mm-thick rolled Silastic sheeting) to stent the common frontal sinus ostia after endoscopic modified Lothrop procedures [24]. The stent was removed in the office at the 2-month postoperative visit. A patency rate of 60% was achieved, while 32% remained stenotic, and symptom improvement was achieved in 72% at a mean follow-up of 22 months (range 6–75 months). However, it is important to note that these results did not differ statistically from a comparison group of nonstented patients undergoing the same Draf III procedure.

Temporary short-term stenting may also play a role in revision frontal sinus surgery. In cases of extensive sinonasal polyposis, hyperplastic mucosa, or after technically demanding FSOT dissections where the mucosa is inevitably traumatized and bone exposed, placement of a soft Silastic stent may aid limiting the amount of postoperative crusting and/or endoscopic identification of the FSOT during postoperative endoscopy. The presence of a stent inherently limits the amount of FSOT probing necessary to debride the operative cavity. Removal of the stent at the first or second postoperative visit when the operative cavity is clean and mucosal inflammation controlled may enhance long-term results.

Surgical Technique

- Most commercially available frontal sinus stents can be easily placed via an endoscopic approach.
- Inadvertent displacement of mucosal flaps into the frontal sinus itself during stent placement should be avoided.

After creation of a frontal sinusotomy, the stent is grasped at the end with the flanges using a 90 side-to-side giraffe forceps (Fig. 34.3). The stent is then introduced into the FSOT under endoscopic visualization with a 70 rigid endoscope. The forceps are released and the instrument is gently maneuvered out of the nose. The stent can then be manipulated with an angled frontal sinus seeker. The stent should move freely within the FSOT and the flanges should be deployed beyond the internal frontal sinus ostium. In addition, the mucosa of the FSOT should lay flush around the stent and inadvertent displacement of mucosal flaps into the frontal sinus itself should be avoided. If the stent does not meet these requirements, then it should be removed and replaced properly. The stent should then

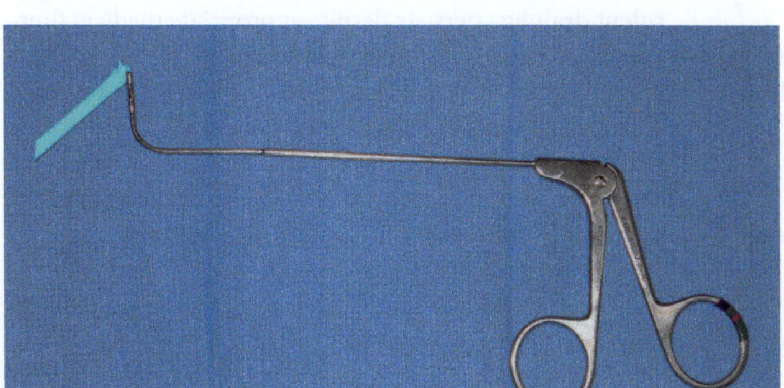

Fig. 34.3 90-degree side-to-side giraffe forceps grasping a Parrell frontal sinus stent (Medtronic, Minneapolis, MN, USA). The flanges are grasped within the forceps to allow for easier endoscopic placement

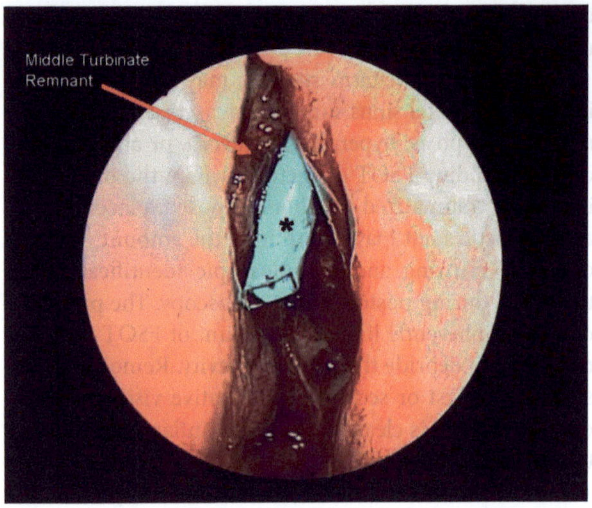

Fig. 34.4 Endoscopic view of a Parrell frontal sinus stent (*; Medtronic) in the left frontal sinus outflow tract (FSOT) placed during revision endoscopic frontal sinusotomy. The middle turbinate had been previously resected and the remnant fragment was destabilized and scarred to the lateral nasal wall

be positioned within the anterior ethmoid cavity between the lateral nasal wall and vertical strut of the middle turbinate or middle turbinate remnant (Fig. 34.4). Proper positioning is best achieved using a 0 or 30 rigid endoscope and Blakesley forceps. This technique can also be applied to rolled Silastic sheeting; however, the stent needs to be fixed to the septum with nondissolvable through-and-through sutures to prevent extrusion.

Postoperative Stent Management

Expert opinion and experience indicates that regular debridement of the nasal cavity and stent itself is warranted. Regular nasal irrigations also play a key role in limiting the buildup of debris.

- Routine care of the stent, regardless of the material and placement technique, are necessary to maintain stent patency, minimize scarring, crusting, and adhesions, and improve long-term results.
- Use topical and/or oral steroids to reduce postoperative inflammation and scar formation around the stent.
- Routine empiric antibiotic coverage for the duration of the stenting is not recommended. Culture-directed antibiotics are used if purulent drainage occurs postoperatively.
- Stents aggregate biofilms given time.
- If purulent drainage persists despite appropriate medical therapy, consider removing the stent.

Even during the early days of frontal sinus stenting, Goodale and Harris routinely probed and cleaned the tantalum tubes with a curved suction [7, 8, 10].

Depending on surgeon preferences, nasal irrigation usually begins within the first few postoperative days and is maintained for at least the duration of stenting. Large-volume irrigations (50 ml twice daily) with a Toomey syringe are employed to manually dislodge crusts. Routine postoperative endoscopic removal of blood clots, crusting, dried secretions, and granulation tissue from within the nasal cavity and within the stent itself, should be performed in the office on a scheduled basis.

The use of topical and/or oral steroids is recommended to reduce postoperative inflammation and scar formation around the stent. Weber and Rains both employed topical inhaled nasal steroids as part of their postoperative medical regimen. [20, 23] However, in the absence of other sinonasal indications for oral or topical steroid use (i.e., sinonasal polyposis, mucosal edema, allergic fungal sinusitis), the presence of a healthy stent alone is not an absolute indication for utilization of these medications.

Routine empiric antibiotic coverage for the duration of the stenting is not recommended. However, appropriate culture-directed antibiotic therapy to control purulent drainage identified during routine endoscopy or as part of an episode of acute frontal sinusitis is warranted. If purulent drainage persists despite appropriate medical therapy, the stent may act as a foreign body or reservoir for biofilms, and consideration should be given to removing it. In a pilot study by Perloff and Palmer, six frontal sinus stents removed 1–4 weeks after functional endoscopic sinus surgery (FESS) and examined by scanning electron microscopy demonstrated evidence of bacterial biofilms [19]. In five of six of their patients, various staphylococcal species were cultured from the sinuses at the time of FESS.

FSOT stenting is an extremely safe procedure when performed by experienced endoscopic surgeons. No cases of orbital penetration, CSF leaks, or skull-base violations have been reported in the literature to date. In rare instances, some stents have required removal under general anesthesia due to significant scarring that obscures visualization and instrumentation in an office setting [3, 5, 6, 24]. However, one case of toxic shock syndrome due to frontal sinus stenting, despite 7 days of postoperative antibiotic prophylaxis, has been reported [4].

Conclusion

Frontal sinus stenting may play a role in specific cases of revision frontal sinus surgery. In cases of extensive mucosal trauma, bone exposure, or destabilized middle turbinate, stenting may improve long-term FSOT patency and enhance mucosalization. Regardless of the specific stent chosen, those made of soft Silicone are preferred to more rigid materials. Stenting may be employed during revision external or endoscopic frontal sinus surgery and is at the discretion of the surgeon. The appropriate duration of stenting has not been defined in the literature and should be determined on a case-by-case basis based upon patient characteristics, findings on CT imaging, and intraoperative observations. Appropriate postoperative stent management is crucial in maintaining long-term stent patency and consists of routine irrigation, endoscopic debridement, and appropriate antibiotic therapy for evidence of purulence. If granulation tissue and purulence persist despite adequate medical therapy, then consideration should be given to stent removal.

Acknowledgments

The authors would like to thank Martin J. Citardi, MD and Pete S. Batra, MD for providing clinical images for the figures.

References

1. Amble FR, Kern EB, Neel B, et al. (1996) Nasofrontal duct reconstruction with silicone rubber sheeting for inflammatory frontal sinus disease: analysis of 164 cases. Laryngoscope 106:809–815
2. Barton RT (1972) Dacron prosthesis in frontal sinus surgery. Laryngoscope 82:1795–1802
3. Benoit CM, Duncavage JA (2001) Combined external and endoscopic frontal sinusotomy with stent placement: a retrospective review. Laryngoscope 111:1246–1249
4. Chadwell JS, Gustafson LM, Tami TA (2001) Toxic shock syndrome associated with frontal sinus stents. Otolaryngol Head Neck Surg 124:573–574
5. Dubin MG, Kuhn FA (2006) Preservation of natural frontal sinus outflow in the management of frontal sinus osteomas. Otolaryngol Head Neck Surg 134:18–24
6. Freeman SB, Blom ED (2000) Frontal sinus stents. Laryngoscope 110:1179–1182
7. Goodale RL (1945) The use of tantalum in radical frontal sinus surgery. Ann Otol Rhinol Laryngol 45:757–762
8. Goodale RL (1954) Ten years' experience in the use of tantalum in frontal sinus surgery. Laryngoscope 64:65–72
9. Har El G, Lucente FE (1995) Endoscopic intranasal frontal sinusotomy. Laryngoscope 105:440–443
10. Harris HE (1948) The use of tantalum tubes in frontal sinus surgery. Cleve Clin Q 15:129–133
11. Hosemann W, Kuhnel TH, Held P, et al. (1997) Endonasal frontal sinusotomy in surgical management of chronic sinusitis: A critical evaluation. Am J Rhinol 11:1–19
12. Hoyt WH (1993) Endoscopic stenting of nasofrontal communication in frontal sinus disease. Ear Nose Throat J 72:596–597
13. Ingals EE (1905) New operation and instruments for draining the frontal sinus. Trans Am Laryngol Rhinol Otol Soc 11:183–189
14. Jacobs JB (1997) 100 years of frontal sinus surgery. Laryngoscope 107:1–36
15. Lynch RC (1921) The technique of radical frontal sinus surgery operation which has given me the best results. Laryngoscope 31:1–5
16. Mirza S, Johnson AP (2000) A simple and effective frontal sinus stent. J Laryngol Otol 114:955–956
17. Neel HB, Whicker JH, Lake CF (1976) Thin rubber sheeting in frontal sinus surgery: animal and clinical studies. Laryngoscope 86:524–536
18. Neel HB, McDonald TJ, Facer GW (1987) Modified Lynch procedure for chronic frontal sinus diseases: rationale, technique, and long-term results. Laryngoscope 97:1274–1279
19. Perloff JR, Palmer JN (2004) Evidence of bacterial biofilms on frontal recess stents in patients with chronic rhinosinusitis Am J Rhinol 18:377–380
20. Rains BM (2001) Frontal sinus stenting. Otolaryngol Clin North Am 34:101–110
21. Schaefer SD, Close LG (1990) Endoscopic management of frontal sinus disease. Laryngoscope 100:155–160
22. Scharfe ED (1953) The use of tantalum in otolaryngology. Arch Otolaryngol 58:133–140
23. Weber R, Mai R, Hosemann W, et al. (2000) The success of 6-month stenting in endonasal frontal sinus surgery. Ear Nose Throat J 79:930–932, 934, 937–938, 940–941
24. Wish B, Dargi Z, Collins W, et al. (2006) Long-term effect of stenting after endoscopic modified Lothrop procedure. Am J Rhinol 20:595–599
25. Yamasoba T, Kikuchi S, Higo R (1994) Transient positioning of a silicone T tube in frontal sinus surgery. Otolaryngol Head Neck Surg 111:776–780

Chapter 35

Use of Intravenous Antibiotics in Sinus Surgery Failures

35

Seth M. Brown, Abtin Tabaee, and Vijay K. Anand

Core Messages

- The management of patients with refractory chronic rhinosinusitis despite adequate surgical and medical treatment remains challenging.
- Intravenous antibiotics may play a role in patients who are considered "surgical failures," particularly in those who demonstrate hyperostosis on imaging.
- Intravenous antibiotics are also indicated in intraorbital and intracranial complications of sinusitis in both adult and pediatric patients.
- Methicillin-resistant *Staphylococcus aureus* is increasing in prevalence as a pathogen in community-acquired sinusitis.
- The trend in intravenous antibiotics is toward home therapy with peripherally inserted central catheters.
- Preliminary studies support the cost-effectiveness and safety of home intravenous antibiotic treatment.

Contents

Introduction

Despite advances in the medical and surgical management of chronic rhinosinusitis (CRS), a subset of patients continues to have refractory symptoms despite "maximal therapy." This group of patients represents a significant management challenge in the field of rhinology. Multiple treatment modalities are described including long-term broad-spectrum oral antibiotics, topical antibiotics, and anti-inflammatory medications [1]. For the patient with recalcitrant disease, this involves additional cost and potential treatment-related complications, with limited overall efficacy. The goal of this chapter is to describe the indications, safety, and outcomes of intravenous antibiotics in this cohort of patients. Given the significant incidence in the general population, negative impact on quality of life, and health-care expenditure associated with CRS, a critical examination of any treatment modality is required prior to widespread adoption.

Indications for Intravenous Antibiotics

1. Refractory rhinossinusitis.
2. Hyperostotic rhinossinusitis.
3. Extranasal complications from rhinossinusitis.
4. Resistant pathogens to oral antibiotics.
5. Patient intolerance to oral antibiotics.
6. Surgical alternative.
7. Failure of surgical therapy.

The indications for intravenous antibiotics in sinonasal disorders are currently in evolution. Traditional indications have included rhinossinusitis with intraorbital or intracranial complications and microbial resistance to oral antibiotics on sinonasal cultures, including methicillin-resistant *Staphylococcus aureus* (MRSA). Additional indications may include patients with medical comorbidities who are not medically fit for surgery and patients who have failed traditional medical and surgical therapy [8]. The use of antibiotics in the latter group remains controversial. The refractory nature of CRS in this cohort is evidenced by the typical history of multiple courses of oral antibiotics and surgical procedures with persistent symptoms [14, 18]. The potential benefits of intravenous therapy in this group of patients have been described in a limited number of studies [8, 13, 18]. Intravenous antibiotics may be initiated independently or as an adjunct to surgical treatment with placement of a peripherally inserted central catheter (PICC) line in the early postoperative period [8]. In this model, treatment is initiated based on the intraoperative cultures and may include combinations of vancomycin, ceftriaxone, ceftazidime, and ciprofloxacin [8].

- Obtaining and reviewing a computed tomography (CT) scan is essential in those patients that have failed surgery.
- The presence of hyperostosis on CT scan may suggest the need for intravenous antibiotics.

For patients with persistent symptoms following surgery, a critical evaluation of a CT scan is necessary to identify mucosal thickening, persistent obstruction of outflow tracts, and diffuse bony changes, termed hyperostosis (Fig. 35.1). The latter finding is felt to result from periosteal reactions, chronic inflammatory cell infiltrates, bony resorption, and osteoneogenesis [12]. Although bacteria have not been identified within the bone to date, these changes have been found to correlate with persistent sinusitis symptoms resistant to conventional medical management, including oral antibiotics [12].

The CT scan in patients with refractory CRS allows the surgeon to determine whether a patient would benefit from additional surgery in cases of polypoid disease or sinonasal obstruction. The role of surgery in hyperostosis alone is unclear. In cases of hyperostosis, often the mucosal disease is limited, although patients may report localized pain to the areas of bony abnormalities. Hyperostosis has also been found to correlate strongly with the presence of massive polyposis (Fig. 35.2) [12]. The presence of hyperostosis may also be a marker of refractory disease. In a retrospective review of a single surgical series, Kacker et al. identified hyperostosis in 65% of patients undergoing revision surgery, compared to 20% in patients undergoing primary surgery [12]. In another multi-institutional study of patients treated with intravenous home-based antibiotic administration for rhinosinusitis, 44 out of 52 had undergone previous sinus surgery [2]. Looking at symptom analysis, significant improvement was seen in these patients when previous treatment with oral antibiotics and/or surgery had failed [2].

- Intravenous antibiotics may represent a safe and effective treatment alternative for patients with MRSA sinusitis.

The increasing incidence of microbial pathogens resistant to currently available oral antibiotics, typically MRSA, represents a major public health concern. The majority of patients with MRSA sinusitis have a known risk factor including a history of hospitalization and multiple treatments including antibiotics and surgeries. The incidence of MRSA in patients with refractory CRS is currently estimated to be 2–15% and is likely increasing [10, 11, 14]. In a study of all sinonasal cultures taken in the senior author's tertiary referral rhinology practice, 9.2% of patients were found to have MRSA [14]. The treatment options for medical therapy in this cohort are limited. In a subsequent study of intravenous antibiotics for treatment of MRSA sinusitis in this group, negative cultures were achieved in five of six patients at last follow up after a 6- to 8-week treatment course. The single patient with persistent cultures was noted to have improvement in clinical and endoscopic disease, suggesting the possibility of MRSA colonization without pathogenicity [18]. These results are further supported when looking at 20-item Sinonasal Outcome Test (SNOT-20) scores. In a study by Tabaee et al., SNOT-20 scores improved from a pretreatment median of 62, to 42 after a 6- to 8-week course of intravenous antibiotics for MRSA [18].

The role of intravenous therapy in the treatment of MRSA sinusitis is currently unclear. We advocate a treatment algorithm based on culture-directed sensitivities (Fig. 35.3). If sensitivity to an oral antibiotic is suggested, this is employed initially, often in combination with a second broad-spectrum antibiotic with anaerobic and Gram-negative coverage. Intravenous antibiotics are initiated if there is persistent clinical disease following a trial of oral therapy, or if the initial culture results show resistance to all oral alternatives. The role of intravenous antibiotics will probably continue to evolve as newer classes of oral antibiotics become available, such as linezolid. Other studies have promoted using mupirocin nasal irrigations for MRSA; however, recurrence rates appear high, with 12 of 24 patients experiencing at least 1 recurrence in 1 series [17]. Finally, despite the potential efficacy of culture-directed therapy for MRSA rhinossinusitis, long-term surveillance for this cohort is required. Repeat cultures should be performed in patients with recurrent disease even if the posttreatment cultures were negative.

Effectiveness of Intravenous Antibiotics

- Intravenous antibiotics appear to be effective for surgical failures or as an adjunct to surgery, but may be far less effective when used as an alternative to surgery.

The efficacy of intravenous antibiotics in conjunction with surgery has been suggested by two recent studies. In a

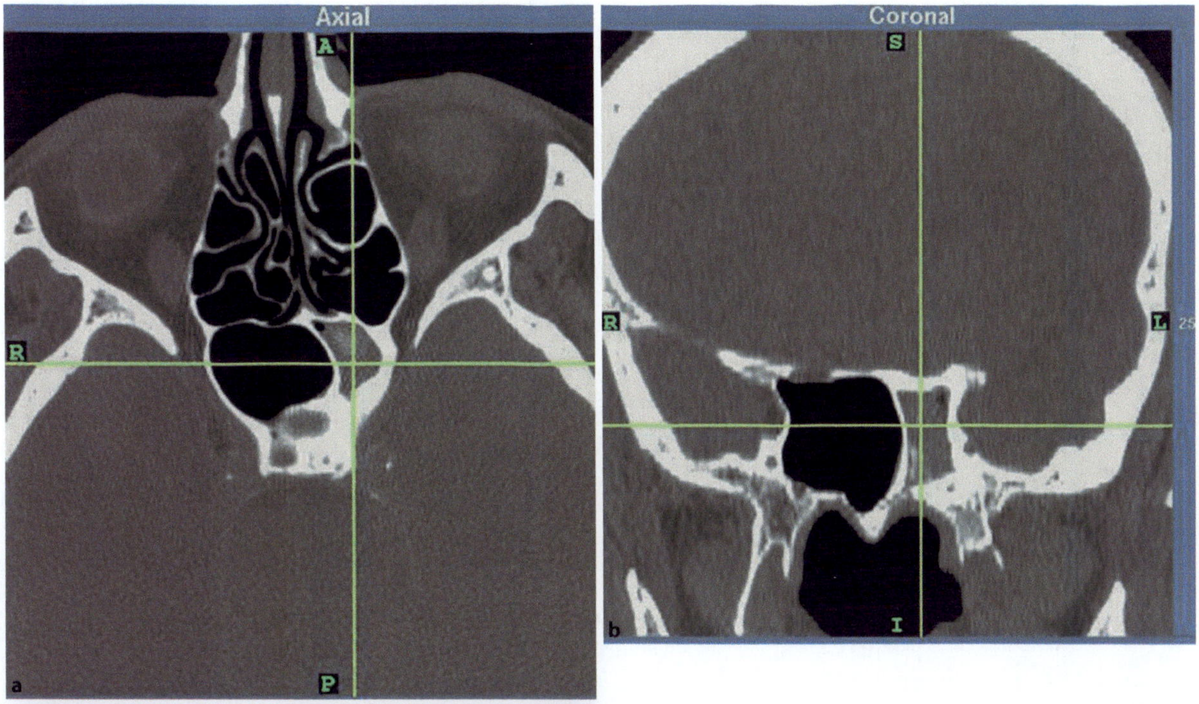

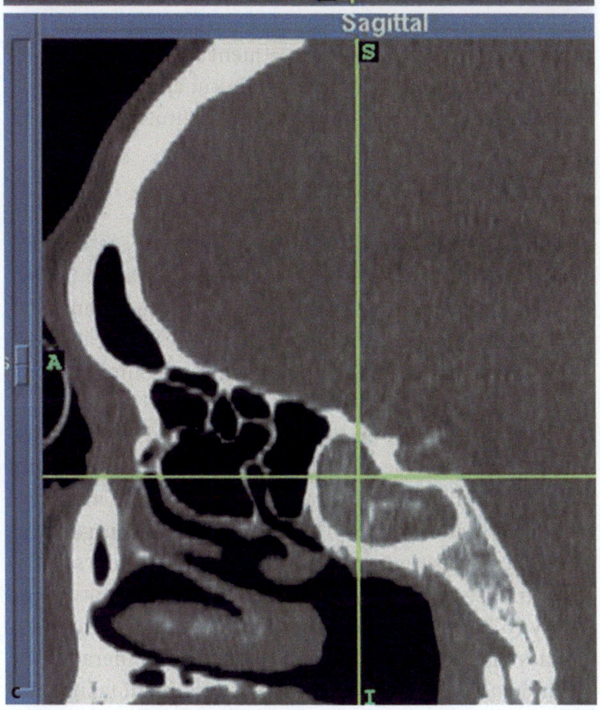

Fig. 35.1 Hyperostosis seen on computed tomography (CT). **a** Axial. **b** Coronal. **c** Sagittal

multi-institutional study of 52 patients with CT evidence of CRS with hyperostosis, Anand et al. reported significant clinical, endoscopic, and radiographic improvement following a course of culture-directed intravenous antibiotics [2]. In this study, the Rhinosinusitis Disability Index was used as one form of assessment and showed an improvement after treatment in average score (from 67.7 to 19.3), physical domain (from 25.4 to 7.7), functional domain (from 23.0 to 6.6), and emotional domain (from 19.3 to 5.0) [2]. In a separate study, Gross et al. showed a partial or complete response in 11 of 14 patients following surgery and culture-directed intravenous antibiotics [8]. Interestingly, the use of culture-directed intravenous antibiotics as an alternative to surgery is not supported

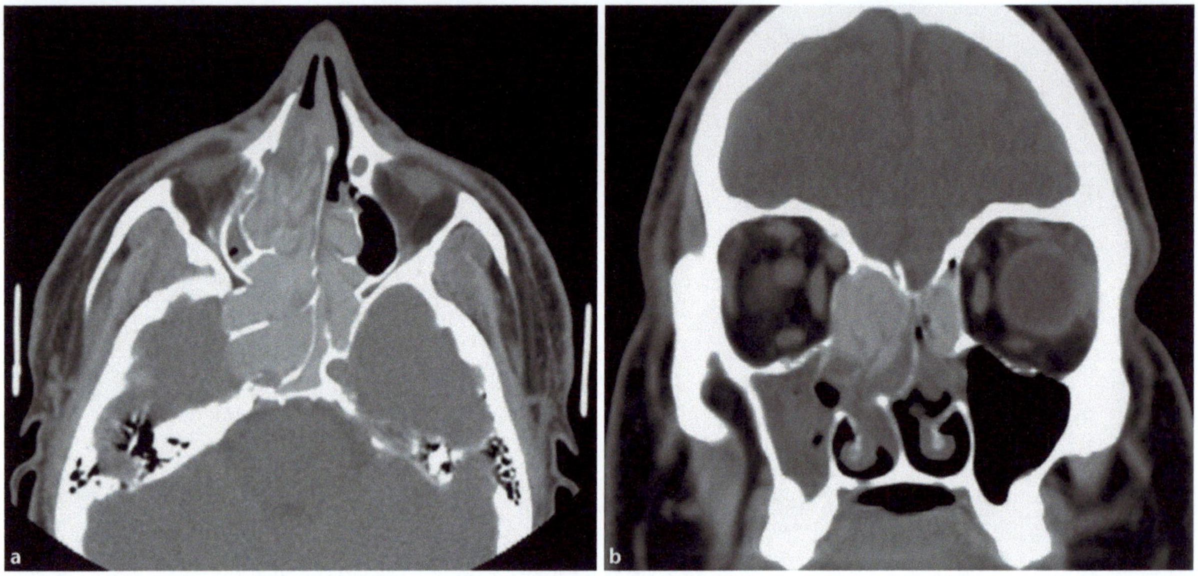

Fig. 35.2 Hyperostosis seen in patient with massive polyposis. **a** Axial CT. **b** Coronal CT

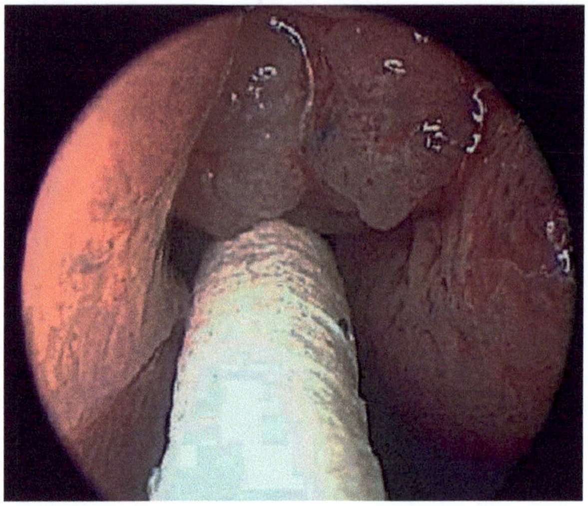

Fig. 35.3 Demonstration of endoscopic-directed culture

by the available literature. In a study of patients receiving a course of intravenous antibiotic therapy without surgery, Fowler et al. found an 89% relapse rate at a mean of 11.5 weeks after treatment [5].

In summary, the available literature, although limited, may support the use of culture-directed intravenous antibiotics in patients with refractory disease following maximal medical therapy and surgery. Treatment duration has been arbitrary in the literature, but for cases of surgical failure with hyperostosis, a 6- to 8-week course may be appropriate, similar to the treatment for osteomyelitis of the extremities [2]. Additional clinical and basic science investigation is required prior to definitive treatment guidelines.

Pediatric Intravenous Antibiotic Treatment

- The limited studies investigating intravenous antibiotics for pediatric rhinossinusitis suggest overall effectiveness, but a significant incidence of complications.

Don et al. reported an 89% success rate in pediatric patients with CRS aged 10 months to 15 years treated with 1–4 weeks of culture-directed intravenous antibiotics and select adenoidectomies [4]. Endoscopic sinus surgery was reserved for patients failing this treatment course. It is also important to note that the majority of patients in the study (67%) had continuation of therapy with oral antibiotics after completion of the intravenous therapy. The authors noted correlations between treatment failure and older patient age, and longer preexisting symptoms [4]. Although the authors did not report data on antibiotic or catheter complications, a separate report suggested higher complication and discontinuation rates for home-based intravenous therapy in children than in adults [7]. However, in the same study they concurred with the high success rates in children, reporting excellent outcomes even in pediatric patients with early discontinuation of treatment [7].

Method of Delivery of Home-Infused Intravenous Antibiotics

Several delivery methods exist for intravenous therapy for CRS. Inpatient, hospital-based treatment, with the use of traditional peripheral intravenous catheters, is significantly limited by the associated health-care cost, negative impact on daily function, and potential for nosocomial complications. Outpatient, home-based therapy, allows for more normal daily patient functioning and avoids the need for prolonged hospitalization. Multiple methods of delivery are available for home therapy. The least invasive and most frequently used is a PICC. The initial placement may be performed by a variety of health-care practitioners, including interventional radiology or dedicated nursing. Insertion of PICC lines has been shown to be highly successful, in one study greater than 96% of patients had a PICC successfully placed; however, 14.6% required a cut-down for successful placement [15]. The line is typically positioned near the antecubital fossa in the upper arm. The position of the distal end of the catheter near the superior vena cava is confirmed with radiographic imaging. In the majority of patients, the line is expected to function without issues and minimal impact on function for the entire duration of therapy, usually 6–8 weeks.

For patients requiring therapy for a greater period of time, such as patients receiving chemotherapy, central venous catheters (CVC) are placed for home therapy. These include such devices as Hickman catheters and portacaths. Care usually requires dressing changes around the insertion site several times a week for both PICC and Hickman catheters, and instruction on attaching the antibiotic up to the intravenous line. This usually requires a visiting nurse in the beginning and occasionally for the entire duration of treatment. Based on evidence from multiple series [2,8,13,18], the majority of patients are able to successfully complete a complete course of outpatient intravenous antibiotic therapy. However, given the potential for significant complications, we recommend a dedicated protocol as outlined below.

Complications of Intravenous Antibiotics

- The potential for both minor and major complications from long-term intravenous antibiotic therapy for sinusitis has been described.
- Most complications appear related to the antibiotic and not the intravenous line.

In the literature, there has been conflicting data regarding the incidence of PICC line complications. This may be due, in part, to the numerous indications for insertion. In addition to antibiotic therapy, PICC lines are often used for home medications including chemotherapy and intravenous hydration or nutrition. Most studies examining PICC lines for long-term antibiotics have reported low complication rates related to the catheter itself, as low as 2% in one study of 177 patients [13]. These complications included line thrombosis and septicemia [13].

Complications can be divided into those related to the catheter, such as catheter failure, thrombosis, or infection, and those related to antibiotic therapy, including allergic reaction, gastrointestinal upset, or rash/flushing. The latter is well documented with the use of vancomycin, and is termed "red-man syndrome." This reaction involves a pruritic and erythematous rash that occurs after infusion of vancomycin (Fig. 35.4). The spectrum of antibiotic-related complications include: neutropenia, elevated liver function tests, allergic reaction, itching, and gastrointestinal upset, and may occur in up to 16% of patients [13]. However, most of these complications are considered minor, as only 9 of the 29 patients with an antibiotic-related complication in a study by Lin et al. required a change in antibiotic [13]. Most reactions are self-limiting and resolve once the antibiotic is switched or stopped. Other studies have seen much lower antibiotic complication rates, only 11 per 10,000 catheter days [15].

One study compared the delivery method of intravenous therapy by comparing PICC to CVC. In this study, PICC lines were found to have a higher complication rate

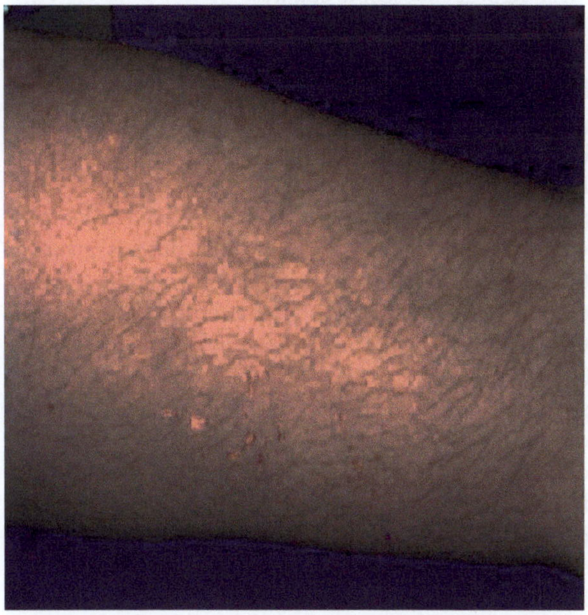

Fig. 35.4 "Red-man syndrome" seen with vancomycin infusion

then CVC. Looking at the specific complications, PICC lines were associated with a statistically significant increase in the incidence of catheter malfunction, thrombophlebitis, and overall complications [16]. Furthermore, the average time period for development of a complication with a PICC was 20 days compared to 281 days for a CVC [16]. Looking specifically at PICC placed for antibiotic therapy, however, no significant difference in complications were noted when compared to CVC [16]. This is more consistent with another study on safety that found 11% complications in CVC compared to only 9% in PICC [9].

Despite the overall safety of outpatient intravenous antibiotic therapy, the potential for major complications do exist. Although complications such as catheter malfunction, thrombophlebitis, and rash may be easily managed, other potential complications are associated with significant morbidity, including neutropenia and anaphylaxis. Additionally, the occurrence of a complication may result in a break or possibly premature termination of therapy, limiting the treatment efficacy. In light of these issues, we recommend a dedicated protocol for patients receiving therapy, with the goals of minimizing the incidence and morbidity of any complications.

- Standard treatment protocol:
  1. Initial consultation with an otolaryngologist and infectious disease specialist.
  2. First antibiotic dose given in the physician's office.
  3. Dedicated visiting nursing at regular intervals.
  4. Weekly office visits.
  5. Regularly scheduled serologic testing.
  6. Repeat endoscopic cultures.

The treatment plan involves initial consultation with both our team and an infectious disease specialist. The patient is counseled regarding the indications, potential benefits, and expected treatment course prior to therapy. Patients are also educated regarding the potential complications of therapy and instructed to contact the team with any concerning issues. The first dose is given in the office to monitor the patient for potential adverse events. The supervision of the first dose by the medical team in the office also increases the patient's emotional comfort with the therapy prior to beginning home infusions. Dedicated visiting nurse services are scheduled during the initial infusions until the patient can reliably demonstrate competence with PICC care and antibiotic infusion. Following this, weekly office visits and home nursing visits are scheduled. Patients are also regularly scheduled for serologic testing of antibiotic levels, when indicated, as well as routine hematological and biochemical testing (given the potential for neutropenia), elevated liver function tests, and renal impairment. The patients are also followed for clinical and endoscopic response throughout the course of therapy. Patients also undergo repeat surveillance sinonasal cultures if there is a history of resistant organisms.

Benefits of Intravenous Antibiotics

- The quality of life associated with home-based intravenous therapy is much higher than with hospital-based treatment.
- The insertion of peripherally inserted catheters, unlike most central catheters, does not require a surgical procedure and is generally well tolerated.

Home-based intravenous therapy requires a dedicated protocol of medical care and the commitment of the patient and family. Although visiting nurse care is often provided initially, the patient is taught how to properly attach the antibiotics and care for the catheter in a sterile fashion. Also, supplies and equipment must be available in the home and the patient's schedule needs to be designed for regular medication delivery. Despite these challenges, the satisfaction and quality of life with home-based intravenous therapy is significant. In one study looking at quality of life on the Short Form-36, significant improvements were found in physical functioning, bodily pain, and emotional/ mental component summary scale scores, in comparing patients on home-based therapy compared to hospital-based treatment [6].

In analyzing direct costs, home-based intravenous therapy appears cost effective compared to hospital treatment. A fivefold decrease in cost is associated with PICC line insertion when compared to CVC [16]. One study estimated a potential saving of approximately $50,000 (US) per patient by using home-based intravenous antibiotic therapy compared to conventional hospital-based treatment [3]. With the rapidly increasing national health care expenditure, the trend toward cost-effective therapy, such as home care, will likely increase over time.

Conclusion

When appropriately indicated, intravenous antibiotic therapy may be beneficial to selected patients with refractory rhinosinusitis.

Tips and Pearls

1. Antibiotics should be considered in those patients with intracranial and intraorbital complications of sinusitis, CRS due to resistant organisms, and refractory CRS following maximal medical and surgical therapy.

2. The presence of hyperostosis on CT scan in patients with refractory CRS may indicate the potential role of intravenous antibiotic therapy.
3. Routine diagnostic and surveillance sinonasal cultures are recommended; choice of medications is largely based on culture and sensitivity information.
4. Pediatric patients may be good candidates for intravenous antibiotics, either as a surgical adjunct or alternative to surgery.
5. PICC lines are well tolerated and less expensive than centrally placed catheters or hospitalized treatment.
6. The majority of complications associated with PICC lines and home-based intravenous antibiotics are minor and easily managed; however, the potential for serious complications does exist.
7. A dedicated protocol is required to manage potential complications and minimize disruption of treatment.
8. The indications for intravenous antibiotic therapy in CRS may be increasing given the rising incidence of resistant organisms and possible role of hyperostosis in refractory sinus disease.

References

1. Anand VK (2004) Epidemiology and economic impact of rhinosinusitis. Ann Otol Rhinol Laryngol 113:3–5
2. Anand V, Levine H, Friedman M, et al. (2003) Intravenous antibiotics for refractory rhinosinusitis in nonsurgical patients: preliminary findings of a prospective study. Am J Rhinol 17:363–368
3. Bernard L, El-hajj, Pron B, et al. (2001) Outpatient parenteral antimicrobial therapy (OPAT) for the treatment of osteomyelitis: evaluation of efficacy, tolerance and cost. J Clin Pharm Ther 26:445–451
4. Don DM, Yellow RF, Casselbrant ML, et al. (2001) Efficacy of a stepwise protocol that includes intravenous antibiotic therapy for the management of chronic sinusitis in children and adolescents. Arch Otolaryngol Head Neck Surg 127:1093–1098
5. Fowler KC, Duncavage JA, Murray JJ, et al. (2003) Chronic sinusitis and intravenous antibiotic therapy: resolution, recurrent and adverse events. J Allergy Clin Immunol 111: s85
6. Goodfellow AF, Wai AO, Frighetto L, et al. (2002) Quality-of-life assessment in an outpatient parental antibiotic program. Ann Pharmacother 36:1851–1855
7. Gomez M, Maraqa N, Alvarez A, et al. (2001) Complications of outpatient parenteral antibiotic therapy in childhood. Pediatr Infect Dis J 20:541–543
8. Gross ND, McInnes RJ, Hwang PH (2002) Outpatient intravenous antibiotics for chronic rhinosinusitis. Laryngoscope 112:1758–1761
9. Hoffman-Terry ML, Fraimow HS, Fox TR, et al. (1999) Adverse effects of outpatient parenteral antibiotic therapy. Am J Med 106:44–49
10. Huang WH, Hung PK (2006) Methicillin-resistant *Staphylococcus aureus* infections in acute rhinosinusitis. Laryngoscope 116:288–291
11. Jiang RS, Jang JW, Hsu CY (1999) Post-functional endoscopic sinus surgery methicillin-resistant *Staphylococcus aureus* sinusitis. Am J Rhinol 13:273–277
12. Kacker A, Huang C, Anand V (2002) Incidence of chronic hyperostotic rhinosinusitis in patients undergoing primary sinus surgery compared to revision surgery. Rhinol 40:80–82
13. Lin JW, Kacker A, Anand VK, et al. (2005) Catheter- and antibiotic-related complications of ambulatory intravenous antibiotic therapy for chronic rhinosinusitis. Am J Rhinol 19:365–369
14. Manarey CR, Anand VK, Huang C (2004) Incidence of methicillin-resistant *Staphylococcus aureus* causing chronic rhinosinusitis. Laryngoscope 114:939–941
15. Ng PK, Ault MJ, Ellrodt AG, et al. (1997) Peripherally inserted central catheters in general medicine. Mayo Clin Proc 72:225–233
16. Smith JR, Friedell ML, Cheatham ML, et al. (1998) Peripherally inserted central catheters revisited. Am J Surg 176:208–211
17. Solares CA, Batra PS, Hall GS, et al. (2006) Treatment of chronic rhinosinusitis exacerbations due to methicillin-resistant *Staphylococcus aureus* with mupirocin irrigations. Am J Otolaryngol 27:161–165
18. Tabaee A, Anand VK, Yoon C (2007) Outpatient intravenous antibiotics for methicillin-resistant *Staphylococcus aureus* sinusitis. Am J Rhinol 21:154–158

Chapter 36

Objective and Subjective Outcomes after Revision Sinus Surgery

36

Michael G. Stewart and Scott M. Rickert

Core Messages

- Assessment of outcome in revision sinus surgery is multifactorial.
- There are several ways to assess both objective and subjective outcomes.
- In revision surgery, and in chronic disease, the definition of a "successful" outcome likely differs from that of success after an acute or resolving process.
- Existing tools developed for chronic rhinosinusitis should be adequate for use in revision surgery.

Contents

Introduction

Assessment of outcome after any type of sinus surgery has not been uniformly defined or standardized, and assessment is likely multifactorial. Objective outcomes, such as endoscopic examination findings, computed tomography (CT) scan findings, need for medical treatment, or surgical revision rate, are important to assess. Subjective outcomes, such as symptoms and quality of life (QOL), are also important. Furthermore, there is good evidence that the objective and subjective data in chronic rhinosinusitis do not always correlate well. Therefore, the assessment of both outcomes is important. After sinus surgery – and particularly revision sinus surgery – these issues are particularly salient, since the anatomy is invariably altered and may remain "abnormal" even with complete resolution of symptoms.

- In addition to discussing *how* to assess outcome, we should consider *when* to assess outcome. In certain diseases (for example, cancer), long-term outcomes are invariably preferred over short-term outcomes. In other chronic diseases, improvement in short-term status can be quite beneficial and should be recommended, even if long-term outcomes are predictably poor. This may be of particular importance in revision surgery for problems such as nasal polyposis

Outcomes Assessment in Rhinosinusitis

Much work has gone into classification and outcomes assessment in chronic rhinosinusitis, and this will be reviewed later in the chapter. However, there is a lack of material specifically focusing on revision surgery. Despite the fact that there are some potential challenges, there is no reason that existing outcome tools cannot be used. Symptoms and QOL should still be important outcomes to assess, and are likely a major driver of patient behavior after surgery – similar to before surgery. In addition, the impact of sinusitis on the symptoms and severity of other diseases, such as asthma, is likely as important after revision surgery as any other time. Objective outcome assessment, in particular CT scan findings, might require a modified interpretation after revision surgery, however. There is limited data on CT mucosal changes that should be expected after surgical intervention. Landmarks have been removed and anatomy altered, but in fact the degree of mucosal changes, and the response to medical treatment, may be different in postsurgical sinuses. For example, some degree of underlying mucosal thickening might be expected and should perhaps be graded as "normal."

In addition, the timing of outcome assessment is important, and we should consider a different model in revision surgery – with respect to long-term outcome as well as "absolute" outcome. In many chronic diseases, the patient will never return to a normal state. In fact, gradual worsening in QOL might be expected. Therefore, successful treatment could limit the reduction in QOL (even though it still declines), or prolong the time before reaching a certain level. For example, a patient with chronic renal failure may always require dialysis, but additional treatment could still improve QOL and be a desirable adjunct. Similarly, in patients with polyposis or other chronic mucosal diseases such as cystic fibrosis, need for revision surgery should not necessarily be counted as "failure," and short-term improvements in health status or QOL could be considered successful outcomes. On the other hand, revision surgery can still result in disease resolution in many cases, so chronic status and eventual failure is not necessarily the norm.

- Outcomes assessed in chronic rhinosinusitis can be divided into two general categories: subjective and objective. Both have been reported frequently in the literature, and clinicians typically use both types of outcome in their everyday evaluations.

Subjective Outcomes

Symptoms are a key issue in rhinosinusitis, and are often the primary reason that patients seek initial medical attention and return for further treatment. In fact, at one time, an international task force on rhinosinusitis used the presence of symptoms as the definition of the disease [15]. This was problematic, however, because some patients with symptoms do not actually have rhinosinusitis. Subsequent publications have moved away from the concept of symptoms as definitional, but nevertheless symptoms are a key component of the disease and a major driver of patient's behavior. There is currently no standardized, validated tool to measure symptom burden in rhinosinusitis, although some tools have been reported [4].

An additional assessment of subjective outcome is QOL, which is measured using validated instruments. QOL instruments are generally divided into two types – global (or "generic"), and disease-specific. Both global and disease-specific instruments have advantages and disadvantages. Global instruments have the advantage of being comparable between diseases and can be used for "benchmarking" against known problems, but have the disadvantage of being less sensitive to the effects of a particular disease. For example, even the very successful treatment of specific problems like hearing loss or visual loss may result in only small changes on a global QOL instrument. Disease-specific instruments are designed with content that addresses the disease of interest, and are much more sensitive to changes in disease status; however, they have the disadvantage of not being comparable across disease states and therefore they can be difficult to interpret. In other words, what does an increase of 21 points on scale X actually *mean* to a patient or interpreting physician?

- In the assessment of symptoms or QOL, it is also important to keep in mind that patients without disease will usually not score 0 (or 100) on scales.

As an example, in one study of the Sino-Nasal Outcome Tool – 16 items, patients with rhinosinusitis scored an average of 22.4 (on a scale of 0–48), and patients with ear disease scored a mean of 10.5. Other studies have shown similar results. So, the baseline or "normal" score should be taken into account when reviewing results in any population.

- The popularity and use of QOL tools has grown significantly, and in general the systematic assessment of QOL yields important information about what patients are feeling, and the true effects of many treatments.
- Most QOL instruments are validated to measure QOL in populations, not individual patients.
- QOL instruments might not be the best tools for assessment of outcome after changes in treatment – particularly in the very short term.

However, the use of QOL instruments is often not fully understood. For example, most QOL instruments are validated to measure QOL in *populations*, not individual patients. The statistical criteria for discrimination between individual patients are more stringent. In addition, many instruments are designed to measure QOL averaged over a recent period of time, not day-to-day changes. For example, items on the SF-36 global instrument ask about the previous 4 weeks, and items on the Chronic Sinusitis Survey ask about the previous 8 weeks. Therefore, QOL instruments might not be the best tools for assessment of outcome after changes in treatment – particularly in the very short term. In such cases, the presence and severity of symptoms might be more useful. However, there needs to be some agreement on exactly which symptoms are important to measure. A simple listing of potential symptoms will not suffice, because it will give equal "weight" to each symptom. For example, if there are ten possible symptoms listed, then each symptom counts for 1/10 (10%) of the total "symptom score." Rhinologists would probably agree that purulent rhinorrhea, for example, is a more important and predictive symptom of sinusitis than, say, headache. If each were on the same list, however, then changes in each would be counted similarly. Some work is needed to define and validate a symptom tool for use as an outcome measure in rhinosinusitis [16, 21].

Despite the obvious importance of symptoms and subjective outcomes, there are problems with using them in isolation – a large problem being that some symptoms and QOL changes will be due to other diseases besides rhinosinusitis. Therefore, subjective outcomes are only part of the overall picture. A review of subjective outcomes instruments follows in a later section.

Objective Outcomes

- CT staging systems are classificatory systems and were designed to allow standardization, classification, and a common language (Fig. 36.1).
- CT staging systems were not designed to predict outcome.
- There is a high correlation between endoscopic stage and CT stage in patients with chronic rhinosinusitis.
- CT staging may be more appropriate than endoscopic staging for frontal sinus disease, due to the remote location of the frontal sinus.

There are several objective outcomes that can be assessed after sinus surgery and revision sinus surgery. CT scan

CT Staging Systems for Chronic Sinusitis

Kennedy		Friedman	
Stage 0	Normal	Stage 0	Normal
Stage I	Anatomic abnormalities All unilateral sinus disease Bilateral disease limited to ethmoid sinuses	Stage I	Single focus disease (involving a single focus or sinus unit)
Stage II	Bilateral ethmoid disease with involvement of one dependent sinus	Stage II	Multifocal disease (includes bilateral or multiple areas of disease which are not confluent or diffuse throughout the ethmoid labyrinth. bileral middle meatal polyps)
Stage III	Bilateral ethmoid disease with involvement of two or more dependent sinuses on each side	Stage III	Diffuse disease (extensive bilateral involvement of multiple sinuses) without bony changes
Stage IV	Diffuse sinonasal polyposis	Stage IV	Diffuse disease associated with body changes

Levine and May		Harvard System	
Stage 0	Normal	Stage 0	Normal (<2mm mucosal thickening on any sinus wall)
Stage I	Disease limited to ostiomeatal complex	Stage I	All unilateral disease or anatomic abnormality
Stage II	Incomplete opacification of one or More major sinuses (frontal. maxillary, sphenoid)	Stage II	Bilateral disease limited to ethmoid or maxillary sinuses
Stage III	Complete opacification of one or more major sinuses, but not all	Stage III	Bilateral disease with involvement of at lease one sphenoid or frontal sinus
Stage IV	Total opacification of all sinuses	Stage IV	Pansinusitus

From: Gliklich. RE. Metson. R. A comparison of sinus computed tomography (CT) staging systems for outcomes research. Am J Rhinology 1994:8:291-297.

Fig. 36.1 Computed tomography (CT) staging systems for chronic rhinosinusitis findings are very important as an assessment of mucosal thickening, ostia obstruction, fluid level, and anatomic extent of disease, as well as demonstrating other important information such as bony dehiscence and presence of extrasinus extension of disease, for example. There are several staging systems that have been proposed for sinus CT scans; among the most popular are the Lund-MacKay, Kennedy, and Harvard systems [17]. These staging systems were designed to allow standardization, classification, and a common language – in other words they are classificatory systems. They were not designed to predict outcome (prognostic systems), although it is possible that they do so. Potential problems with any CT staging system include missing sinuses, the effect of previous surgical sinus dissection, and difficulty in differentiating mucosal thickening from retained secretions [17]. In revision surgery, these issues can be particularly difficult because of the changed anatomy of the ostiomeatal complex. Despite these issues, however, the CT scan is easily available, gives useful anatomic information, and is a widely used technique for assessing the sinus mucosa and anatomy.

There is a staging system for endoscopic findings [17]. Since endoscopic examination and the CT scan are both used to assess anatomy and mucosal status, not surprisingly there is a high correlation between endoscopic stage and CT stage. This is likely particularly true after revision sinus surgery, where the ostia have been opened and tissue removed, making endoscopic evaluation of most of the sinuses even easier. However, even after successful surgery, there are some sinuses, in particular the frontal, which might be difficult to assess with endoscopy alone, and CT scans still play an important role.

Other objective outcomes of potential use in revision sinus surgery include culture results, olfactory testing, and the presence and severity of related diseases such as asthma. In addition, if one of the complaints is nasal obstruction, then acoustic rhinometry or rhinomanometry can yield objective data [18]. However, neither of those tests is widely accepted in clinical practice and there is debate about the techniques of testing and interpretation. Nevertheless, they do provide objective data on the anatomy of the nasal airway.

Bacteriology, and in particular the presence of resistant bacteria, or fungus, can be important outcomes in revision sinus surgery. However, many patients are on long-term antibiotics, making culture results possibly less reliable, and there is always the possibility of sampling error and differences in laboratory techniques when reviewing culture results. Olfactory testing is beyond the scope of this chapter, but there are reproducible tests of olfaction. One obvious caveat is that olfactory function may be impaired before treatment, or as a result of another disease.

Another potential "objective" outcome is the need for oral or topical medications, with the theory being that successful surgery might reduce the need for extensive medical treatment. However, use of that as an outcome may be problematic for a few reasons. The use of medications to control persistent disease or prevent recurrent disease may be desirable, and should not necessarily represent "failure." In addition, medications are often taken for related problems (such as allergies or pulmonary disease). Finally, use of medication is volitional, and patients may use or not use them for different reasons, making medication frequency of use less "objective" than it might initially seem.

Association Between Objective and Subjective Outcomes

- It is now well-established that symptoms and QOL do not correlate with CT scan findings in chronic rhinosinusitis [7, 8, 11, 14, 24, 27, 28].
- This does not mean that CT scan findings are not important, or that symptoms are not important, but it does mean that they are not measuring the same thing, and that you cannot predict one simply by knowing the other.

While it is clear that CT scan findings do not predict symptoms at any given point in time, there is conflicting evidence on whether or not CT findings might actually predict *changes* in symptoms or QOL after surgery or other treatment. One prospective study found that the CT scan stage was a significant independent predictor of improvement in symptoms after sinus surgery [26]. In that study, patients with higher-stage disease on CT (i.e., worse mucosal disease) had larger proportional improvements in disease-specific QOL after surgery. Another prospective study also found that CT stage approached significance as a predictor of outcome [25]. Other prospective studies however found that CT stage was *not* an independent predictor of change in disease-specific QOL or symptom severity after surgery [6, 8]. All studies have shown large overall improvements in disease-specific QOL after endoscopic sinus surgery.

In addition, one study has shown that objective findings may predict the need for revision sinus surgery [12]. Specifically, patients from a tertiary referral practice who eventually required revision endoscopic surgery were statistically more likely to have an abnormal endoscopic examination at 18 months after the initial surgery. Interestingly, in that series symptom severity at 18 months was *not* predictive of needing eventual surgical revision.

Available Validated Health Status Instruments for Use in Rhinosinusitis

Global QOL Instruments

There are hundreds of validated global QOL instruments, any of which could be potentially used as an outcome assessment in revision surgery. The Short Form 36-item Health Survey (SF-36) has been used in studies of chronic rhinosinusitis and the effect of sinus surgery, and it is clearly sensitive to the impact of chronic rhinosinusitis. The instrument comprises 36 questions that are scored into 8 general health domains, such as, for example, bodily pain, vitality, and social functioning. A shortened version, the SF-12, is also a global instrument, and it is scored into only two subscales – physical health component and mental health component. One desirable characteristic of the SF-36 and SF-12 are that they have both been used extensively, and there are good benchmark comparison data for healthy individuals and also multiple diseases.

Many other global QOL instruments can be used. However, when using any global instrument, it is possible that the scale will not be sensitive to the effects of a specific disease. So, lack of response on a global QOL instrument does not necessarily mean lack of effectiveness.

Disease-Specific Instruments

There are several validated disease-specific instruments for rhinosinusitis in adults, and in fact all have been used successfully in studies. Content, length, period of symptom recall, and scoring are different for each, so there are several potential options [21].

The Chronic Sinusitis Survey (CSS; Fig. 36.2) [10] was designed for chronic rhinosinusitis, contains six items, and was validated for a symptom recall period of 8 weeks. There are two subscales: medication and symptom. The CSS is very sensitive to change over time, although its limited content might exclude some aspects of sinusitis in some patients.

The Rhinosinusitis Outcome Measure (RSOM-31; Fig. 36.3) [22] was originally developed as a 31-question comprehensive assessment of sinusitis-specific symptoms with some general health assessment included. Since its initial inception, this particular instrument has been simplified and revalidated to be shorter and more sinusitis-specific. The current widely used version is the Sinonasal Outcome Test-20 items (SNOT-20; Fig. 36.4), which contains 20 items, with no designated period of symptom recall. The SNOT-20 is scored as a single scale.

The Rhinosinusitis Disability Index (RSDI; Fig. 36.5) [3] is a validated instrument with items written in the first person, and it relates symptoms to limitations on daily life. It was designed for CRS, contains 30 items, and has no designated period of symptom recall. It is scored into three subscales: emotional, physical, and functional. The content of some of the items cover more global QOL issues than other disease-specific instruments.

The Rhinosinusitis Quality of Life Survey (RhinoQOL; Fig. 36.6) [2] is a validated instrument that was designed to be used for both acute and chronic rhinosinusitis. It contains 17 items and uses a recall period of 7 days. It is scored into three subscales: symptom frequency, symptom bother, and symptom effect. While the authors report that the instrument can be used in acute or chronic sinusitis, there is some potential concern that the content for those diseases will not be identical.

Results after Revision Endoscopic Sinus Surgery

Compared to the volume of literature on primary sinus surgery, there are fewer reports on outcomes after revision sinus surgery. Many of the published reports on revision surgery address indications and techniques, but not outcomes. Others report outcome only as success or failure rate, usually defined as the need for further revision surgery. As we have discussed earlier, this is probably not the ideal outcome to assess in this group of patients. We briefly describe the results from selected series below; this is not an exhaustive list.

One study of 125 patients over a 3-year period undergoing revision endoscopic sinus surgery reported both objective and subjective outcomes [19]. In that series, objective outcomes were CT scan findings, assessed using the Lund-MacKay system, and endoscopy score, assessed using a scoring system described by the 1997 Rhinosinusitis Task Force [17]. Subjective outcomes were SNOT-20 score, and individual symptoms measured on a visual analog scale. The mean number of prior surgical procedures was 1.9. The authors found significant and sustained improvements in both objective and subjective outcomes after revision surgery. In particular, mean SNOT-20 scores improved from 30.7 to 7.7 at 2 years of follow-up, and mean endoscopy scores improved from 7.3 to 2.1 at 2-years follow-up. Six individual symptoms were measured using Likert scales (nasal obstruction, congestion, rhinorrhea, postnasal drip, facial pain/pressure, olfactory dysfunction), and all six showed large-magnitude and statistically significant improvements at 2 years. Of the 125 patients, 59 had nasal polyposis; those 59 patients also had more prior surgeries, higher CT scores (worse disease), but lower (better) SNOT-20 scores. The authors did not report postoperative CT scores.

In another report from a subset ($n=80$) of the same

CHRONIC SINUSITIS SURVEY

Please answer every question by circling the appropriate number. If you are unsure about how to answer a question, please give the best answer you can.

1. During the past 8 *weeks*, how many *weeks* have you had: (circle one answer in each row)

a. Sinus headaches, facial pain or pressure — 1a

0 weeks | *1-2 weeks* | *3-4 weeks* | *5-6 weeks* | *7-8 weeks*

b. Nasal drainage or postnasal drip — 1b

0 weeks | *1-2 weeks* | *3-4 weeks* | *5-6 weeks* | *7-8 weeks*

c. Nasal congestion or difficulty breathing through your nose — 1c

0 weeks | *1-2 weeks* | *3-4 weeks* | *5-6 weeks* | *7-8 weeks*

2. During the past 8 *weeks*, how many *weeks* have you taken: (circle one answer in each row)

a. Antibiotics — 2a

0 weeks | *1-2 weeks* | *3-4 weeks* | *5-6 weeks* | *7-8 weeks*

b. Nasal sprays prescribed by your doctor — 2b

0 weeks | *1-2 weeks* | *3-4 weeks* | *5-6 weeks* | *7-8 weeks*

c. Sinus medications in pill form (such as antihistamines, decongestants) — 2c

0 weeks | *1-2 weeks* | *3-4 weeks* | *5-6 weeks* | *7-8 weeks*

3. What is your overall state of health? (circle one) — 3

excellent | *very good* | *good* | *fair* | *poor*

4. How much do sinus symptoms contribute to your overall health problems? (circle one) — 4

not at all | *a little bit* | *moderate amount* | *a lot* | *severely affected*

5. How much improvement in your sinus symptoms do you expect after treatment? (circle one) — 5

no change | *a little better* | *moderately better* | *a lot better* | *totally improved*

Fig. 36.2 Chronic sinusitis survey

RHINOSINUSITIS OUTCOME MEASURE (RSOM-31)

To let us know more about your nose and sinus disease, please answer the following questions about the consequences of your nose and sinus disease. There are no "right" or "wrong" answers, and only ***you*** *can provide this information. For each of the statements listed please indicate* ***how much of a problem*** *it is to you. If a statement does not apply to you, please circle 0 and go to the next statement.*

Thank you for your time and participation.

	Not present / No problem	Very mild problem	Mild or slight problem	Moderate problem	Severe problem	Problem is as "bad as can be"
1. Stuffy / blocked nose	0	1	2	3	4	5
2. Runny nose	0	1	2	3	4	5
3. Sneezing	0	1	2	3	4	5
4. Decreased sense of taste or smell	0	1	2	3	4	5
5. Postnasal discharge	0	1	2	3	4	5
6. Thick nasal discharge / debris	0	1	2	3	4	5
7. Itchy or watery eyes	0	1	2	3	4	5
8. Sore or swollen eyes	0	1	2	3	4	5
9. Difficulty getting to sleep	0	1	2	3	4	5
10. Wake up during the night	0	1	2	3	4	5
11. Lack of a good night's sleep	0	1	2	3	4	5
12. Wake up tired	0	1	2	3	4	5
13. Fullness in ears	0	1	2	3	4	5
14. Ringing in ears	0	1	2	3	4	5
15. Dizziness	0	1	2	3	4	5
16. Pain in ears	0	1	2	3	4	5
17. Decreased hearing	0	1	2	3	4	5
18. Fatigue / being worn out	0	1	2	3	4	5
19. Reduced productivity	0	1	2	3	4	5
20. Poor concentration	0	1	2	3	4	5
21. Headache	0	1	2	3	4	5
22. Facial pain / pressure	0	1	2	3	4	5
23. Cough	0	1	2	3	4	5
24. Short of breath	0	1	2	3	4	5
25. Inconvenience of having to carry tissues	0	1	2	3	4	5
26. Need to rub nose / eyes	0	1	2	3	4	5
27. Need to blow nose repeatedly	0	1	2	3	4	5
28. Bad breath	0	1	2	3	4	5
29. Frustrated, impatient, or irritable	0	1	2	3	4	5
30. Feeling depressed or sad	0	1	2	3	4	5
31. Embarrassed by your symptoms	0	1	2	3	4	5

Fig. 36.3 Rhinosinusitis outcome measure (RSOM-31)

patient population, patients for revision surgery who also had asthma had significantly worse CT scan findings than patients without asthma (mean Lund-MacKay scores of 18.6 vs. 11.7) [13]. However, disease-specific QOL before revision surgery was not significantly different (mean SNOT-20 scores of 49.6 vs. 44.9). Patients with and without asthma both had highly significant – but statistically indistinguishable – improvements in SNOT-20 score (70% improvement vs. 72.6% improvement) compared to preoperative scores. Therefore, despite worse CT scan findings, patients with asthma had equivalent significant improvement in symptoms after revision surgery compared to patients without asthma.

Another prospective study on revision sinus surgery reported changes in symptoms using the Rhinosinusitis Symptom Inventory, which is a summation of individual

I.D.:________ **SINO-NASAL OUTCOME TEST** DATE:________

Below you will find a list of symptoms and social/emotional consequences of your rhinosinusitis. We would like to know more about these problems and would appreciate your answering the following questions to the best of your ability. There are no right or wrong answers, and only you can provide us with this information. Please rate your problems as they have been over the past two weeks. Thank you for your participation. Do not hesitate to ask for assistance if necessary.

Considering how severe the problem is when you experience it and how frequently it happens, please rate each item below on how "bad" it is by circling the number that corresponds with how you feel using this scale: →	*No Problem*	*Mild or Slight Problem*	*Moderate Problem*	*Severe Problem*
1. Need to blow nose	0	1	2	3
2. Sneezing	0	1	2	3
3. Runny nose	0	1	2	3
4. Cough	0	1	2	3
5. Post-nasal discharge	0	1	2	3
6. Thick nasal discharge	0	1	2	3
7. Ear fullness	0	1	2	3
8. Dizziness	0	1	2	3
9. Ear pain	0	1	2	3
10. Facial pain/pressure	0	1	2	3
11. Difficult	0	1	2	3
12. Wake up at night	0	1	2	3
13. Lack of a good night's sleep	0	1	2	3
14. Wake up tired	0	1	2	3
15. Fatigue	0	1	2	3
16. Reduced productivity	0	1	2	3
17. Reduced concentration	0	1	2	3
18. Frustrated/restless/irritable	0	1	2	3
19. Sad	0	1	2	3
20. Embarrassed	0	1	2	3

Fig. 36.4 Sinonasal outcome test

symptoms (12 in all) from the 1997 Task Force list of major and minor symptoms [5]. A total of 21 patients with a mean follow-up of 12.4 months after revision surgery were reported. The author converted raw symptom score changes into effect sizes to make interpretation easier; the effect size is a *relative* measure of change calculated by dividing actual change by the standard deviation of the baseline value. In this study, all symptoms improved after revision surgery. Substantial improvement was seen in the individual symptoms of "nasal obstruction" and "hyposmia," and moderate improvements were seen in symptoms "facial pressure," "rhinorrhea," "headache," "fatigue," and "ear pain." When grouped into four content domains (nasal, facial, oropharyngeal, systemic), all domains showed at least moderate improvement in effect size. These improvements were statistically similar in magnitude to changes in a group of patients after primary endoscopic sinus surgery. This series also reported on

RHINOSINUSITIS DISABILITY INDEX (RSDI)

*The purpose of this scale is to identify difficulties that you may be experiencing because of your nose or sinus problems. Please answer: **Never, Almost Never, Sometimes, Almost Always, Always** to each item. Answer each item as it pertains to your nose and sinus problem only.*	***Never***	***Almost Never***	***Sometimes***	***Almost Always***	***Always***
Emotional					
1. Because of my problem I feel stressed in relationships with friends and family.	☐	☐	☐	☐	☐
2. Because of my problem I feel confused.	☐	☐	☐	☐	☐
3. Because of my problem I have difficulty paying attention.	☐	☐	☐	☐	☐
4. Because of my problem I avoid being around people.	☐	☐	☐	☐	☐
5. Because of my problem I am frequently angry.	☐	☐	☐	☐	☐
6. Because of my problem I do not like to socialize.	☐	☐	☐	☐	☐
7. Because of my problem I frequently feel tense.	☐	☐	☐	☐	☐
8. Because of my problem I frequently feel irritable.	☐	☐	☐	☐	☐
9. Because of my problem I am depressed.	☐	☐	☐	☐	☐
10. My problem places stress on my relationships with members of my family or friends.	☐	☐	☐	☐	☐
Functional					
11. Because of my problem I feel handicapped.	☐	☐	☐	☐	☐
12. Because of my problem I feel restricted in performance of my routine daily activities.	☐	☐	☐	☐	☐
13. Because of my problem I restrict my recreational activities.	☐	☐	☐	☐	☐
14. Because of my problem I feel frustrated.	☐	☐	☐	☐	☐
15. Because of my problem I feel fatigued.	☐	☐	☐	☐	☐
16. Because of my problem I avoid travelling.	☐	☐	☐	☐	☐
17. Because of my problem I miss work or social activities.	☐	☐	☐	☐	☐
18. My outlook on the world is affected by my problem.	☐	☐	☐	☐	☐
19. Because of my problem I find it difficult to focus my attention away from my problem and on other things.	☐	☐	☐	☐	☐
Physical					
20. The pain or pressure in my face makes it difficult for me to concentrate.	☐	☐	☐	☐	☐
21. The pain in my eyes makes it difficult for me to read.	☐	☐	☐	☐	☐
22. I have difficulty stooping over to lift objects because of face pressure.	☐	☐	☐	☐	☐
23. Because of my problem I have difficulty with strenuous yard work and housework.	☐	☐	☐	☐	☐
24. Straining increases or worsens my problem.	☐	☐	☐	☐	☐
25. I am inconvenienced by my chronic runny nose.	☐	☐	☐	☐	☐
26. Food does not taste good because of my change in smell.	☐	☐	☐	☐	☐
27. My frequent sniffing is irritating to my friends and family.	☐	☐	☐	☐	☐
28. Because of my problem I don't sleep well.	☐	☐	☐	☐	☐
29. I have difficulty with exertion due to my nasal obstruction.	☐	☐	☐	☐	☐
30. My sexual activity is affected by my problem.	☐	☐	☐	☐	☐

Fig. 36.5 Rhinosinusitis disability index (RSDI)

RHINOSINUSITIS QOL INSTRUMENT

YOUR RECENT SINUS / NASAL SYMPTOMS

Answer questions by checking the box to the right of your answer.

► You are sometimes told to skip over some questions. When this happens, you will see a note that tells you what question to answer next, like this: ***If None of the time, go to #3.***

		None of the time	*A little of the time*	*Some of the time*	*Most of the time*	*All of the time*
1.	In the last 7 days, how much of the time did you have sinus headaches, facial pain or facial pressure? ***If None of the time, go to #2.***	☐	☐	☐	☐	☐
1a.	On a scale of 0 to 10, where 0 is not bothered at all and 10 is bothered a lot, how much were you bothered by the sinus headaches, facial pain or facial pressure? 0☐ 1☐ 2☐ 3☐ 4☐ 5☐ 6☐ 7☐ 8☐ 9☐ 10☐					
2.	In the last 7 days, how much of the time did you have a blocked or stuffy nose? ***If None of the time, go to #3.***	☐	☐	☐	☐	☐
2a.	On a scale of 0 to 10, where 0 is not bothered at all and 10 is bothered a lot, how much were you bothered by having a blocked or stuffy nose? 0☐ 1☐ 2☐ 3☐ 4☐ 5☐ 6☐ 7☐ 8☐ 9☐ 10☐					
3.	In the last 7 days, how much of the time did you have post-nasal drip? ***If None of the time, go to #4.***	☐	☐	☐	☐	☐
3a.	On a scale of 0 to 10, where 0 is not bothered at all and 10 is bothered a lot, how much were you bothered by this post-nasal drip? 0☐ 1☐ 2☐ 3☐ 4☐ 5☐ 6☐ 7☐ 8☐ 9☐ 10☐					
4.	In the last 7 days, how much of the time did you have a thick nasal discharge?	☐	☐	☐	☐	☐
5.	In the last 7 days, how much of the time did you have a runny nose?	☐	☐	☐	☐	☐
	For these next questions, please think about all the nasal symptoms you've recently experienced.					
6.	In the last 7 days, how much of the time did you have trouble sleeping because of your nasal symptoms?	☐	☐	☐	☐	☐
7.	In the last 7 days, how much of the time did you feel it was harder to concentrate because of your nasal symptoms?	☐	☐	☐	☐	☐
8.	In the last 7 days, how much of the time did you feel it was harder to do the things you normally do because of your nasal symptoms?	☐	☐	☐	☐	☐
9.	In the last 7 days, how much of the time did you feel embarrassed because of your nasal symptoms?	☐	☐	☐	☐	☐
10.	In the last 7 days, how much of the time did you feel frustrated because of your nasal symptoms?	☐	☐	☐	☐	☐
11.	In the last 7 days, how much of the time did you feel irritable because of your nasal symptoms?	☐	☐	☐	☐	☐
12.	In the last 7 days, how much of the time did you feel sad or depressed because of your nasal symptoms?	☐	☐	☐	☐	☐
13.	In the last 7 days, how much of the time did you think about your nasal symptoms?	☐	☐	☐	☐	☐

Fig. 36.6 Rhinosinusitis quality of life (QOL) instrument

medication use after revision sinus surgery; use of nasal steroids, antihistamines, and antibiotics did not show statistically significant changes.

Other studies have shown significant improvement in disease-specific QOL and in frontal recess patency in patients undergoing revision frontal sinus endoscopic surgery using image guidance [9]. QOL scores were noted to be clinically as well as statistically significantly improved.

Patients with massive nasal polyposis have been reported to have a high rate of revision surgery (47%), and in one study, a history of prior sinus surgery or the presence of asthma predicted a higher rate of revision surgery [29]. Whether or not the presence of asthma predicts poorer outcome after ESS is controversial, and many studies have not found a significant association [25].

One retrospective study noted that patients with classic Samter's triad (asthma, nasal polyposis, aspirin sensitivity) had more extensive disease on CT scan scores than patients with chronic rhinosinusitis without Samter's triad. In addition, the Samter's triad patients required a larger number of revision surgeries [1]. However, patients seem to benefit from improved QOL and improved control of asthma – even if repeated revision surgery is needed [20, 23]. So the presence of Samter's triad should not deter the surgeon from pursuing revision surgery if it is indicated.

- Difficulties in assessing outcomes in patients undergoing revision sinus surgery include the lack of a control group. So, even though large improvements were identified, it is not clear that they were necessarily due to the intervention. However, given the nature of revision surgery, in particular the fact that it is usually only performed when other treatment options have been exhausted, it would be difficult to perform a study with a true control group. Therefore, uncontrolled studies might be the best evidence possible in this disease.

Conclusions

Outcomes after revision sinus surgery can be divided into subjective and objective findings. In general, patients with rhinosinusitis had significant improvements in objective outcomes such as endoscopy score, and subjective outcomes such as QOL and symptom burden, after revision sinus surgery. In fact, outcomes after revision surgery seem to be equivalent to outcomes after successful primary surgery in some cases.

The CT scan is an important indicator of the anatomic extent of disease and severity of mucosal change. However, CT findings after revision surgery are not well described, and surgical changes can modify the interpretation of anatomic findings. Therefore, symptoms and QOL might be somewhat more important as outcome measures after surgery or revision surgery. However, it is generally best to consider subjective and objective outcomes as complimentary. Researchers and clinicians should choose from a variety of outcomes tools in the evaluation of patients being considered for revision sinus surgery.

References

1. Amar YG, Frenkiel S, Sobol SE (2000) Outcome analysis of endoscopic sinus surgery for chronic sinusitis in patients having Samter's triad. J Otolaryngol 29:7–12
2. Atlas SJ, Metson RB, Singer DE, Wu YA, Gliklich RE (2005) Validity of a new health-related quality of life instrument for patients with chronic sinusitis. Laryngoscope 115:846–854
3. Benninger MS, Senior BA (1997) The development of the Rhinosinusitis Disability Index. Arch Otolaryngol Head Neck Surg 123:1175–1179
4. Bhattacharyya N (2003) The economic burden and symptom manifestations of chronic rhinosinusitis. Am J Rhinol 17:27–32
5. Bhattacharyya N (2004) Clinical outcomes after revision endoscopic sinus surgery. Arch Otolaryngol Head Neck Surg 130:975–978
6. Bhattacharyya N (2006) Radiographic stage fails to predict symptom outcomes after endoscopic sinus surgery for chronic rhinosinusitis. Laryngoscope 116:18–22
7. Bhattacharyya T, Piccirillo JF, Wippold FJ 2nd (1997) Relationship between patient-based descriptions of sinusitis and paranasal sinus computed tomographic findings. Arch Otolaryngol Head Neck Surg 123:1189–1192
8. Bradley DT, Kountakis SE (2005) Correlation between computed tomography scores and symptomatic improvement after endoscopic sinus surgery. Laryngoscope 115:466–469
9. Chiu AG, Vaughan WC (2004) Revision endoscopic frontal sinus surgery with surgical navigation. Otolaryngol Head Neck Surg 130:312–318
10. Gliklich RE, Metson R (1995) Techniques for outcomes research in chronic sinusitis. Laryngoscope 105:387–390
11. Hwang PH, Irwin SB, Griest SE, Caro JE, Nesbit GM (2003) Radiologic correlates of symptom-based diagnostic criteria for chronic rhinosinusitis. Otolaryngol Head Neck Surg 128:489–496
12. Kennedy DW, Wright ED, Goldberg AN (2000) Objective and subjective outcomes in surgery for chronic sinusitis. Laryngoscope 110:29–31
13. Kountakis SE, Bradley DT (2003) Effect of asthma on sinus computed tomography grade and symptom scores in patients undergoing revision functional endoscopic sinus surgery. Am J Rhinol 17:215–219
14. Krouse JH (2000) Computed tomography stage, allergy testing, and quality of life in patients with sinusitis. Otolaryngol Head Neck Surg 123:389–392
15. Lanza DC, Kennedy DW (1997) Adult rhinosinusitis defined. Otolaryngol Head Neck Surg 117:S1–S7
16. Ling FT, Kountakis SE (2007) Important clinical symptoms in patients undergoing functional endoscopic sinus surgery for chronic rhinosinusitis. Laryngoscope. 117(6):1090–1093
17. Lund VJ, Kennedy DW (1997) Staging for rhinosinusitis. Otolaryngol Head Neck Surg 117:S35–S40
18. Mamikoglu B, Houser SM, Corey JP (2002) An interpretation method for objective assessment of nasal congestion with acoustic rhinometry. Laryngoscope 112:926–929
19. McMains KC, Kountakis SE (2005) Revision functional endoscopic sinus surgery: objective and subjective surgical outcomes. Am J Rhinol 19:344–347
20. McMains KC, Kountakis SE (2006) Medical and surgical considerations in patients with Samter's triad. Am J Rhinol 20:573–576
21. Meltzer EO, Hamilos DL, Hadley JA, Lanza DC, Marple BF, Nicklas RA, Adinoff AD, Bachert C, Borish L, Chinchilli VM, Danzig MR, Ferguson BJ, Fokkens WJ, Jenkins SG, Lund VJ, Mafee MF, Naclerio RM, Pawankar R, Ponikau JU, Schubert MS, Slavin RG, Stewart MG, Togias A, Wald ER, Winther B; The Rhinosinusitis Initiative (2006) Rhinosinusitis: developing guidance for clinical trials. Otolaryngol Head Neck Surg 135:S31–S80

22. Piccirillo JF, Merritt MG, Richards ML (2002) Psychometric and clinimetric validity of the 20-item Sino-Nasal Outcome Test (SNOT-20). Otolaryngol Head Neck Surg 126:41–47
23. Robinson JL, Griest S, James KE, Smith TL (2007) Impact of aspirin intolerance on outcomes of sinus surgery. Laryngoscope 117:825–830
24. Smith TL, Rhee JS, Loehrl TA, Burzynski ML, Laud PW, Nattinger AB (2003) Objective testing and quality-of-life evaluation in surgical candidates with chronic rhinosinusitis. Am J Rhinol 17:351–356
25. Smith TL, Mendolia-Loffredo S, Loehrl TA, Sparapani R, Laud PW, Nattinger AB (2005) Predictive factors and outcomes in endoscopic sinus surgery for chronic rhinosinusitis. Laryngoscope 115:2199–2205
26. Stewart MG, Donovan DT, Parke RB, Bautista MH (2000) Does the severity of sinus computed tomography findings predict outcome in chronic sinusitis? Otolaryngol Head Neck Surg 123:81–84
27. Stewart MG, Sicard MW, Piccirillo JF, Diaz-Marchan PJ (1999) Severity staging in chronic sinusitis: are CT scan findings related to patient symptoms? Am J Rhinol 13:161–167
28. Stewart MG, Smith TL (2005) Objective versus subjective outcomes assessment in rhinology. Am J Rhinol 19:529–535
29. Wynn R, Har-El G (2004) Recurrence rates after endoscopic sinus surgery for massive sinus polyposis. Laryngoscope 114:811–813

Chapter 37

Bioabsorbable Materials in Revision Sinus Surgery

37

Rakesh K. Chandra and Robert C. Kern

Core Messages

- A spectrum of absorbable biomaterials is available for revision endoscopic sinus surgery.
- Each of these agents has unique properties that impact on both the mode of application and mucosal healing.
- The anatomy of revision sinonasal cavities exhibits significant variability depending upon the extent of previous surgery and the healing process.
- The mucosa of patients with recalcitrant disease undergoing revision sinus surgery may exhibit significant qualitative differences compared to that of primary cases.
- Roles of absorbable biomaterials include potential impact on hemostasis as well as mucosal healing.
- Properties differ between the available products.
- A complete understanding of the unique features of available bioabsorbable agents and their tissue effects is crucial, so that the appropriate material may be selected for a particular revision surgery.

Contents

Introduction

A variety of individual factors may be associated with the need for revision endoscopic sinus surgery (ESS). Some of these reflect recurrence (or reexacerbation) of the underlying inflammatory disease process, such as regrowth of polyposis or localized sinus ostial obstruction secondary to mucosal edema. Other causes of primary surgical failure may be anatomic in nature, reflecting the quality of healing or retained anatomy after initial surgery. These conditions include the development of synechiae or fixed ostial stenosis. Certainly any combination of inflammatory, anatomic, and infectious etiologies may exist in any one patient. As our understanding of chronic rhinosinusitis has continued to evolve, it has also become clear that patients with recalcitrant rhinosinusitis may exhibit histologic and ultrastructural abnormalities including deficiencies of ciliary density, anatomy, and function [1,2,7]. Other factors may include biofilm formation [19] and osteitis of the underlying bone [14].

Our understanding of the pathophysiology of recurrent or recalcitrant sinus disease has paralleled an increase in the application of revision surgery. This, in turn, has been facilitated by continued evolution in surgical instrumentation, medical therapies, and intranasal dressings.

- Packing agents have been applied after primary and revision ESS to attain three objectives:
  1. Hemostasis.
  2. Stenting to support the middle turbinate in a medial position.
  3. Spacers to prevent the accumulation of blood and mucus in the surgical cavity.

Ideally, absorbable biomaterials should attain these goals with optimal patient comfort. Such agents also report theoretical enhancements in postoperative mucosal healing. These are worthy objectives because conventional packing may be associated with significant patient discomfort while in place and during removal potentially leading to patient dissatisfaction and increases in oral analgesic use [13]. This fact has been established in controlled studies comparing absorbable agents to tampon packing [3].

Other investigations have revealed that some forms of nonabsorbable packing are associated with untoward tissue effects. One such study using a sheep model demonstrated that Neuropatties were associated with loss of up to 50% of the ciliated mucosal surface [23]. In contrast, the same group later demonstrated that foam tampons are not associated with ineffective mucociliary function following removal [17].

Regardless of the packing method and material used, mucosal healing properties will vary substantially. Furthermore, recent studies have underscored that these principles are maintained when absorbable dressings are utilized. The unique properties of the various available agents must therefore be understood in the context of recalcitrant sinus disease and the challenges encountered during revision ESS.

The goal of the present chapter is to present a framework for rational selection and application of absorbable biomaterials.

Classification of Absorbable Biomaterials

Absorbable materials may be classified according to molecular composition, which significantly affects the biological properties.

- Classification of absorbable biomaterials used in sinus surgery:
  1. Collagen/gelatin based:
     a. Gelfoam – sponge composed of porcine collagen.
     b. Gelfilm – sheet composed of porcine collagen.
     c. SurgiFlo – microfibrillar porcine collagen prepared with saline or thrombin to create an injectable paste.
     d. FloSeal – bovine-derived gelatin matrix prepared with thrombin to create an injectable paste.
     e. Avitene – microfibrillar bovine collagen powder prepared with saline or thrombin to create a slurry or injectable paste.
  2. Hyaluronic acid based:
     a. SepraPack – wafer composed of hyaluronic acid carboxymethyl cellulose.
     b. Sepragel – hyaluronic acid carboxymethyl cellulose injectable gel.
     c. Merogel – hyaluronic acid ester fabric.
     d. Merogel injectable – hyaluronic acid ester injectable gel.
  3. Cellulose based:
     a. Surgicel – oxidized cellulose fabric.
     b. Sinu-Knit – carboxymethyl cellulose fabric.
     c. Sinu-Foam – carboxymethyl cellulose injectable.

Selection of Material

Collagen or Gelatin Based

- Main role is as a topical hemostat.
- Possible fibrogenic effect.

These agents were introduced primarily for their hemostatic properties and were initially utilized in cardiovascular applications. Only later were they adapted for rhinologic surgery. The hemostatic effect of these agents is considered acceptable to manage mild to moderate bleeding, where the primary mechanism of action is to provide a matrix for platelet aggregation of fibrin deposition [3,5,6,9,12]. The latter can be facilitated by addition of thrombin solution, usually at a concentration of 1000 U/ml. Although this class of materials does have significant value in otolaryngology and ESS, known effects on mucosal healing must be examined.

Gelfoam and Gelfilm were both widely utilized in middle-ear applications prior to adaptation to ESS. The first report to illustrate that absorbable biomaterials were not inert was published in 1997, where Tom et al. assessed healing in cavities managed with and without Gelfilm in a population of children who underwent a planned second-look 2–3 weeks after ESS [26]. In this investigation, Gelfilm was associated with adverse healing with increased granulation tissue. Gelfoam appears to have more benign effects on the healing of sinonasal mucosa, at least when compared to FloSeal. Randomized prospective evaluation comparing these agents revealed that the latter was associated with greater prevalence of granulation tissue and adhesions at 6–8 weeks postoperatively [5]. These findings must, however, be interpreted in the context of additional studies suggesting that crusting and synechiae were no different at a 1- to 3-month follow-up when FloSeal is compared to an unpacked control [12].

Nonetheless, long-term evaluation of the FloSeal versus Gelfoam cohort at 2 years postoperatively demonstrated that FloSeal was associated with greater prevalence of adhesions and an increased incidence of the need to surgically remove adhesions [6]. These observations suggest that collagen-based hemostats, particularly FloSeal, may function as a scaffold for in-growth of granulation tissue and eventually scar. Foreign material has been noted to incorporate into healing mucosa [5,6,16]. It should be noted that in this series of studies, the absorbable hemostatic material was left in place filling the sinus cavity, even after cessation of bleeding (Fig. 37.1). This contradicts the initial descriptions for use of these agents, where removal of excess product was advocated after achieving hemostasis.

The role for these agents appears to be for use as a topical hemostat rather than as a surgical stent. Although

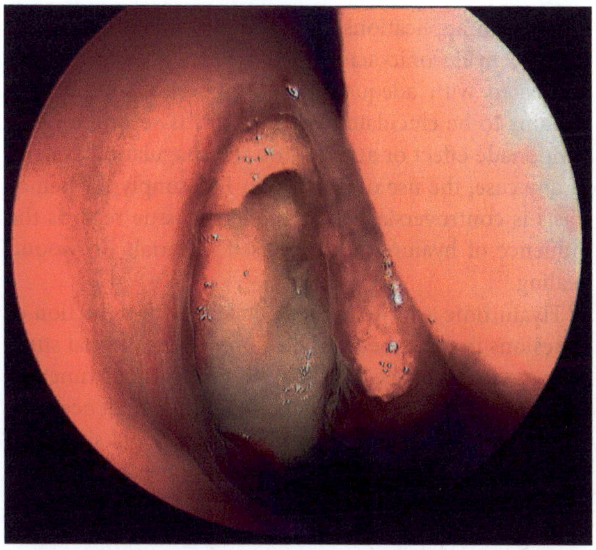

Fig. 37.1 Ethmoid cavity filled with FloSeal. Note the particulate nature of the material, which has the consistency of a paste. Leaving the cavity in this manner may predispose to adhesions

studies have introduced the possibility of adverse healing, the hemostatic role may be of significant value in scenarios encountered during revision surgery. First, it may be advisable to limit the application of cautery in revision surgery, as thermal effects are destructive to the ciliated mucosal surface. Such treatment potentially impairs recovery of optimal mucociliary clearance in this difficult patient population. Second, revision surgery often includes dissection and exposure of the skull base and regions near the orbital apex, such as the sphenoid and posterior ethmoid region. Use of cautery may be inadvisable in these anatomic sites given their proximity to intracranial structures and the optic nerve. In these situations, an absorbable hemostatic agent should be applied precisely to the bleeding focus (Fig. 37.2), and the excess should be suctioned or irrigated from the cavity following attainment of hemostasis. Leaving the material in situ (as shown in Fig. 37.1) potentially results in significant fibrin accumulation within 1 week postoperatively (Fig. 37.3), potentially leading to meatal stenosis.

Hyaluronic Acid Based

- Associated with adequate hemostasis.
- Some preparations may augment optimal healing.
- Composition affects healing properties.

Active research is ongoing for an absorbable biomaterial with ideal properties of simultaneously providing hemostasis and functioning as a stent to support the middle

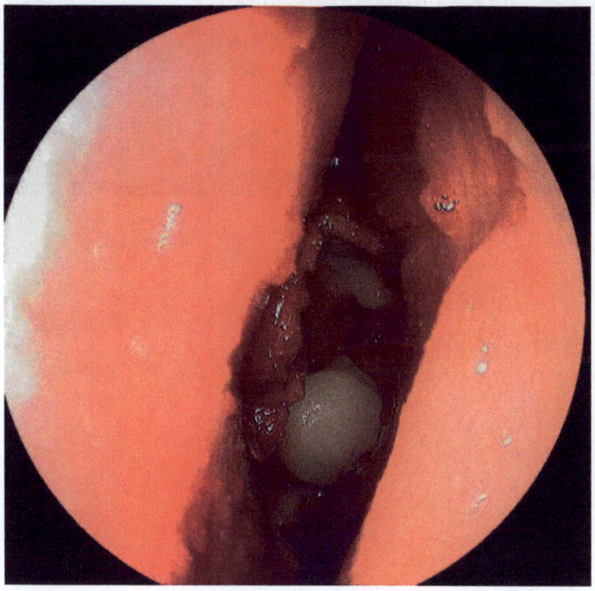

Fig. 37.2 Focal application of SurgiFlo to a bleeding focus in the region of the sphenopalatine artery. The excess material should be suctioned or irrigated from the cavity after cessation of bleeding

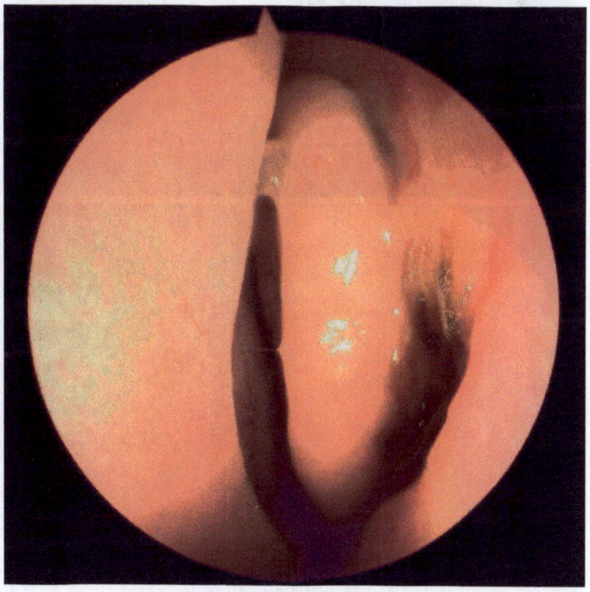

Fig. 37.3 One week postoperatively following filling of the ethmoid cavity with FloSeal for stenting of the middle meatus (as shown in Fig. 37.1). The middle turbinate has lateralized with significant fibrin deposition and early adhesions within the ethmoid cavity, requiring extensive debridement

turbinate while occluding the ethmoid cavity to prevent accumulation of blood and mucus, thus avoiding the promotion of fibrosis. Recent trends have included the use of materials based on hyaluronic acid, or hyaluronan, a glycosaminoglycan found in the extracellular milieu. Physiologically, this molecule interacts with water to give viscosity to extracellular fluids and has cellular effects in epithelial proliferation and possibly immune regulation. Hyaluronic acid has been implicated in the nearly scarless healing observed in fetal wounds [15]. Polymers of hyaluronic acid were initially utilized to prevent adhesions in abdominopelvic surgery [4]. Because of these properties, preparations have been subsequently developed for use in sinonasal surgery (Fig. 37.4), but most of the research studying the biologic effects of this molecule have been in abdominal models.

Unlike collagen-based materials (FloSeal, Surgiflo, Avitene), hyaluronic acid is not a vigorous promoter of coagulation, and in fact, it has even been utilized in cardiovascular applications to reduce platelet adhesion [10]. In ESS, hyaluronic-acid-based biomaterials have been associated with adequate hemostatic effects [8], but it remains to be elucidated whether this is secondary to a tamponade effect or an effect on the coagulation system. In any case, the use of packing in ESS simply for hemostasis is controversial. Thus, the larger issue regards the influence of hyaluronic-acid-based materials on wound healing.

Hyaluronic acid was first associated with reduction of adhesions in peritoneal applications, where animal studies suggested that the primary effect is due to its function as a barrier that attracts water [25]. This evidence provided justification for the use of this material in sinonasal applications, where additional studies have investigated the influence of hyaluronic acid on the biology of wound healing in respiratory mucosa. Early data from animal models has suggested that the composition of hyaluronic acid does have a significant effect on healing. Proctor et

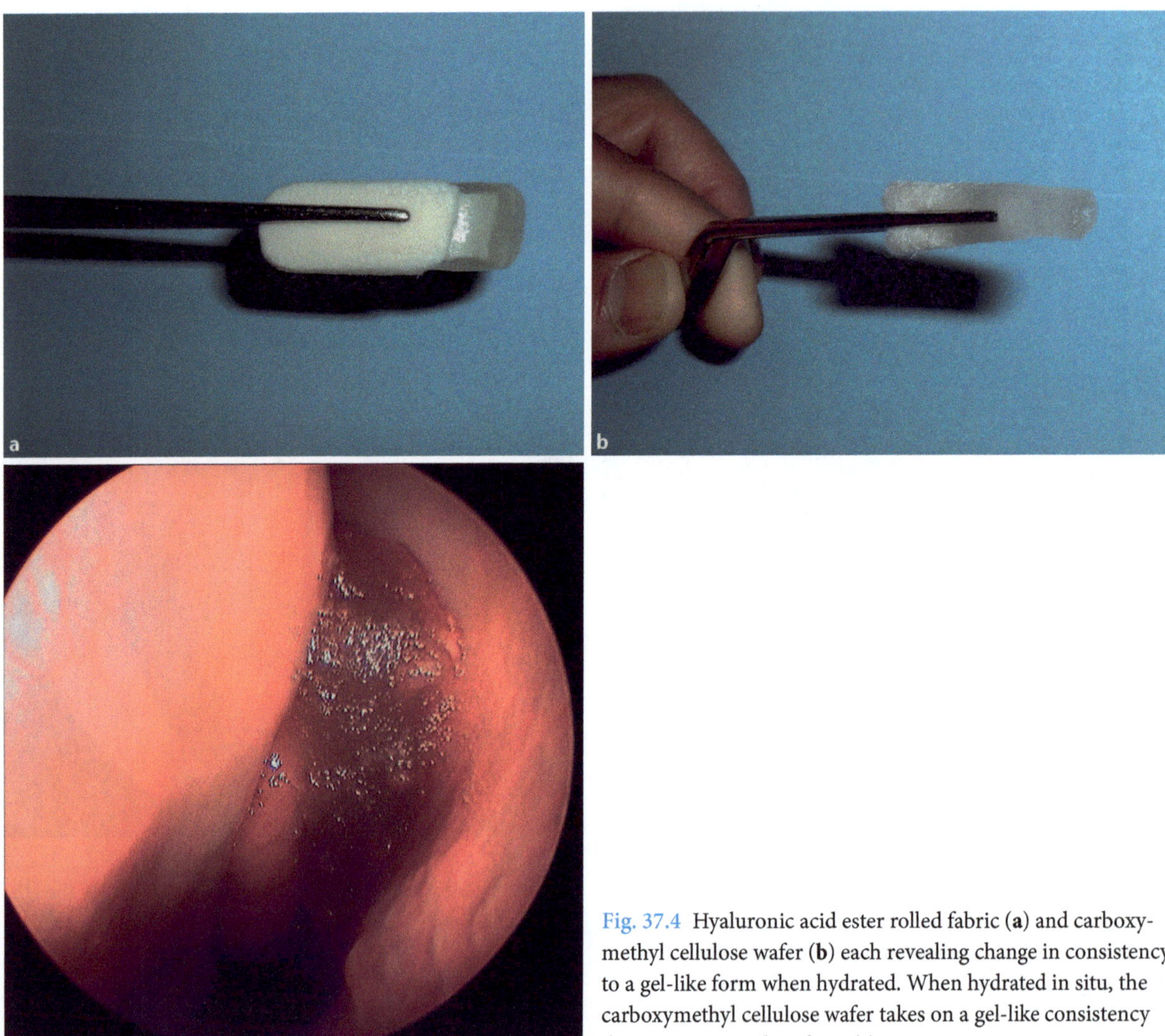

Fig. 37.4 Hyaluronic acid ester rolled fabric (**a**) and carboxymethyl cellulose wafer (**b**) each revealing change in consistency to a gel-like form when hydrated. When hydrated in situ, the carboxymethyl cellulose wafer takes on a gel-like consistency that coats mucosal surfaces (**c**)

al. [20] demonstrated in a rabbit model that woven hyaluronic acid ester (Merogel) is associated with increased foamy macrophages, granulation tissue, and ostial stenosis when compared to cross-linked hyaluronic acid gel or hyaluronic acid conjugated with mitomycin C. The latter two preparations exhibited greater ostial diameter than untreated controls. In this investigation, biomaterials were applied following creation of an antrostomy with a 4-mm otologic drill. Another rabbit model, where the maxillary sinus was stripped of its mucosa, also revealed that the woven hyaluronic acid ester was associated with incorporation into regenerating mucosa [16].

Sheep models have suggested that hyaluronic acid ester may augment epithelialization of experimentally induced mucosal wounds in healthy sheep, when examined 12 weeks postinjury [17]. This material, however, had no beneficial influence on promotion of reepithelialization or reduction of synechiae in these animal models [22]. The same group investigated a preparation of hyaluronic acid impregnated with insulin-like growth factor 1 (IGF-1) in a sheep model, where improved reepithelialization was observed in healthy sheep. However, this composite material actually had an adverse effect on ciliary regeneration in wounds of sheep with chronic rhinosinusitis [21]. This series of animal studies demonstrates that mucosal healing after ESS is affected not only by the biomaterial that is applied, but also by the underlying inflammatory state.

Wormald et al. explored the effects of hyaluronic acid ester on mucosal healing in patients with chronic rhinosinusitis undergoing ESS [28]. No influence was observed on synechiae or mucosal edema when comparing treated and unpacked cavities. Others have compared tissue healing between hyaluronic acid ester and a nonabsorbable tampon, where no significant differences were discovered [18]. It should be noted, however, that need for lysis of adhesions during the 8-week study period was less in the latter group (8% vs. 14%), although the difference did not reach statistical significance.

There are fewer available studies investigating hyaluronic acid carboxymethyl cellulose preparations (Sepragel, SepraPack) in animal models. Ongoing work from our group utilizing a rabbit model (unpublished data) compared mucosal regeneration after maxillary sinus stripping in sinuses packed with hyaluronic acid carboxymethyl cellulose to those packed with hyaluronic acid ester. Blinded evaluation by a pathologist revealed more untoward healing characteristics in the latter group. In contrast, regenerated mucosa in the hyaluronic acid carboxymethyl cellulose group was similar to unstripped mucosa and to unpacked controls.

Initial studies using hyaluronic acid carboxymethyl cellulose gel (Sepragel) compared to an untreated control in patients undergoing ESS revealed that the former is associated with reduction of synechiae. This study however, included only ten patients with a short follow-up. A randomized controlled multicenter trial [27] comparing hyaluronic acid carboxymethyl cellulose wafer (SepraPack) to no packing in 53 patients followed over 8 weeks suggested that SepraPack was associated with significantly less synechiae at 2 weeks. A trend was also observed toward decreased synechiae at 8 weeks, although this did not reach significance. This study also demonstrated improved patient comfort with the biomaterial, as patients reported significantly less congestion in experimental sides at 4 and 8 weeks postoperatively. This is an interesting finding given that patients were blinded to which was the experimental versus control side.

Although there was no difference in final cavity status between packed and unpacked sides, this data suggests that hyaluronic acid carboxymethyl cellulose wafer is associated with more favorable postoperative recovery secondary to decreased congestive symptoms and less need for aggressive debridement. Overall, studies of hyaluronic acid carboxymethyl cellulose materials support the principle that composition of hyaluronic acid has a measurable impact on the quality of healing after ESS. Use of this material should be considered in patients where significant postoperative hemorrhage is not a concern, but the patient would benefit from an agent to support the middle turbinate, particularly in those who exhibit significant apprehension about nonabsorbable packing from untoward experiences during previous procedures.

Cellulose Based

- Adequate hemostatic effect.
- Paucity of data regarding tissue healing characteristics.

The use of Surgicel in multiple surgical applications is well known where the primary role has been to augment hemostasis, particularly around vascular anastomoses. In otolaryngology, Surgicel is commonly used in the management of epistaxis, and data has also demonstrated that this agent is associated with improved comfort compared to tampon packing after ESS [24]. In that study, patients described less discomfort while the packing material was in place and during removal; in addition, the use of Surgicel was associated with less bleeding upon removal. Subsequently, other cellulose-based materials (Surgicel, Sinu-Knit, Sinu-Foam) have been released specifically for sinonasal application. A possible advantage of cellulose-based fabrics (Surgicel, Sinu-Knit) is that these agents are less likely to disturb a clot during pack removal, as is often observed when a sponge tampon is utilized. Unfortunately, there is a paucity of data examining the efficacy of these agents in mucosal healing after ESS when left in situ. Given that these materials promote platelet aggregation and are formulated primarily for hemostasis, it would appear prudent to avoid leaving these materials in the cavity, as the fabric/platelet plug may be a matrix for fibrosis. In contrast, the Sinu-Foam dressing consists of high-viscosity, injectable cellulose-based material that can be instilled as a paste and may be more amenable to clearance though mucociliary flow and/or irrigation. Both animal and human studies are necessary to investigate the effects of these materials on mucosal healing after ESS.

Additional Considerations and Future Directions

Following application of an absorbable biomaterial in the form of a fabric or wafer, it is important that the agent is deliberately hydrated with saline. This allows the material to convert to a more gel-like consistency that can be dissolved by mucociliary clearance and/or by the application of saline via spray or irrigation (Fig. 37.3). In reality, these "bioabsorbable" agents are more likely to dissolve rather than undergo true absorption by the surrounding tissues. Allowing the material to hydrate with ambient blood in the cavity may result in the formation of a plug consisting of fibrin and platelets, which may subsequently form a matrix for deposition of a collagen scar. In addition, allowing the material to persist in the cavity may result in frank incorporation of particles into the scar tissue or the regenerated mucosa, as studies have demonstrated [16]. This observation underscores the importance of ongoing postoperative management with endoscopic surveillance, debridement, and medical management.

Use of biomaterials does not apparently compensate for mucosal stripping during surgery, and in fact, murine studies have even demonstrated that hyaluronic acid ester is associated with significant osteoneogenesis if applied directly to denuded bone [11]. The use of absorbable biomaterials may be associated with significant patient comfort compared to a traditional pack and in some cases may augment healing, but does not replace the roles of mucosal preservation during surgery and meticulous postoperative care. It should also be stressed that no studies have demonstrated improved long-term outcome between the use of an absorbable and a traditional tampon pack; therefore, if there is potential for severe postoperative bleeding or if the middle turbinate is highly destabilized, use of a nonabsorbable spacer should be considered.

Future directions include conjugation or impregnation of the current molecules (i.e., hyaluronic acid) with antibiotics, anti-inflammatory medications (e.g,. steroids), compounds that dissolve biofilms, mediators that promote epithelialization (as was attempted with IGF-1), and those that prevent fibrosis (e.g., mitomycin-C). Furthermore, it is clear that agents composed of the same fundamental molecule, such as hyaluronic acid, may exhibit differential properties based on the material composition (polymerized as an ester versus carboxymethyl cellulose). The search goes on for the ideal preparation of the ideal molecule. In summary, these materials play a significant role in the armamentarium of the revision endoscopic sinus surgeon, but their strengths and shortcomings must be considered so the appropriate material can be selected for the given clinical scenario.

References

1. Asai K, Haruna S, Otori N, Yanagi K, Fukami M, Moriyama H (2000) Saccharin test of maxillary sinus mucociliary function after endoscopic sinus surgery. Laryngoscope 110:117–122
2. Bassiouny A, Abd El Raouf M, Atef A, Nasr S, Talaat S, Nasr M, Ayad E (2005) A comparative study between ciliary count and the degree of opacity of paranasal sinus CT scans in chronic rhinosinusitis pre and post FESS. J Laryngol Otol 119:950–954
3. Baumann A, Caversaccio M (2003) Hemostasis in endoscopic sinus surgery using a specific gelatin-thrombin based agent (FloSeal) Rhinology 41:244–249
4. Beck DE, Cohen Z, Fleshman JW, Kaufman HS, van Goor H, Wolff BG (2003) A prospective, randomized, multicenter, controlled study of the safety of Seprafilm adhesion barrier in abdominopelvic surgery of the intestine. Dis Colon Rectum 46:1310–1319
5. Chandra RK, Conley DB, Kern RC (2003) The effect of FloSeal on mucosal healing after endoscopic sinus surgery: a comparison with thrombin-soaked gelatin foam. Am J Rhinol 17:51–55
6. Chandra RK, Conley DB, Haines GK 3rd, Kern RC (2005) Long-term effects of FloSeal packing after endoscopic sinus surgery. Am J Rhinol 19:240–243
7. Cohen NA (2006) Sinonasal mucociliary clearance in health and disease. Ann Otol Rhinol Laryngol Suppl 196:20–26
8. Frenkiel S, Desrosiers MY, Nachtigal D (2002) Use of hylan B gel as a wound dressing after endoscopic sinus surgery. J Otolaryngol 31:S41–S44
9. Gall RM, Witterick IJ, Shargill NS, Hawke M (2002) Control of bleeding in endoscopic sinus surgery: use of a novel gelatin-based hemostatic agent. J Otolaryngol 31:271–274
10. Gunaydin S, Mccusker K, Vijay V (2005) Clinical performance and biocompatibility of novel hyaluronan-based heparin-bonded extracorporeal circuits. J Extra Corpor Technol 37:290–295

11. Jacob A, Faddis BT, Chole RA (2002) MeroGel hyaluronic acid sinonasal implants: osteogenic implications. Laryngoscope 112:37–42
12. Jameson M, Gross CW, Kountakis SE (2006) FloSeal use in endoscopic sinus surgery: effect on postoperative bleeding and synechiae formation. Am J Otolaryngol 27:86–90
13. Kuo MJ, Zeitoun H, Macnamara M, Wagstaff K, Carlin WV, Turner N (1995) The use of topical 5% lignocaine ointment for the relief of pain associated with post-operative nasal packing. Clin Otolaryngol Allied Sci 20:357–359
14. Lee JT, Kennedy DW, Palmer JN, Feldman M, Chiu AG (2006) The incidence of concurrent osteitis in patients with chronic rhinosinusitis: a clinicopathological study. Am J Rhinol 20:278–282
15. Longaker MT, Chiu ES, Adzick NS, Stern M, Harrison MR, Stern R (1991) Studies in fetal wound healing. V. A prolonged presence of hyaluronic acid characterizes fetal wound fluid. Ann Surg 213:292–296
16. Maccabee MS, Trune DR, Hwang PH (2003) Effects of topically applied biomaterials on paranasal sinus mucosal healing. Am J Rhinol 17:203–207
17. McIntosh D, Cowin A, Adams D, Wormald PJ (2005) The effect of an expandable polyvinyl acetate (Merocel) pack on the healing of the nasal mucosa of sheep. Am J Rhinol 19:577–581
18. Miller RS, Steward DL, Tami TA, Sillars MJ, Seiden AM, Shete M, Paskowski C, Welge J (2003) The clinical effects of hyaluronic acid ester nasal dressing (Merogel) on intranasal wound healing after functional endoscopic sinus surgery. Otolaryngol Head Neck Surg 128:862–869
19. Palmer J (2006) Bacterial biofilms in chronic rhinosinusitis. Ann Otol Rhinol Laryngol Suppl 196:35–39
20. Proctor M, Proctor K, Shu XZ, McGill LD, Prestwich GD, Orlandi RR (2006) Composition of hyaluronan affects wound healing in the rabbit maxillary sinus. Am J Rhinol 20:206–211
21. Rajapaksa S, McIntosh D, Cowin A, Adams D, Wormald PJ (2005) The effect of insulin-like growth factor 1 incorporated into a hyaluronic acid-based nasal pack on nasal mucosal healing in a healthy sheep model and a sheep model of chronic rhinosinusitis. Am J Rhinol 19:251–256
22. Rajapaksa SP, Cowin A, Adams D, Wormald PJ (2005) The effect of a hyaluronic acid–based nasal pack on mucosal healing in a sheep model of rhinosinusitis. Am J Rhinol 19:572–576
23. Shaw CL, Dymock RB, Cowin A, Wormald PJ (2000) Effect of packing on nasal mucosa of sheep. J Laryngol Otol 114:506–509
24. Shinkwin CA, Beasley N, Simo R, Rushton L, Jones NS (1996) Evaluation of Surgicel Nu-knit, Merocel and Vasolene gauze nasal packs: a randomized trial. Rhinology 34:41–43
25. Tarhan OR, Eroglu A, Cetin R, Y Nce A, Bulbul M, Altuntas YR (2005) Effects of seprafilm on peritoneal fibrinolytic system. ANZ J Surg 75:690–692
26. Tom LW, Palasti S, Potsic WP, Handler SD, Wetmore RF (1997) The effects of gelatin film stents in the middle meatus. Am J Rhinol 11:229–232
27. Woodworth BA, Chandra RK, Hoy M, Schlosser RJ, Gillespie MB (2006) SepraPack dressing after sinus surgery: a randomized trial. Arch Otolaryngol Head Neck Surg 135: P74–P75
28. Wormald PJ, Boustred RN, Le T, Hawke L, Sacks R (2006) A prospective single-blind randomized controlled study of use of hyaluronic acid nasal packs in patients after endoscopic sinus surgery. Am J Rhinol 20:7–10

Chapter 38

Endoscopic Approach after Failure of Open Sinus Procedures

38

Raymond Sacks and Larry Kalish

Core Messages

- Surgeons need to be familiar with the external surgical approaches including the indications and techniques in order to perform revision cases safely.
- Every effort should be made to obtain a detailed knowledge of the previous surgery.
- Potential for complications is greater due to the disruption of normal anatomy and pathways and greater likelihood of osteoneogenesis, adhesions, and breech of sinus boundaries compared to endoscopic surgery.
- Image guidance is useful but does not compensate for lack of preoperative planning.
- Always operate from known to unknown and always be vigilant that significant surgical defects can be found behind normal anatomy.

Contents

Introduction

External approaches to the sinuses were refined in the preantibiotic era when intervention was focused primarily on saving lives rather than improving quality of life. As our knowledge and ability has improved, so has our preference for endonasal techniques. Revising open surgical approaches presents some unique challenges. Many surgeons today have limited experience with open procedures and many open procedures have been significantly refined to reduce morbidity and complement endoscopic techniques rather than supplant them. The role of the open procedure after failed endoscopic techniques has been addressed in Chap. 31. The present chapter will focus on some of the challenges and consequences associated with failure of the open sinus approach. We will focus on the open procedures, which most commonly remain in the armamentarium of the modern-day rhinologist [29], and discuss the implications of their failures for the endoscopic approach (Table 38.1).

Revision endoscopic sinus surgery is often substantially more complex than primary surgery because essential landmarks are drastically altered [6]. This is especially true following open surgery. The surgeon should be intimately familiar with concepts involved in external sinus surgery in order to facilitate a safe approach during revision surgery [6, 17, 38, 39].

Table 38.1 External approaches to the paranasal sinuses [29]

- Caldwell-Luc procedure
- External ethmoidectomy
- Lynch procedure
- Frontal trephine
- Osteoplastic frontal sinus surgery ± obliteration

Indications

Indications for endoscopic revision after open surgery of the:

1. Maxilla:
   a. Persistent inflammatory mucosal disease after failed medical management.
   b. Recurrent benign neoplasms including inverted papilloma, juvenile nasopharyngeal angiofibroma (JNA).
   c. Oroantral fistulae aggravated by maxillary pathology.
   d. Orbital decompression.
   e. Access to the pterygomaxillary fissure and/or infratemporal fossa.
2. Ethmoids:
   a. Persistent inflammatory mucosal disease after failed medical management.
   b. Recurrent benign neoplasms including inverted papilloma and JNA.
   c. Mucocele of an ethmoid sinus cell.
   d. Access to orbital pathology.
3. Frontal:
   a. Persistent inflammatory mucosal disease after failed medical management.
   b. Frontal mucocele – recurrent or complication of a frontal sinus obliteration procedure.
   c. Recurrent benign neoplasms including osteoma and inverted papilloma.

Contraindications

1. A surgically unfit patient.
2. Unrealistic expectations.
3. Appropriate instrumentation and/or imaging not available.
4. Surgical inexperience.
5. Extensive osteoneogenesis.
6. Limited dimensions of the frontal recess.

Preoperative Workup

This is an essential component of successful revision surgery.

Patient Factors

The patient's *principal* concern and a symptom profile, both current and initial need to be established [26]. Undiagnosed medical conditions may have contributed to failure of the initial procedures and need to be addressed prior to further management [45].

Anatomical Considerations

- The Caldwell-Luc (C-L) procedure will result in distorted maxillary anatomy, but this is obscured by a normal uncinate, especially if no inferior antrostomy was performed.
- Similarly, after external ethmoidectomy physical findings on rhinoscopy and nasendoscopy may be deceptively normal.

Computed tomography (CT) is the diagnostic modality of choice [31]. Bony window (wide window 4000 setting) fine cuts in coronal, axial, and parasagittal planes are obtained ideally with soft-tissue views (narrow window 150–250 setting) with intravenous contrast.

Magnetic resonance imaging (MRI) is particularly important when CT reveals opacification adjacent to a dehiscent skull base. In this situation, MRI identifies whether the erosion is secondary to sinus disease or secondary to a prior skull-base erosion or trauma with resultant meningoencephalocele (Fig. 38.1) [6]. T1- and T2-weighted MRI images with intravenous gadolinium in axial, coronal, and parasagittal planes are obtained.

The surgeon should have an appreciation of the three-dimensional nature of the sinuses and pay particular attention to areas of maximal risk. These include:

1. The skull base, with attention to erosions or thinning, slope, symmetry, and height of the lateral lamella as per the Keros classification [18].
2. The medial orbital wall with attention to overall shape, dehiscence, and possible orbital prolapse obstructing the frontal recess, the relation to the uncinate process, and adjacent Haller cells.
3. The maxillary sinus and the presence of accessory ostia, previous inferior antrostomy, anterior and lateral wall neo-osteogenesis, and synechiae following open surgery, integrity of the orbital floor and bone surrounding the nasolacrimal duct.

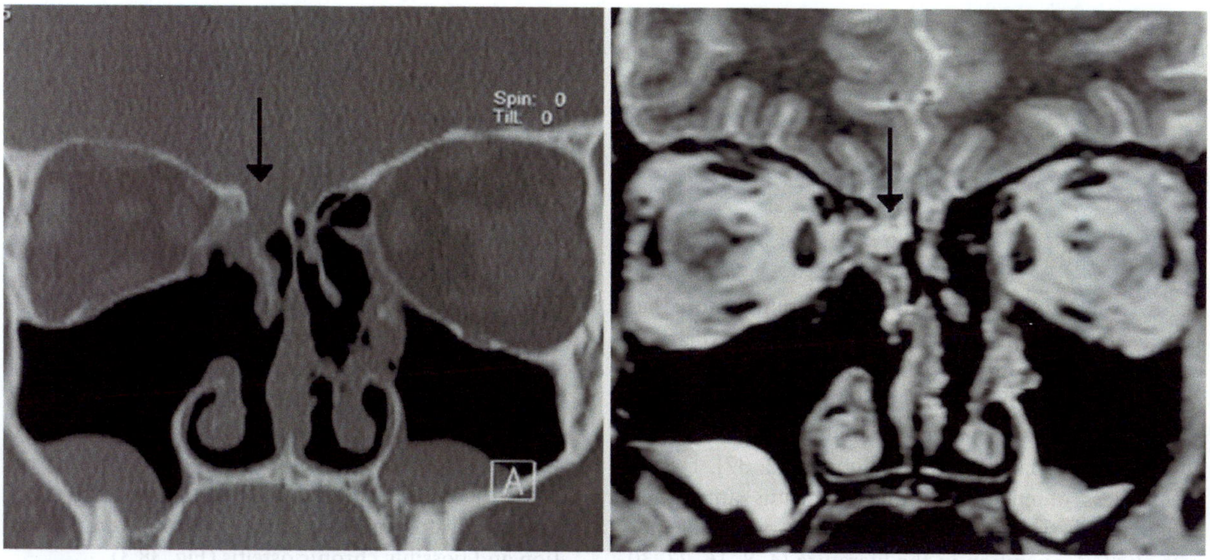

Fig. 38.1 **a** Dehiscent cribriform fossae on computed tomography (CT; arrow) confirmed as meningoencephalocele on magnetic resonance imaging (**b**, *arrow*)

4. The ethmoid vessels – assessing the relationship to the skull base and evidence of previous clip ligation.
5. Presence of Onodi cells (posterior ethmoid cells with pneumatization superior to the sphenoid) and a possible exposed optic nerve and susceptible skull base.
6. The internal carotid artery and the cavernous sinus with respect to the sphenoid sinus.
7. The degree of frontal sinus pneumatization with emphasis on anteroposterior dimension as well as distance from lamina to lamina. The presence of frontoethmoidal cells, the specific anatomy of the frontal recess, and the presence of septation.

Image guidance has been discussed in Chap. 29. It plays an increasingly important role in revision surgery and may reduce the complication rate [5, 11]. It is, however, no substitute for a thorough preoperative assessment, detailed knowledge of the anatomy, and a cautious respectful approach.

Pathological Factors

Current indications for open surgical approaches as described above largely incorporate recalcitrant inflammatory disease of the frontal sinus and less frequently the maxillary sinus, and then a variety of neoplasms including inverted papilloma, osteomas, and recurrent JNA. Prior to any revision surgery, maximal medical management needs to be instituted [3]. In order to do this effectively, a clear understanding of the pathology is required. An individualized medical treatment plan should be formulated for each patient. Atypical facial pain should be further assessed and treated prior to any surgical intervention. Other disorders that cause facial pain should be considered [44]. A trial management of the neuropathic pain with carbamazepine or amitriptyline, should preceed surgical intervention [52]. This can also include patients who have small mucoceles after frontal sinus obliteration in order to distinguish symptomatic recurrences from atypical pain syndromes.

Identification and treatment of infection preoperatively aids revision surgery, reduces intraoperative blood loss and enhances postoperative care. Staphylococcus aureus and Gram-negative organisms such as Pseudomonas are recovered most commonly in patients presenting for revision surgery [32]. Both have been implicated in the pathogenesis of chronic rhinosinusitis either as a superantigen stimulus or in biofilm formation [36, 43].

Symptomatic mucoceles occurring after obliteration procedures require surgical intervention. These can be geographically removed from the natural sinus; image guidance may be required. Benign tumors recurring after failed open procedures may act differently from the primary tumor. The recurrent JNA is frequently fibrosed and may bleed less. Planes of dissection are more indistinct and invasion into vital structures may occur. The possibility of malignant transformation in inverted papillomas needs to always be carefully considered. Recurrence can occur directly onto the periorbita or dura.

Patients are counseled on the importance of continuing medical therapy before, during, and after their operation.

Surgical Techniques

Revising the C-L Procedure

Caldwell and Luc described the C-L operation more than 100 years ago as the surgical treatment for maxillary sinus disease [24]. During the last decades, less radical interventions using the endoscopic approach have mainly replaced the classical procedures performed for chronic and recurrent maxillary rhinossinusitis [2, 37]. Despite the success of endoscopic middle-meatus antrostomy coupled with the reports of fairly high morbidity rates with the C-L operation in the literature [4, 8, 16, 23, 30, 33, 40, 54], several indications remain, and still many surgeons advocate the use of this procedure for endoscopic failures with irreversible mucosal disease [7, 25].

38

Comparative studies of endoscopic sinus surgery and C-L have largely favored the endoscopic approach, demonstrating better ostial patency rates and overall patient symptomatic control [37, 49]. This has been attributed by some to the increased fibrosis and abnormal bony changes of the maxillary sinus that are encountered in a higher proportion of open procedures compared to endoscopic approaches (Fig. 38.2) [49]. However, select patients seem to benefit from radical removal of diseased and condemned mucosa through a C-L or one of its modified procedures, such as the canine fossa puncture [9, 10, 42].

The concepts that one needs to consider specific to the endoscopic revision of previously performed C-L surgery include:

1. It is not a physiological procedure.
2. The inferior meatal antrostomy does not surgically address the physiologic drainage tract of the maxillary sinus, which is directed to the middle meatus through the infundibulum and hiatus semilunaris [46].
3. The term "mucus recirculation phenomenon" is used to describe an antrostomy that did not accurately include the natural ostium of the maxillary sinus at the middle meatus and can predispose to chronic infection and possibly chronic osteitis (Fig. 38.3).
4. The natural ostium may be patent behind a completely intact uncinate; however, significant synechiae may lie just beyond, necessitating a wide appropriate antrostomy.
5. Synechiae and osteoneogenesis may result in abnormal barriers preventing access to all of the diseased mucosa in the maxillary sinus, and may interfere with disease monitoring.
6. With angled scopes and instrumentation, endoscopic repair of oroantral fistulae and retrieval of foreign

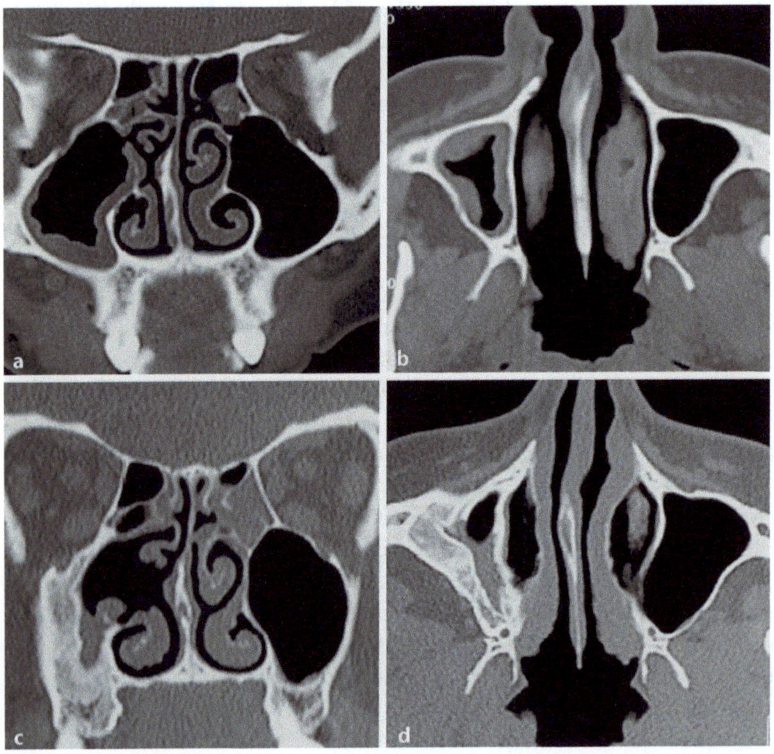

Fig. 38.2a–d **a, b** Preoperative CT scan axial and coronal views; **c, d** CT scan post-Caldwell-Luc procedure showing significant osteoneogenesis

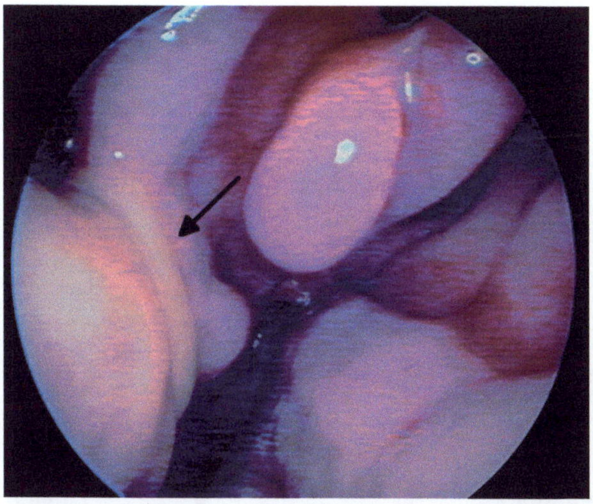

Fig. 38.3 Post-Caldwell-Luc mucus recirculation (*arrow*) from maxillary antrostomy to inferior antrostomy (not seen)

bodies is often safely and expediently achieved [22]. Following previous C-L procedures, the inferior antrostomy can be utilized for better access for scopes or instruments; however, synechiae and neo-osteogenesis can again slow progress and present potential traps.

7. The ethmoid complex is seldom addressed and recurrence from missed adjacent disease may need to be treated prior to revising the maxillary disease.
8. Postoperative debridement and monitoring is not always possible through the inferior antrostomy.

Endoscopic Revision of the C-L Procedure

The patient is appropriately positioned; the nose is then prepared with injection of lidocaine 2% + 1:100,000 epinephrine using a dental syringe and needle. The points of infiltration are at the axillae of the middle turbinate, the anterior end of the middle turbinate, and the lateral nasal wall. Neuropatties (1 × 1.5-inch) soaked with a mixture of 4% xylocaine solution, epinephrine 1:1000, and oxymetazoline are carefully placed into the sphenoethmoidal recess, lateral to the middle turbinate in the middle meatal recess, medial to the middle turbinate, and along the inferior turbinate.

An uncinectomy is performed by carefully identifying the free edge of the uncinate with a ball-tipped, right-angled probe, always being vigilant of potential synechiae and lamina dehiscence from the previous open surgery. Once the free edge is established, a Microfrance back-biting instrument is used to make the inferior cut of the uncinate. Care is taken to not to drop bony fragments inadvertently into the maxilla. A ball-tipped, right-angled probe is passed through the inferior incision and slid anteriorly as close as possible to the uncinate's insertion into the lateral nasal wall. We then palpate using the ball probe for synechiae resulting from the original C-L procedure. The probe is then pulled anteriorly, gently breaking down any synechiae and fracturing the uncinate at its insertion. A 45°, upturned, through-cutting Blakesley forceps is used to cut the middle portion of the uncinate flush with the frontal process of the maxilla. The superior edge of the uncinate is then divided using a straight, through-cutting Blakesley forceps. A complete uncinectomy assists in exposing the natural maxillary ostium, accessory ostia, and surgically created ostia following the previous C-L procedure. A 45°, angled endoscope is used while performing a wide maxillary antrostomy to confirm that the natural ostium has been incorporated into the surgical antrostomy, and to adequately assess the post-C-L antrum.

Careful assessment of preoperative imaging will direct the surgeon to potential areas of pathology behind newly formed bone and scar bands resulting from the previous C-L. Angled endoscopes, 45° and sometimes 75°, together with angled microdebriders assist in locating and managing problem areas. Positioning instruments or endoscopes through a patent inferior antrostomy may also be useful. Care is taken to identify the infraorbital nerve and appreciate floor or orbit dehiscence. Pressure over the patient's cheek will identify lateral sinus defects and aid in medializing pathological mucosa for debridement. The ethmoid sinuses are then addressed by performing complete anterior and posterior ethmoidectomies.

Revision of the External Ethmoidectomy

Although rarely used these days for inflammatory sinus disease, the external approach to the ethmoids is still encountered in the management of subperiosteal orbital abscesses, ligation of the ethmoid arteries, and as part of a skull-base approach [29, 35, 41]. Of particular concern when revising these procedures is medial orbital bone removal, which may allow the orbital contents to collapse into the ethmoid cavity, resulting in ethmoid and frontal recess obstruction (Fig. 38.4) [34]. Injury to the nasolacrimal duct occurs at a slightly higher rate with revision surgery following previous radical ethmoidectomy [20].

Endoscopic Revision of the External Ethmoidectomy

A complete uncinectomy and maxillary antrostomy is performed. Care is taken when performing the uncinectomy to avoid dehiscence of the lamina by gently palpat-

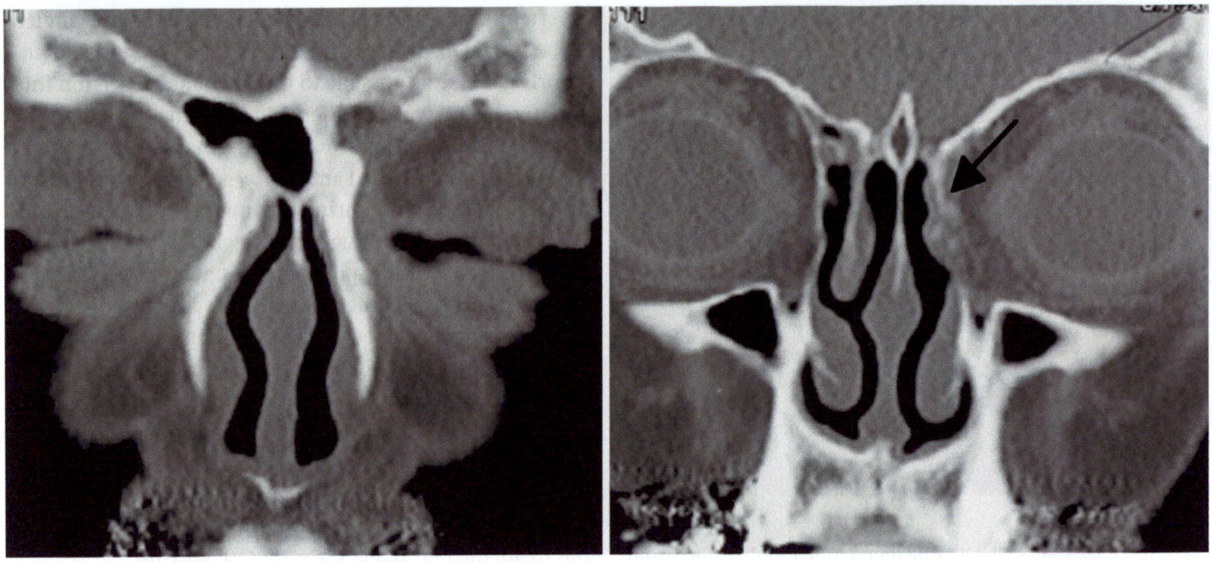

Fig. 38.4 Post-external-ethmoidectomy demonstrating dehiscent lamina, fused middle turbinate to the periorbita (*arrow*), and obstructed frontal recess

ing with a ball-tipped, right-angled probe. Intact lamina is identified as soon as possible and correlation made with preoperative imaging. The scrub assistant performs frequent balloting of the ipsilateral orbit so that any dehiscence is recognized early.

The ethmoid bulla may be intact after an open ethmoidectomy, but the surgeon should be cautious as dehiscent orbital contents may lie just beyond. We minimize the use of microdebriders and advocate careful curettage by placing the angled curette medial to the ethmoid bulla between the bulla and middle turbinate, palpating for a natural ostium, rotating the curette laterally, and pulling it anteriorly. Similar technique is used throughout the revision case to prevent inadvertent trauma to the periorbita or skull base.

The skull base is identified ideally after performing a sphenoidotomy and then followed anteriorly, this allows the surgeon to identify the skull base posterior to the previous surgery; this is important as the external ethmoidectomy can remove bone flush with the skull base, leading to the inadvertent breech when revising the case endoscopically.

Revision of the Frontal Sinus Trephine

Like many external procedures, the frontal trephine has evolved from a potentially cosmetically deforming procedure to a minimally invasive adjunct to endoscopic surgery [12, 28]. Its original description involved removal of enough bone to allow adequate visualization into the sinus and for placement of a drainage tube in order to avoid mucosal necrosis, osteomyelitis, and intracranial complications [19]. When the frontal trephine fails, endoscopic frontal sinus surgery is performed as described in Chap. 14.

Revision of the Lynch-Howarth Procedure

In 1921, Lynch in the USA and Howarth in the United Kingdom popularized a procedure to remove the frontal sinus floor but with preservation of the anterior wall, which included removal of the frontal sinus mucosa, dealing with any intranasal obstruction and antral disease and creating a large frontonasal drainage via an ethmoidectomy [19]. Although multiple techniques to address the frontal recess have been described over the years, the Lynch-Howarth procedure has remained a viable alternative. In a severely scarred frontal recess with osteitic bone after multiple endoscopic surgical approaches, the Lynch-Howarth approach may still be a procedure worth considering, along with modified endoscopic Lothrop approaches and osteoplastic flap with or without obliteration (Fig. 38.5).

Endoscopic Revision of the Lynch-Howarth Procedure

Positioning and preparation of the patient as described above. Image guidance is recommended if available. Careful assessment of the preoperative imaging is made to determine the best approach. The options usually include a

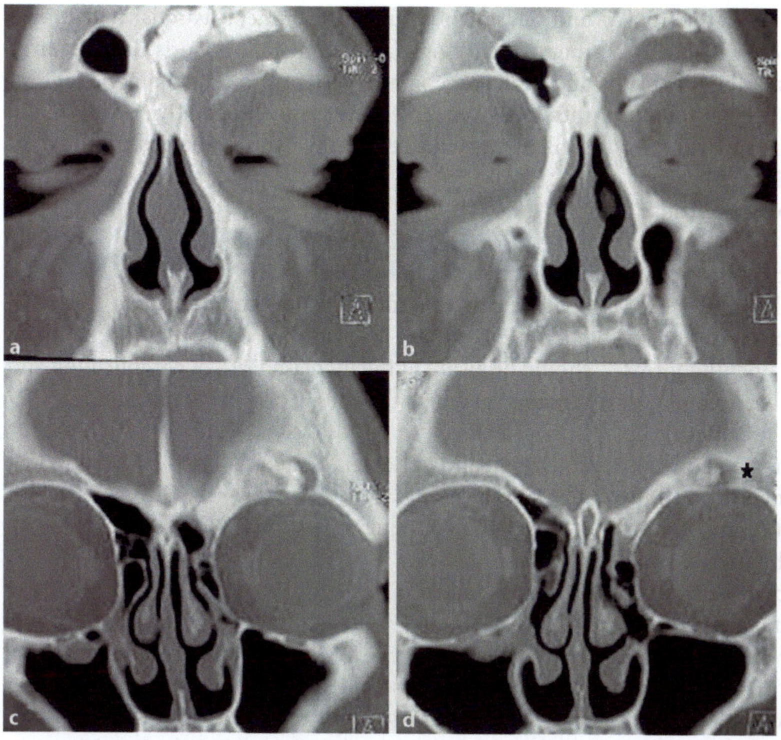

Fig. 38.5 **a–d** Coronal CT from anterior to posterior showing postoperative external Lynch-Howarth procedure to drain an anterolateral mucocele (indicated by "*" in **d**) caused by a frontal osteoma

Draf IIb procedure or an endoscopic modified Lothrop procedure (Draf III; see below). This is often determined by the degree of orbital content prolapse, the presence of a middle turbinate, and the underlying pathology. For example, a frontal mucocele secondary to frontal recess obstruction with an intact middle turbinate may be adequately treated by a Draf IIb, whereas a recurrent frontal sinus osteoma in a patient with only a remnant middle turbinate will do better with a more aggressive endoscopic modified Lothrop procedure.

Osteoplastic Frontal Sinus Surgery with and Without Obliteration

This can be a useful procedure and can be associated with short- and long-term complications [1, 14, 21, 50]. Mucoceles can occur centrally within the obliterated sinus cavity and are separated from the nasal cavity by bone and thick fibrous tissue, resulting in no communication between the mucocele and the nasal cavity, and consequently no pathway for the surgeon to follow [51, 52]. Obliterated frontal sinuses are frequently smaller than their unobliterated counterparts, and adequate drainage is only achieved by drilling a wide communication, thereby creating a circumferential injury [47]. Surgeons have to allow for significant (30–55%) contracture of the neo-ostium, and physical space is limited especially in the anteroposterior dimension [21]

Endoscopic Revision of the Failed Osteoplastic Flap Procedure with or Without Obliteration

Infiltration with lidocaine and epinephrine is performed above the axilla of the middle turbinate and on both sides of the midseptum adjacent to the middle turbinate. The soft tissue is removed with a microdebrider from the axilla of the middle turbinate to the roof of the nose, exposing the underlying bone. The microdebrider is utilized to remove all mucosa of the septum anterior to the attachment of the middle turbinate, and an area approximately 2.5 × 2.0 cm of mucosa is removed from both sides of the septum. The visible septal bone and cartilage is removed completely to create a wide window through which one can operate on both sides of the nose simultaneously. The septal window should be low enough that one can clearly see the axilla of the middle turbinate with a 0° telescope from the opposite nasal cavity. Frontal trephines have limited usefulness when an obliteration procedure has been performed, but in an osteoplastic procedure without obliteration there may be an indication to perform frontal trephine at this stage for fluorescein guidance.

The axilla of the middle turbinate on both sides is extended superiorly using a Hajek-Koeffler punch or a Kerrison rongeur. A 3.2-mm cutting burr is then used to remove the hardened frontal process of the maxilla above the axilla until a small amount of skin is exposed, thus defining the lateral anterior extent of the dissection. The procedure is performed on the opposite side and the frontal sinus cavity is entered. The floor between the frontal sinus openings on both sides is removed with further removal of the beak of the frontal process of the maxilla. This limits the anterior dissection. It is important to note that the dissection is only performed in the superior and lateral direction until the frontal sinus cavity has been entered, so as not to damage the olfactory fossa and cause a cerebrospinal fluid (CSF) leak.

Once the frontal sinus has been entered on both sides, the dissection can now be brought medially until the intersinus septum is seen. The intersinus septum is then removed and at this stage, the frontal sinus opening forms a horseshoe appearance. Once this has been achieved, the frontal bone is removed until there is no anterior lip of bone separating the frontal sinus from the nasal cavity. The posterior projection is then thinned down until the first olfactory neuron is identified. Fat or any fibrous tissue needs to be gently removed from the frontal sinus cavity in order to create a continuous cavity from the frontal sinus into the nose. Malleable frontal curettes and suction are critical in order to clear fat or other obliterative tissue from the sinus cavity. A 45° or 70° endoscope is typically required in order to achieve complete clearance of diseased tissue.

The use of packing material such as bismuth-iodoform-paraffin paste or absorbable packs such as oxidized cellulose, is controversial and studies are currently underway to look at the long-term results of these packing materials.

Postoperative Care

Absorbable packing such as Surgicel Fibrillar (Ethicon) oxidized regenerated cellulose or Nasopore (Polyganics) biodegradable fragmentable foam, are preferred for postoperative hemostasis in order to maximize patient comfort and minimize adhesions and bleeding. Vigorous hypertonic, buffered-saline sinus irrigation using a bulb syringe or sinus rinse bottle, in the nasal douche position, is encouraged to optimize irrigation of the frontal recess and maxillary sinuses [53]. After frontal sinus surgery, the "mini trephines" are left in situ and 4-hourly flushes with dexamethasone, normal saline, and an antibiotic solution is given for 1–5 days postoperatively. Instruction sheets are given to the patient detailing postoperative care. Medical management is reinstituted on an individual basis and may include short course oral antibiotics, longer-term macrolide antibiotics, topical and systemic steroids, or recommencement of aspirin desensitization. All patients are seen in clinic 1 week postoperatively for endoscopic debridement of residual packing, crust, and division of any potential early adhesions, and then on a weekly or fortnightly basis for endoscopic surveillance and debridement until the surgeon is satisfied with the mucosal healing. Long-term follow up is also required and both surgeon and patient should remain vigilant for the signs of recurrence, as a good operative result should facilitate easier access to the sinuses for medical therapy.

Complications and Outcomes

Specific concerns during endoscopic revision following open surgery have been discussed herein. The surgeon should be aware of the increased risk of complication and remain vigilant at all times. Complications include:

1. CSF leak.
2. Orbital and optic nerve injury.
3. Major bleeding.
4. Nasolacrimal injury.
5. Anosmia.
6. Neural injury.

There have been very few papers directly addressing the outcome of endoscopic sinus surgery following open surgery. In a retrospective review, post-C-L failures had similar clinical improvements with either revision endoscopic surgery or revision C-L, 67% and 60%, respectively, and required similar number of revisions, 1.7±1.0 and 1.3±0.5, respectively [13]. However, the operative morbidity and potential sequelae of open surgery significantly favored an endoscopic approach.

Experimental studies have indicated that mucosal stripping leads to regeneration of mucosa that bears patchy, dysmorphic, and dyskinetic cilia [13, 14]. Thus, for endoscopic revision to be successful it depends on the regeneration of mucociliary function or residual mucosa left behind after the original open surgery. The persistence of maxillary sinus disease despite endoscopic evidence of complete uncinectomy and wide patency of the ostial outflow tract is likely to occur after complete mucosal stripping and may require a more aggressive endoscopic approach including an mega-antrostomy or an endoscopic medial maxillectomy approach [13].

Few studies have addressed endoscopic revision of open frontal sinus surgery including obliteration [15, 27, 48, 51]. A significant number of patients with persistent frontal sinusitis after obliteration can be successfully managed endoscopically. It is important to select patients carefully. Disease localized in the frontal recess or inferomedial frontal sinus is more likely to be successful than superior and lateral frontal disease, which may be best approached externally [15]. MRI and CT can be helpful in guiding the selection of the surgical approach. However, when radiological findings are equivocal, the surgeon must be aware of possible occult disease beyond the reach of endoscopic techniques. Patients undergoing endoscopic salvage should be counseled about the possible need for repeat obliteration if clinical symptoms persist [15, 48, 51].

Tips and Pearls

1. Patient selection – beware of facial pain syndromes of potential nonrhinological origin. Patients with realistic expectations.
2. Preoperative antibiotics and steroids in revision inflammatory surgery.
3. Hypotensive bradycardic anesthesiae to minimize intraoperative bleeding.
4. Experienced scrub nurse familiar with endoscopic instrumentation.
5. Constant balloting of the eye during ethmoid dissection.
6. Frequent correlation with imaging and image guidance is required.
7. Blunt dissection using probes and curette.
8. Judicious use of powered instrumentation.
9. Avoid tight packing material.
10. Postoperative aggressive and meticulous debridement.

References

1. Alsarraf R, Kriet J, Weymuller EA Jr (1999) Quality-of-life outcomes after osteoplastic frontal sinus obliteration. Otolaryngol Head Neck Surg 121:435–4340
2. Barzilai G, Greenberg E, Uri N (2005) Indications for the Caldwell-Luc approach in the endoscopic era. Otolaryngol Head Neck Surg 132:219–220
3. Benninger MS, Ferguson BJ, Hadley JA, et al. (2003) Adult chronic rhinosinusitis: definitions, diagnosis, epidemiology, and pathophysiology. Otolaryngol Head Neck Surg Supp 129:S1–S32
4. Blitzer A, Lawson W (1991) The Caldwell-Luc procedure in 1991. Otolaryngol Head Neck Surg 105:717–722
5. Chiu AG, Vaughan WC (2004) Revision endoscopic frontal sinus surgery with surgical navigation. Otolaryngol Head Neck Surg 130:312–318
6. Cohen NA, Kennedy DW (2006) Revision endoscopic sinus surgery. Otolaryngol Clin North Am 39:417–435
7. Cutler JL, Duncavage JA, Matheny K, et al. (2003) Results of Caldwell-Luc after failed endoscopic middle meatus antrostomy in patients with chronic sinusitis. Laryngoscope 113:2148–2150
8. DeFreitas J, Lucente FE (1988) The Caldwell-Luc procedure: institutional review of 670 cases: 1975–1985. Laryngoscope 98:1297–1300
9. Forsgren K, Stierna P, Kumlien J, et al. (1993) Regeneration of maxillary sinus mucosa following surgical removal. Experimental study in rabbits. Ann Otol Rhinol Laryngol 102:459–466
10. Forsgren K, Fukami M, Penttila M, et al. (1995) Endoscopic and Caldwell-Luc approaches in chronic maxillary sinusitis: a comparative histopathologic study on preoperative and postoperative mucosal morphology. Ann Otol Rhinol Laryngol 104:350–335
11. Fried MP, Moharir VM, Shin J, et al. (2002) Comparison of endoscopic sinus surgery with and without image guidance. Am J Rhinol 16:193–197
12. Gallagher RM, Gross CW (1999) The role of mini-trephination in the management of frontal sinusitis. Am J Rhinol 13:289–293
13. Han JK, Smith TL, Loehrl TA, et al. (2005) Surgical revision of the post-Caldwell-Luc maxillary sinus. Am J Rhinol 19:478–482
14. Hardy JM, Montgomery WW (1976) Osteoplastic frontal sinusotomy: an analysis of 250 operations. Ann Otol Rhinol Laryngol 85:523–532
15. Hwang PH, Han JK, Bilstrom EJ, et al. (2005) Surgical revision of the failed obliterated frontal sinus. Am J Rhinol 19:425–429
16. Ikeda K, Hirano K, Oshima T, et al. (1996) Comparison of complications between endoscopic sinus surgery and Caldwell-Luc operation. Tohoku J Exp Med 180:27–31
17. Kennedy DW, Senior BA, Gannon FH, et al. (1998) Histology and histomorphometry of ethmoid bone in chronic rhinosinusitis. Laryngoscope 108:502–507
18. Keros P (1962) On the practical value of differences in the level of the lamina cribrosa or the ethmoid. Z Laryngol Rhinol Otol 41:809–813
19. Kerr AG, Groves J (eds) (1987) Scott-Brown's Otolaryngology – Rhinology. Butterworth-Heinneman, Boston
20. Kerrebijn JD, Drost HE, Spoelstra HA, et al. (1996) If functional sinus surgery fails: a radical approach to sinus surgery. Otolaryngol Head Neck Surg 114:745–747
21. Langton-Hewer CD, Wormald PJ (2005) Endoscopic sinus surgery rescue of failed osteoplastic flap with fat obliteration. Curr Opin Otolaryngol Head Neck Surg 13:45–49
22. Lopatin AS, Sysolyatin SP, Sysolyatin PG, et al. (2002) Chronic maxillary sinusitis of dental origin: is external surgical approach mandatory? Laryngoscope 112:1056–1059
23. Low WK (1995) Complications of the Caldwell-Luc operation and how to avoid them. Aust N Z J Surg 65:582–584
24. Macbeth R (1971) Caldwell, Luc, and their operation. Laryngoscope 81:1652–1657
25. Matheny KE, Duncavage JA (2003) Contemporary indications for the Caldwell-Luc procedure. Curr Opin Otolaryngol Head Neck Surg 11:23–26
26. Meltzer EO, Hamilos DL, Hadley JA, et al. (2004) Rhinosinusitis: establishing definitions for clinical research and patient care. Otolaryngol Head Neck Surg 131:S1–S62

27. Mendians AE, Marks SC (1999) Outcome of frontal sinus obliteration. Laryngoscope 109:1495–1498
28. Mortimore S, Wormald PJ (1999) Management of acute complicated sinusitis: a 5-year review. Otolaryngol Head Neck Surg 121:639–642
29. Murr AH (2004) Contemporary indications for external approaches to the paranasal sinuses. Otolaryngol Clin North Am 37:423–434
30. Murray JP (1983) Complications after treatment of chronic maxillary sinus disease with Caldwell-Luc procedure. Laryngoscope 93:282–284
31. Musy PY, Kountakis SE (2004) Anatomic findings in patients undergoing revision endoscopic sinus surgery. Am J Otolaryngol 25:418–422
32. Nadel DM, Lanza DC, Kennedy DW (1998) Endoscopically guided cultures in chronic sinusitis. Am J Rhinol 12:233–241
33. Narkio-Makela M, Qvarnberg Y (1997) Endoscopic sinus surgery or Caldwell-Luc operation in the treatment of chronic and recurrent maxillary sinusitis. Acta Otolaryngol Suppl 529:177–180
34. Neil GD (1985) External ethmoidectomy. Otolaryngol Clin North Am 18:55–60
35. Noordzij JP, Harrison SE, Mason JC, et al. (2002) Pitfalls in the endoscopic drainage of subperiosteal orbital abscesses secondary to sinusitis. Am J Rhinol 16:97–101
36. Palmer JN (2005) Bacterial biofilms: do they play a role in chronic sinusitis? Otolaryngol Clin North Am 38:1193–1201
37. Penttila MA, Rautiainen ME, Pukander JS, et al. (1994) Endoscopic versus Caldwell-Luc approach in chronic maxillary sinusitis: comparison of symptoms at one-year follow-up. Rhinology 32:161–165
38. Perloff JR, Gannon FH, Bolger WE, et al. (2000) Bone involvement in sinusitis: an apparent pathway for the spread of disease. Laryngoscope 110:2095–2099
39. Richtsmeier WJ (2001) Top 10 reasons for endoscopic maxillary sinus surgery failure. Laryngoscope 111:1952–1956
40. Romagnoli R, Aimetti M, Secco F, et al. (1998) The Caldwell-Luc procedure in the management of maxillary sinusitis. Long-term results. Minerva Stomatol 47:143–147
41. Sargent LA, Rogers GF (1999) Nasoethmoid orbital fractures: diagnosis and management. J Craniomaxillofac Trauma 5:19–27
42. Sathananthar S, Nagaonkar S, Paleri V, et al. (2005) Canine fossa puncture and clearance of the maxillary sinus for the severely diseased maxillary sinus. Laryngoscope 115:1026–1029
43. Seiberling KA, Grammer L, Kern RC (2005) Chronic rhinosinusitis and superantigens. Otolaryngol Clin North Am 38:1215–1236
44. Seiden AM, Martin VT (2001) Headache and the frontal sinus. Otolaryngol Clin North Am 34:227–241
45. Sonnenburg RE, Senior BA (2004) Revision endoscopic frontal sinus surgery. Curr Opin Otolaryngol Head Neck Surg 12:49–52
46. Stammberger H (1991) Functional Endoscopic Sinus Surgery: The Messerklinger Technique. BC Decker, Philadelphia
47. Stankiewicz JA, Wachter B (2003) The endoscopic modified Lothrop procedure for salvage of chronic frontal sinusitis after osteoplastic flap failure. Otolaryngol Head Neck Surg 129:678–683
48. Ulualp SO, Carlson TK, Toohill RJ (2000) Osteoplastic flap versus modified endoscopic Lothrop procedure in patients with frontal sinus disease. Am J Rhinol 14:21–26
49. Unlu HH, Caylan R, Nalca Y, et al. (1994) An endoscopic and tomographic evaluation of patients with sinusitis after endoscopic sinus surgery and Caldwell-Luc operation: a comparative study. J Otolaryngol 23:197–203
50. Weber R, Draf W, Keerl R, et al. (2000) Osteoplastic frontal sinus surgery with fat obliteration: technique and long-term results using magnetic resonance imaging in 82 operations. Laryngoscope 110:1037–1044
51. Wormald PJ (2003) Salvage frontal sinus surgery: the endoscopic modified Lothrop procedure. Laryngoscope 113:276–283
52. Wormald PJ, Ananda A, Nair S (2003) Modified endoscopic Lothrop as a salvage for the failed osteoplastic flap with obliteration. Laryngoscope 113:1988–1992
53. Wormald PJ, Cain T, Oates L, et al. (2004) A comparative study of three methods of nasal irrigation. Laryngoscope 114:2224–2227
54. Yarington CT (1984) The Caldwell-Luc operation revisited. Ann Otol Rhinol Laryngol 93:380–384

Subject Index

MIX
Papier aus verantwortungsvollen Quellen
Paper from responsible sources
FSC® C105338

If you have any concerns about our products,
you can contact us on
ProductSafety@springernature.com

In case Publisher is established outside the EU,
the EU authorized representative is:
Springer Nature Customer Service Center GmbH
Europaplatz 3, 69115 Heidelberg, Germany

Printed by Libri Plureos GmbH
in Hamburg, Germany